Exploring the Gut Microbiome in Cancer

This book explores the relationship between the gut microbiome and cancer, illuminating various facets from fundamental roles to personalized therapies. It provides a comprehensive overview of the impact of the gut microbiome on cancer development, offering potential for innovative diagnostic and treatment approaches.

- The book discusses the role of dysbiosis in cancer development, the influence of the microbiome on treatment responses, and strategies to modulate the microbiome for enhanced therapies.
- It reviews the influence of the gut microbiome on immunotherapy resistance and chemoresistance in cancer patients.
- Additionally, the book presents gut microbiome biomarkers for cancer diagnosis and prognosis, the implication of the gut–brain axis on cancer development and progression, and the impact of diet and lifestyle on the microbiome.

Towards the end, the book investigates the role of the gut microbiome in pediatric cancer and provides an outlook on the future challenges, technological advancements, and ethical considerations of gut microbiome research in the context of personalized cancer therapies. This book is intended for cancer researchers, medical oncologists, clinicians, pharmacologists, translational investigators, and medical students.

Exploring the Gut Microbiome in Cancer

From Biomarkers to Personalized Therapies

Edited by
Zodwa Dlamini

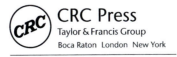

CRC Press
Taylor & Francis Group
Boca Raton London New York

CRC Press is an imprint of the
Taylor & Francis Group, an **informa** business

Designed cover image: Shutterstock

First edition published 2025
by CRC Press
2385 NW Executive Center Drive, Suite 320, Boca Raton, FL 33431

and by CRC Press
4 Park Square, Milton Park, Abingdon, Oxon, OX14 4RN

CRC Press is an imprint of Taylor & Francis Group, LLC

© 2025 selection and editorial matter, Zodwa Dlamini; individual chapters, the contributors

Reasonable efforts have been made to publish reliable data and information, but the author and publisher cannot assume responsibility for the validity of all materials or the consequences of their use. The authors and publishers have attempted to trace the copyright holders of all material reproduced in this publication and apologize to copyright holders if permission to publish in this form has not been obtained. If any copyright material has not been acknowledged please write and let us know so we may rectify in any future reprint.

Except as permitted under U.S. Copyright Law, no part of this book may be reprinted, reproduced, transmitted, or utilized in any form by any electronic, mechanical, or other means, now known or hereafter invented, including photocopying, microfilming, and recording, or in any information storage or retrieval system, without written permission from the publishers.

For permission to photocopy or use material electronically from this work, access www.copyright.com or contact the Copyright Clearance Center, Inc. (CCC), 222 Rosewood Drive, Danvers, MA 01923, 978-750-8400. For works that are not available on CCC please contact mpkbookspermissions@tandf.co.uk

Trademark notice: Product or corporate names may be trademarks or registered trademarks and are used only for identification and explanation without intent to infringe.

Library of Congress Cataloging-in-Publication Data
Names: Dlamini, Zodwa, editor.
Title: Exploring the gut microbiome in cancer : from biomarkers to personalized therapies / Zodwa Dlamini.
Description: First edition. | Boca Raton : CRC Press, 2024. | Includes bibliographical references and index. |
Summary: "This book explores the relationship between the gut microbiome and cancer, illuminating various facets from fundamental roles to personalized therapies. It provides a comprehensive overview of the impact of the gut microbiome on cancer development, offering potential for innovative diagnostic and treatment approaches"– Provided by publisher.
Identifiers: LCCN 2024008691 (print) | LCCN 2024008692 (ebook) | ISBN 9781032706429 (hardback) | ISBN 9781032706443 (paperback) | ISBN 9781032706450 (ebook)
Subjects: MESH: Gastrointestinal Microbiome | Neoplasms | Tumor Microenvironment | Biomarkers, Tumor | Antineoplastic Agents | Precision Medicine
Classification: LCC RC268.57 (print) | LCC RC268.57 (ebook) | DDC 616.99/4071–dc23/eng/20240522
LC record available at https://lccn.loc.gov/2024008691
LC ebook record available at https://lccn.loc.gov/2024008692

ISBN: 9781032706429 (hbk)
ISBN: 9781032706443 (pbk)
ISBN: 9781032706450 (ebk)

DOI: 10.1201/9781032706450

Typeset in Times
by Newgen Publishing UK

Contents

About the Editor..vii
List of Contributors..ix

Chapter 1 Introduction to the Gut Microbiome and Cancer 1

Rodney Hull, Brhanu Teka, Nkhensani Chauke-Malinga, and Zodwa Dlamini

Chapter 2 Gut Microbiome Dysbiosis and Cancer Risk 14

Demetra Demetriou, Georgios Lolas, Benny Mosoane, and Zodwa Dlamini

Chapter 3 Gut Microbiome and Cancer Treatment Response..26

Thulo Molefi, Talent Chipiti, Benny Mosoane, Ravi Mehrotra, and Zodwa Dlamini

Chapter 4 Gut Microbiome Modulation for Personalized Cancer Therapies 40

Lloyd Mabonga, Godfrey Grech, and Zodwa Dlamini

Chapter 5 Gut Microbiome and Immunotherapy Resistance...57

Botle Precious Damane, Lorraine Tshegofatso Maebele, Ramsey Maluleke, Melvin Anyani Ambele, Thanyani Mulaudzi, Jyotsna Batra, and Zodwa Dlamini

Chapter 6 Gut Microbiome and Chemotherapy Resistance 69

Sikhumbuzo Z. Mbatha, Botle Precious Damane, Kevin Gaston, and Zodwa Dlamini

Chapter 7 Gut Microbiome Biomarkers for Colorectal Cancer Diagnosis and Prognosis 82

Rahaba Marima, Afra Basera, Patrick T. Dumakude, Olalekan Fadebi, Linomtha Gabada, Amahle Nyalambisa, Lydia Mphahlele, Egnesious Sambo, Kamal S. Saini, and Zodwa Dlamini

Chapter 8 Microbial Metabolites and Cancer 93

Benny Mosoane, Masibulele Nonxuba, Jessica McIntyre, Meshack Bida, Tsholofelo Kungoane, and Zodwa Dlamini

Chapter 9 Gut–Brain Axis and Cancer: Delving into the Intricate Connection Between the Gut and the Brain 107

Rodney Hull, Georgios Lolas, and Zodwa Dlamini

Chapter 10 Gut Microbiome and Cancer-Related Inflammation 122

Meshack Bida, Masibulele Nonxuba, Benny Mosoane, Tsholofelo Kungoane, Victoria P. Belancio, and Zodwa Dlamini

Chapter 11 Diet, Lifestyle, and the Gut Microbiome 134

Thabiso Victor Miya, Zukile Mbita, Suzana Savkovic, and Zodwa Dlamini

Chapter 12 Microbiome Dynamics in Pediatric Solid Tumors: Challenges and Opportunities 153

Michelle McCabe, Dineo Disenyane, Lindie Lamola, Botle Precious Damane, Demetra Demetriou, Thabiso Victor Miya, Talent Chipiti, Lloyd Mabonga, Ellen Mapunda, and Zodwa Dlamini

Chapter 13 Gut Microbiome and Systemic Side Effects of Cancer Therapies 169

Richard Khanyile, Lloyd Mabonga, and Zodwa Dlamini

Chapter 14 Gut Microbiome and Precision Medicine in Cancer 179

Langanani Mbodi, Aristotelis Chatziioannou, and Zodwa Dlamini

Chapter 15 Therapeutic Potential of the Gut Virome in Cancer 188

Zilungile Mkhize-Kwitshana, Pragalathan Naidoo, Rene Khan, Andreas M. Kaufmann, and Zodwa Dlamini

Chapter 16 Microbiome-Based Cancer Therapeutics 208

Thifhelimbilu Luvhengo, Thabiso Victor Miya, Demetra Demetriou, Kim R.M Blenman, and Zodwa Dlamini

Chapter 17 Gut Microbiome Engineering for Cancer Therapies 227

Talent Chipiti, Elisa Marie Ledet, Amanda Skepu, and Zodwa Dlamini

Chapter 18 Conclusion, Future Perspectives, and Challenges in Gut Microbiome Cancer Research 238

Zodwa Dlamini, Rodney Hull, Serwalo Ramagaga, and Alexandre Kokoua

Index 243

About the Editor

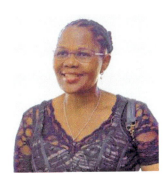

Zodwa Dlamini is a Professor of Molecular Oncology known for her unwavering commitment to advancing precision oncology. At the core of her career is her pivotal role as the Founding Director of the Pan African Cancer Research Institute (PACRI). Additionally, as the Director of the SAMRC Precision Oncology Research Unit (PORU) and a DSI/NRF SARChI Chair in Precision Oncology and Cancer Prevention (POCP), she is fully committed to advancing precision medicine in the battle against cancer. Beyond her institutional leadership, Professor Dlamini also serves as a distinguished member of the American Association for Cancer Research (AACR) Regional Advisory Committee on sub-Saharan Africa. She additionally guides the AACR Pathology Resources in Africa Advisory Group, actively identifying strategies to address gaps in cancer pathology services across the African continent. Professor Dlamini extends her contributions to the African Organisation for Research and Training in Cancer (AORTIC), where she actively influences the organization's strategic direction and mission as a member of the Research Committee Scientific Advisory Board. Her dedication to advancing cancer research in Africa was honored with a Special Award from the Council and Executive of the African Society of Morphology and she was then admitted as an "Honorary Fellow" of the West African College of Morphologists. Moreover, she is an Overseas Fellow of the Royal Society of Medicine (London), Professional Member of the New York Academy of Sciences (USA), and a member of the Academy of Science of South Africa, highlighting her contributions to the field of science. Through her multifaceted efforts, Professor Zodwa Dlamini remains steadfast in her commitment to shaping the ever-evolving landscape of cancer research and her journey is driven by an unshakable belief that cancer can be conquered, paving the way for a healthier and more equitable world.

Contributors

Melvin Anyani Ambele
Department of Oral and Maxillofacial Pathology
Institute for Cellular and Molecular Medicine
Faculty of Health Sciences ure
University of Pretoria
Pretoria, South Africa

Afra Basera
SAMRC Precision Oncology Research Unit (PORU)
DSI/NRF SARChI Chair in Precision Oncology and Cancer Prevention (POCP)
Pan African Cancer Research Institute (PACRI)
University of Pretoria
Pretoria, South Africa

Steve Biko Academic Hospital
University of Pretoria
Pretoria, South Africa

Jyotsna Batra
Queensland University of Technology
Brisbane, Australia

Victoria P. Belancio
Tulane Cancer Center
Tulane University
New Orleans, Louisiana, USA

Meshack Bida
National Health Laboratory Services (NHLS)
University of Pretoria
Pretoria, South Africa

SAMRC Precision Oncology Research Unit (PORU)
DSI/NRF SARChI Chair in Precision Oncology and Cancer Prevention (POCP)
Pan African Cancer Research Institute (PACRI)
University of Pretoria
Pretoria, South Africa

Kim R.M. Blenman
Yale University
New Haven, Connecticut, USA

Aristotelis Chatziioannou
Center of Systems Biology Biomedical Research Foundation of the Academy of Athens
Athens, Greece

e-NIOS Applications PC
Kallithea, Greece

Nkhesani Chauke-Malinga
Papillon Aesthetics, Netcare
Linksfield, South Africa

Talent Chipiti
SAMRC Precision Oncology Research Unit (PORU)
DSI/NRF SARChI Chair in Precision Oncology and Cancer Prevention (POCP)
Pan African Cancer Research Institute (PACRI)
University of Pretoria
Pretoria, South Africa

Botle Precious Damane
Steve Biko Academic Hospital
University of Pretoria
Pretoria, South Africa

Demetra Demetriou
SAMRC Precision Oncology Research Unit (PORU)
DSI/NRF SARChI Chair in Precision Oncology and Cancer Prevention (POCP)
Pan African Cancer Research Institute (PACRI)
University of Pretoria
Pretoria, South Africa

Dineo Disenyane
National Health Laboratory Service (NHLS)
Pretoria, South Africa

Patrick T. Dumakude
SAMRC Precision Oncology Research Unit (PORU)
DSI/NRF SARChI Chair in Precision Oncology and Cancer Prevention (POCP)
Pan African Cancer Research Institute (PACRI)
University of Pretoria
Pretoria, South Africa

Steve Biko Academic Hospital
University of Pretoria
Pretoria, South Africa

Olalekan Fadebi
SAMRC Precision Oncology Research Unit (PORU)
DSI/NRF SARChI Chair in Precision Oncology and Cancer Prevention (POCP)
Pan African Cancer Research Institute (PACRI)
University of Pretoria
Pretoria, South Africa

Steve Biko Academic Hospital
University of Pretoria
Pretoria, South Africa

Linomtha Gabada
SAMRC Precision Oncology Research Unit (PORU)
DSI/NRF SARChI Chair in Precision Oncology and Cancer Prevention (POCP)
Pan African Cancer Research Institute (PACRI)
University of Pretoria
Pretoria, South Africa

Steve Biko Academic Hospital
University of Pretoria
Pretoria, South Africa

Kevin Gaston
University of Nottingham
Nottingham, UK

Godfrey Grech
Department of Pathology, Faculty of Medicine and Surgery
University of Malta
Malta, Malta

Rodney Hull
SAMRC Precision Oncology Research Unit (PORU)
DSI/NRF SARChI Chair in Precision Oncology and Cancer Prevention (POCP)
Pan African Cancer Research Institute (PACRI)
University of Pretoria
Pretoria, South Africa

Andreas M. Kaufmann
Charité – Universitätsmedizin Berlin
Berlin, Germany

Rene Khan
University of KwaZulu-Natal
Durban, South Africa

Richard Khanyile
SAMRC Precision Oncology Research Unit (PORU)
DSI/NRF SARChI Chair in Precision Oncology and Cancer Prevention (POCP)
Pan African Cancer Research Institute (PACRI)
University of Pretoria
Pretoria, South Africa

Steve Biko Academic Hospital
University of Pretoria
Pretoria, South Africa

Alexandre Kokoua
University of Félix Houphouët-Boigny
Abidjan, Côte d'Ivoire

Tsholofelo Kungoane
University of Pretoria
Pretoria, South Africa

Lindie Lamola
National Health Laboratory Service (NHLS)
Johannesburg, South Africa

Elisa Marie Ledet
Tulane University
New Orleans, Louisiana, USA

Georgios Lolas
SAMRC Precision Oncology Research Unit (PORU)
DSI/NRF SARChI Chair in Precision Oncology and Cancer Prevention (POCP)
Pan African Cancer Research Institute (PACRI)
University of Pretoria
Pretoria, South Africa

Integrate Computational & Mathematical Modelling Approaches (InCELLiA)
Amarousion, Greece

National and Kapodistrian
University of Athens
Athens, Greece

Thifhelimbilu Luvhengo
SAMRC Precision Oncology Research Unit (PORU)
DSI/NRF SARChI Chair in Precision Oncology and Cancer Prevention (POCP)
Pan African Cancer Research Institute (PACRI)
University of Pretoria
Pretoria, South Africa

University of Witwatersrand
Johannesburg, South Africa

Lloyd Mabonga
SAMRC Precision Oncology Research Unit (PORU)
DSI/NRF SARChI Chair in Precision Oncology and Cancer Prevention (POCP)
Pan African Cancer Research Institute (PACRI)
University of Pretoria
Pretoria, South Africa

Lorraine Tshegofatso Maebele
Steve Biko Academic Hospital
University of Pretoria
Pretoria, South Africa

Ramsey Maluleke
Steve Biko Academic Hospital
University of Pretoria
Pretoria, South Africa

Ellen Mapunda
Charlotte Maxeke Johannesburg Academic Hospital
University of Witwatersrand
Johannesburg, South Africa

List of Contributors

Rahaba Marima
SAMRC Precision Oncology Research Unit (PORU)
DSI/NRF SARChI Chair in Precision Oncology and Cancer Prevention (POCP)
Pan African Cancer Research Institute (PACRI)
University of Pretoria
Pretoria, South Africa

Sikhumbuzo Z. Mbatha
University of Pretoria
Pretoria, South Africa

Zukile Mbita
University of Limpopo
Polokwane, South Africa

Langanani Mbodi
Charlotte Maxeke Johannesburg Academic Hospital
University of Witwatersrand
Johannesburg, South Africa

Michelle McCabe
National Health Laboratory Service (NHLS)
Pretoria, South Africa

Jessica McIntyre
National Health Laboratory Services (NHLS)
University of Pretoria
Pretoria, South Africa

Ravi Mehrotra
Indian Cancer Genome Atlas
Maharashtra, India

Centre for Health Innovation and Policy (CHIP) Foundation
Uttar Pradesh, India

Thabiso Victor Miya
SAMRC Precision Oncology Research Unit (PORU)
DSI/NRF SARChI Chair in Precision Oncology and Cancer Prevention (POCP)
Pan African Cancer Research Institute (PACRI)
University of Pretoria
Pretoria, South Africa

Zilungile Mkhize-Kwitshana
University of KwaZulu-Natal
Durban, South Africa

South African Medical Research Council
Cape Town, South Africa

Thulo Molefi
SAMRC Precision Oncology Research Unit (PORU)
DSI/NRF SARChI Chair in Precision Oncology and Cancer Prevention (POCP)
Pan African Cancer Research Institute (PACRI)
University of Pretoria
Pretoria, South Africa

Steve Biko Academic Hospital
University of Pretoria
Pretoria, South Africa

Benny Mosoane
National Health Laboratory Services (NHLS)
University of Pretoria
Pretoria, South Africa

Lydia Mphahlele
SAMRC Precision Oncology Research Unit (PORU)
DSI/NRF SARChI Chair in Precision Oncology and Cancer Prevention (POCP)
Pan African Cancer Research Institute (PACRI)
University of Pretoria
Pretoria, South Africa

Steve Biko Academic Hospital
University of Pretoria
Pretoria, South Africa

Thanyani Mulaudzi
Steve Biko Academic Hospital
University of Pretoria
Pretoria, South Africa

Pragalathan Naidoo
University of KwaZulu-Natal
Durban, South Africa

South African Medical Research Council
Cape Town, South Africa

Masibulele Nonxuba
University of Pretoria
Pretoria, South Africa

Amahle Nyalambisa
SAMRC Precision Oncology Research Unit (PORU)
DSI/NRF SARChI Chair in Precision Oncology and Cancer Prevention (POCP)
Pan African Cancer Research Institute (PACRI)
University of Pretoria
Pretoria, South Africa

Steve Biko Academic Hospital
University of Pretoria
Pretoria, South Africa

Serwalo Ramagaga
Steve Biko Academic Hospital
University of Pretoria
Pretoria, South Africa

Kamal S. Saini
Fortrea Inc.
Durham, North Carolina, USA

Addenbrooke's Hospital
Cambridge University
Cambridge, UK

Egnesious Sambo
SAMRC Precision Oncology Research Unit (PORU)
DSI/NRF SARChI Chair in Precision Oncology and Cancer Prevention (POCP)
Pan African Cancer Research Institute (PACRI)
University of Pretoria
Pretoria, South Africa

Steve Biko Academic Hospital
University of Pretoria
Pretoria, South Africa

Suzana Savkovic
Tulane University
New Orleans, Louisiana, USA

Amanda Skepu
Council for Scientific and Industrial Research (CSIR)
Pretoria, South Africa

Brhanu Teka
Addis Ababa University
Tikur Anbesa Hospital
Addis Ababa Ethiopia

1 Introduction to the Gut Microbiome and Cancer

Rodney Hull, Brhanu Teka, Nkhensani Chauke-Malinga, and Zodwa Dlamini

INTRODUCTION

The human microbiome consists of a multitude of different microorganisms including bacteria, viruses, fungi, protozoa, and archaea. Every surface of the human body and every cavity that connects to the outside is populated by an ecosystem of microorganisms (Ağagündüz et al., 2023). These microorganisms have a large influence on their human hosts (Sender et al., 2016). It is estimated that these microbes contributed to the development of cancer in at least 2.2 million cancer cases worldwide in 2018 (de Martel et al., 2020). The International Agency for Research on Cancer (IARC) has classified 11 of these microorganisms as being Group 1 carcinogens. This list is made up of the bacteria *Helicobacter pylori,* and three species of parasitic worms, *Opisthorchis viverrini, Clonorchis sinensis,* and *Schistosoma haematobium.* The majority of these microorganisms are viruses. The seven viruses include Epstein-Barr virus, hepatitis B virus, hepatitis C virus, Kaposi sarcoma virus, human immunodeficiency virus-1, human papillomaviruses, and human T-cell lymphotropic virus. Other microorganisms have been classified as group 2A carcinogens, or those that are probably carcinogenic. These include *Plasmodium falciparum* as well as various polyomaviruses (IARC, 2019). Other microorganisms are suspected of being carcinogenic, but studies are still underway to verify this. These include the bacteria *Salmonella typhi,* the human cytomegalovirus, hepatitis D virus, and the parasitic worms *Schistosoma mansoni* and *Opisthorchis felineus* (IARC, 2019). Apart from these, there are many microbes that may promote cancer development and progression indirectly (Figure 1.1). Apart from these pathogens, dysbiosis in any form is thought to contribute to conditions that may lead to the development of cancer and could contribute to carcinogenesis in a multitude of ways. The prevalence of cancers caused by various microbes and the abundance of microorganisms in the human body has led some to suggest that polymorphic microbes should be added to the list of the hallmarks of cancer (Hanahan, 2022).

Various regions of the human body are rich in microbes and are also common sites for the development of cancer. These include the mouth, respiratory system, skin, breast, gastrointestinal tract, and urogenital areas. The area with the most microbes that has received the most attention is undoubtedly the gut, which has been implicated in the development and progression of cancers (Rooks and Garrett, 2016).

GUT MICROBIOME DYSBIOSIS AND CANCER

Dysbiosis refers to a change in the population, types, or species of microorganisms within an individual's natural microbiota relative to microbiota found in healthy individuals. This results in an imbalance that could result in disease (Figure 1.2). In the gut, the altered interaction between the intestinal epithelium, the immune system, and this dysbiosis of microbiota may lead to inflammation, altered metabolism, and ultimately cancer (Rea et al., 2018). This dysbiosis of the gut microbiota can lead to tumors within the gastrointestinal system or distal tumors that arise far from the gut (Sheflin et al., 2014). Multiple studies using mouse models have found that gut dysbiosis can drive the development and progression of a variety of different cancers (Bhatt et al., 2017; Arthur et al., 2012).

It has been shown that different stages of gastric cancer were associated with changes in bacterial interactions, and changes in the numbers of specific species of bacteria. Specifically, the bacterial species associated with the development and progression of gastric cancer include *P. stomatitis, D. pneumosintes, S. exigua, P. micra,* and *S. anginosus* (Coker et al., 2018). Pathogenic infections are a common cause of dysbiosis as infections result in the growth of new species of bacteria or alternatively can change the levels of certain populations of microorganisms. Pathogenic infections can also occur as a result of dysbiosis

DOI: 10.1201/9781032706450-1

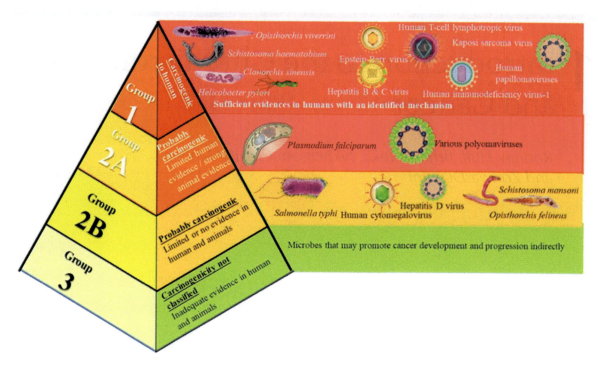

FIGURE 1.1   **The microbes categorized by the IARC carcinogen classification.** Currently only 11 microorganisms are classified as known carcinogen to humans (Class 1). Most of these are viruses but also include *H. pylori* and certain parasitic worms. Those microorganisms that are probably carcinogenic (Class 2) once again mostly include viruses as well as the bacteria *S. typhi*.

as changes in the microbiome allow for the colonization of new, sometimes pathogenic microbiota. This leads to the release of toxins. The effect of these toxins on DNA replication and integrity has been the goal of multiple studies (Kim et al., 2002; Toller et al., 2011; Grasso and Frisan, 2015). It is now known that some of these toxins can damage DNA causing genomic instability as well as tumor initiation and progression (Yao and Dai, 2014; Frisan, 2016; Zhang et al., 2021a). An example of this is the contribution of *Escherichia coli* to the development of colorectal cancer, where it has been found that the bacteria produce the compound colibactin (Pleguezuelos-Manzano et al., 2020). Colibactin causes double-stranded DNA breaks, chromosomal instability, and DNA alkylation (Nougayrède et al., 2006). The DNA damage caused by this compound, as well as another compound, cytolethal distending toxin (CDT), also produced by *E. coli,* results in transient cell cycle arrests. This cell cycle arrest can in turn lead to genomic mutations and carcinogenesis (Lara-Tejero and Galán, 2000). Other bacteria such as *Shigella flexneri* can promote DNA damage by interfering with the DNA damage response pathway by promoting p53 degradation. The bacteria accomplish this through the synthesis and secretion of enzymes such as inositol phosphate phosphatase D (IpgD) and cysteine protease-like virulence gene A (VirA) (Bergounioux et al., 2012). *H. pylori* is a class I carcinogen and one of the factors that contributes to this is the expression of the bacterial protein CagA by *H. pylori*. This protein is known to be associated with and contribute to the development of human cancers. CagA interferes with the AKT pathway, which results in p53 degradation in gastric epithelial cells (Hatakeyama, 2017).

Apart from initiating DNA damage or preventing DNA repair, dysbiosis can also lead bacteria to produce increased levels of metabolites that affect proliferative and survival pathways. *Fusobacterium nucleatum* produces FadA, while *Bacteroides frag* produces MP. Both these compounds interact with E-cadherin, disrupting intercellular junctions between epithelial cells. This results in the activation of β-catenin signaling, promoting proliferation and leading to carcinogenesis (Murata-Kamiya et al., 2007; Wu et al., 2007; Rubinstein et al., 2013).

Bacteria have received the most attention in research surrounding the role of the gut microbiome in cancer. However, the microbiome also consists of viruses and the virome. The human virome is made up of all the viruses that infect not only human cells but also those that infect bacteria and other microorganisms, such as protozoa, within the human host. It also includes genetic elements derived from viruses (Virgin, 2014). Like dysbiosis with other microorganisms, virome imbalance is associated with multiple diseases including cancer (Santiago-Rodriguez and Hollister, 2019; Spencer et al., 2022; Bai et al., 2022). For instance, colorectal cancer patients were found to have an altered gut virome compared to healthy patients, with some viruses only being present in the cancer patients (Chen et al., 2023). Oncolytic phages have been investigated as a means of targeting and killing cancer cells (Zheng et al., 2019; Shi et al., 2020; Kaufman et al., 2015; Twumasi-Boateng et al., 2018). The viruses in the virome are also responsible for the development and activity of the host's immune system. As such they may help to modulate

Introduction to the Gut Microbiome and Cancer

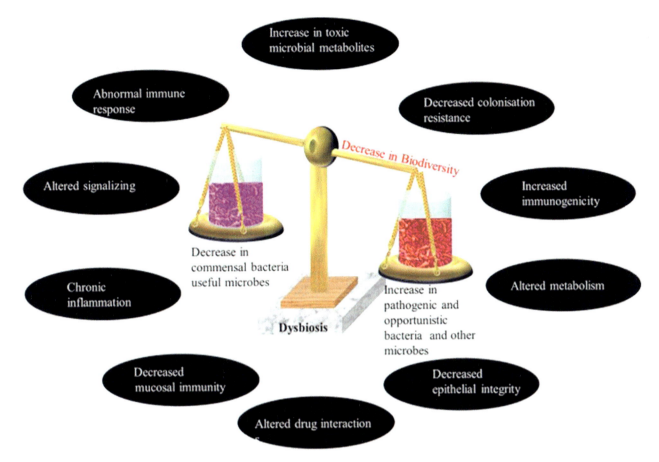

FIGURE 1.2 Dysbiosis of the gut microbiome and its consequences. Dysbiosis of the gut microbiome occurs when the composition of the microbial population shifts from commensal beneficial microbes to more pathogenic or harmful ones. This is accompanied by a decrease in the biodiversity of the gut microbiome. Dysbiosis can lead to changes that promote the development and progression of cancer. These are indicated by the black circles and include alterations in immune signaling, chronic inflammation, decreased epithelial integrity, and the release of bioactive metabolites from bacteria.

the immune response to cancer cells or the effectiveness of immunotherapy (Virgin, 2014).

FACTORS GOVERNING THE MAKEUP OF THE GUT MICROBIOME AND ITS RELATION TO CANCER

The makeup of the gut microbiota is determined by both host genetics and environmental factors. Initially, it is acquired by an individual from their mother during delivery and lactation. The host's gut is then further colonized until 3 years of age whereafter the composition remains stable in the absence of disturbances. Further alterations can occur as the result of external environmental factors (Koenig et al., 2011; Mulder et al., 2009; Bäckhed et al., 2015). The association between gut microbiome dysbiosis and cancer in children is demonstrated by the link between the changing risks of malignancy and the type of birth. Developing studies are showing that cesarean section children have a higher risk of developing acute lymphocytic leukemia (ALL) (Wang et al., 2017), perhaps because these children are not exposed to or colonized by the maternal vaginal microbiome. Breastfeeding has been shown to reduce the risk of the development of the most common malignancies in children. This is due to the immunomodulating role played by the mother's milk, which includes nutrients, antibodies, or anti-inflammatory factors (Amitay and Keinan-Boker, 2015). Other factors which contribute to the formation of a child's microbiome include hospitalization at birth and the use of antibiotics. Children with ALL had a lower DNA content in their stool, indicating a decreased biodiversity and microbe levels in these children. Specifically, they had lower levels of *Bifidobacterium*, *Lactobacillus*, and *E. coli* (Huang et al., 2012).

Diet-cancer-microbiome interactions are known to play an important role in determining the composition of an individual's microbiome. A high-fat, low-fiber protein-based diet is a risk factor for cancer and results in lower short-chain fatty acids (SCFA) by gut microbes (Ou et al., 2012), with SCFAs like butyrate being associated with enhanced activation of irinotecan (Encarnação et al., 2018). The fact that many cancer patients are cachexic, or experience loss of appetite, means that altering their nutrition to encourage the desired changes in their microbiome becomes complex and difficult (Vernieri et al., 2022). Antibiotic-induced alterations in microbial composition can have deleterious effects on human health, such as decreased microbial diversity, modifications to the microbiota's functional characteristics, and the emergence and selection of antibiotic-resistant strains that increase susceptibility of hosts to pathogen infection. There is evidence that treatment of infants with antibiotics can cause lifelong phenotypic changes (Mu and Zhu, 2019).

The gut microbiome is also able to influence other regions of the body. These include the lungs (Dang and Marsland, 2019), skin (Sinha et al., 2021), and brain (Hull et al., 2021). These communications systems are known as axes and the gut–brain axis is especially important in the development and progression of cancer. The gut microbiome is able to release signals in the form of metabolites or neuroactive proteins and peptides that influence the nervous system (Carabotti et al., 2015; Rubinstein et al., 2013). The interactions between the gut microbiome and the immune system can also influence the nervous system through immune signaling (Arthur et al., 2012). The blood-brain barrier (BBB) normally protects the central nervous system from many of these signals, but the presence of specific bacteria in abnormally high numbers changes the permeability of the BBB resulting in the transmission of these signaling molecules to the CNS (Kuwahara et al., 2020; Braniste et al., 2014). The gut and the brain are connected by the vagus nerve and dysbiosis in the gut microbiome changes the signals sent to this nerve (Travagli and Anselmi, 2016). These aberrant signals to the nervous system can lead to cancer through assisting tumor cells to evade the immune system, increase proliferation, bypass cell cycle checkpoints, and increase cell survival. These signals may also stimulate neurogenesis which supports cancer cell growth in a similar way as angiogenesis. These new nerve fibers connect the cancer cells to the nervous system, giving them a path to travel along and imitate metastasis and cell migration.

THE EFFECT OF THE MICROBIOME ON CANCER THERAPY

Multimodal treatment strategies are the optimal therapeutic choice for most solid cancers and include surgery immunotherapy, radiotherapy, and chemotherapy (Pan et al., 2020). The microbiome of a patient will change significantly due not only to the disease but also due to the changes caused by the therapeutic interventions, changes in diet, radiotherapy and various chemotherapeutic, neoadjuvant, and adjuvant agents which can all contribute to dysbiosis. This dysbiosis can affect patient outcomes by altering the effectiveness of the treatment. The gut microbiome influences drug metabolism and affects the tumor microenvironment and the immune system (Sánchez-Alcoholado et al., 2020). The effect of the microbiome on cancer treatment and the effect of the treatment on the microbiome can be summarized by the TIMER hypothesis. TIMER stands for Translocation, Immunomodulation, Metabolism, Enzymatic degradation, and Reduced diversity (Alexander et al., 2017).

Dysbiosis caused by chemotherapy can drive drug toxicity and decrease drug efficacy and gut microbiome diversity can be used as a predictor of chemotoxicity (Forsgård et al., 2017).

Resistance to Immunotherapy

The gut microbiome strongly influences host immunity, and therefore cancer immunotherapy (Zheng et al., 2020). The mucosal immune system in the gut comprises a layer of mucus secreted by goblet cells, which are rich in antimicrobial peptides and immunoglobulin A secreted by intestinal epithelial cells and B cells. This system forms a physical barrier between the host and microbiome that is able to inhibit adhesion and colonization of bacteria (Caballero and Pamer, 2015). Dysbiosis is also associated with changes in the immune system which can result in resistance of cancers to immunotherapy. Dysbiosis is known to cause altered immune pathway signaling, such as increased levels pf prostaglandin E2, resulting in greater levels of M2-macrophage differentiation. This can lead to autoimmune responses allergy and inflammation (Sekirov et al., 2010).

Immunotherapy for cancer involves treatments such as the use of Toll-like receptor (TLR) agonists, vaccines, immune checkpoint inhibitors (ICIs), and adoptive T-cell therapy (ACT) (Lee et al., 2016). ICIs specifically include the use of antibodies that block signaling via the programmed cell death protein 1/programmed cell death 1 ligand 1 (PD-1/PD-L1) and the cytotoxic T-lymphocyte antigen-4 (CTLA-4) (Lee et al., 2016). Cytotoxic T-lymphocyte–associated antigen 4 (CTLA-4) and programmed cell death protein 1 (PD-1) are both immune checkpoints that inhibit T-cell function. Antibodies against these checkpoint proteins have been developed as cancer therapies and include Ipilimumab. The efficacy of this monoclonal antibody against CTLA-4, relies on the gut microbiota's interactions with the immune system. The sensitivity of tumors to this antibody is reduced in germ-free carcinoma mouse models or those treated with antibiotics. This is because the anti-CTLA-4 treatment relies on IL-12-dependent Th1 immune signaling, This signaling was found to be dependent on the presence of bacteria such as *Bacteroides fragilis*, *Bacteroides thetaiotaomicron*, and Burkholderiales in mice (Vétizou et al., 2015). The PD-1/PD-L1 pathway suppresses T effector cells promoting immune evasion by tumor cells leading to tumor growth and metastasis (Bardhan et al., 2016). It also promotes the activity of immunosuppressive Tregs (Ohaegbulam et al., 2015). Mice models have shown that bacteria from the taxon *Bifidobacterium* increase the efficacy of PD-L1 blocking therapies (Sivan et al., 2015), while increased numbers of species from *Akkermansia muciniphila* and *Enterococcus hirae* were isolated from human cancer patients who responded well to this immunotherapy (Gopalakrishnan et al., 2018). Additionally, an analysis of lung cancer patients from China showed that a more diverse and stable gut microbiome was associated with better outcomes following ICI treatment (Jin et al., 2019).

CpG oligodeoxynucleotides are unmethylated CG dinucleotides that enhance antineoplastic therapies, by stimulating the immune system (Zhang et al., 2021b). The gut microbiome is known to affect the function of CpGs as treatment of EL4-bearing mice with antibiotics increased CpG efficacy. This was due to increased levels of tumor necrosis factor expression. The increased levels of TNF can be reversed in both these germ-free or antibiotic-treated mice by inoculating them with *Alistipes shahii* (Iida et al., 2013).

CHEMOTHERAPY RESISTANCE

The microbiome, dysbiosis, and a loss of gut microbiota diversity can affect chemotherapy treatment in a number of ways. These include changing the efficacy of the drug negating the anticancer effect of the drug or even altering the drug toxicity (Ma et al., 2019). The response to, efficacy, and toxicity of chemotherapy can be greatly affected by the enzymatic activity of the organisms that make up the gut microbiome. These enzymes, mostly from bacteria, can then degrade or alter these compounds (Pollet et al., 2017).

E. coli is able to metabolize and inactivate a multitude of drugs, including cladribine, vidarabine, doxorubicin, idarubicin, daunorubicin, etoposide phosphate, mitoxantrone, and β-lapachone (Lehouritis et al., 2015). Many chemotherapy drugs require the presence of specific microorganisms to stimulate immune responses required for the efficacy of the drug (Matson et al., 2021; Viaud et al., 2013). The gut microbiome may also decrease the toxicity of drugs, such as the antimetabolite chemotherapy agent, methotrexate. This drug prevents DNA replication and repair. The drug causes intestinal mucositis, leading to diarrhea (Chrysostomou et al., 2023); the gut microbiota inhibits this toxicity.

The alkylating agent cyclophosphamide (CTX), which is used to treat hematological cancers and various solid tumors, disrupts the gut epithelial barrier. This results in the translocation of specific Gram-positive bacteria from the intestine into the lymphoid organs, activating T-helper cells resulting in the drug's antitumor activity (Helmink et al., 2019). This anticancer effect can therefore be diminished through the use of broad-spectrum antibiotics (Goubet et al., 2018). As such dysbiosis can greatly affect the efficacy of this chemotherapeutic drug (Goubet et al., 2018). Platinum derivative chemotherapeutic drugs, such as oxaliplatin, form DNA adducts, damaging DNA leading to apoptosis (Alcindor and Beauger, 2011). The efficacy of these drugs is enhanced in mice with a healthy gut microbiome. This is due to the microbes enhancing the release of reactive oxygen species from myeloid cells, leading to enhanced inflammation and cytokine production. Once again broad-spectrum antibiotics are able to decrease the effectiveness of these drugs (Iida et al., 2013). Anthracyclines, which disrupt DNA replication by intercalating between the base pairs of DNA (or RNA), are synthesized by some bacterial strains such as *Streptomyces* strains. These drugs act as antibiotics and therefore alter the gut microbiome composition. However, some bacterial species are able to detoxify these drugs (Mikó et al., 2019). One of these drugs, doxorubicin, is known to be inactivated by the gut bacteria *Raoultella planticola* (Yan et al., 2018). Gemcitabine, a pyrimidine nucleoside antimetabolite, is used to treat pancreatic or biliary tract cancer (Ciccolini et al., 2016). The efficacy of gemcitabine can be reduced by specific microbiota (Geller et al., 2017). This is due to the ability of these bacteria to produce cytidine deaminase (CDD), an enzyme that processes gemcitabine into its metabolite 2′,2′-difluoro-2′-deoxyuridine (dFdU) (Vande Voorde et al., 2014). This resistance can be reduced using antibiotics such as ciprofloxacin (Geller et al., 2017; Choy et al., 2018). The pyrimidine analogue Ahyuj9jf6/23 5-Fluorouracil (5-FU) (Peters, 2014) is one of the most commonly used chemotherapies. The efficacy of this drug can be reduced by certain gut microbes, especially mycoplasma species or bacteria. This occurs via upregulation in the expression of Baculoviral IAP Repeat Containing 3 (BIRC3). BIRC3 inhibits apoptosis by inhibiting apoptotic protein (IAP) (Deng et al., 2018).

These enzymes can also alter the drug, leading it to become more dangerous or toxic to the patient, resulting in either the reduction of the drug dosage or even suspension of its use (Vanhoefer et al., 2001). For example, the topoisomerase inhibitor irinotecan is an inactive prodrug that is processed into its active form through the activity of the hepatic carboxylesterases. This active form, SN38, is toxic and is detoxified in the liver. However, bacterial β-glucuronidases in the gut convert it back into the toxic form, leading to diarrhea (Wallace et al., 2010).

TARGETING THE MICROBIOME FOR THE TREATMENT AND MANAGEMENT OF CANCER

The link between chemotherapy drug activity and dysbiosis means that the microbiome can be targeted to improve treatment response. For instance, treatment of mice models with 5-FU led to an increase in the number of *Staphylococcus* and *Clostridium* species and a decrease in the number of *Bacteroides* and *Lactobacillus* species. Therefore, the administration of probiotics may be used to restore the microbiome or increase the abundance of bacteria that promote antitumor activity of these drugs (Nakayama et al., 1997).

The microbiome can also be influenced through the use of prebiotics, probiotics, symbiotic, and postbiotics. Prebiotics are nondigestible dietary fibers, which microorganisms can ferment, and selectively favor the growth of commensal microbes (Raman et al., 2013). Prebiotics have been shown to have anticancer effects, as demonstrated in tumor models where a prebiotic increased the ability of various chemotherapy agents to decrease tumor development and metastasis (Taper and Roberfroid, 2000). Probiotics are live microorganisms that can colonize the gut and alter the gut microbiome, consequently they can also alter the gut metabolome and change the interactions between the gut microbiome and the immune system. Probiotics have been shown to decrease colon cancer development and progression in animal models (Górska et al., 2019). Synbiotics are a mixture of pro- and prebiotics (Geier et al., 2006). Postbiotics are a collection of molecules, such as cell metabolites metabolic byproducts, as well as cell types, such as nonfunctioning microbial cells (Homayouni Rad et al., 2021). It is common for cancer patients undergoing chemotherapy/immunotherapy to receive antibiotics in order to protect them from infections that could result from a suppressed immune system. However, they may also be used to target the microbiome and alter the makeup of the gut microbiome to act as an adjunct to cancer therapy (Kong et al., 2014). Antibiotics can also be used to alter the relative abundance of certain bacteria and alter treatment response (Viaud et al., 2013). For example, treatment with cisplatin often leads to nephrotoxicity. When rats being treated with cisplatin were given probiotics containing *Lactobacillus reuteri* and *Clostridium butyricum*, they showed reduced renal inflammation, oxidative stress, fibrosis, and apoptosis (Hsiao et al., 2021). Cisplatin was also shown to be less effective in germ-free mice models of lung cancer (Gui et al., 2015). Bacterial strains can also be engineered to enhance the immune response in order to induce tumor regression (Chowdhury et al., 2019).

One of the methods to manipulate the makeup of the microbiome is through the use of fecal microbiota transplant, which can rapidly and dramatically alter the host microbiome, improving therapy outcomes (Chen et al., 2019a; Chen et al., 2019b). The effectiveness of this method has been demonstrated in mice models. Fecal transplant from mice that were responding to anti-PD-L1 treatment improved the efficacy of immunotherapy in germ-free mice being treated with anti-PD-L1 therapy (Routy et al., 2018).

PERSONALIZED MEDICINE AND THE MICROBIOME

With the development of techniques such as next-generation sequencing (NGS), it has become possible to determine the makeup of an individual's microbiome (Kau et al., 2011; Russo et al., 2016; Tyler et al., 2014). This would allow the microbiome to be used as a diagnostic biomarker or therapeutic target (Morgan and Huttenhower, 2012). Personalized medicine is concerned with tailor-making medical solutions to an individual or group of individuals based on their personal characteristics such as genetic makeup or individual lifestyle. Personalized medicine is a promising solution for the treatment of many diseases, especially cancer (Cho et al., 2012). By understanding a tumor's molecular patterns, therapies and diagnostic tools can be fine-tuned to target or identify these specific molecular patterns. In the same way, an individual's microbiome can be analyzed using NGS or mass spectroscopy to identify the species present in the microbiome. This will give the personalized microbiome of an individual. Changes to the microbiome can be associated with specific diseases (Ling et al., 2010) or disease outcomes. In addition to this, the makeup of the microbiome can be manipulated for therapeutic applications. For instance, the ability of the microbiome to influence the outcome of immunotherapies means that establishing the makeup of an individual's microbiome can be used to ascertain if the treatment will be effective before it is attempted, thereby saving time and money (Gopalakrishnan et al., 2018; Routy et al., 2018). The microbiome can also be used to assess treatment response. For instance, patients that were responding well to anti-PD1 treatment, could be identified by the increased presence of *Faecalibacterium*, while those that were responding poorly show higher numbers of Bacteroidales (Sivan et al., 2015).

Since the microbiome undergoes changes in the composition of the microbial population and structure as cancer is developing, progressing, and being treated, it can be used as a biomarker for the diagnosis, characterization, prognosis, and response of cancer. Fecal samples can be used to diagnose early-stage colorectal cancer. CRC patients show changes in their microbiome as the disease progresses or responds to treatment, associated with CRC stage (Yachida et al., 2019; Mori et al., 2018). Apart from fecal samples, samples can be collected from blood and tissues (Figure 1.3). This is due to the horizontal and vertical translocation of gut microbiome. Horizontal translocation describes the gut microbiome spreading throughout the digestive tract, whereas vertical translocation occurs when microorganisms from the gut are transferred from the intestinal lumen through the deep mucosa and even through the entire host (Jiayi and Lei, 2021).

CONCLUSION

The microbiome is known to play an important role in cancer development and progression. On the other hand, the microbiome and its metabolites can act as cancer inhibitors. Many of the mechanisms involved in this process have been uncovered (Figure 1.4), however, much remains unknown. This book presents our current knowledge on the role played by the microbiome in carcinogenesis and how this knowledge can be used to aid in the treatment and management of a wide variety of cancers. The second chapter will examine the role played by dysbiosis in the gut microbiota in the development of various cancers in more detail, with a focus on the resulting disruption of the delicate equilibrium within the gut. This chapter will explore the mechanisms behind the cancer promoting effect of dysbiosis, including the effects on the immune system, inflammation, and metabolism. Chapter 3 will focus on the influence the gut microbiome has on the response of cancer to treatment and explore the interplay between specific bacteria and various cancer therapies. It will discuss how the efficacy of various treatments can be impacted by the microbiome. This includes the ability of the microbiome to modulate chemotherapy efficacy, affect drug metabolism, modulate the immune response, and alter the tumor microenvironment. Chapter 4 discusses the modulation of the gut microbiome as a strategy to enhance personalized medicine. It will discuss the use of changes to the diet as a means to initiate changes in the microbiome. These include dietary alterations such as a fiber-rich diet or a diet rich in specific nutrients. It will review how these changes to the diet of the patient aim to promote a healthy gut microbial composition. The chapter will also discuss the role and use of probiotics prebiotics,

Introduction to the Gut Microbiome and Cancer

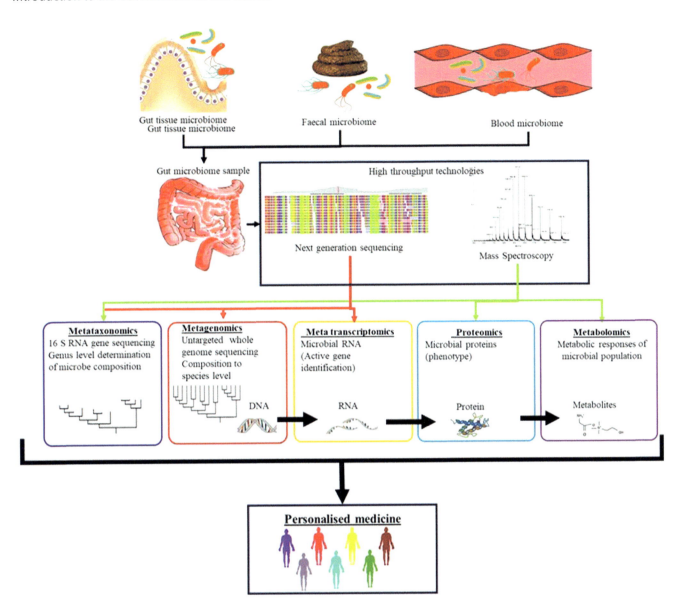

FIGURE 1.3 **The use of the microbiome in personalized medicine.** Samples of the gut microbiome can be collected from various sources, including fecal samples, gut tissue samples, or even blood. This is due to the ability of the microflora to translocate both horizontally and vertically. These samples can be analyzed in numerous ways using next-generation sequencing or mass spectroscopy. The species composition of the microbiome can be determined using whole-genome sequencing or 16S RNA gene sequencing. The genes being expressed by the microbiome can be determined through transcriptomic analysis and the active proteins through mass spectrophotometry. Finally, the pattern of metabolites produced by the microbiome can be determined using mass spectrophotometry. These patterns or the changes in these patterns can be used to make diagnoses, prognostic predictions or even track the course of a disease.

antibiotics, and fecal microbiota transplantation as methods to alter the gut microbiome population, Finally, this chapter will examine case studies as examples of personalized therapeutic approaches.

Chapter 5 will discuss the influence of the gut microbiome on immunotherapy resistance in cancer patients, examining how specific bacterial species modulate immune checkpoint inhibitors response and expel the mechanisms underlying these responses. The chapter will also examine how microbiome-based interventions can be used to overcome immunotherapy resistance and enhance treatment efficacy. This will be followed by Chapter 6 which meticulously examines the interplay between the gut microbiome and chemotherapy, more specifically the impact the microbiome has on chemotherapy resistance. The chapter will delve into the complex dynamics between gut bacteria and cancer treatment efficacy to illuminate how the composition and function of the gut microbiome might contribute to variations in chemotherapy response. The chapter will offer novel insights into potential strategies for enhancing treatment outcomes in cancer patients. Chapter 7 examines the emerging field of gut microbiome biomarkers for cancer diagnosis and prognosis. It will discuss the use of specific microbial signatures as indicators of different cancer types and stages. The chapter

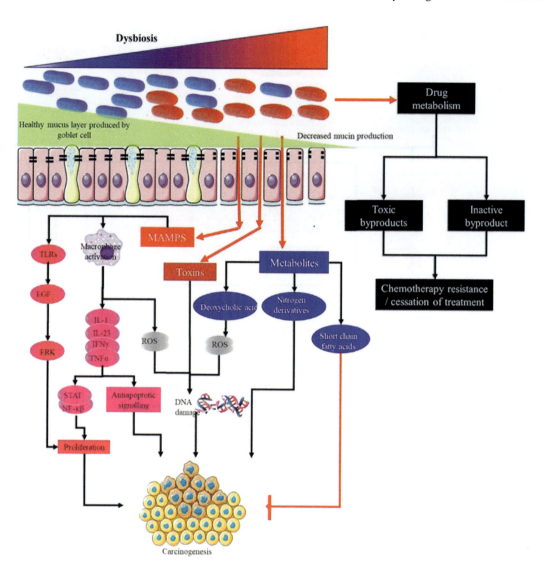

FIGURE 1.4 **The role of the gut microbiome in the development and progression of cancer.** Dysbiosis leads to an increase in pathogenic or potentially harmful bacteria which secrete MAMPS, toxins, or metabolites that lead to a breakdown of the mucosa barrier and decreased secretion of mucins. MAMPS lead to immune signaling which can lead to increased proliferation, decreased apoptosis, and higher levels of reactive oxygen species, which results in DNA damage, and toxins secreted by these microbes can lead to increased DNA damage. These processes and signaling pathways can all lead to increased carcinogenesis. The secondary metabolites released by the gut microbiota can both promote or inhibit carcinogenesis and the change in the population of microbes secreting these substances can result in increased or decreased levels of carcinogenesis. Chemotherapeutic drugs can also be metabolized leading to their detoxification or increased toxicity.

will also highlight the potential of microbial biomarkers in predicting treatment responses and patient outcomes and discuss how this will aid in the development of personalized cancer management.

Chapter 8 focuses on microbial metabolites, exploring the bioactive compounds produced by gut bacteria and their impact on cancer development and progression. It will review the ability of microbial metabolites to modulate immune responses as well as their ability to promote or inhibit tumor growth, angiogenesis, and drug metabolism. The chapter will then highlight the therapeutic potential of targeting specific microbial metabolites. Chapter 9 will examine the implications the gut–brain axis has on the development and progression of cancer. It will examine how immune signaling initiated by the gut microbiome is able to affect the nervous system and the brain and how the metabolites and neurotransmitters released by the gut microbiome are able to influence signaling in the nervous system to initiate neurogenesis and the resulting impact on cancer development and progression. Finally, the chapter highlights the potential for targeting the gut–brain axis as a therapeutic avenue in cancer treatment. Chapter 10 will discuss the role of the gut microbiome in cancer-related inflammation and will explore how specific gut bacteria contribute to chronic inflammation thereby promoting cancer growth and metastasis. It discusses the complex interactions between gut microbes, immune cells, and inflammatory mediators, and highlights potential strategies for modulating inflammation-associated cancer risks. Chapter 11 explores the impact of diet on the gut microbiome and how different diets and lifestyles including exercise and stress influence the composition of the microbiome and therefore influence cancer development and progression. It explores the potential of dietary interventions, such as plant-based diets, probiotics, and fermented foods, in modulating the gut microbiome and reducing cancer risk. The chapter emphasizes the importance of adopting a healthy lifestyle for a diverse and balanced gut microbiome.

Chapter 12 focuses on the role played by the gut microbiome in pediatric cancers. It will examine the unique aspects of the gut microbial community in children, its impact on cancer susceptibility, treatment response, and long-term outcomes. It will then discuss how this knowledge can be used to tailor microbiome-based interventions to the pediatric population in order to improve treatment efficacy and reduce treatment-related complications. Chapter 13 will examine the ways in which the gut microbiome influences the systemic side effects of cancer therapies. This includes the role played by the gut microbiome in chemotherapy-induced toxicity, the response to radiation therapy and treatment-associated complications, including mucositis and gastrointestinal disorders. Chapter 14 will discuss the use of the microbiome in personalized cancer therapy, this includes the use of microbiome profiling to enhance the selection of the correct treatment for patients through microbiome profiling-assisted patient stratification. It will also discuss the development of personalized therapeutic strategies involving the microbiome of an individual patients. It will also discuss the tools and expertise required from multiple fields in order to achieve these goals. This includes collaboration between oncologists, microbiologists, and bioinformaticians. This will be followed by Chapter 15 that reviews the therapeutic potential of the gut virome, which consists of viruses inhabiting the gut, in cancer treatment. This includes the roles that phage therapy, oncolytic viruses, and the manipulation of the virome to modulate antitumor immune responses can play in treating various cancers. The chapter will highlight current research and the problems facing these virome-based strategies. Chapter 16 will review the current cutting-edge research into microbiome-based cancer therapeutics. The chapter will examine the role of gut bacteria, immune modulation, and tumor microenvironment interactions in order to treat cancer. It will also discuss the methods to harness the microbiome to enhance the efficacy of cancer therapies. This includes a review of innovative approaches as well as the challenges and opportunities in translating microbiome research into effective cancer treatments. The final chapter will examine the approaches that can be used to optimize cancer therapies, including the use of microbiome engineering and other innovative approaches. The chapter also highlights the challenges and future directions in gut microbiome engineering research. The role played by the gut microbiome in cancer development and progression and the roles that it could play in improving cancer treatments and outcomes are an exciting topic which we hope this book will assist the reader in understanding.

REFERENCES

AĞAGÜNDÜZ, D., COCOZZA, E., CEMALI, Ö., BAYAZIT, A. D., NANÌ, M. F., CERQUA, I., MORGILLO, F., SAYGILI, S. K., BERNI CANANI, R., AMERO, P., CAPASSO, R. 2023. Understanding the role of the gut microbiome in gastrointestinal cancer: a review. *Front Pharmacol*, 14, 1130562.

ALCINDOR, T. & BEAUGER, N. 2011. Oxaliplatin: a review in the era of molecularly targeted therapy. *Curr Oncol*, 18, 18–25.

ALEXANDER, J. L., WILSON, I. D., TEARE, J., MARCHESI, J. R., NICHOLSON, J. K. & KINROSS, J. M. 2017. Gut microbiota modulation of chemotherapy efficacy and toxicity. *Nat Rev Gastroenterol Hepatol*, 14, 356–365.

AMITAY, E. L. & KEINAN-BOKER, L. 2015. Breastfeeding and childhood leukemia incidence: a meta-analysis and systematic review. *JAMA Pediatr*, 169, e151025.

ARTHUR, J. C., PEREZ-CHANONA, E., MÜHLBAUER, M., TOMKOVICH, S., URONIS, J. M., FAN, T. J., CAMPBELL, B. J., ABUJAMEL, T., DOGAN, B., ROGERS, A. B., RHODES, J. M., STINTZI, A., SIMPSON, K. W., HANSEN, J. J., KEKU, T. O., FODOR, A. A. & JOBIN, C. 2012. Intestinal inflammation targets cancer-inducing activity of the microbiota. *Science*, 338, 120–123.

BÄCKHED, F., ROSWALL, J., PENG, Y., FENG, Q., JIA, H., KOVATCHEVA-DATCHARY, P., LI, Y., XIA, Y., XIE, H., ZHONG, H., KHAN, M. T., ZHANG, J., LI, J., XIAO, L., AL-AAMA, J., ZHANG, D., LEE, Y. S., KOTOWSKA, D., COLDING, C., TREMAROLI, V., YIN, Y., BERGMAN, S., XU, X., MADSEN, L., KRISTIANSEN, K., DAHLGREN, J. & WANG, J. 2015. Dynamics and stabilization of the human gut microbiome during the first year of life. *Cell Host Microbe*, 17, 690–703.

BAI, G. H., LIN, S. C., HSU, Y. H. & CHEN, S. Y. 2022. The human virome: viral metagenomics, relations with human diseases, and therapeutic applications. *Viruses*, Jan 28;14(2):278.

BARDHAN, K., ANAGNOSTOU, T. & BOUSSIOTIS, V. A. 2016. The PD1: PD-L1/2 pathway from discovery to clinical implementation. *Front Immunol*, 7, 550.

BERGOUNIOUX, J., ELISEE, R., PRUNIER, A. L., DONNADIEU, F., SPERANDIO, B., SANSONETTI, P. & ARBIBE, L. 2012. Calpain activation by the Shigella flexneri effector VirA regulates key steps in the formation and life of the bacterium's epithelial niche. *Cell Host Microbe*, 11, 240–252.

BHATT, A. P., REDINBO, M. R. & BULTMAN, S. J. 2017. The role of the microbiome in cancer development and therapy. *CA: Cancer J Clin*, 67, 326–344.

BRANISTE, V., AL-ASMAKH, M., KOWAL, C., ANUAR, F., ABBASPOUR, A., TÓTH, M., KORECKA, A., BAKOCEVIC, N., NG, L. G., KUNDU, P., GULYÁS, B., HALLDIN, C., HULTENBY, K., NILSSON, H., HEBERT, H., VOLPE, B. T., DIAMOND, B. & PETTERSSON, S. 2014. The gut microbiota influences blood-brain barrier permeability in mice. *Sci Transl Med*, 6, 263ra158.

CABALLERO, S. & PAMER, E. G. 2015. Microbiota-mediated inflammation and antimicrobial defense in the intestine. *Ann Rev Immunol*, 33, 227–256.

CARABOTTI, M., SCIROCCO, A., MASELLI, M. A. & SEVERI, C. 2015. The gut-brain axis: interactions between enteric microbiota, central and enteric nervous systems. *Ann Gastroenterol*, 28, 203–209.

CHEN, D., WU, J., JIN, D., WANG, B. & CAO, H. 2019a. Fecal microbiota transplantation in cancer management: current status and perspectives. *Int J Cancer*, 145, 2021–2031.

CHEN, F., LI, S., GUO, R., SONG, F., ZHANG, Y., WANG, X., HUO, X., LV, Q., ULLAH, H., WANG, G., MA, Y., YAN, Q. & MA, X. 2023. Meta-analysis of fecal viromes demonstrates high diagnostic potential of the gut viral signatures for colorectal cancer and adenoma risk assessment. *J Adv Res,* 49, 103–114.

CHEN, M. X., WANG, S. Y., KUO, C. H. & TSAI, I. L. 2019b. Metabolome analysis for investigating host-gut microbiota interactions. *J Formos Med Assoc,* 118(Suppl 1), S10–S22.

CHO, S. H., JEON, J. & KIM, S. I. 2012. Personalized medicine in breast cancer: a systematic review. *J Breast Cancer,* 15, 265–272.

CHOWDHURY, S., CASTRO, S., COKER, C., HINCHLIFFE, T. E., ARPAIA, N. & DANINO, T. 2019. Programmable bacteria induce durable tumor regression and systemic antitumor immunity. *Nat Med,* 25, 1057–1063.

CHOY, A. T. F., CARNEVALE, I., COPPOLA, S., MEIJER, L. L., KAZEMIER, G., ZAURA, E., DENG, D. & GIOVANNETTI, E. 2018. The microbiome of pancreatic cancer: from molecular diagnostics to new therapeutic approaches to overcome chemoresistance caused by metabolic inactivation of gemcitabine. *Expert Rev Mol Diagn,* 18, 1005–1009.

CHRYSOSTOMOU, D., ROBERTS, L. A., MARCHESI, J. R. & KINROSS, J. M. 2023. Gut microbiota modulation of efficacy and toxicity of cancer chemotherapy and immunotherapy. *Gastroenterology,* 164, 198–213.

CICCOLINI, J., SERDJEBI, C., PETERS, G. J. & GIOVANNETTI, E. 2016. Pharmacokinetics and pharmacogenetics of Gemcitabine as a mainstay in adult and pediatric oncology: an EORTC-PAMM perspective. *Cancer Chemother Pharmacol,* 78, 1–12.

COKER, O. O., DAI, Z., NIE, Y., ZHAO, G., CAO, L., NAKATSU, G., WU, W. K., WONG, S. H., CHEN, Z., SUNG, J. J. Y. & YU, J. 2018. Mucosal microbiome dysbiosis in gastric carcinogenesis. *Gut,* 67, 1024–1032.

DANG, A. T. & MARSLAND, B. J. 2019. Microbes, metabolites, and the gut-lung axis. *Mucosal Immunol,* 12, 843–850.

DE MARTEL, C., GEORGES, D., BRAY, F., FERLAY, J. & CLIFFORD, G. M. 2020. Global burden of cancer attributable to infections in 2018: a worldwide incidence analysis. *Lancet Glob Health,* 8, e180–e190.

DENG, X., LI, Z., LI, G., LI, B., JIN, X. & LYU, G. 2018. Comparison of microbiota in patients treated by surgery or chemotherapy by 16S rRNA sequencing reveals potential biomarkers for colorectal cancer therapy. *Front Microbiol,* 9, 1607.

ENCARNAÇÃO, J. C., PIRES, A. S., AMARAL, R. A., GONÇALVES, T. J., LARANJO, M., CASALTA-LOPES, J. E., GONÇALVES, A. C., SARMENTO-RIBEIRO, A. B., ABRANTES, A. M. & BOTELHO, M. F. 2018. Butyrate, a dietary fiber derivative that improves irinotecan effect in colon cancer cells. *J Nutr Biochem,* 56, 183–192.

FORSGÅRD, R. A., MARRACHELLI, V. G., KORPELA, K., FRIAS, R., COLLADO, M. C., KORPELA, R., MONLEON, D., SPILLMANN, T. & ÖSTERLUND, P. 2017. Chemotherapy-induced gastrointestinal toxicity is associated with changes in serum and urine metabolome and fecal microbiota in male Sprague-Dawley rats. *Cancer Chemother Pharmacol,* 80, 317–332.

FRISAN, T. 2016. Bacterial genotoxins: the long journey to the nucleus of mammalian cells. *Biochim Biophys Acta,* 1858, 567–575.

GEIER, M. S., BUTLER, R. N. & HOWARTH, G. S. 2006. Probiotics, prebiotics and synbiotics: a role in chemoprevention for colorectal cancer? *Cancer Biol Ther,* 5, 1265–1269.

GELLER, L. T., BARZILY-ROKNI, M., DANINO, T., JONAS, O. H., SHENTAL, N., NEJMAN, D., GAVERT, N., ZWANG, Y., COOPER, Z. A., SHEE, K., THAISS, C. A., REUBEN, A., LIVNY, J., AVRAHAM, R., FREDERICK, D. T., LIGORIO, M., CHATMAN, K., JOHNSTON, S. E., MOSHER, C. M., BRANDIS, A., FUKS, G., GURBATRI, C., GOPALAKRISHNAN, V., KIM, M., HURD, M. W., KATZ, M., FLEMING, J., MAITRA, A., SMITH, D. A., SKALAK, M., BU, J., MICHAUD, M., TRAUGER, S. A., BARSHACK, I., GOLAN, T., SANDBANK, J., FLAHERTY, K. T., MANDINOVA, A., GARRETT, W. S., THAYER, S. P., FERRONE, C. R., HUTTENHOWER, C., BHATIA, S. N., GEVERS, D., WARGO, J. A., GOLUB, T. R. & STRAUSSMAN, R. 2017. Potential role of intratumor bacteria in mediating tumor resistance to the chemotherapeutic drug gemcitabine. *Science,* 357, 1156–1160.

GOPALAKRISHNAN, V., SPENCER, C. N., NEZI, L., REUBEN, A., ANDREWS, M. C., KARPINETS, T. V., PRIETO, P. A., VICENTE, D., HOFFMAN, K., WEI, S. C., COGDILL, A. P., ZHAO, L., HUDGENS, C. W., HUTCHINSON, D. S., MANZO, T., PETACCIA DE MACEDO, M., COTECHINI, T., KUMAR, T., CHEN, W. S., REDDY, S. M., SZCZEPANIAK SLOANE, R., GALLOWAY-PENA, J., JIANG, H., CHEN, P. L., SHPALL, E. J., REZVANI, K., ALOUSI, A. M., CHEMALY, R. F., SHELBURNE, S., VENCE, L. M., OKHUYSEN, P. C., JENSEN, V. B., SWENNES, A. G., MCALLISTER, F., MARCELO RIQUELME SANCHEZ, E., ZHANG, Y., LE CHATELIER, E., ZITVOGEL, L., PONS, N., AUSTIN-BRENEMAN, J. L., HAYDU, L. E., BURTON, E. M., GARDNER, J. M., SIRMANS, E., HU, J., LAZAR, A. J., TSUJIKAWA, T., DIAB, A., TAWBI, H., GLITZA, I. C., HWU, W. J., PATEL, S. P., WOODMAN, S. E., AMARIA, R. N., DAVIES, M. A., GERSHENWALD, J. E., HWU, P., LEE, J. E., ZHANG, J., COUSSENS, L. M., COOPER, Z. A., FUTREAL, P. A., DANIEL, C. R., AJAMI, N. J., PETROSINO, J. F., TETZLAFF, M. T., SHARMA, P., ALLISON, J. P., JENQ, R. R. & WARGO, J. A. 2018. Gut microbiome modulates response to anti-PD-1 immunotherapy in melanoma patients. *Science,* 359, 97–103.

GÓRSKA, A., PRZYSTUPSKI, D., NIEMCZURA, M. J. & KULBACKA, J. 2019. Probiotic bacteria: a promising tool in cancer prevention and therapy. *Curr Microbiol,* 76, 939–949.

GOUBET, A. G., DAILLÈRE, R., ROUTY, B., DEROSA, L., Roberti, P. M. & ZITVOGEL, L. 2018. The impact of the intestinal microbiota in therapeutic responses against cancer. *C R Biol,* 341, 284–289.

GRASSO, F. & FRISAN, T. 2015. Bacterial genotoxins: merging the DNA damage response into infection biology. *Biomolecules,* 5, 1762–1782.

GUI, Q. F., LU, H. F., ZHANG, C. X., XU, Z. R. & YANG, Y. H. 2015. Well-balanced commensal microbiota contributes to anti-cancer response in a lung cancer mouse model. *Genet Mol Res,* 14, 5642–5651.

HANAHAN, D. 2022. Hallmarks of cancer: new dimensions. *Cancer Discov,* 12, 31–46.

HATAKEYAMA, M. 2017. Structure and function of Helicobacter pylori CagA, the first-identified bacterial protein involved in human cancer. *Proc Jpn Acad Ser B Phys Biol Sci,* 93, 196–219.

HELMINK, B. A., KHAN, M. A. W., HERMANN, A., GOPALAKRISHNAN, V. & WARGO, J. A. 2019. The microbiome, cancer, and cancer therapy. *Nat Med,* 25, 377–388.

HOMAYOUNI RAD, A., AGHEBATI MALEKI, L., SAMADI KAFIL, H., FATHI ZAVOSHTI, H. & ABBASI, A. 2021. Postbiotics as promising tools for cancer adjuvant therapy. *Adv Pharm Bull,* 11, 1–5.

HSIAO, Y. P., CHEN, H. L., TSAI, J. N., LIN, M. Y., LIAO, J. W., WEI, M. S., KO, J. L. & OU, C. C. 2021. Administration of Lactobacillus reuteri combined with clostridium butyricum attenuates cisplatin-induced renal damage by gut microbiota reconstitution, increasing butyric acid production, and suppressing renal inflammation. *Nutrients,* Aug 15;13(8):2792

HUANG, Y., YANG, W., LIU, H., DUAN, J., ZHANG, Y., LIU, M., LI, H., HOU, Z. & WU, K. K. 2012. Effect of high-dose methotrexate chemotherapy on intestinal Bifidobacteria, Lactobacillus and Escherichia coli in children with acute lymphoblastic leukemia. *Exp Biol Med (Maywood),* 237, 305–311.

HULL, R., LOLAS, G., MAKROGKIKAS, S., JENSEN, L. D., SYRIGOS, K. N., EVANGELOU, G., PADAYACHY, L., EGBOR, C., MEHROTRA, R., MAKHAFOLA, T. J., OYOMNO, M. & DLAMINI, Z. 2021. Microbiomics in collusion with the nervous system in carcinogenesis: diagnosis, pathogenesis and treatment. *Microorganisms,* Aug 15;13(8):2792.

IARC. 2019. Advisory group recommendations on priorities for the IARC monographs. *Lancet Oncol,* 20, 763–764.

IIDA, N., DZUTSEV, A., STEWART, C. A., SMITH, L., BOULADOUX, N., WEINGARTEN, R. A., MOLINA, D. A., SALCEDO, R., BACK, T., CRAMER, S., DAI, R. M., KIU, H., CARDONE, M., NAIK, S., PATRI, A. K., WANG, E., MARINCOLA, F. M., FRANK, K. M., BELKAID, Y., TRINCHIERI, G. & GOLDSZMID, R. S. 2013. Commensal bacteria control cancer response to therapy by modulating the tumor microenvironment. *Science,* 342, 967–970.

JIAYI, H. & LEI, C. 2021. Research progress of intestinal flora imbalance and colorectal cancer. *Transl Med J,* 10 (4).

JIN, Y., DONG, H., XIA, L., YANG, Y., ZHU, Y., SHEN, Y., ZHENG, H., YAO, C., WANG, Y. & LU, S. 2019. The diversity of gut microbiome is associated with favorable responses to anti-programmed death 1 immunotherapy in Chinese patients with NSCLC. *J Thorac Oncol,* 14, 1378–1389.

KAU, A. L., AHERN, P. P., GRIFFIN, N. W., GOODMAN, A. L. & GORDON, J. I. 2011. Human nutrition, the gut microbiome and the immune system. *Nature,* 474, 327–336.

KAUFMAN, H. L., KOHLHAPP, F. J. & ZLOZA, A. 2015. Oncolytic viruses: a new class of immunotherapy drugs. *Nat Rev Drug Discov,* 14, 642–662.

KIM, J. J., TAO, H., CARLONI, E., LEUNG, W. K., GRAHAM, D. Y. & SEPULVEDA, A. R. 2002. Helicobacter pylori impairs DNA mismatch repair in gastric epithelial cells. *Gastroenterology,* 123, 542–553.

KOENIG, J. E., SPOR, A., SCALFONE, N., FRICKER, A. D., STOMBAUGH, J., KNIGHT, R., ANGENENT, L. T. & LEY, R. E. 2011. Succession of microbial consortia in the developing infant gut microbiome. *Proc Natl Acad Sci USA,* 108 Suppl 1, 4578–4585.

KONG, R., LIU, T., ZHU, X., AHMAD, S., WILLIAMS, A. L., PHAN, A. T., ZHAO, H., SCOTT, J. E., YEH, L. A. & WONG, S. T. 2014. Old drug new use--amoxapine and its metabolites as potent bacterial β-glucuronidase inhibitors for alleviating cancer drug toxicity. *Clin Cancer Res,* 20, 3521–3530.

KUWAHARA, A., MATSUDA, K., KUWAHARA, Y., ASANO, S., INUI, T. & MARUNAKA, Y. 2020. Microbiota-gut-brain axis: enteroendocrine cells and the enteric nervous system form an interface between the microbiota and the central nervous system. *Biomed Res,* 41, 199–216.

LARA-TEJERO, M. & GALÁN, J. E. 2000. A bacterial toxin that controls cell cycle progression as a deoxyribonuclease I-like protein. *Science,* 290, 354–357.

LEE, L., GUPTA, M. & SAHASRANAMAN, S. 2016. Immune checkpoint inhibitors: an introduction to the next-generation cancer immunotherapy. *J Clin Pharmacol,* 56, 157–169.

LEHOURITIS, P., CUMMINS, J., STANTON, M., MURPHY, C. T., MCCARTHY, F. O., REID, G., URBANIAK, C., BYRNE, W. L. & TANGNEY, M. 2015. Local bacteria affect the efficacy of chemotherapeutic drugs. *Sci Rep,* 5, 14554.

LING, Z., KONG, J., LIU, F., ZHU, H., CHEN, X., WANG, Y., LI, L., NELSON, K. E., XIA, Y. & XIANG, C. 2010. Molecular analysis of the diversity of vaginal microbiota associated with bacterial vaginosis. *BMC Genomics,* 11, 488.

MA, W., MAO, Q., XIA, W., DONG, G., YU, C. & JIANG, F. 2019. Gut microbiota shapes the efficiency of cancer therapy. *Front Microbiol,* 10, 1050.

MATSON, V., CHERVIN, C. S. & GAJEWSKI, T. F. 2021. Cancer and the microbiome-influence of the commensal microbiota on cancer, immune responses, and immunotherapy. *Gastroenterology,* 160, 600–613.

MIKÓ, E., KOVÁCS, T., SEBŐ, É., TÓTH, J., CSONKA, T., UJLAKI, G., SIPOS, A., SZABÓ, J., MÉHES, G. & BAI, P. 2019. Microbiome-microbial metabolome-cancer cell interactions in breast cancer-familiar, but unexplored. *Cells,* Mar 29;8(4):293.

MORGAN, X. C. & HUTTENHOWER, C. 2012. Chapter 12: human microbiome analysis. *PLoS Comput Biol,* 8, e1002808.

MORI, G., RAMPELLI, S., ORENA, B. S., RENGUCCI, C., DE MAIO, G., BARBIERI, G., PASSARDI, A., CASADEI GARDINI, A., FRASSINETI, G. L., GAIARSA, S., ALBERTINI, A. M., RANZANI, G. N., CALISTRI, D. & PASCA, M. R. 2018. Shifts of faecal microbiota during sporadic colorectal carcinogenesis. *Sci Rep,* 8, 10329.

MU, C. & ZHU, W. 2019. Antibiotic effects on gut microbiota, metabolism, and beyond. *Appl Microbiol Biotechnol,* 103, 9277–9285.

MULDER, I. E., SCHMIDT, B., STOKES, C. R., LEWIS, M., BAILEY, M., AMINOV, R. I., PROSSER, J. I., GILL, B. P., PLUSKE, J. R., MAYER, C. D., MUSK, C. C. & KELLY, D. 2009. Environmentally-acquired bacteria influence microbial diversity and natural innate immune responses at gut surfaces. *BMC Biol,* 7, 79.

MURATA-KAMIYA, N., KURASHIMA, Y., TEISHIKATA, Y., YAMAHASHI, Y., SAITO, Y., HIGASHI, H., ABURATANI, H., AKIYAMA, T., PEEK, R. M., JR., AZUMA, T. & HATAKEYAMA, M. 2007. Helicobacter pylori CagA interacts with E-cadherin and deregulates the beta-catenin signal that promotes intestinal transdifferentiation in gastric epithelial cells. *Oncogene,* 26, 4617–4626.

NAKAYAMA, H., KINOUCHI, T., KATAOKA, K., AKIMOTO, S., MATSUDA, Y. & OHNISHI, Y. 1997. Intestinal anaerobic bacteria hydrolyse sorivudine, producing the high blood concentration of 5-(E)-(2-bromovinyl)uracil that increases the level and toxicity of 5-fluorouracil. *Pharmacogenetics,* 7, 35–43.

NOUGAYRÈDE, J. P., HOMBURG, S., TAIEB, F., BOURY, M., BRZUSZKIEWICZ, E., GOTTSCHALK, G., BUCHRIESER, C., HACKER, J., DOBRINDT, U. & OSWALD, E. 2006. Escherichia coli induces DNA double-strand breaks in eukaryotic cells. *Science*, 313, 848–851.

OHAEGBULAM, K. C., ASSAL, A., LAZAR-MOLNAR, E., YAO, Y. & ZANG, X. 2015. Human cancer immunotherapy with antibodies to the PD-1 and PD-L1 pathway. *Trends Mol Med*, 21, 24–33.

OU, J., DELANY, J. P., ZHANG, M., SHARMA, S. & O'KEEFE, S. J. 2012. Association between low colonic short-chain fatty acids and high bile acids in high colon cancer risk populations. *Nutr Cancer*, 64, 34–40.

PAN, C., LIU, H., ROBINS, E., SONG, W., LIU, D., LI, Z. & ZHENG, L. 2020. Next-generation immuno-oncology agents: current momentum shifts in cancer immunotherapy. *J Hematol Oncol*, 13, 29.

PETERS, G. J. 2014. Novel developments in the use of antimetabolites. *Nucleosides Nucleotides Nucl Acids*, 33, 358–374.

PLEGUEZUELOS-MANZANO, C., PUSCHHOF, J., ROSENDAHL HUBER, A., VAN HOECK, A., WOOD, H. M., NOMBURG, J., GURJAO, C., MANDERS, F., DALMASSO, G., STEGE, P. B., PAGANELLI, F. L., GEURTS, M. H., BEUMER, J., MIZUTANI, T., MIAO, Y., VAN DER LINDEN, R., VAN DER ELST, S., GARCIA, K. C., TOP, J., WILLEMS, R. J. L., GIANNAKIS, M., BONNET, R., QUIRKE, P., MEYERSON, M., CUPPEN, E., VAN BOXTEL, R. & CLEVERS, H. 2020. Mutational signature in colorectal cancer caused by genotoxic pks(+) E. coli. *Nature*, 580, 269–273.

POLLET, R. M., D'AGOSTINO, E. H., WALTON, W. G., XU, Y., LITTLE, M. S., BIERNAT, K. A., PELLOCK, S. J., PATTERSON, L. M., CREEKMORE, B. C., ISENBERG, H. N., BAHETHI, R. R., BHATT, A. P., LIU, J., GHARAIBEH, R. Z. & REDINBO, M. R. 2017. An Atlas of β-glucuronidases in the human intestinal microbiome. *Structure*, 25, 967–977.e5.

RAMAN, M., AMBALAM, P., KONDEPUDI, K. K., PITHVA, S., KOTHARI, C., PATEL, A. T., PURAMA, R. K., DAVE, J. M. & VYAS, B. R. 2013. Potential of probiotics, prebiotics and synbiotics for management of colorectal cancer. *Gut Microbes*, 4, 181–192.

REA, D., COPPOLA, G., PALMA, G., BARBIERI, A., LUCIANO, A., DEL PRETE, P., ROSSETTI, S., BERRETTA, M., FACCHINI, G., PERDONÀ, S., TURCO, M. C. & ARRA, C. 2018. Microbiota effects on cancer: from risks to therapies. *Oncotarget*, 9, 17915–17927.

ROOKS, M. G. & GARRETT, W. S. 2016. Gut microbiota, metabolites and host immunity. *Nat Rev Immunol*, 16, 341–352.

ROUTY, B., LE CHATELIER, E., DEROSA, L., DUONG, C. P. M., ALOU, M. T., DAILLÈRE, R., FLUCKIGER, A., MESSAOUDENE, M., RAUBER, C., ROBERTI, M. P., FIDELLE, M., FLAMENT, C., POIRIER-COLAME, V., OPOLON, P., KLEIN, C., IRIBARREN, K., MONDRAGÓN, L., JACQUELOT, N., QU, B., FERRERE, G., CLÉMENSON, C., MEZQUITA, L., MASIP, J. R., NALTET, C., BROSSEAU, S., KADERBHAI, C., RICHARD, C., RIZVI, H., LEVENEZ, F., GALLERON, N., QUINQUIS, B., PONS, N., RYFFEL, B., MINARD-COLIN, V., GONIN, P., SORIA, J. C., DEUTSCH, E., LORIOT, Y., GHIRINGHELLI, F., ZALCMAN, G., GOLDWASSER, F., ESCUDIER, B., HELLMANN, M. D., EGGERMONT, A., RAOULT, D., ALBIGES, L., KROEMER, G. & ZITVOGEL, L. 2018. Gut microbiome influences efficacy of PD-1-based immunotherapy against epithelial tumors. *Science*, 359, 91–97.

RUBINSTEIN, M. R., WANG, X., LIU, W., HAO, Y., CAI, G. & HAN, Y. W. 2013. Fusobacterium nucleatum promotes colorectal carcinogenesis by modulating E-cadherin/β-catenin signaling via its FadA adhesin. *Cell Host Microbe*, 14, 195–206.

RUSSO, E., TADDEI, A., RINGRESSI, M. N., RICCI, F. & AMEDEI, A. 2016. The interplay between the microbiome and the adaptive immune response in cancer development. *Therap Adv Gastroenterol*, 9, 594–605.

SÁNCHEZ-ALCOHOLADO, L., RAMOS-MOLINA, B., OTERO, A., LABORDA-ILLANES, A., ORDÓÑEZ, R., MEDINA, J. A., GÓMEZ-MILLÁN, J. & QUEIPO-ORTUÑO, M. I. 2020. The role of the gut microbiome in colorectal cancer development and therapy response. *Cancers (Basel)*, May 29;12(6):1406.

SANTIAGO-RODRIGUEZ, T. M. & HOLLISTER, E. B. 2019. Human virome and disease: high-throughput sequencing for virus discovery, identification of phage-bacteria dysbiosis and development of therapeutic approaches with emphasis on the human gut. *Viruses*, 11. Jul 18;11(7):656.

SEKIROV, I., RUSSELL, S. L., ANTUNES, L. C. & FINLAY, B. B. 2010. Gut microbiota in health and disease. *Physiol Rev*, 90, 859–904.

SENDER, R., FUCHS, S. & MILO, R. 2016. Revised estimates for the number of human and bacteria cells in the body. *PLoS Biol*, 14, e1002533.

SHEFLIN, A. M., WHITNEY, A. K. & WEIR, T. L. 2014. Cancer-promoting effects of microbial dysbiosis. *Curr Oncol Rep*, 16, 406.

SHI, T., SONG, X., WANG, Y., LIU, F. & WEI, J. 2020. Combining oncolytic viruses with cancer immunotherapy: establishing a new generation of cancer treatment. *Front Immunol*, 11, 683.

SINHA, S., LIN, G. & FERENCZI, K. 2021. The skin microbiome and the gut-skin axis. *Clin Dermatol*, 39, 829–839.

SIVAN, A., CORRALES, L., HUBERT, N., WILLIAMS, J. B., AQUINO-MICHAELS, K., EARLEY, Z. M., BENYAMIN, F. W., LEI, Y. M., JABRI, B., ALEGRE, M. L., CHANG, E. B. & GAJEWSKI, T. F. 2015. Commensal Bifidobacterium promotes antitumor immunity and facilitates anti-PD-L1 efficacy. *Science*, 350, 1084–1089.

SPENCER, L., OLAWUNI, B. & SINGH, P. 2022. Gut virome: role and distribution in health and gastrointestinal diseases. *Front Cell Infect Microbiol*, 12, 836706.

TAPER, H. S. & ROBERFROID, M. B. 2000. Nontoxic potentiation of cancer chemotherapy by dietary oligofructose or inulin. *Nutr Cancer*, 38, 1–5.

TOLLER, I. M., NEELSEN, K. J., STEGER, M., HARTUNG, M. L., HOTTIGER, M. O., STUCKI, M., KALALI, B., GERHARD, M., SARTORI, A. A., LOPES, M. & MÜLLER, A. 2011. Carcinogenic bacterial pathogen Helicobacter pylori triggers DNA double-strand breaks and a DNA damage response in its host cells. *Proc Natl Acad Sci USA*, 108, 14944–14949.

TRAVAGLI, R. A. & ANSELMI, L. 2016. Vagal neurocircuitry and its influence on gastric motility. *Nat Rev Gastroenterol Hepatol*, 13, 389–401.

TWUMASI-BOATENG, K., PETTIGREW, J. L., KWOK, Y. Y. E., BELL, J. C. & NELSON, B. H. 2018. Oncolytic viruses as engineering platforms for combination immunotherapy. *Nat Rev Cancer,* 18, 419–432.

TYLER, A. D., SMITH, M. I. & SILVERBERG, M. S. 2014. Analyzing the human microbiome: a "how to" guide for physicians. *Am J Gastroenterol,* 109, 983–993.

VANDE VOORDE, J., SABUNCUOĞLU, S., NOPPEN, S., HOFER, A., RANJBARIAN, F., FIEUWS, S., BALZARINI, J. & LIEKENS, S. 2014. Nucleoside-catabolizing enzymes in mycoplasma-infected tumor cell cultures compromise the cytostatic activity of the anticancer drug gemcitabine. *J Biol Chem,* 289, 13054–13065.

VANHOEFER, U., HARSTRICK, A., ACHTERRATH, W., CAO, S., SEEBER, S. & RUSTUM, Y. M. 2001. Irinotecan in the treatment of colorectal cancer: clinical overview. *J Clin Oncol,* 19, 1501–15018.

VERNIERI, C., FUCÀ, G., LIGORIO, F., HUBER, V., VINGIANI, A., IANNELLI, F., RAIMONDI, A., RINCHAI, D., FRIGÈ, G., BELFIORE, A., LALLI, L., CHIODONI, C., CANCILA, V., ZANARDI, F., AJAZI, A., CORTELLINO, S., VALLACCHI, V., SQUARCINA, P., COVA, A., PESCE, S., FRATI, P., MALL, R., CORSETTO, P. A., RIZZO, A. M., FERRARIS, C., FOLLI, S., GARASSINO, M. C., CAPRI, G., BIANCHI, G., COLOMBO, M. P., MINUCCI, S., FOIANI, M., LONGO, V. D., APOLONE, G., TORRI, V., PRUNERI, G., BEDOGNETTI, D., RIVOLTINI, L. & DE BRAUD, F. 2022. Fasting-mimicking diet is safe and reshapes metabolism and antitumor immunity in patients with cancer. *Cancer Discov,* 12, 90–107.

VÉTIZOU, M., PITT, J. M., DAILLÈRE, R., LEPAGE, P., WALDSCHMITT, N., FLAMENT, C., RUSAKIEWICZ, S., ROUTY, B., ROBERTI, M. P., DUONG, C. P., POIRIER-COLAME, V., ROUX, A., BECHAREF, S., FORMENTI, S., GOLDEN, E., CORDING, S., EBERL, G., SCHLITZER, A., GINHOUX, F., MANI, S., YAMAZAKI, T., JACQUELOT, N., ENOT, D. P., BÉRARD, M., NIGOU, J., OPOLON, P., EGGERMONT, A., WOERTHER, P. L., CHACHATY, E., CHAPUT, N., ROBERT, C., MATEUS, C., KROEMER, G., RAOULT, D., BONECA, I. G., CARBONNEL, F., CHAMAILLARD, M. & ZITVOGEL, L. 2015. Anticancer immunotherapy by CTLA-4 blockade relies on the gut microbiota. *Science,* 350, 1079–1084.

VIAUD, S., SACCHERI, F., MIGNOT, G., YAMAZAKI, T., DAILLÈRE, R., HANNANI, D., ENOT, D. P., PFIRSCHKE, C., ENGBLOM, C., PITTET, M. J., SCHLITZER, A., GINHOUX, F., APETOH, L., CHACHATY, E., WOERTHER, P. L., EBERL, G., BÉRARD, M., ECOBICHON, C., CLERMONT, D., BIZET, C., GABORIAU-ROUTHIAU, V., CERF-BENSUSSAN, N., OPOLON, P., YESSAAD, N., VIVIER, E., RYFFEL, B., ELSON, C. O., DORÉ, J., KROEMER, G., LEPAGE, P., BONECA, I. G., GHIRINGHELLI, F. & ZITVOGEL, L. 2013. The intestinal microbiota modulates the anticancer immune effects of cyclophosphamide. *Science,* 342, 971–976.

VIRGIN, H. W. 2014. The virome in mammalian physiology and disease. *Cell,* 157, 142–150.

WALLACE, B. D., WANG, H., LANE, K. T., SCOTT, J. E., ORANS, J., KOO, J. S., VENKATESH, M., JOBIN, C., YEH, L. A., MANI, S. & REDINBO, M. R. 2010. Alleviating cancer drug toxicity by inhibiting a bacterial enzyme. *Science,* 330, 831–835.

WANG, R., WIEMELS, J. L., METAYER, C., MORIMOTO, L., FRANCIS, S. S., KADAN-LOTTICK, N., DEWAN, A. T., ZHANG, Y. & MA, X. 2017. Cesarean section and risk of childhood acute lymphoblastic leukemia in a population-based, record-linkage study in California. *Am J Epidemiol,* 185, 96–105.

WU, S., RHEE, K. J., ZHANG, M., FRANCO, A. & SEARS, C. L. 2007. Bacteroides fragilis toxin stimulates intestinal epithelial cell shedding and gamma-secretase-dependent E-cadherin cleavage. *J Cell Sci,* 120, 1944–1952.

YACHIDA, S., MIZUTANI, S., SHIROMA, H., SHIBA, S., NAKAJIMA, T., SAKAMOTO, T., WATANABE, H., MASUDA, K., NISHIMOTO, Y., KUBO, M., HOSODA, F., ROKUTAN, H., MATSUMOTO, M., TAKAMARU, H., YAMADA, M., MATSUDA, T., IWASAKI, M., YAMAJI, T., YACHIDA, T., SOGA, T., KUROKAWA, K., TOYODA, A., OGURA, Y., HAYASHI, T., HATAKEYAMA, M., NAKAGAMA, H., SAITO, Y., FUKUDA, S., SHIBATA, T. & YAMADA, T. 2019. Metagenomic and metabolomic analyses reveal distinct stage-specific phenotypes of the gut microbiota in colorectal cancer. *Nat Med,* 25, 968–976.

YAN, A., CULP, E., PERRY, J., LAU, J. T., MACNEIL, L. T., SURETTE, M. G. & WRIGHT, G. D. 2018. Transformation of the anticancer drug doxorubicin in the human gut microbiome. *ACS Infect Dis,* 4, 68–76.

YAO, Y. & DAI, W. 2014. Genomic instability and cancer. *J Carcinog Mutagen,* 5.

ZHANG, W., AN, Y., QIN, X., WU, X., WANG, X., HOU, H., SONG, X., LIU, T., WANG, B., HUANG, X. & CAO, H. 2021a. Gut microbiota-derived metabolites in colorectal cancer: the bad and the challenges. *Front Oncol,* Feb 25;11, 739648.

ZHANG, Z., KUO, J. C., YAO, S., ZHANG, C., KHAN, H. & LEE, R. J. 2021b. CpG oligodeoxynucleotides for anticancer monotherapy from preclinical stages to

ZHENG, D., LIWINSKI, T. & ELINAV, E. 2020. Interaction between microbiota and immunity in health and disease. *Cell Res,* 30, 492–506.

ZHENG, M., HUANG, J., TONG, A. & YANG, H. 2019. Oncolytic viruses for cancer therapy: barriers and recent advances. *Mol Ther Oncolytics,* 15, 234–247.

2 Gut Microbiome Dysbiosis and Cancer Risk

Demetra Demetriou, Georgios Lolas, Benny Mosoane, and Zodwa Dlamini

INTRODUCTION TO THE GUT MICROBIOME DYSBIOSIS

The human gastrointestinal tract harbors approximately 10^{14} bacterial cells of diverse species, primarily Firmicutes and Bacteroidetes (DeGruttola et al., 2016, Faith et al., 2013). However, the gut microbiota extends beyond bacteria to include archaea, fungi, viruses, and protists (Hrncir, 2022), exhibiting a remarkable susceptibility to changes. The prominent phyla within the gut microbiota include Bacteroidetes, Firmicutes, Actinobacteria, Proteobacteria, Verrucomicrobia, and Fusobacteria (Arumugam et al., 2011). The three most common genera are *Bacteroides*, *Prevotella*, and *Ruminococcus* (Arumugam et al., 2011). The term "gut microbiome" (GM) encompasses the collective of all microorganisms present in the environment along with their metabolites and surroundings (Berg et al., 2020) whereas "gut microbiota" (GMB) refers to the microorganisms inhabiting a particular environment (Hou et al., 2022). The microbiome and microbiota are frequently used interchangeably. The GM plays a crucial role in the development of various diseases, including cancer. It consists of about 3 million genes and produces thousands of metabolites that have diverse effects on the host's activities compared to the approximately 23,000 genes found in the human genome (Vyas and Ranganathan, 2012, Shreiner et al., 2015, Rath and Dorrestein, 2012). These interactions impact the health, characteristics, and overall well-being of the host throughout this process (Rath and Dorrestein, 2012).

Diseases are influenced by changes in the GM function and composition, i.e., dysbiosis (Hrncirova et al., 2019, Levy et al., 2017). Dysbiosis refers to the "imbalance" of the gut microbiome (DeGruttola et al., 2016) and is basically the disruption of the delicate equilibrium within the gut. Dysbiosis influences the gastrointestinal, metabolic, neuromusculoskeletal, cardiovascular, and endocrine systems (Figure 2.1). Dysbiosis is characterized by the depletion of beneficial gut microbiota, the proliferation of harmful bacteria, and a decline in microbial diversity (Hrncir, 2022). It occurs as a result of various health factors such as inflammation or infections, lifestyle choices like diet and hygiene practices, and exposure to substances like drugs or food additives (Hrncir, 2022). Imbalances in the composition of gut microorganisms have significant physiological implications within the gastrointestinal tract. For instance, diets high in sugar can disrupt the integrity of the intestinal barrier leading to inflammation and negative metabolic effects on the host (Vrieze et al., 2012).

According to the American Cancer Society (ACS), colorectal cancer (CRC) is ranked as the third most common type of cancer in the United States, while recent research has shown a connection between dysbiosis and CRC development (DeGruttola et al., 2016). CRC patients have shown a decrease in butyrate-producing bacteria while there is an increase in pathogenic bacteria (Schulz et al., 2014, Castellarin et al., 2012). The composition and quantity of microbial species in dysbiosis associated with CRC vary based on the state and the severity of the tumor. For instance, CRC patients with tumors exhibited an elevated presence of Enterobacteriaceae in the mucosa compared to patients with polyps. Additionally, Bacteroidetes were found to be increased in CRC tumor tissue when compared to non-tumor tissues (Sobhani et al., 2011). In a study conducted by Zackular et al., it was demonstrated that the rate of tumorigenesis significantly rose in germ-free (GF) mice when they received gut microbiome transplants from mice carrying tumors (Zackular et al., 2013). GF mice lack an intestinal microbiome and are frequently used to study the effects of gut microbiomes. The modulation of the gut microbiota using antibiotics has demonstrated the importance of the microbiota in tumor development, as evidenced by a decrease in both size and quantity of tumors observed in mice susceptible to CRC following antibiotic treatment (Zackular et al., 2013, Schulz et al., 2014). Schulz et al. also demonstrated that mice deficient in myeloid differentiation factor 88 (MyD88) exhibit reduced neoplastic development and tumor progression, suggesting a potential carcinogenic role of MyD88 in CRC tumorigenesis (Huikuan et al., 2019). The GMB can contribute to the progression and development of CRC through immune responses and ongoing inflammatory conditions that affect host metabolism, alter stem cell dynamics, and modulate the biosynthesis of genotoxic and toxic metabolites (Cani et al., 2016, Tsilimigras et al., 2017).

Intracellular pathogens have also been the subject of thorough investigation in the realm of infectious diseases. In the case of numerous bacterial pathogens, residing within host cells is a vital, and at times, necessary aspect of their lifestyle

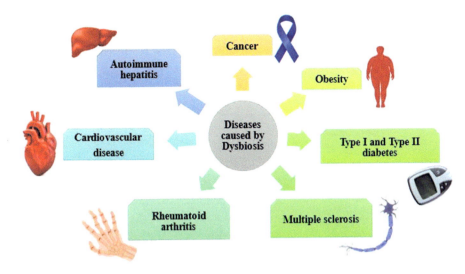

FIGURE 2.1 Effects of dysbiosis on gastrointestinal, metabolic, neuromusculoskeletal, cardiovascular, and endocrine systems. Dysbiosis leads to multiple disorders within the body and can lead to cancer development.

(Schorr et al., 2023). As an illustration, specific bacteria found within tumors, like enterotoxigenic *Bacteroides fragilis* (*B. fragilis*) and genotoxic *Escherichia coli* (*E. coli*), have been associated with the generation of metabolites that foster inflammation and DNA damage. These factors contribute to the commencement and progression of tumors (Dejea et al., 2018, Nougayrède et al., 2006, Arthur et al., 2012) and can influence the response of tumors to immunotherapy and chemotherapy (Yu et al., 2017, Gharaibeh and Jobin, 2019). A subset of bacteria has the capacity to influence the immune response, particularly when it comes to immune checkpoint blockade, thereby affecting the response to immunotherapy (Choi et al., 2023, Mager et al., 2020). Bacteria within tumors could potentially serve as viable targets for cancer treatment. To illustrate, when mice transplanted with patient-derived colorectal cancer xenografts that tested positive for *Fusobacterium nucleatum* were treated with antibiotics, it resulted in a reduction in tumor size and a decrease in cancer cell proliferation. This suggests that inhibiting bacterial presence may contribute to suppressing tumor growth (Bullman et al., 2017).

Hallmarks of Cancer

The "hallmarks of cancer" were introduced as a collection of functional attributes that human cells acquire as they transition from a normal state to neoplastic growth, specifically traits essential for their capacity to develop malignant tumors (Hanahan, 2022). The hallmarks serve as a structured framework for comprehending the intricacies of neoplastic diseases. They encompass maintaining proliferative signaling, bypassing growth inhibitory mechanisms, thwarting cell death, enabling continuous replication, promoting angiogenesis, and triggering invasion and metastasis. At the core of these hallmarks are genome instability, which leads to the genetic diversity that accelerates their acquisition, and inflammation, which promotes various hallmark functions (Hanahan and Weinberg, 2011). Microbes can contribute to the advancement and progression of cancer either through direct or indirect means (Hull et al., 2021).

Figure 2.2 illustrates the various ways in which the microbiota within the body can impact different cancer hallmarks.

Gut–Brain Axis

The significant impact of an individual's emotional state on digestion is a well-established fact, revealing the integral role the nervous system plays in the gut, and vice versa. This mutual relationship has been termed the gut–brain axis (Rhee et al., 2009, Heym et al., 2019). The microbiota-gut-brain axis encompasses the brain, gut, glands, immune cells, and gut microbiota (Cryan and Dinan, 2012). Communication between the gastrointestinal tract and the brain is regulated by both the enteric nervous system (Kuwahara et al., 2020) and central nervous system (Ma et al., 2019). In addition to the nervous system, this axis is also influenced by hormonal and immunological signaling (Sherman et al., 2015, Carabotti et al., 2015). The gut–brain axis is discussed in Chapter 9.

DYSBIOSIS AND CANCER

Maintaining gut homeostasis and the integrity of the gut barrier are critical for overall health. The disruption of the intestinal barrier has been linked to various diseases, including cancer. Dysbiosis, which affects immune function, inflammation, and metabolism, plays a significant role in promoting cancer development. Certain bacteria have been found to negatively impact metabolism, immune response, and gut functionality, potentially contributing to the progression of cancer (Rea et al., 2018). It should be noted that dysbiosis within the

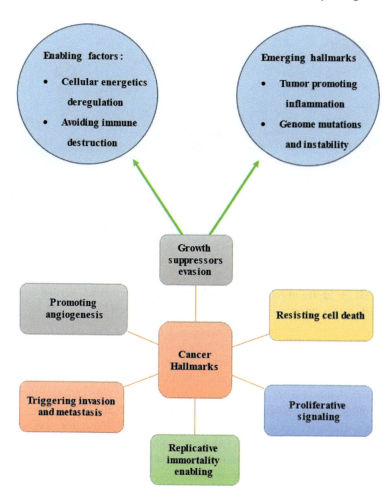

FIGURE 2.2 **The influence of the microbiome on cancer hallmarks**. The hallmarks of cancer consist of distinct biological traits that propel the development of malignancy. These core hallmarks encompass sustained evasion of growth suppressors, enabling replicative immortality, proliferative signaling, resisting cell death, triggering invasion and metastasis, and promoting angiogenesis. Enabling factors, such as the disruption of cellular energetics and evading immune responses, bolster these hallmarks. Furthermore, emerging hallmarks like tumor-promoting inflammation and genome instability play a role in the advancement and progression of cancer. An understanding of these hallmarks facilitates the development of more precise and efficacious cancer therapies.

gastrointestinal system can lead to both local and remote development of malignancies (Sheflin et al., 2014).

Dysbiosis Effects on the Immune System and Inflammation

The delicate balance of the gut microbiome mirrors the fragile equilibrium of the immune system. The body's well-being relies on preserving this balance: warding off harmful pathogens while also maintaining self-tolerance to prevent autoimmunity. The gut microbiota plays a vital role in regulating the body's immune system, having evolved alongside the host over millennia. Its functions include immune regulation, digestion, nutrition synthesis, safeguarding against infections, and detoxification (Finke, 2009, Ley et al., 2006, Hill and Artis, 2009, Bäckhed et al., 2005, Ley et al., 2008). By ensuring a harmonious coexistence between tolerance for healthy self-tissue and the elimination of invasive pathogens, the immune system actively contributes to the overall health of the body. However, patients with autoimmune disorders experience failure in the process of preserving self-tolerance. This failure leads the immune system to erroneously target and destroy health self-tissue (Westerberg et al., 2008, Goodnow et al., 2005).

The interaction between microorganisms and host's immune system is a continuous process that primarily takes place in the gastrointestinal area. (Cani et al., 2016). Not only is the gut an important location for absorption and digestion but it is also the largest immunological bodily organ. The gut contains 60–80% of the common immune structures and cells that maintain the equilibrium of the gut immune system (McDermott and Huffnagle, 2014). Gut microbiota influences the therapeutic response and cancer development (Elinav et al., 2019). Microbiota-derived molecules can modulate the host immune system through nucleotide-binding oligomerization (NOD)-like receptor (NLR) signaling, toll-like receptor (TLR), inflammasome signaling, or the shift in the regulatory and proinflammatory immune cells balance

(Hrncir, 2022). Additionally, the gut microbiota influences distal mucosal sites, primarily through immunomodulation, systemic metabolic pathways, and the circulatory system (Asseri et al., 2023).

The interaction between the host's immune system and tumorigenicity can be categorized into three stages: (i) Elimination phase: during this stage, the host's immune surveillance identifies and eliminates the tumor; (ii) Equilibrium phase: in this phase, the tumor is unable to proliferate or be completely eradicated by the immune system due to the host's immune checkpoints regulation; (iii) Immunological escape phase: in this stage, tumor cells can evade immune monitoring, enabling them to grow devoid of host immune protection (Zhao et al., 2022, Yang et al., 2013). An important characteristic of intestinal antigen-presenting cells (APCs), which co-evolve with the microbiota, is their ability to maintain immune tolerance towards the normal gut flora while also safeguarding the body from infections. Dendritic cells (DCs) of Peyer's patches, which are lymphoid nodules implanted in the gut wall, produce large quantities of interleukin-10 (IL-10) compared to splenic DCs activated under specific conditions (Iwasaki and Kelsall, 1999). Similarly, gut macrophages, like DCs, adopt a specific phenotype termed "inflammation anergy" when they come into contact with microbial stimuli in homeostatic circumstances, which alludes to the intestine macrophages' non-inflammatory nature (Smythies et al., 2005). These intestinal macrophages do not release pro-inflammatory cytokines in response to microbial stimuli like TLR ligands (Smythies et al., 2010).

During the inflammation process, leukocytes undergo changes allowing DCs, macrophages, neutrophils, and natural killer (NK) cells to generate reactive oxygen species (ROS), which harm intestinal epithelial cells' DNA and raise the amounts of enzymes like cyclooxygenase-2 (COX-2). The induction of mucosal cancer depends on these occurrences (Savari et al., 2014). Dysbiosis and the increased immune response to antigens can contribute to amplified chronic inflammation, which is suggested to be a cause of colitis-associated development of CRC (Elinav et al., 2013, Strober et al., 2002). Ulcerative colitis, Crohn's disease, and inflammatory bowel disease (IBD) are inflammatory diseases that affect the small intestine and colon. Patients with IBD often exhibit elevated levels of proteobacteria, reduced levels of Bacteroidetes and Firmicutes species (Sokol et al., 2006, Frank et al., 2007), and face a higher risk of around 10–15%, of developing CRC (Loddo and Romano, 2015).

Crucial components of the immune system, known as pattern recognition receptors (PRRs), have the ability to identify GMB based on their chemical structures (Thaiss et al., 2016). Sentinel cells express a set of proteins called TLRs that are designed to recognize pathogens and trigger an immune response. There are two key TLR pathways, one is the TIR-domain-containing adapter-inducing interferon-β (TRIF)-dependent pathway and the other is the MyD88 adaptor proteins pathway (O'Neill et al., 2013, Abreu, 2010). During the MyD88-dependent pathway, upon TLR activation, the downstream factors, which include mitogen-activated protein kinases (MAPK), interferon regulatory factors (IRF), and NF-kB, are activated (O'Neill et al., 2013). A phosphatase responsible for the nuclear factor activation of the activated T cells (NFAT) family, Calcineurin (Cn), is significantly expressed in CRC and has been linked to the growth and spread of tumors (Peuker et al., 2016). The DNA binding activity of NFAT and intracellular Cabb are both elevated following the stimulation of TLR4 and TLR2 by gut bacteria, which affects CRC carcinogenesis (Peuker et al., 2016).

Regulatory T cells, such as Forkhead box P3 (Foxp3) regulatory T (Treg) cells and type 1 regulatory T cells (Tr1) that produce IL-10, are also responsible for maintaining intestinal homeostasis. Round et al. showed that *B. fragilis* can control Foxp3 Treg cells, demonstrating the impact of microbiota homeostasis through the TLR2-dependent signaling pathway (Lowe et al., 2010, Round et al., 2011). TLR4 can bind bacterial lipopolysaccharide which leads to the activation of inflammatory gene expression via the NF-KB signaling pathway (Zou et al., 2018). By specifically activating TLR4, as demonstrated by Van Helden et al., Gram-negative bacteria can promote DC migration, leading to persistent infections (van Helden et al., 2010). Round et al. also demonstrated that the binding of MyD88 and TLR4 plays a key role in carcinogenesis by inducing tumor invasion, cell proliferation, tumor migration, developing chemoresistance, and escaping from the immunosurveillance (Round et al., 2011). TLRs can also be used as a biomarker for colorectal carcinogenesis, for example, TLR4 overexpression can promote NF-kB activation resulting in Cyclooxygenase 2 (COX-2) expression induction (Yesudhas et al., 2014). The NF-kB signaling pathway is a key mechanism in immunity and regulates gene expression involved with inflammation and immune responses (Figure 2.3). Dysbiosis induces the expression of TLR4 resulting in the activation of NF-kB leading to miRNA expression changes and the promotion of tumor growth (Figure 2.3).

Given the continuous presence of antigens and immunomodulators derived from both the diet and commensal microbiota, it is important to note that the intestine also acts as a gateway for various pathogens. Consequently, the immune processes within the intestines have been increasingly implicated in regulating the development of diseases in other parts of the body (Coombes and Powrie, 2008). Due to the variety of gut microbiota and different locations of activity, an alternative approach to study the gut microbiota and mechanisms of action must be used. Transcriptomics is used to study differences in gene expression profiles and the functional components of the genome and this has led to spatial transcriptomics (ST) (Cao et al., 2023). ST enables the visualization of transcriptional patterns within specific geographical regions that play a crucial role in development. These regions are essential for organogenesis, as they are responsible for shaping organ development through the establishment of distinct patterns and location-specific morphogen gradients (Asp et al., 2019). ST integrates high-resolution tissue imaging with unbiased spatially localized RNA sequencing (RNA-seq) through the utilization of

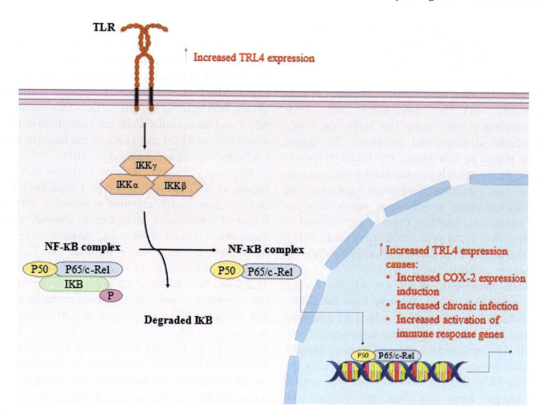

FIGURE 2.3 **The role of Toll-like receptors on the NF-kB signaling pathway and effect on expression.** A crucial component of immunity, the NF-kB signaling system controls the expression of genes related to inflammation and immunological responses. Dysbiosis causes an increase in the expression of TLR4, which activates NF-kB and causes alterations in the expression of miRNA, increased immune response activation, increased chronic inflammation, and increased COX-2 expression, all of which can encourage the growth of tumors.

barcoded spots on glass slides (Ståhl et al., 2016). This approach is quite appealing for elucidating variations in gene expression across distinct regions, providing a significantly more extensive and diverse dataset compared to conventional transcriptome analyses (Parigi et al., 2022).

Targeted cancer therapies, such as immunotherapy, focus on specific malignant cells, aiming to minimize side effects and enhance patient's life quality and overall survival (Dy and Adjei, 2013). However, tumors exhibit heterogeneity adding a layer of genetic complexity. Tumor heterogeneity refers to the differences in genotypic and phenotypic characteristics between cancers of the same histological type or between a primary tumor and its metastases. Tumor heterogeneity is the process by which the first tumor cell, which was created by a chance occurrence of driving mutation(s) in the genes, gives rise to multiple clones, each displaying varying innate sensitivity to the anti-cancer therapy (Bhang et al., 2015). Therefore, it is essential to comprehend the tumor heterogeneity complexity to enhance patient outcomes and to create efficient treatment plans.

Immunotherapy presents innovative approaches for treating tumors by reversing the tumor-immune loop and restoring the host's antitumor immune responses (Asseri et al., 2023). Immunotherapy targets recurrence mechanisms, cancer resistance (Emens et al., 2017) and affects the microbiomes of patients, thereby impacting their response to treatments (Roy and Trinchieri, 2017). The primary immune-targeted tumor therapies are TLR agonists, immune checkpoint inhibitors (ICIs), adoptive T-cell therapy, and vaccines (Pandey and Khan, 2023). The discovery of ICIs marked the beginning of the use of the immune system against cancer, primarily because of their effectiveness against metastatic tumors and bioactivity against cancers with unique histopathologies (Pitt et al., 2016, Belkaid and Naik, 2013).

The most important immune checkpoints are inhibitors of programmed cell death ligand 1 (PD-L1), cytotoxic T lymphocyte-associated protein 4 (CTLA-4) and programmed cell death 1 (PD-1), which enables malignant tumors to avoid the host's immune surveillance (Marincola et al., 2003). The immune system's defense against the cancer cells is triggered by their suppression. Therefore, in several advanced cancers like kidney cancer, lymphoma, non-small cell lung cancer (NSCLC), melanoma, prostate cancer, bladder cancer, and head and neck cancer, antibodies targeting these checkpoints, such as PD-1 and PD-L1 targeting antibodies and CTLA-4 blocker targeting antibodies, can be thought of as a standard of care (Yu et al., 2019). As a result of its potential to provide targeted and long-lasting anti-cancer effects, the development of novel medications that target immunological checkpoints is viewed in this context as a promising strategy in treating CRC. Numerous cancer types have benefited clinically from immunotherapy (Singh et al., 2015). In comparison to conventional therapy, immunotherapy has fewer side effects

Gut Microbiome Dysbiosis and Cancer Risk

and demonstrates superior efficacy in eradicating malignancies (Pandey and Khan, 2023).

It is now recognized that the gut microbiome significantly affects the effectiveness of cancer immunotherapy. Numerous studies have shown that particular microorganism species are connected to the response or lack thereof to immune checkpoint inhibitors (ICIs), such as anti-PD-1/PD-L1 monoclonal antibodies (Gopalakrishnan et al., 2018, Hodi et al., 2010, Rosenberg et al., 2016, Topalian et al., 2012). Exploring the gut microbiota offers a viable avenue for developing diagnostic biomarkers and therapeutic strategies for cancer immunotherapy. Modifying the function and composition of the gut microbiome can enhance treatment outcomes and patient responses to ICIs.

Dysbiosis Effects on Nutrition and Metabolism

Two examples of non-digestible substrates that can be fermented by the gut microbiota are dietary fibers and endogenous intestinal mucus. The host and gut microorganisms coexist in a commensal manner. On the one hand, the bacteria can produce vitamin K, provide important nutrients, support angiogenesis and enteric nerve function, and aid in cellulose digestion (Guarner and Malagelada, 2003, Hill and Artis, 2009, Müller and Macpherson, 2006). Probiotics and commensal bacteria can also strengthen the barrier and keep infections and allergens out of the mucosal tissues (Ulluwishewa et al., 2011) and assist the host defense by maintaining the immune system's homeostasis (Macfarlane and Cummings, 1999). In exchange, commensal bacteria benefit from the host's protective and nutrient-rich environment (Tsuji et al., 2008).

In order to improve treatment outcomes and lessen the negative effects of microbial modifications during anticancer therapy, nutrition is thought to be one of the main drivers for altering microbial activity and structure before or during anticancer treatment (Rinninella et al., 2021). Prebiotics such as fructo-oligosaccharides (FOS), galactooligosaccharides (GOS), and insulin are essential for the growth of a particular type of anaerobic colon-dwelling bacteria (Aravind et al., 2021). These are mostly digested in the colon by bacteria, which effectively encourages the growth of beneficial bacteria (Zwartjes et al., 2021, Gibson et al., 1995). The therapeutic effect of the anticancer medications has been discovered to be significantly impacted by both inulin and oligofructose as an in vivo investigation showed the effects of 15% inulin and oligo-fructose given to the animals' basal diets throughout chemotherapy (Witczak et al., 2020, Taper and Roberfroid, 2005).

Metabolism is a powerful process influenced by gut microbiota and responds to diets and environmental signals. The gut microbiota produces metabolites that signal and communicate with various organs and tissues and impact overall health (Figure 2.4).

The gut microbiota can create metabolites or genotoxic stress to cause genetic and/or epigenetic changes resulting in cancer (Belcheva et al., 2015). Diet plays a key role in the carcinogenesis of CRC. High intake of processed meat can increase the CRC risk while the increased intake of total dietary fiber can decrease the risk of CRC (Bernstein et al., 2015). The effects on the host metabolic system are moderated by the production of dietary fiber SCFAs, conversion of choline to trimethylamine (TMA), and/or changes in bile acid composition (Huikuan et al., 2019). The increase of this fermentation is beneficial to bacteria that produce short-chain fatty acids (SCFA) and gas (Wong et al., 2006). Butyrate, propionate, and acetate are the main SCFAs generated and are synthesized by various microorganisms including *Propionibacterium, Bacteroides, Prevotella, Bifidobacterium*, and others. The microbiota ferments dietary fiber to create SCFAs through an enzymatic mechanism in the metabolism of SCFAs. SCFAs are metabolized through a variety of metabolic pathways in organic acids with fewer than six carbons, where they either help to synthesize necessary molecules or are turned into energy. Small amounts of unmetabolized SCFAs make their way to the systemic circulation from the liver's portal circulation (Figure 2.5). The metabolism of SCFAs is essential for preserving energy homeostasis and general metabolic health. Various studies have linked SCFA levels and gut microorganisms to colorectal cancer mortality differentials (Bultman and Jobin, 2014, Hester et al., 2015, Russell et al., 2013).

Butyrate serves as the principal energy source for human colonocytes. Additionally, it has the capacity to induce intestinal gluconeogenesis and induce death in colon cancer

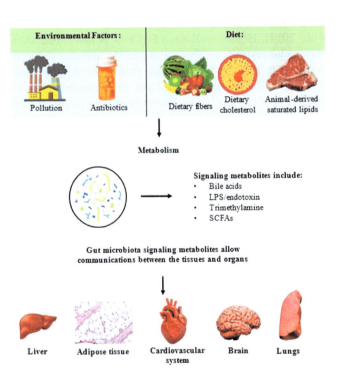

FIGURE 2.4 Gut microbiota metabolites organ communication. Metabolism responds to diets and environmental signals. The gut microbiota produces metabolites, for example, endotoxins, bile acids, and short-chain fatty acids (SCFA), that signal and communicate with various organs, tissues, and systems.

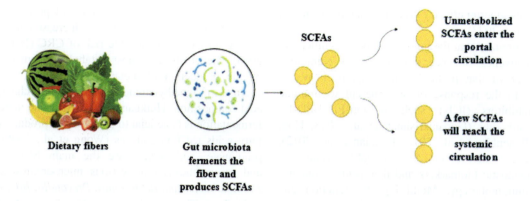

FIGURE 2.5 **SCFA metabolism and circulation.** SCFAs metabolism involves enzymatic processes where the microbiota ferments dietary fiber to produce SCFAs. Organic acids with fewer than six carbons undergo multiple metabolic pathways where SCFAs contribute to the synthesis of essential molecules or are converted into energy. Small amounts of unmetabolized SCFAs make their way to the systemic circulation from the liver's portal circulation. The metabolism of SCFAs is crucial for preserving energy and general metabolic health.

cells, both of which have favorable effects on glucose and energy homeostasis (De Vadder et al., 2014). Butyrate is necessary for the production of a condition of hypoxia by epithelial cells that protect against gut microbial dysbiosis and maintain the balance of oxygen in the gut (Byndloss et al., 2017). To regulate gluconeogenesis and satiety signals, propionate is delivered to the liver where it interacts with gut fatty acid receptors (De Vadder et al., 2014). Acetate, the most common SCFA, enters peripheral tissues where it is used in cholesterol metabolism and lipogenesis. It may also have an effect on central appetite control. Another crucial chemical for the development of more bacteria is acetate (Frost et al., 2014). Higher synthesis of SCFAs is associated with less insulin resistance (Zhao et al., 2018) and diet-induced obesity (Lin et al., 2012). In mice propionate and butyrate appear to regulate gut hormones and curb hunger and food intake (Lin et al., 2012). Gut microbial enzymes support bile acid metabolism by generating secondary and unconjugated bile acids, which act as metabolic regulators and signaling molecules to influence important host pathways (Long et al., 2017).

CHALLENGES OF GUT DYSBIOSIS AND CANCER RISKS

The intricacy of the microbiome's makeup results in datasets that require advanced statistical techniques for analysis and do not lend themselves to industrial applications, which contributes to the challenge of turning research into medicinal treatments (Brüssow, 2020). Treatment development into commercially available products have also encountered challenges due to the complexity of dysbiosis and the financial implications (Verbeke et al., 2017, Vyas et al., 2015). The definitions of "dysbiosis" have also been under scrutiny. Dysbiosis is frequently used in microbiome research publications without even a cursory description or clarification. This disregard not only demonstrates a lack of scientific rigor, but it may also impede the transition of the field of the microbiome from a descriptive to a translational science (Brüssow, 2020). Standardization is thus an important challenge to overcome.

The loss of microbial diversity leading to dysbiosis is also another challenge that must be overcome. The reduction of overall microbial diversity and a simultaneous expansion of species known as pathobionts, which are genetic variations of the "pathogenic" microbiota, are signs of dysbiosis (Schippa et al., 2012, Myers and Hawrelak, 2004, Petersen and Round, 2014, Carding et al., 2015). The environment and dietary intake are also factors that can cause dysbiosis and lead to increased risk of cancer and other diseases (Putignani and Dallapiccola, 2016). Rebuilding the microbiotic ecosystem can overcome dysbiosis and decrease the risk of cancer. The strategies to overcome dysbiosis include fecal transplantation, probiotic, prebiotic, and synbiotic supplementation, bacterial consortium transplantation, and phage therapy (Gagliardi et al., 2018). Probiotics, which function as anti-mutagens and have effects at different stages of carcinogenesis, have also been linked to having anticancer potential (Raman et al., 2013). The challenge, however, is the availability of probiotics or other treatments and the financial implications. Additionally, each patient's gut microbiota must be carefully considered when prescribing precision medicines for dysbiosis and the uniqueness of gut microbiota structure must be investigated based on all the data from integrated "omic" platforms. This is challenging as it involves large data sets and countless pieces of information leading to very time-consuming research. Improved technology and the use of artificial intelligence can decrease this burden. Considering intracellular bacteria, the quantity of research studies dedicated specifically to intracellular bacteria within the context of cancer is still quite limited, and there is often a lack of clear differentiation between the effects occurring within the tumor and those taking place inside host cells (Schorr et al., 2023).

CONCLUSION

The microbial ecology of the intestine has a profound impact on human physiology, influencing metabolic and immunological functions. The GM, particularly when in a dysbiosis state, plays an important role in various aspects of cancer development. Specific bacterial species have been found to influence both the risk and progression of cancer. Understanding how commensal bacteria modulate immune function is capturing scientific interest and presenting potential therapeutic opportunities for improving health outcomes. The development of an exhaustive and culture-independent method to characterize gut microbial communities has undergone a revolution as a result of recent advances in "next-generation" sequencing. It is now understood that the gut microbiota significantly influences the human immune system and impacts autoimmune-related illnesses both inside and outside the gut. Dysbiosis, which influences the microbiota and contributes to the emergence and spread of cancer, is influenced by environmental factors in addition to genetic ones.

REFERENCES

ABREU, M. T. 2010. Toll-like receptor signalling in the intestinal epithelium: how bacterial recognition shapes intestinal function. *Nat Rev Immunol,* 10, 131–144.

ARAVIND, S. M., WICHIENCHOT, S., TSAO, R., RAMAKRISHNAN, S. & CHAKKARAVARTHI, S. 2021. Role of dietary polyphenols on gut microbiota, their metabolites and health benefits. *Food Res Int,* 142, 110189.

ARTHUR, J. C., PEREZ-CHANONA, E., MÜHLBAUER, M., TOMKOVICH, S., URONIS, J. M., FAN, T.-J., CAMPBELL, B. J., ABUJAMEL, T., DOGAN, B. & ROGERS, A. B. 2012. Intestinal inflammation targets cancer-inducing activity of the microbiota. *Science,* 338, 120–123.

ARUMUGAM, M., RAES, J., PELLETIER, E., LE PASLIER, D., YAMADA, T., MENDE, D. R., FERNANDES, G. R., TAP, J., BRULS, T. & BATTO, J.-M. 2011. Enterotypes of the human gut microbiome. *Nature,* 473, 174–180.

ASP, M., GIACOMELLO, S., LARSSON, L., WU, C., FÜRTH, D., QIAN, X., WÄRDELL, E., CUSTODIO, J., REIMEGÅRD, J. & SALMÉN, F. 2019. A spatiotemporal organ-wide gene expression and cell atlas of the developing human heart. *Cell,* 179, 1647–1660.

ASSERI, A. H., BAKHSH, T., ABUZAHRAH, S. S., ALI, S. & RATHER, I. A. 2023. The gut dysbiosis-cancer axis: illuminating novel insights and implications for clinical practice. *Front Pharmacol,* 14.

BÄCKHED, F., LEY, R. E., SONNENBURG, J. L., PETERSON, D. A. & GORDON, J. I. 2005. Host-bacterial mutualism in the human intestine. *Science,* 307, 1915–1920.

BELCHEVA, A., IRRAZABAL, T. & MARTIN, A. 2015. Gut microbial metabolism and colon cancer: can manipulations of the microbiota be useful in the management of gastrointestinal health? *Bioessays,* 37, 403–412.

BELKAID, Y. & NAIK, S. 2013. Compartmentalized and systemic control of tissue immunity by commensals. *Nat Immunol,* 14, 646–653.

BERG, G., RYBAKOVA, D., FISCHER, D., CERNAVA, T., VERGÈS, M. C., CHARLES, T., CHEN, X., COCOLIN, L., EVERSOLE, K., CORRAL, G. H., KAZOU, M., KINKEL, L., LANGE, L., LIMA, N., LOY, A., MACKLIN, J. A., MAGUIN, E., MAUCHLINE, T., MCCLURE, R., MITTER, B., RYAN, M., SARAND, I., SMIDT, H., SCHELKLE, B., ROUME, H., KIRAN, G. S., SELVIN, J., SOUZA, R. S. C., VAN OVERBEEK, L., SINGH, B. K., WAGNER, M., WALSH, A., SESSITSCH, A. & SCHLOTER, M. 2020. Microbiome definition re-visited: old concepts and new challenges. *Microbiome,* 8, 103.

BERNSTEIN, A. M., SONG, M., ZHANG, X., PAN, A., WANG, M., FUCHS, C. S., LE, N., CHAN, A. T., WILLETT, W. C., OGINO, S., GIOVANNUCCI, E. L. & WU, K. 2015. Processed and unprocessed red meat and risk of colorectal cancer: analysis by tumor location and modification by time. *PLoS One,* 10, e0135959.

BHANG, H.-E. C., RUDDY, D. A., KRISHNAMURTHY RADHAKRISHNA, V., CAUSHI, J. X., ZHAO, R., HIMS, M. M., SINGH, A. P., KAO, I., RAKIEC, D. & SHAW, P. 2015. Studying clonal dynamics in response to cancer therapy using high-complexity barcoding. *Nat Med,* 21, 440–448.

BRÜSSOW, H. 2020. Problems with the concept of gut microbiota dysbiosis. *Microb Biotechnol,* 13, 423–434.

BULLMAN, S., PEDAMALLU, C. S., SICINSKA, E., CLANCY, T. E., ZHANG, X., CAI, D., NEUBERG, D., HUANG, K., GUEVARA, F. & NELSON, T. 2017. Analysis of Fusobacterium persistence and antibiotic response in colorectal cancer. *Science,* 358, 1443–1448.

BULTMAN, S. J. & JOBIN, C. 2014. Microbial-derived butyrate: an oncometabolite or tumor-suppressive metabolite? *Cell Host Microbe,* 16, 143–145.

BYNDLOSS, M. X., OLSAN, E. E., RIVERA-CHÁVEZ, F., TIFFANY, C. R., CEVALLOS, S. A., LOKKEN, K. L., TORRES, T. P., BYNDLOSS, A. J., FABER, F. & GAO, Y. 2017. Microbiota-activated PPAR-γ signaling inhibits dysbiotic Enterobacteriaceae expansion. *Science,* 357, 570–575.

CANI, P. D., PLOVIER, H., VAN HUL, M., GEURTS, L., DELZENNE, N. M., DRUART, C. & EVERARD, A. 2016. Endocannabinoids — at the crossroads between the gut microbiota and host metabolism. *Nat Rev Endocrinol,* 12, 133–143.

CAO, M., XUE, T., HUO, H., ZHANG, X., WANG, N. N., YAN, X. & LI, C. 2023. Spatial transcriptomes and microbiota reveal immune mechanism that respond to pathogen infection in the posterior intestine of Sebastes schlegelii. *Open Biol,* 13, 220302.

CARABOTTI, M., SCIROCCO, A., MASELLI, M. A. & SEVERI, C. 2015. The gut-brain axis: interactions between enteric microbiota, central and enteric nervous systems. *Annu Gastroenterol,* 28, 203.

CARDING, S., VERBEKE, K., VIPOND, D. T., CORFE, B. M. & OWEN, L. J. 2015. Dysbiosis of the gut microbiota in disease. *Microbial Ecol Health Dis,* 26, 26191.

CASTELLARIN, M., WARREN, R. L., FREEMAN, J. D., DREOLINI, L., KRZYWINSKI, M., STRAUSS, J., BARNES, R., WATSON, P., ALLEN-VERCOE, E., MOORE, R. A. & HOLT, R. A. 2012. Fusobacterium nucleatum infection is prevalent in human colorectal carcinoma. *Genome Res,* 22, 299–306.

CHOI, Y., LICHTERMAN, J. N., COUGHLIN, L. A., POULIDES, N., LI, W., DEL VALLE, P., PALMER, S. N., GAN, S., KIM, J. & ZHAN, X. 2023. Immune checkpoint blockade induces gut microbiota translocation that augments extraintestinal antitumor immunity. *Sci Immunol,* 8, eabo2003.

COOMBES, J. L. & POWRIE, F. 2008. Dendritic cells in intestinal immune regulation. *Nat Rev Immunol,* 8, 435–446.

CRYAN, J. F. & DINAN, T. G. 2012. Mind-altering microorganisms: the impact of the gut microbiota on brain and behaviour. *Nat Rev Neurosci,* 13, 701–712.

DE VADDER, F., KOVATCHEVA-DATCHARY, P., GONCALVES, D., VINERA, J., ZITOUN, C., DUCHAMPT, A., BÄCKHED, F. & MITHIEUX, G. 2014. Microbiota-generated metabolites promote metabolic benefits via gut-brain neural circuits. *Cell,* 156, 84–96.

DEGRUTTOLA, A. K., LOW, D., MIZOGUCHI, A. & MIZOGUCHI, E. 2016. Current understanding of dysbiosis in disease in human and animal models. *Inflamm Bowel Dis,* 22, 1137–1150.

DEJEA, C. M., FATHI, P., CRAIG, J. M., BOLEIJ, A., TADDESE, R., GEIS, A. L., WU, X., DESTEFANO SHIELDS, C. E., HECHENBLEIKNER, E. M. & HUSO, D. L. 2018. Patients with familial adenomatous polyposis harbor colonic biofilms containing tumorigenic bacteria. *Science,* 359, 592–597.

DY, G. K. & ADJEI, A. A. 2013. Understanding, recognizing, and managing toxicities of targeted anticancer therapies. *CA: A Cancer J Clin,* 63, 249–279.

ELINAV, E., GARRETT, W. S., TRINCHIERI, G. & WARGO, J. 2019. The cancer microbiome. *Nat Rev Cancer,* 19, 371–376.

ELINAV, E., NOWARSKI, R., THAISS, C. A., HU, B., JIN, C. & FLAVELL, R. A. 2013. Inflammation-induced cancer: crosstalk between tumours, immune cells and microorganisms. *Nat Rev Cancer,* 13, 759–771.

EMENS, L. A., ASCIERTO, P. A., DARCY, P. K., DEMARIA, S., EGGERMONT, A. M. M., REDMOND, W. L., SELIGER, B. & MARINCOLA, F. M. 2017. Cancer immunotherapy: opportunities and challenges in the rapidly evolving clinical landscape. *Eur J Cancer,* 81, 116–129.

FAITH, J. J., GURUGE, J. L., CHARBONNEAU, M., SUBRAMANIAN, S., SEEDORF, H., GOODMAN, A. L., CLEMENTE, J. C., KNIGHT, R., HEATH, A. C., LEIBEL, R. L., ROSENBAUM, M. & GORDON, J. I. 2013. The long-term stability of the human gut microbiota. *Science,* 341, 1237439.

FINKE, D. 2009. *Induction of intestinal lymphoid tissue formation by intrinsic and extrinsic signals.* Seminars in Immunopathology. Springer, 151–169. https://doi.org/10.1007/s00281-009-0163-6

FRANK, D. N., ST. AMAND, A. L., FELDMAN, R. A., BOEDEKER, E. C., HARPAZ, N. & PACE, N. R. 2007. Molecular-phylogenetic characterization of microbial community imbalances in human inflammatory bowel diseases. *Proc Natl Acad Sci,* 104, 13780–13785.

FROST, G., SLEETH, M. L., SAHURI-ARISOYLU, M., LIZARBE, B., CERDAN, S., BRODY, L., ANASTASOVSKA, J., GHOURAB, S., HANKIR, M. & ZHANG, S. 2014. The short-chain fatty acid acetate reduces appetite via a central homeostatic mechanism. *Nat Commun,* 5, 3611.

GAGLIARDI, A., TOTINO, V., CACCIOTTI, F., IEBBA, V., NERONI, B., BONFIGLIO, G., TRANCASSINI, M., PASSARIELLO, C., PANTANELLA, F. & SCHIPPA, S. 2018. Rebuilding the gut microbiota ecosystem. *Int J Environ Res Public Health,* 15(8), 1679.

GHARAIBEH, R. Z. & JOBIN, C. 2019. Microbiota and cancer immunotherapy: in search of microbial signals. *Gut,* 68, 385–388.

GIBSON, G. R., BEATTY, E. R., WANG, X. I. N. & CUMMINGS, J. H. 1995. Selective stimulation of bifidobacteria in the human colon by oligofructose and inulin. *Gastroenterology,* 108, 975–982.

GOODNOW, C. C., SPRENT, J., DE ST GROTH, B. F. & VINUESA, C. G. 2005. Cellular and genetic mechanisms of self tolerance and autoimmunity. *Nature,* 435, 590–597.

GOPALAKRISHNAN, V., SPENCER, C. N., NEZI, L., REUBEN, A., ANDREWS, M. C., KARPINETS, T., PRIETO, P. A., VICENTE, D., HOFFMAN, K. & WEI, S. C. 2018. Gut microbiome modulates response to anti–PD-1 immunotherapy in melanoma patients. *Science,* 359, 97–103.

GUARNER, F. & MALAGELADA, J.-R. 2003. Gut flora in health and disease. *The Lancet,* 361, 512–519.

HANAHAN, D. 2022. Hallmarks of cancer: new dimensions. *Cancer Discovery,* 12, 31–46.

HANAHAN, D. & WEINBERG, ROBERT A. 2011. Hallmarks of cancer: the next generation. *Cell,* 144, 646–674.

HESTER, C. M., JALA, V. R., LANGILLE, M. G., UMAR, S., GREINER, K. A. & HARIBABU, B. 2015. Fecal microbes, short chain fatty acids, and colorectal cancer across racial/ethnic groups. *World J Gastroenterol,* 21, 2759–2769.

HEYM, N., HEASMAN, B. C., HUNTER, K., BLANCO, S. R., WANG, G. Y., SIEGERT, R., CLEARE, A., GIBSON, G. R., KUMARI, V. & SUMICH, A. L. 2019. The role of microbiota and inflammation in self-judgement and empathy: implications for understanding the brain-gut-microbiome axis in depression. *Psychopharmacology,* 236, 1459–1470.

HILL, D. A. & ARTIS, D. 2009. Intestinal bacteria and the regulation of immune cell homeostasis. *Ann Rev Immunol,* 28, 623–667.

HODI, F. S., O'DAY, S. J., MCDERMOTT, D. F., WEBER, R. W., SOSMAN, J. A., HAANEN, J. B., GONZALEZ, R., ROBERT, C., SCHADENDORF, D. & HASSEL, J. C. 2010. Improved survival with ipilimumab in patients with metastatic melanoma. *N Engl J Med,* 363, 711–723.

HOU, K., WU, Z.-X., CHEN, X.-Y., WANG, J.-Q., ZHANG, D., XIAO, C., ZHU, D., KOYA, J. B., WEI, L., LI, J. & CHEN, Z.-S. 2022. Microbiota in health and diseases. *Signal Trans Targeted Ther,* 7, 135.

HRNCIR, T. 2022. Gut microbiota dysbiosis: triggers, consequences, diagnostic and therapeutic options. *Microorganisms,* 10(3), 578. doi: 10.3390/microorganisms10030578. PMID: 35336153; PMCID: PMC8954387.

HRNCIROVA, L., MACHOVA, V., TRCKOVA, E., KREJSEK, J. & HRNCIR, T. 2019. Food preservatives induce proteobacteria dysbiosis in human-microbiota associated Nod2-deficient mice. *Microorganisms,* 7(10), 83.

HUIKUAN, C., YI, D., LING, Y. & BERND, S. 2019. Small metabolites, possible big changes: a microbiota-centered view of non-alcoholic fatty liver disease. *Gut,* 68, 359.

HULL, R., LOLAS, G., MAKROGKIKAS, S., JENSEN, L. D., SYRIGOS, K. N., EVANGELOU, G., PADAYACHY, L., EGBOR, C., MEHROTRA, R., MAKHAFOLA, T. J., OYOMNO, M. & DLAMINI, Z. 2021. Microbiomics in collusion with the nervous system in carcinogenesis: diagnosis, pathogenesis and treatment. *Microorganisms,* 9(10), 2129.

IWASAKI, A. & KELSALL, B. L. 1999. Freshly isolated Peyer's patch, but not spleen, dendritic cells produce interleukin 10 and induce the differentiation of T helper type 2 cells. *J Exp Med,* 190, 229–240.

KUWAHARA, A., MATSUDA, K., KUWAHARA, Y., ASANO, S., INUI, T. & MARUNAKA, Y. 2020. Microbiota-gut-brain axis: enteroendocrine cells and the enteric nervous system form an interface between the microbiota and the central nervous system. *Biomed Res*, 41, 199–216.

LEVY, M., KOLODZIEJCZYK, A. A., THAISS, C. A. & ELINAV, E. 2017. Dysbiosis and the immune system. *Nat Rev Immunol*, 17, 219–232.

LEY, R. E., LOZUPONE, C. A., HAMADY, M., KNIGHT, R. & GORDON, J. I. 2008. Worlds within worlds: evolution of the vertebrate gut microbiota. *Nat Rev Microbiol*, 6, 776–788.

LEY, R. E., PETERSON, D. A. & GORDON, J. I. 2006. Ecological and evolutionary forces shaping microbial diversity in the human intestine. *Cell*, 124, 837–848.

LIN, H. V., FRASSETTO, A., KOWALIK JR, E. J., NAWROCKI, A. R., LU, M. M., KOSINSKI, J. R., HUBERT, J. A., SZETO, D., YAO, X. & FORREST, G. 2012. Butyrate and propionate protect against diet-induced obesity and regulate gut hormones via free fatty acid receptor 3-independent mechanisms. *PloS One*, 7, e35240.

LODDO, I. & ROMANO, C. 2015. Inflammatory Bowel disease: genetics, epigenetics, and pathogenesis. *Front Immunol*, 6, 551.

LONG, S. L., GAHAN, C. G. M. & JOYCE, S. A. 2017. Interactions between gut bacteria and bile in health and disease. *Mol Aspects Med*, 56, 54–65.

LOWE, E. L., CROTHER, T. R., RABIZADEH, S., HU, B., WANG, H., CHEN, S., SHIMADA, K., WONG, M. H., MICHELSEN, K. S. & ARDITI, M. 2010. Toll-like receptor 2 signaling protects mice from tumor development in a mouse model of colitis-induced cancer. *PLoS One*, 5, e13027.

MA, Q., XING, C., LONG, W., WANG, H. Y., LIU, Q. & WANG, R.-F. 2019. Impact of microbiota on central nervous system and neurological diseases: the gut-brain axis. *J Neuroinflamm*, 16, 1–14.

MACFARLANE, G. T. & CUMMINGS, J. H. 1999. Probiotics and prebiotics: can regulating the activities of intestinal bacteria benefit health? *BMJ*, 318, 999–1003.

MAGER, L. F., BURKHARD, R., PETT, N., COOKE, N. C. A., BROWN, K., RAMAY, H., PAIK, S., STAGG, J., GROVES, R. A. & GALLO, M. 2020. Microbiome-derived inosine modulates response to checkpoint inhibitor immunotherapy. *Science*, 369, 1481–1489.

MARINCOLA, F. M., WANG, E., HERLYN, M., SELIGER, B. & FERRONE, S. 2003. Tumors as elusive targets of T-cell-based active immunotherapy. *Trends Immunol*, 24, 334–341.

MCDERMOTT, A. J. & HUFFNAGLE, G. B. 2014. The microbiome and regulation of mucosal immunity. *Immunology*, 142, 24–31.

MÜLLER, C. & MACPHERSON, A. J. 2006. Layers of mutualism with commensal bacteria protect us from intestinal inflammation. *Gut*, 55, 276–284.

MYERS, S. P. & HAWRELAK, J. 2004. The causes of intestinal dysbiosis: a review. *Altern Med Rev*, 9, 180–197.

NOUGAYRÈDE, J.-P., HOMBURG, S., TAIEB, F., BOURY, M., BRZUSZKIEWICZ, E., GOTTSCHALK, G., BUCHRIESER, C., HACKER, J. R., DOBRINDT, U. & OSWALD, E. 2006. Escherichia coli induces DNA double-strand breaks in eukaryotic cells. *Science*, 313, 848–851.

O'NEILL, L. A. J., GOLENBOCK, D. & BOWIE, A. G. 2013. The history of Toll-like receptors — redefining innate immunity. *Nat Rev Immunol*, 13, 453–460.

PANDEY, P. & KHAN, F. 2023. Gut microbiome in cancer immunotherapy: current trends, translational challenges and future possibilities. *Biochim Biophys Acta, Gen Subj*, 1867, 130401.

PARIGI, S. M., LARSSON, L., DAS, S., RAMIREZ FLORES, R. O., FREDE, A., TRIPATHI, K. P., DIAZ, O. E., SELIN, K., MORALES, R. A. & LUO, X. 2022. The spatial transcriptomic landscape of the healing mouse intestine following damage. *Nat Commun*, 13, 828.

PETERSEN, C. & ROUND, J. L. 2014. Defining dysbiosis and its influence on host immunity and disease. *Cell Microbiol*, 16, 1024–1033.

PEUKER, K., MUFF, S., WANG, J., KÜNZEL, S., BOSSE, E., ZEISSIG, Y., LUZZI, G., BASIC, M., STRIGLI, A., ULBRICHT, A., KASER, A., ARLT, A., CHAVAKIS, T., VAN DEN BRINK, G. R., SCHAFMAYER, C., EGBERTS, J. H., BECKER, T., BIANCHI, M. E., BLEICH, A., RÖCKEN, C., HAMPE, J., SCHREIBER, S., BAINES, J. F., BLUMBERG, R. S. & ZEISSIG, S. 2016. Epithelial calcineurin controls microbiota-dependent intestinal tumor development. *Nat Med*, 22, 506–515.

PITT, J. M., VÉTIZOU, M., DAILLÈRE, R., ROBERTI, M. P., YAMAZAKI, T., ROUTY, B., LEPAGE, P., BONECA, I. G., CHAMAILLARD, M. & KROEMER, G. 2016. Resistance mechanisms to immune-checkpoint blockade in cancer: tumor-intrinsic and -extrinsic factors. *Immunity*, 44, 1255–1269.

PUTIGNANI, L. & DALLAPICCOLA, B. 2016. Foodomics as part of the host-microbiota-exposome interplay. *J Proteomics*, 147, 3–20.

RAMAN, M., AMBALAM, P., KONDEPUDI, K. K., PITHVA, S., KOTHARI, C., PATEL, A. T., PURAMA, R. K., DAVE, J. M. & VYAS, B. R. M. 2013. Potential of probiotics, prebiotics and synbiotics for management of colorectal cancer. *Gut Microbes*, 4, 181–192.

RATH, C. M. & DORRESTEIN, P. C. 2012. The bacterial chemical repertoire mediates metabolic exchange within gut microbiomes. *Curr Opin Microbiol*, 15, 147–154.

REA, D., COPPOLA, G., PALMA, G., BARBIERI, A., LUCIANO, A., DEL PRETE, P., ROSSETTI, S., BERRETTA, M., FACCHINI, G. & PERDONÀ, S. 2018. Microbiota effects on cancer: from risks to therapies. *Oncotarget*, 9, 17915.

RHEE, S. H., POTHOULAKIS, C. & MAYER, E. A. 2009. Principles and clinical implications of the brain–gut–enteric microbiota axis. *Nat Rev Gastroenterol Hepatol*, 6, 306–314.

RINNINELLA, E., RAOUL, P., CINTONI, M., PALOMBARO, M., PULCINI, G., GASBARRINI, A. & MELE, M. C. 2021. Nutritional interventions targeting gut microbiota during cancer therapies. *Microorganisms*, 9, 1469.

ROSENBERG, J. E., HOFFMAN-CENSITS, J., POWLES, T., VAN DER HEIJDEN, M. S., BALAR, A. V., NECCHI, A., DAWSON, N., O'DONNELL, P. H., BALMANOUKIAN, A. & LORIOT, Y. 2016. Atezolizumab in patients with locally advanced and metastatic urothelial carcinoma who have progressed following treatment with platinum-based chemotherapy: a single-arm, multicentre, phase 2 trial. *The Lancet*, 387, 1909–1920.

ROUND, J. L., LEE, S. M., LI, J., TRAN, G., JABRI, B., CHATILA, T. A. & MAZMANIAN, S. K. 2011. The Toll-like receptor 2 pathway establishes colonization by a commensal of the human microbiota. *Science*, 332, 974–977.

ROY, S. & TRINCHIERI, G. 2017. Microbiota: a key orchestrator of cancer therapy. *Nat Rev Cancer*, 17, 271–285.

RUSSELL, W. R., HOYLES, L., FLINT, H. J. & DUMAS, M. E. 2013. Colonic bacterial metabolites and human health. *Curr Opin Microbiol,* 16, 246–254.

SAVARI, S., VINNAKOTA, K., ZHANG, Y. & SJÖLANDER, A. 2014. Cysteinyl leukotrienes and their receptors: bridging inflammation and colorectal cancer. *World J Gastroenterol,* 20, 968–977.

SCHIPPA, S., IEBBA, V., TOTINO, V., SANTANGELO, F., LEPANTO, M., ALESSANDRI, C., NUTI, F., VIOLA, F., DI NARDO, G. & CUCCHIARA, S. 2012. A potential role of Escherichia coli pathobionts in the pathogenesis of pediatric inflammatory bowel disease. *Can J Microbiol,* 58, 426–432.

SCHORR, L., MATHIES, M., ELINAV, E. & PUSCHHOF, J. 2023. Intracellular bacteria in cancer—prospects and debates. *NPJ Biofilms Microbiomes,* 9, 76.

SCHULZ, M. D., ATAY, Ç., HERINGER, J., ROMRIG, F. K., SCHWITALLA, S., AYDIN, B., ZIEGLER, P. K., VARGA, J., REINDL, W., POMMERENKE, C., SALINAS-RIESTER, G., BÖCK, A., ALPERT, C., BLAUT, M., POLSON, S. C., BRANDL, L., KIRCHNER, T., GRETEN, F. R., POLSON, S. W. & ARKAN, M. C. 2014. High-fat-diet-mediated dysbiosis promotes intestinal carcinogenesis independently of obesity. *Nature,* 514, 508–512.

SHEFLIN, A. M., WHITNEY, A. K. & WEIR, T. L. 2014. Cancer-promoting effects of microbial dysbiosis. *Current Oncol Rep,* 16, 1–9.

SHERMAN, M. P., ZAGHOUANI, H. & NIKLAS, V. 2015. Gut microbiota, the immune system, and diet influence the neonatal gut–brain axis. *Ped Res,* 77, 127–135.

SHREINER, A. B., KAO, J. Y. & YOUNG, V. B. 2015. The gut microbiome in health and in disease. *Curr Opin Gastroenterol,* 31, 69.

SINGH, P. P., SHARMA, P. K., KRISHNAN, G. & LOCKHART, A. C. 2015. Immune checkpoints and immunotherapy for colorectal cancer. *Gastroenterol Rep,* 3, 289–297.

SMYTHIES, L. E., SELLERS, M., CLEMENTS, R. H., MOSTELLER-BARNUM, M., MENG, G., BENJAMIN, W. H., ORENSTEIN, J. M. & SMITH, P. D. 2005. Human intestinal macrophages display profound inflammatory anergy despite avid phagocytic and bacteriocidal activity. *J Clin Invest,* 115, 66–75.

SMYTHIES, L. E., SHEN, R., BIMCZOK, D., NOVAK, L., CLEMENTS, R. H., ECKHOFF, D. E., BOUCHARD, P., GEORGE, M. D., HU, W. K. & DANDEKAR, S. 2010. Inflammation anergy in human intestinal macrophages is due to Smad-induced IκBα expression and NF-κB inactivation. *J Biol Chem,* 285, 19593–19604.

SOBHANI, I., TAP, J., ROUDOT-THORAVAL, F., ROPERCH, J. P., LETULLE, S., LANGELLA, P., CORTHIER, G., TRAN VAN NHIEU, J. & FURET, J. P. 2011. Microbial dysbiosis in colorectal cancer (CRC) patients. *PLoS One,* 6, e16393.

SOKOL, H., SEKSIK, P., RIGOTTIER-GOIS, L., LAY, C., LEPAGE, P., PODGLAJEN, I., MARTEAU, P. & DORÉ, J. 2006. Specificities of the fecal microbiota in inflammatory bowel disease. *Inflammatory Bowel Dis,* 12, 106–111.

STÅHL, P. L., SALMÉN, F., VICKOVIC, S., LUNDMARK, A., NAVARRO, J. F., MAGNUSSON, J., GIACOMELLO, S., ASP, M., WESTHOLM, J. O. & HUSS, M. 2016. Visualization and analysis of gene expression in tissue sections by spatial transcriptomics. *Science,* 353, 78–82.

STROBER, W., FUSS, I. J. & BLUMBERG, R. S. 2002. The immunology of mucosal models of inflammation. *Annu Rev Immunol,* 20, 495–549.

TAPER, H. S. & ROBERFROID, M. B. 2005. Possible adjuvant cancer therapy by two prebiotics-inulin or oligofructose. *in vivo,* 19, 201–204.

THAISS, C. A., LEVY, M., KOREM, T., DOHNALOVÁ, L., SHAPIRO, H., JAITIN, D. A., DAVID, E., WINTER, D. R., GURY-BENARI, M., TATIROVSKY, E., TUGANBAEV, T., FEDERICI, S., ZMORA, N., ZEEVI, D., DORI-BACHASH, M., PEVSNER-FISCHER, M., KARTVELISHVILY, E., BRANDIS, A., HARMELIN, A., SHIBOLET, O., HALPERN, Z., HONDA, K., AMIT, I., SEGAL, E. & ELINAV, E. 2016. Microbiota diurnal rhythmicity programs host transcriptome oscillations. *Cell,* 167, 1495–1510.e12.

TOPALIAN, S. L., HODI, F. S., BRAHMER, J. R., GETTINGER, S. N., SMITH, D. C., MCDERMOTT, D. F., POWDERLY, J. D., CARVAJAL, R. D., SOSMAN, J. A. & ATKINS, M. B. 2012. Safety, activity, and immune correlates of anti–PD-1 antibody in cancer. *N Engl J Med,* 366, 2443–2454.

TSILIMIGRAS, M. C., FODOR, A. & JOBIN, C. 2017. Carcinogenesis and therapeutics: the microbiota perspective. *Nat Microbiol,* 2, 17008.

TSUJI, M., SUZUKI, K., KINOSHITA, K. & FAGARASAN, S. 2008. *Dynamic interactions between bacteria and immune cells leading to intestinal IgA synthesis.* Seminars in Immunology. Elsevier, 20(1), 59–66.

ULLUWISHEWA, D., ANDERSON, R. C., MCNABB, W. C., MOUGHAN, P. J., WELLS, J. M. & ROY, N. C. 2011. Regulation of tight junction permeability by intestinal bacteria and dietary components. *J Nutri,* 141, 769–776.

VAN HELDEN, S. F., VAN DEN DRIES, K., OUD, M. M., RAYMAKERS, R. A., NETEA, M. G., VAN LEEUWEN, F. N. & FIGDOR, C. G. 2010. TLR4-mediated podosome loss discriminates gram-negative from gram-positive bacteria in their capacity to induce dendritic cell migration and maturation. *J Immunol,* 184, 1280–1291.

VERBEKE, F., JANSSENS, Y., WYNENDAELE, E. & DE SPIEGELEER, B. 2017. Faecal microbiota transplantation: a regulatory hurdle? *BMC Gastroenterol,* 17, 1–11.

VRIEZE, A., VAN NOOD, E., HOLLEMAN, F., SALOJÄRVI, J., KOOTTE, R. S., BARTELSMAN, J. F. W. M., DALLINGA-THIE, G. M., ACKERMANS, M. T., SERLIE, M. J., OOZEER, R., DERRIEN, M., DRUESNE, A., VAN HYLCKAMA VLIEG, J. E. T., BLOKS, V. W., GROEN, A. K., HEILIG, H. G. H. J., ZOETENDAL, E. G., STROES, E. S., DE VOS, W. M., HOEKSTRA, J. B. L. & NIEUWDORP, M. 2012. Transfer of intestinal microbiota from lean donors increases insulin sensitivity in individuals with metabolic syndrome. *Gastroenterology,* 143, 913–916.e7.

VYAS, D., AEKKA, A. & VYAS, A. 2015. Fecal transplant policy and legislation. *World J Gastroenterol: WJG,* 21, 6.

VYAS, U. & RANGANATHAN, N. 2012. Probiotics, prebiotics, and synbiotics: gut and beyond. *Gastroenterol Res Pract,* 2012. doi: 10.1155/2012/872716. Epub 2012 Sep 19. PMID: 23049548; PMCID: PMC3459241

WESTERBERG, L. S., KLEIN, C. & SNAPPER, S. B. 2008. Breakdown of T cell tolerance and autoimmunity in primary immunodeficiency—lessons learned from monogenic disorders in mice and men. *Curr Opin Immunol,* 20, 646–654.

WITCZAK, M., JAWORSKA, G. & WITCZAK, T. 2020. Influence of inulin and oligofructose on the sensory properties and antioxidant activity of apple jelly. *Slovak J Food Sci,* 14, 774–780.

WONG, J. M. W., DE SOUZA, R., KENDALL, C. W. C., EMAM, A. & JENKINS, D. J. A. 2006. Colonic health: fermentation and short chain fatty acids. *J Clin Gastroenterol,* 40, 235–243.

YANG, J., LIU, K.-X., QU, J.-M. & WANG, X.-D. 2013. The changes induced by cyclophosphamide in intestinal barrier and microflora in mice. *Eur J Pharmacol,* 714, 120–124.

YESUDHAS, D., GOSU, V., ANWAR, M. A. & CHOI, S. 2014. Multiple roles of toll-like receptor 4 in colorectal cancer. *Front Immunol,* 5, 334.

YU, J. X., HUBBARD-LUCEY, V. M. & TANG, J. 2019. Immuno-oncology drug development goes global. *Nat Rev Drug Discov,* 18, 899–900.

YU, T., GUO, F., YU, Y., SUN, T., MA, D., HAN, J., QIAN, Y., KRYCZEK, I., SUN, D. & NAGARSHETH, N. 2017. Fusobacterium nucleatum promotes chemoresistance to colorectal cancer by modulating autophagy. *Cell,* 170, 548–563.

ZACKULAR, J. P., BAXTER, N. T., IVERSON, K. D., SADLER, W. D., PETROSINO, J. F., CHEN, G. Y. & SCHLOSS, P. D. 2013. The gut microbiome modulates colon tumorigenesis. *mBio,* 4, e00692–e00713.

ZHAO, H., LYU, Y., ZHAI, R., SUN, G. & DING, X. 2022. Metformin mitigates sepsis-related neuroinflammation via modulating gut microbiota and metabolites. *Front Immunol,* 13, 797312.

ZHAO, L., ZHANG, F., DING, X., WU, G., LAM, Y. Y., WANG, X., FU, H., XUE, X., LU, C. & MA, J. 2018. Gut bacteria selectively promoted by dietary fibers alleviate type 2 diabetes. *Science,* 359, 1151–1156.

ZOU, S., FANG, L. & LEE, M. H. 2018. Dysbiosis of gut microbiota in promoting the development of colorectal cancer. *Gastroenterol Rep (Oxf),* 6, 1–12.

ZWARTJES, M. S. Z., GERDES, V. E. A. & NIEUWDORP, M. 2021. The role of gut microbiota and its produced metabolites in obesity, dyslipidemia, adipocyte dysfunction, and its interventions. *Metabolites,* 11, 531.

3 Gut Microbiome and Cancer Treatment Response

Thulo Molefi, Talent Chipiti, Benny Mosoane, Ravi Mehrotra, and Zodwa Dlamini

INTRODUCTION

A staggering amount of microorganisms live in the human body. There are over 40 trillion microorganisms, which include around 3000 distinct types of bacteria, fungi, and viruses (Zhao et al., 2023). The bacterial makeup differs from person to person and is critical for maintaining a healthy and stable system. The bacteria that exist in the gastrointestinal system, primarily the colon, are referred to as the gut microbiota (Sender et al., 2016). The gut microbiota has been intensively researched and discovered to have a significant role in the regulation of a wide range of physiological roles, notably immune system development and nutrition generation (Adak and Khan, 2019; Gensollen et al., 2016a). Gut dysbiosis can occur when the microbiota and the human host are out of balance. Taxonomic changes, metabolic products, and secretory vesicles can all ensue, and have been linked to a variety of physiological illnesses, including cancer (Ma et al., 2018; Meisel et al., 2018; Parida et al., 2021; Tilg et al., 2018). While scientists have long studied microorganisms in the digestive system, there is a growing interest in the intratumoral microbiota in the era of targeted therapy. This is due to the fact that bacteria in the tumor microenvironment (TME) can influence cancer growth and therapeutic efficacy (Cogdill et al., 2018; LaCourse et al., 2022; Liou et al., 2020).

Despite being identified more than a century ago, the local diversity and relevance of intratumoral microorganisms have only lately been investigated because of advances in next- and third-generation sequencing (Stearn et al., 1925; Zhao et al., 2023). The characterization of the intratumoral microbiota, in contrast to the intestinal microbiota, is still in its early phases. Although some understanding of its influence on carcinogenesis and treatment efficacy has been achieved, its roles have not yet been fully defined (Fu et al., 2022; Narunsky-Haziza et al., 2022; Nejman et al., 2020). This could be because intratumoral germs are mostly intracellular and can be detected in the surrounding immune cells of cancer cells as well. As a result, it is necessary to use more sensitive observation techniques in order to identify the location of intracellular bacteria. Moreover, the TME microbial biomass is very low in comparison to gut microorganisms, with just one microbial cell found for every 10^4 tumor cells (Dohlman et al., 2022). This makes studying the intratumoral microbiota difficult.

GUT DYSBIOSIS IN CANCER

The balance of microorganisms in the gastrointestinal tract is essential. When it is disrupted, a condition called gut dysbiosis occurs, which can cause the microbiota to become less stable and diverse, and more pathogenic. This condition adversely affects the natural processes of the body and can contribute to various health issues. This may negatively affect cancer development and treatment. Therefore, understanding the molecular mechanisms underlying tumors and normal epithelia involves studying microbes in their microenvironment (Amabebe et al., 2020; Mousa et al., 2022). The presence of microbes on the mucosal surface or TME can affect cancer in various ways (Łaniewski et al., 2020; Sadrekarimi et al., 2022). Contact-dependent and contact-independent impacts are the two different categories of impact. The processes underlying contact-independent effects might be far more intricate than those driving contact-dependent effects, which are well understood. Negative molecules originating from the gut microbiota can penetrate the bloodstream through capillaries and cause contact-independent effects. These effects can contribute either directly to the development of distant cancer or indirectly, through a reduction in the host ability to fight against cancer (Garrett, 2015; Zitvogel et al., 2016). Two metabolites of Gram-positive gut bacteria, lipideichoic acid (LTA) and deoxycholic acid (DCA), have been found to accelerate the development of hepatocellular carcinomas following liver translocation through the use of enterohepatic circulation. This is a common non-contact influence of gut microorganisms on cancer (Loo et al., 2017; Yoshimoto et al., 2013; Zhao et al., 2023). This chapter will look at the influence of bacteria on cancer development from these two perspectives.

MICROBES AND THE TUMOR MICROENVIRONMENT (TME) INTERACTIONS

The TME, or tumor microenvironment, is a complex internal environment that provides the necessary conditions for cancer cells to survive and multiply. Tumor cells, stromal cells, immunological cells such as T lymphocytes, B lymphocytes, natural killer cells, and tumor-associated macrophages, as well as a dense network of microvessels, form the TME (Hui and Chen, 2015). It has been recently discovered that bacteria can also be found within the TME, living inside cancer cells and immune cells, and affecting the biological phenotype of cancer cells and the local immunological microenvironment within the TME (Fu et al., 2022; Nejman et al., 2020). Tumors have several intrinsic properties that make them conducive to microbial invasion, colonization, and proliferation. For instance, angiogenic substances generated by tumor cells during carcinogenesis cause vascularization, which facilitates the invasion of distant microorganisms into the TME (Lugano et al., 2020). Additionally, tumors have innate immunological privilege, which means that bacteria within the TME can potentially operate as immune inhibitors, promoting intratumoral microbial colonization and proliferation (Joyce and Fearon, 2015; Ma et al., 2021).

Elements inside the tumor microenvironment (TME), such as the local oxygen level, might potentially impact the makeup of the tumor microbiota. An abundance of microaerophilic and anaerobic bacteria inside the TME, such as *Bacteroides fragilis* and *Enterococcus faecalis* in colorectal cancer, is linked to the hypoxic and anoxic zones found in many solid tumors. There is a spatial variation of oxygen content within the tumor, but it is unclear if this unequal oxygen distribution results in distinct microbial members throughout different parts of the TME (Milotti et al., 2020; Vaupel and Harrison, 2004). Furthermore, varied microbiome compositions have been discovered across distinct tumor types, which may be the consequence of complicated interactions but require further investigation (Nejman et al., 2020). Intratumoral bacteria can alter cancer features, such as increasing malignant cell spreadability. Tumor-resident bacteria have been detected in high numbers in cancer cells cytoplasm, and these bacteria can promote metastasis in breast cancer by altering the cellular cytoskeleton and increasing resistance to mechanical stress (Fu et al., 2022). In human breast cancer, a conserved intracellular bacterial profile represented by *Enterococcus* and *Streptococcus* was discovered, demonstrating that microorganisms exist and may support cancer progression. Similarly, *Fusobacterium. nucleatum* can promote the proliferative and invasive features of CRC, increasing its metastatic potential (Chen et al., 2020; Xu et al., 2021). Clinical studies targeting the microorganisms within breast cancer should be carried out in the future to prevent breast cancer metastasis.

Bacterial signals may promote cancer growth by decreasing antitumor immunity in the local environment (Ma et al., 2021). The presence of *F. nucleatum* in CRC is negatively associated with the density of CD3+ T-cell infiltration in the TME, resulting in antitumor adaptive immunity downregulation (Mima et al., 2015). Bacteria that induce immunosuppression in the TME might enter the body through the digestive tract or the oral cavity. Intratumoral microorganisms impacts on tumors are quite complex, and the same bacterium may have various effects on different malignancies (Abed et al., 2020; Pushalkar et al., 2018). *F. nucleatum* is favorably linked with tumor-infiltrating lymphocytes in colorectal cancer with low levels of microsatellite instability (MSI) (Hamada et al., 2018). Hence, it can be inferred that additional host parameters other than the MSI level may impact the involvement of microbes inside the TME, although further study is required. Microbes can affect the TME through their OMVs or metabolites. OMVs allow bacteria to deliver virulent factors, proteins, and genetic elements throughout the body. The contents of OMVs can have a negative impact on the TME. For example, *H. pylori* OMVs contain active CagA, which stimulates the TLR and NF-κB pathways in gastric cells, reinforcing inflammation and cell proliferation linked to carcinogenesis (Chmiela et al., 2018; González et al., 2021). Moreover, by activating vascular endothelial growth factor receptor 2, certain microbial metabolites, like DCA produced by gut bacteria following the metabolism of primary bile acids, might encourage vasculogenic mimicry and the epithelial-mesenchymal transition (EMT). The malignant transformation of intestinal epithelial cells requires this receptor (Song et al., 2022).

The TME has also been shown to include fungi. Because pancreatic ductal adenocarcinoma cells contain glycans that bind to mannose-binding lectins, *Malassezia* species present in these tumors have the ability to activate the complement cascade and promote tumor development (Aykut et al., 2019). In cancer patients, the presence of *Candida* species in gastrointestinal malignancies may be associated with poor prognoses, pro-inflammatory gene expression, and metastasis (Dohlman et al., 2022). The connection between fungal and bacterial populations inside the TME is often peaceful rather than competitive. However, it is unknown whether this peaceful association indicates a synergistic cancer-promoting function.

TUMOR MICROBIOME IN TUMORIGENESIS

Cancer-promoting microorganisms can contribute to oncogenesis via several molecular pathways, and four major methods are outlined below in Figure 3.1: (1) abnormalities in DNA damage and epigenetics; (2) interference with the DNA damage response (DDR); (3) aberrant signaling pathways; and (4) immunological suppression (Zhao et al., 2023).

INDUCTION OF DNA DAMAGE AND EPIGENETICS ALTERATIONS

Cancer is a genetic illness that develops at the genetic level of cells, and microorganisms involved in tumor development and progression may induce mutations that manifest as cellular DNA damage (Barrett et al., 2020). Many bacteria have the intrinsic capacity to cause or assist DNA damage, which has been linked to cancer onset. Genotoxic compounds from bacteria like *Morganella morganii*, such as colibactin, have been found to cause DNA damage in colonic epithelial cells, causing double-strand breaks and interference with DNA replication and transcription (Cao et al., 2022). Additionally, contaminated cell-autonomous mechanisms that respond to bacterial infections or their byproducts, including reactive oxygen species (ROS), can indirectly cause damage to DNA (Vizcaino and Crawford, 2015). Epigenetic modifications, such as DNA methylation, histone posttranslational modification, chromatin remodeling, and control by noncoding RNAs, have also been linked to cancer development. Recent research has

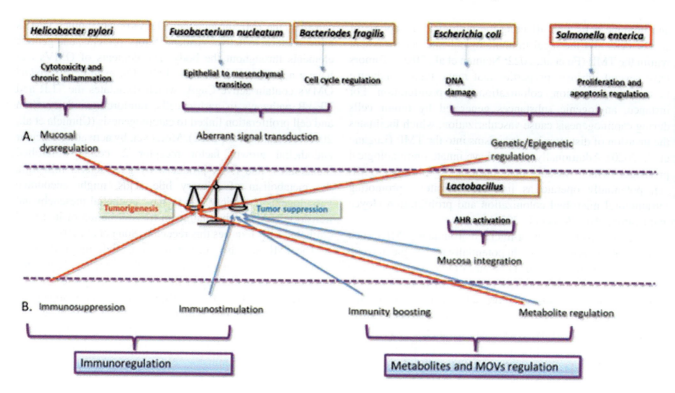

FIGURE 3.1 **Mechanisms of microbial tumorigenesis and tumor suppression.** (A) Shows mechanisms by which microbes trigger tumorigenesis and tumor suppression in the gut in the tumor microenvironment (TME). The microbiome plays an important role in carcinogenesis and tumor suppression. This can be grouped as follows: (1) Mucosal dysregulations, such as the virulence factor CagA, can enter mucosal cells via T4SS, encouraging cell proliferation and increasing the pace at which tumor cells convert. (2) *F. nucleatum* Fap2 and OMVs stimulate colonic epithelial cells, generating TNF and IL-8, and FadA interacts with E-cadherin, leading to carcinogenesis via the NF-B pathway. (3) Genotoxin-mediated mutagenesis can promote cancer by causing DNA damage and genetic/epigenetic changes, while PRR ligation can impair immunosurveillance, leading to tumor development and metastasis. (4) Immune suppression: boosting immunity, metabolic modulation in anticancer activity, and sIgA production from B cells are all mechanisms of microorganisms that trigger carcinogenesis and tumor suppression in the TME. (B) Microbes in the tumor microenvironment (TME) can influence carcinogenesis or tumor suppression in two ways: (1) enhancing immunity through bacterial metabolites, such as CD8+ T cells that generate IFN- κB; (2) controlling anticancer metabolites through SCFAs, such as butyrate from commensal bacteria. TNF, IL-8, Treg regulatory T cells, TILs, and the TME tumor microenvironment are all engaged in these pathways (Zhao et al., 2023).

shown that bacteria *F. nucleatum* and *Hungatella hathewayi* induce hypermethylation, which fuels the development of intestinal tumors (Tse et al., 2017).

INTERFERENCE WITH THE DNA DAMAGE RESPONSE (DDR)

There is always a chance that the human genome might be harmed by pathogenic microbes or endogenous genotoxic stress. This damage activates the DNA damage response (DDR), which locates harmful mutations and helps to restore damaged DNA regions (Ciccia and Elledge, 2010; Tubbs and Nussenzweig, 2017). Microbes can, however, also obstruct the DDR, encouraging the spread of deleterious mutations to offspring cells and perhaps resulting in oncogenesis (Harper and Elledge, 2007). The MRN complex initiates the DDR in response to DSBs by recruiting and activating ataxia-telangiectasia mutated kinase (ATM), an essential component of DNA repair (Lee and Paull, 2005). *C. trachomatis*, a pathogen linked to ovarian and cervical cancer, induces ROS generation and prevents MRE11, ATM, and 53BP1 from activating and recruiting at damaged DNA locations, hence contributing to DNA damage. *H. pylori* causes DSDs and tampers with different DDR. Higher point mutation frequencies and an elevated risk of carcinogenesis result from *H. pylori* induction of DSBs and disruption of many DDR pathways (Lavin, 2007; Lee and Paull, 2007).

H. pylori inhibits homologous recombination (HR) and promotes the error-prone DSB pathway known as non-homologous end-joining (NHEJ). Because NHEJ is promoted and HR is inhibited, an overactive NHEJ pathway may be linked to cancers (Koeppel et al., 2015; Li and Heyer, 2008). An important DDR regulator that either stimulates cell repair or death is the p53 protein. Nevertheless, *H. pylori* has the ability to cause p53 degradation in order to obstruct the DDR process. This increases resistance to apoptosis and Hp colonization, making the host more vulnerable to malignant transformation (Buti et al., 2011; Kastenhuber and Lowe, 2017; Williams and Schumacher, 2016).

TRIGGERING ABERRANT SIGNALING PATHWAYS

Microbes can accelerate the growth of cancer by disrupting DDR pathways and negatively affecting other signaling pathways. An essential signaling system that controls a variety of biological processes, including the determination of cell destiny throughout embryonic development, is Wnt/-catenin signaling (Clevers, 2006). Wnt signaling activity is associated with cancer initiation and progression (Gregorieff and Clevers, 2005; Zhan et al., 2017). Bacteria have the ability to alter the Wnt pathway, resulting in malignant transformation. ETBF-secreted *Fusobacterium* adhesin A (FadA) and BFT may stimulate Wnt signaling (Rubinstein et al., 2013). Certain bacteria can also use mitogen-activated protein kinases (MAPK) to induce carcinogenesis (Fang and Richardson, 2005). Through contact with GRB2, Hp-derived CagA may activate T cell factor (TCF), triggering the ERK signaling cascade (Mimuro et al., 2007). TCF increases the expression of the induced myeloid leukemia cell differentiation protein 1 (MCL1), which may protect gastric epithelial cells against apoptosis. *Salmonella typhi*, a risk factor for gallbladder carcinoma, can cause gallbladder cancer.

ELICITING IMMUNOSUPPRESSIVE EFFECTS

When it comes to identifying and getting rid of aberrant cells, immunosurveillance relies heavily on the human immune system. Cancer cells need to evade being discovered and dying in order to initiate carcinogenesis. Bacteria such as *F. nucleatum* have been shown to shield cancer cells from immunosurveillance, which may be connected to cancer formation, by binding to the inhibitory receptor TIGIT on human NK cells and other T cells (Gur et al., 2015). *F. nucleatum* can suppress the assault of natural killer (NK) lymphocytes on tumor cells. Gut microorganisms can also promote pancreatic ductal adenocarcinoma by lowering intratumoral NK cell infiltration and activity (Yu and Schwabe, 2017). *F. nucleatum* may preferentially attract tumor-infiltrating myeloid-derived suppressor cells (MDSCs), which may aid in the development and spread of intestinal tumors (Gabrilovich, 2017; Kostic et al., 2013). Gut Gram-negative bacteria/lipopolysaccharides drive hepatocytes to recruit MDSCs in the liver, causing liver cancer by establishing an immunosuppressive microenvironment (Zhang et al., 2021). During malignant transformation, *H. pylori* aids precancerous cells in evading immunosurveillance (Holokai et al., 2019). Indole compounds decrease antitumor immunity by activating the aryl hydrocarbon receptor in tumor-associated macrophages (Hezaveh et al., 2022). Pathogenic fungi can also disrupt immune surveillance, impacting cancer progression (Rieber et al., 2015).

MECHANISMS OF MICROBES IN TUMOR SUPPRESSION

Microbes can cause cancer or repress it, both during the start and promotion phases. This can occur in one of two ways: direct destruction of tumor cells or positive immunoregulatory effects.

DIRECT TUMOR-SUPPRESSIVE EFFECTS

Bacterial genotoxins can cause and promote cancer initiation and progression, although other toxins have anticancer characteristics and may be used as anticancer agents (Sharma et al., 2022). *Clostridium perfringens* enterotoxin (CPE) is a virulence factor that causes food poisoning; however, on a positive note, it has been found to inhibit cancer cell growth by interacting with the transmembrane tight junction proteins claudin-3 and -4 (Brynestad and Granum, 2002; Kominsky et al., 2004). *Pseudomonas aeruginosa*, *Salmonella typhimurium*, and *Clostridium difficile* are some more direct anticancer microorganisms. These toxins such as enterotoxin (CPE) or their attenuated derivatives might be used to create future chemotherapeutic treatments. In most situations, genetic engineering approaches are required to overcome systemic toxicity (Zhao et al., 2023).

BENEFICIAL EFFECTS ON IMMUNOREGULATION

Gut bacteria have a major role in the development of the host immune system, which can help prevent and reduce cancer. It improves the development of lymphoid organs and immune cell differentiation, demonstrating the influence of microorganisms on the composition and functionality of the immune system (Gensollen et al., 2016b). The gut microbiota has a significant influence in both the central and peripheral lymphoid organs, which are the two categories of lymphoid tissue (Sommer and Bäckhed, 2013). A recent study has revealed that commensal fungi travel to peripheral lymph nodes and commence their growth via retinoic acid signaling (Zhang et al., 2016). Additionally, the formation of gut-associated lymphoid tissue (GALT) (as illustrated in Figure 3.2b), which improves intestinal homeostasis, depends on gut microbiota. Commensal bacteria can reduce the risk of several cancers, including colorectal cancer, by strengthening the gut mucosa immune system resilience to infections (Zhao et al., 2023).

Based on the anticancer properties of the gut microbiota, specific strains have been demonstrated to tantalizingly treat cancer by raising anticancer immunity. Eleven bacterial strains isolated from healthy human donor feces demonstrated promise in stimulating intestinal CD8+ T cells that produce interferon and increasing the efficacy of immune checkpoint inhibitors in tumor-bearing mouse models, indicating a potential role for microorganisms in cancer treatment (Tanoue et al., 2019).

The mucosal surface of the gastrointestinal system can be directly impacted by gut bacteria, which can have genotoxic effects and encourage the growth of epithelial cells. Through RIG-IFN-1 signaling, they can also promote hematopoiesis of the thymic and bone marrow, which makes them radioprotective against radiation. Through immunostimulatory or immunosuppressive effects on T cells and dendritic cells, gut

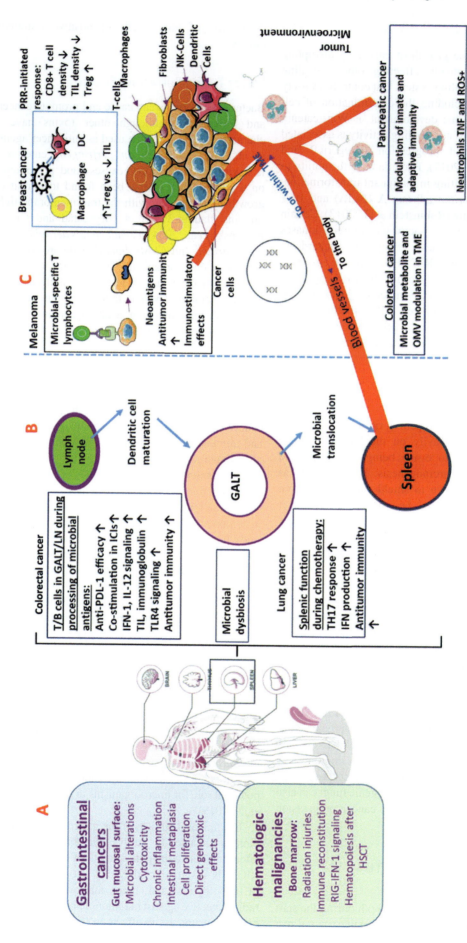

FIGURE 3.2 **The gut microbiome and cancer development.** The gut microbiome may affect cancer in one of three ways: (A) contact-dependent interactions at the mucosal surface or within primary lymphoid organs such as the thymus and bone marrow; (B) secondary lymphoid organs such as the spleen, lymph nodes, and GALT; or (C) TME, which may also expand to contact-independent interactions triggered by circulating microbial metabolites and OMVs (Zhao et al, 2023).

microorganisms and their metabolites interact with the GALT, LN, and spleen. Microbial modulation of the TME includes metabolite release, cargo-carrying OMVs, and the control of neutrophils, TNF, ROS, and adaptive immune responses.

GUT–TUMOR MICROBIOME AXIS: GUT MICROBIOME AS TREATMENT MODALITY

With the established link between the gut microbiome and its relation to the TME, the natural progression is to manipulate this interaction to affect beneficial cancer treatment responses. Fecal microbial transplantation (FMT) is the process of transplanting favorable gut microbiota from healthy donors, into individuals with dysbiosis to alter their gut microbiota as a means of treating a variety of diseases (Wang et al., 2018). In patients who have previously shown resistance to immune checkpoint inhibitors, FMT has been utilized to enhance therapy results. Tyrosine kinase inhibitors and immune checkpoint inhibitors, among other targeted cancer medicines, have also been used to address adverse medication responses. To get beyond the main drawback of FMT, which is the transplanting of both favorable and unfavorable microbiota without selection, specially prepared microbial mixtures have been selected based on their capacity to improve immunological function and microbial homeostasis, both of which have favorable anticancer effects (Cheng et al., 2020; Wang et al., 2018). Antibacterial approaches, such as targeting tumorigenic organisms with antibiotics and the use of bacteriophages and genetically modified bacteria, have been used to modulate the gut microbiota, with varying anticancer results. Often these modalities have unexpected adverse effects which warrant further study. Microbial-inspired drug delivery systems using nanotechnology and dormant microbial spores are showing themselves to be a way of improving drug pharmacokinetics and reducing treatment bystander effects.

MICROBIOME EFFECTS ON TREATMENT RESPONSE (SURGERY, IMMUNOTHERAPY, CHEMOTHERAPY, AND RADIATION)

One approach to think of the gut microbiota as a separate organ is to consider the various ways in which its composition may be changed. More importantly, recent studies on gut microbes have demonstrated a strong correlation between the effectiveness of anticancer therapies and gut microorganisms (Gunjur, 2020; Huang et al., 2022). This has given rise to a new area of promising anticancer research: altering the microbial makeup of the gut to increase the effectiveness and decrease the therapeutic toxicity of traditional anticancer treatments (Lou et al., 2021; Singh et al., 2021). Despite this, a truly effective microbial anticancer drug is still a long way off. Promising connections have been shown between anticancer drugs and gut microbes, as well as between current and novel microbial therapeutics for cancer treatment (Knippel et al., 2021; Zhu et al., 2021). Figure 3.3 summarizes the relationship between several anticancer models and gut flora.

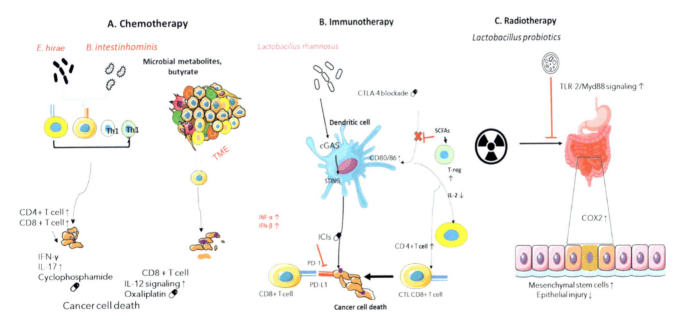

FIGURE 3.3 **Microbiota factors influencing cancer therapy effectiveness.** (A) *Enterococcus hirae* and *Barnesiella intestinhominis* administration can improve the antitumor effectiveness of cyclophosphamide-based treatment by activating tumor-specific T cells and generating IFN-. Butyrate, a dietary fiber fermented by gut bacteria, has been shown to improve the anticancer effects of oxaliplatin-based chemotherapy by modulating CD8+ T cell activity via IL-12 signaling. (B) *Lactobacillus rhamnosus* can boost PD-1 immunotherapy via the cGAS-STING signaling pathway, but short-chain fatty acids (SCFAs) can restrict CTLA-4 blockade anticancer effects by reducing Treg cells. (C) *Lactobacillus* probiotics can protect the gut mucosa from radiation damage by encouraging mesenchymal stem cells to migrate to the crypt.

MICROBIOTA EFFECTS ON IMMUNOTHERAPY

Adoptive T-cell therapy (ACT) and immune checkpoint therapy (CTLA-4 and PD1) are two examples of cancer immunotherapy, which is now an essential part of cancer treatment (Waldman et al., 2020). However, many patients continue to receive immunotherapy with minimal effect, demonstrating primary or acquired resistance to treatment (Fehrenbacher et al., 2016; Sharma et al., 2017). This disparity in effectiveness might be attributed to gut microbes (Derosa et al., 2020; Naqash et al., 2021; Rangan and Mondino, 2022). The most sophisticated kind of cancer therapy is immune checkpoint inhibitors (ICIs), which target coinhibitory molecules like PD-1/PD-L1 to enhance endogenous host immunity and stop tumor cells from eluding immune surveillance (Wei et al., 2018). The gut microbiota may also be implicated in the modification of host immunity, which may alter cancer patients responses to ICIs indirectly. Due to the richness of the gut microbiota, research has demonstrated that gut bacteria have the exact opposite effect, by antagonising the intended efficacy of ICIs (Routy et al., 2018). Certain gut microorganisms, for example, might diminish CTLA-4 blockade antitumor effects, whereas high levels of butyrate in cancer patients can reduce ipilimumab anticancer effectiveness by decreasing the accumulation of associated T cells and IL-2 impregnation (Coutzac et al., 2020). Gut microorganisms also contribute to food metabolism, creating compounds that alter the body immunity and, as a result, the effects of ICIs (Kang, 2012; Leeming et al., 2019).

Gut microbes affect both the efficacy of ICI and ACT. Vancomycin treatment during ACT reduced the growth of tumors in tumor-bearing rats by depleting their gut bacteria; metronidazole and neomycin had no impact. The impact of gut flora on anticancer therapy (ACT) has been confirmed by observational studies, which have found a negative correlation between antibiotic usage and poorer clinical outcomes and prognosis in the four weeks prior to CAR-T-cell treatment (Zhao et al., 2023).

CHEMOTHERAPY AND ITS INTERACTION WITH GUT MICROBIOTA IN CANCER THERAPY

Although chemotherapy is a common cancer treatment, not all individuals benefit from it (Sasako et al., 2011). The variations in the reactions of cancer patients might be attributed to the makeup of the gut flora. The effectiveness of chemotherapy is regulated by certain gut microorganisms, which can have both boosting and inhibiting effects (Lim et al., 2021; Liu et al., 2021). Within the context of pancreatic ductal adenocarcinoma (PDAC), intestinal microbes like *Gammaproteobacteria* (Alexander et al., 2017; Dapito et al., 2012) may have an impact on the chemotherapy drug gemcitabine. Gemcitabine anticancer activity may be enhanced when combined with chemotherapy and antibiotics that target *Gammaproteobacteria*. Butyrate, a dietary fiber product produced by gut microbes, can increase gemcitabine effectiveness by triggering apoptosis (Panebianco et al., 2022). Another immunostimulatory drug used in chemotherapy, cyclophosphamide, has been demonstrated to reduce the antitumor effectiveness in mice treated with antibiotics or kept germ-free because it suppresses Th1- and Th17-related immune responses. However, by stimulating tumor-specific CD8+ and CD4+ T cells as well as Th1 and Th17 cells, the injection of *Enterococcus hirae* and *Barnesiella intestinhominis* can recover the antitumor activity (Heshiki et al., 2020).

Bacteroides xylanisolvens and *Bacteroides ovatus* are two gut bacteria that have been favorably associated with erlotinib, a highly selective tyrosine kinase inhibitor. In a mouse lung cancer model, oral treatment of these bacteria may dramatically increase the effectiveness of erlotinib and promote the expression of IFN-γ and C-X-C motif ligand 9 (CXCL9) (Heshiki et al., 2020; Zhao et al., 2023). Individual oxaliplatin effectiveness varies and may be related to the presence of certain gut bacteria metabolites. Butyrate may enhance oxaliplatin anticancer actions by modulating the activity of CD8+ T lymphocytes in the tumor mesenchymal environment (TME) (He et al., 2021). In conclusion, dysbiosis of the gut microbiota in cancer patients may be one cause of drug resistance, and therapies targeting the gut microbiota might be a potential way to increase cancer chemotherapy effectiveness.

INTERACTIONS BETWEEN RADIOTHERAPY AND THE GUT MICROBIOTA THAT ARE BIDIRECTIONAL

Radiation therapy (RT) has been used to treat cancer for almost a century, with its primary concepts being twofold: directly killing cancer cells by ionizing radiation and indirectly inducing reactive oxygen species-dependent DNA damage (Petroni et al., 2022). However, RT can have a negative impact on normal tissues and commensal microbes, especially in the gut (Oh et al., 2021a). There is a bidirectional link between RT and the gut microbiota, with dysbiosis of the gut microbiota being one of the adverse events (Guo et al., 2020). This dysbiosis reduces the abundance of good microorganisms while increasing the abundance of dangerous ones, which is aggravated by radiation-related diseases such as radiation enteropathy (Poonacha et al., 2022). The presence of commensal microorganisms is crucial for increasing radiation effectiveness and reducing RT-related side events (Oh et al., 2021a). Antibiotic depletion before radiation has been demonstrated in studies to result in quicker tumor development and lower survival in tumor-bearing mice (Shiao et al., 2021). Tumor-bearing mice, on the other hand, developed more slowly than the control group when given antibiotics alone without radiation (Shiao et al., 2021; Zhao et al., 2023). Fungi have also been linked to radiation treatment response, suggesting that additional secondary bacteria in the gut microbiota might impact radiotherapy efficacy, however, this effect may be detrimental. There is a reticular link between gut bacteria, tumors, and radiation, with a large study space (Zhao et al., 2023).

EFFECTS OF TREATMENT ON MICROBIOME DIVERSITY

Chemotherapy, while often effective at killing cancer cells, also has off-target adverse effects, including the killing of favorable intestinal flora. The resultant dysbiosis then promotes further chemotherapy adverse effects (Oh et al., 2021). Radiotherapy has direct and indirect effects on the cancer it is directed towards, including its surrounding tissues. The effect on gut dysbiosis is well established, and probiotics have been used to treat radiation enteropathy (Shiao et al., 2021). Alteration of normal anatomy after surgery to the GIT for cancer has long been recognized as a cause of dysbiosis, with negative surgical and cancer outcomes. Multiple strategies aimed at restoring microbial homeostasis are under investigation to improve postsurgical prognosis. Immunotherapy has been found to reduce the proportion of favorable microbes, such as *Lactobacillus* species (Huang et al., 2022). The replenishment of such organisms has been used to successfully treat immune checkpoint-related colitis. Radiotherapy has divergent effects on gut microbiota and represents an area of growing cancer research.

ROLE OF MICROBIOME ON THE INCIDENCE OF TREATMENT ADVERSE EFFECTS

There are drawbacks to even immunotherapy, which has grown in popularity recently (Palamaris et al., 2022; Yazbeck et al., 2022). Based on observations, the toxicity of conventional anticancer medicines has been linked to the gut microbiota, and it may be lessened by altering the gut microbiome constituent parts (Li et al., 2021). Therefore, for a personalized decrease of these adverse events, it is especially crucial to comprehend the interaction between various microorganisms and the side effects of conventional anticancer therapy. One of the most harmful adverse effects of immune checkpoint therapy is colitis, which may have very significant inflammatory side effects (Khan and Gerber, 2020). Researchers have discovered that the amount of *Lactobacillus* in the gut significantly decreased in patients with severe ICI-related colitis. A subsequent study has verified that this probiotic may be taken orally to mitigate ICI-related colitis (Wang et al., 2019). The inhibition of ICI-related colitis by *L. reuteri* is linked, mechanistically, to a reduction in the distribution of group 3 innate lymphocytes (Wang et al., 2019; Zhao et al., 2023).

Furthermore, a greater abundance of *B. intestinalis* was linked to immunotherapy side effects, according to profiling of the gut microbiota in melanoma patients undergoing combination PD-1 and CTLA-4 inhibition (Andrews et al., 2021). Similarly, the gut microbiota is related to the immunotoxicity of immune agonist antibodies (IAAs), a new immunotherapy medication that targets costimulatory molecules (Blake et al., 2021). In particular, compared to normal or microbially recolonized germ-free mice, animals that were treated with antibiotics and kept germ-free experienced fewer side effects after receiving the IAAs anti-CD40 and anti-CD137 (Blake et al., 2021; Zhao et al., 2023).

When combined, these data show a strong correlation between gut microbiota profiles and ICI toxicity, which may pave the way for the future development of novel treatment approaches.

Chemotherapy can save cancer patients, but it also has a number of negative side effects, such as diarrhea, mucositis, and an imbalance in the gut flora (Akbarali et al., 2022). For instance, the popular chemotherapy medication irinotecan can destroy cancer cells, but it can also kill commensal microbes in the stomach and normal epithelial cells. As a result, intestinal flora imbalance and toxic side effects in the gastrointestinal tract are common with irinotecan. In vivo irinotecan clearance times can be extended by the β-glucuronidase released by gut microorganisms, which can intensify irinotecan-induced gastrointestinal toxicity (Yue et al., 2021). Furthermore, by impairing the intestinal mucosal barrier, irinotecan-induced intestinal dysbiosis may make the drug gastrointestinal toxicity worse. Thus, it is evident that gut bacteria play a role in the processes behind the negative effects of irinotecan. Irinotecan gastrointestinal toxicity may be lessened, and patients quality of life may be enhanced by direct suppression of β-glucuronidase (Kaliannan et al., 2022; Roberts et al., 2013; Zhao et al., 2023). Additionally, using particular probiotics, such as the *E. coli* strain Nissle 1917, might lessen the negative effects of irinotecan by regulating gut barrier epithelial function, easing gut dysbiosis, and eventually reducing intestinal difficulties brought on by irinotecan (Zhao et al., 2023).

In addition to killing cancer cells, radiation therapy (RT) alters the kind and quantity of commensal gut microbes and has variable negative effects on healthy organs (Bai et al., 2021; Oh et al., 2021b). Radiation treatment (RT)-induced dysbiotic gut microbiota hence intensifies the gastrointestinal toxicity (Oh et al., 2021b). On the other hand, some probiotics or probiotic preparations, such as *Lactobacillus*, *Streptococcus*, and *Bifidobacterium* species included in VSL#3 probiotic preparation, may shield the intestinal epithelium from harm and lessen the negative effects of RT (Ciorba et al., 2012; Delia et al., 2007; Touchefeu et al., 2014). Postoperative complications in gastrointestinal cancer surgery, including site infections and anastomotic leaks, can lead to serious consequences. To reduce these risks, patients undergo preoperative bowel preparation and take antibiotics. Changes in microbial activity, including the creation of organic compounds and the transfer of nutrients, are linked to metabolism after gastric surgery (Erawijantari et al., 2020).

The makeup of the intestinal microbiota may be able to predict a patient short-term prognosis following gastrointestinal cancer surgery, according to related research (Zhao et al., 2023). For example, postoperative anastomotic leaks are linked to mucin-degrading members of the *Bacteroideae* and *Lachnospiraceae* families and limited microbial diversity (El Bairi et al., 2020; van Praagh et al., 2019). Several variables, including the use of extended and invasive therapies, antibiotic exposure, and the emergence of virulent and drug-resistant microbes as a result of globalization, can lead to surgical site infections (Alverdy et al., 2017). Some probiotics, such as *Lactobacillus* and *Bifidobacterium* strains, have been found to inhibit pathogenic microorganisms associated with postoperative infections, such as methicillin-resistant *Staphylococcus aureus*, by direct cell competitive exclusion and the production of inhibitors (Sikorska and Smoragiewicz, 2013). Targeting these associated microbes may make it possible in the future to create microbial therapeutics to enhance the postoperative prognosis.

CHALLENGES AND FUTURE OUTLOOK

Cancer treatment has been a long-standing challenge in medical science. Despite significant attempts to maximize the therapeutic effects and minimize harmful toxicity, therapeutic resistance and negative effects remain major obstacles in cancer therapy management. As a result, using cancer-associated microorganisms in the clinic has both opportunities and obstacles that need to be identified and addressed (Jardim et al., 2021). Due to a lack of standardized procedures, it is currently impossible to guarantee the homogeneity and consistency of mechanistic information about microbial effect on cancer. This covers discrepancies in resource analysis, technology, data quality, sample selection, and collecting. The results of multiple samples taken from the same subjects might change significantly because the kind and quantity of bacteria that colonize different bodily areas can differ significantly (Parthasarathy et al., 2016). To obtain objective study outcomes, various sorts of samples should be gathered and studied going forward.

Furthermore, a number of errors may occur during the collection and processing of the sample. Due to the low biomass of tumor microbiota, microbial research can be seriously hampered by sample contamination, which can be brought on by lengthy surgery, cross-contamination from other samples, and a complex laboratory setting (Eisenhofer et al., 2019; Nejman et al., 2020). Several measures must be taken to lower the possibility of sample contamination in order to guarantee accurate study findings. For example, when collecting samples, all exposed human regions should be covered with clean, protective clothing (Eisenhofer et al., 2019). In addition, technical factors like data collection, DNA extraction, sample management, and bioinformatics are available to help identify specific compositional and functional microbial fingerprints. However, using several samples and sequencing technologies can make data resources more heterogeneous and make them harder to access. In the coming years, it may be possible to develop a comprehensive standard operating procedure (SOP) for all methods in order to address these issues (Sinha et al., 2017).

Despite increasing data on human subjects, microbe-targeted therapeutic regimens have not yet been developed into well-established uses for cancer patients. The causes of this phenomenon are incredibly complex, however, individual differences in sensitivity to the same microbial infections may play a role. Is it possible to integrate microbe-targeted medicines with current cancer management approaches to achieve significant and advantageous antitumor effects? Since the issue is unresolved, more preclinical investigations and prospective clinical studies are needed to pinpoint the challenges (Zhao et al., 2023). Ultimately, it is impossible to overstate the importance and promise of the gut microbiota for the creation of cutting-edge anticancer therapies. Changes in the makeup of the gut microbiota can have a major effect on the onset and course of illness. The gut microbiota is crucial for the immune system and metabolic regulation. Thus, it is critical to look into a comprehensive approach that takes microbiological aspects into account, as this will result in the creation of more individualized and effective cancer treatments.

CONCLUSION

This chapter reviewed how the gut microbiome and its link to the TME affects cancer pathogenesis and the response to anticancer therapeutics. The link between the gut microbiome and cancer is no longer merely that of association but has been shown to have a clear causal relation, mostly through animal model studies. The difference between animals and humans can not be understated, however, preclinical data has shown that the multilevel interplay between the microbiome, host, cancer, and cancer-directed therapies can be manipulated to positively alter cancer outcomes. Cancer, being a disease under constant evolution, requires novel treatment approaches and this new field of pharmacomicrobiomics represents an exciting, albeit complicated area of investigation. Identifying critical pathways in the gut-tumor microbial axis is fundamental to developing viable treatment approaches. Studies aimed at defining the exact cancer-impacting mechanisms, whether they be cancer-promoting or suppressive, need to be designed. The human gut microbiome is known to have geographic and regional variations. So, studies investigating their effect on cancer and its treatment, would require standardized microbial analysis to elicit how manipulating its link to cancer can be used to develop predictive models and treatment algorithms to alter clinical care.

Microbial-directed therapy is undoubtedly an exciting anticancer approach to add to the current treatment landscape. However, in light of inter-individual microbial variations, an approach geared towards personalized precision antimicrobial cancer therapy is possibly the most appropriate route to accelerate the use of pharmacomicrobiomics in the oncology clinic.

REFERENCES

Abed, J., Maalouf, N., Manson, A.L., Earl, A.M., Parhi, L., Emgård, J.E.M., Klutstein, M., Tayeb, S., Almogy, G., Atlan, K.A., 2020. Colon cancer-associated Fusobacterium nucleatum may originate from the oral cavity and reach colon tumors via the circulatory system. *Front Cell Infect Microbiol* 10, 400.

Adak, A., Khan, M.R., 2019. An insight into gut microbiota and its functionalities. *Cell Mol Life Sci* 76, 473–493.

Akbarali, H.I., Muchhala, K.H., Jessup, D.K., Cheatham, S., 2022. Chemotherapy induced gastrointestinal toxicities. *Adv Cancer Res* 155, 131–166.

Alexander, J.L., Wilson, I.D., Teare, J., Marchesi, J.R., Nicholson, J.K., Kinross, J.M., 2017. Gut microbiota modulation of chemotherapy efficacy and toxicity. *Nat Rev Gastroenterol Hepatol* 14, 356–365.

Alverdy, J.C., Hyoju, S.K., Weigerinck, M., Gilbert, J.A., 2017. The gut microbiome and the mechanism of surgical infection. *J Br Surg* 104, e14–e23.

Amabebe, E., Robert, F.O., Agbalalah, T., Orubu, E.S.F., 2020. Microbial dysbiosis-induced obesity: role of gut microbiota in homoeostasis of energy metabolism. *Br J Nutri* 123, 1127–1137.

Andrews, M.C., Duong, C.P.M., Gopalakrishnan, V., Iebba, V., Chen, W.-S., Derosa, L., Khan, M.A.W., Cogdill, A.P., White, M.G., Wong, M.C., 2021. Gut microbiota signatures are associated with toxicity to combined CTLA-4 and PD-1 blockade. *Nat Med* 27, 1432–1441.

Aykut, B., Pushalkar, S., Chen, R., Li, Q., Abengozar, R., Kim, J.I., Shadaloey, S.A., Wu, D., Preiss, P., Verma, N., 2019. The fungal mycobiome promotes pancreatic oncogenesis via activation of MBL. *Nature* 574, 264–267.

Bai, J., Barandouzi, Z.A., Rowcliffe, C., Meador, R., Tsementzi, D., Bruner, D.W., 2021. Gut microbiome and its associations with acute and chronic gastrointestinal toxicities in cancer patients with pelvic radiation therapy: a systematic review. *Front Oncol* 11, 5237.

Barrett, M., Hand, C.K., Shanahan, F., Murphy, T., O'Toole, P.W., 2020. Mutagenesis by microbe: the role of the microbiota in shaping the cancer genome. *Trends Cancer* 6, 277–287.

Blake, S.J., James, J., Ryan, F.J., Caparros-Martin, J., Eden, G.L., Tee, Y.C., Salamon, J.R., Benson, S.C., Tumes, D.J., Sribnaia, A., 2021. The immunotoxicity, but not antitumor efficacy, of anti-CD40 and anti-CD137 immunotherapies is dependent on the gut microbiota. *Cell Rep Med* 2. 2(12):100464

Brynestad, S., Granum, P.E., 2002. Clostridium perfringens and foodborne infections. *Int J Food Microbiol* 74, 195–202.

Buti, L., Spooner, E., Van der Veen, A.G., Rappuoli, R., Covacci, A., Ploegh, H.L., 2011. Helicobacter pylori cytotoxin-associated gene A (CagA) subverts the apoptosis-stimulating protein of p53 (ASPP2) tumor suppressor pathway of the host. *Proc Natl Acad Sci* 108, 9238–9243.

Cao, Y., Oh, J., Xue, M., Huh, W.J., Wang, J., Gonzalez-Hernandez, J.A., Rice, T.A., Martin, A.L., Song, D., Crawford, J.M., 2022. Commensal microbiota from patients with inflammatory bowel disease produce genotoxic metabolites. *Science* 378(6618):eabm3233.

Chen, S., Su, T., Zhang, Y., Lee, A., He, J., Ge, Q., Wang, Lan, Si, J., Zhuo, W., Wang, Liangjing, 2020. Fusobacterium nucleatum promotes colorectal cancer metastasis by modulating KRT7-AS/KRT7. *Gut Microbes* 11, 511–525.

Cheng, W.Y., Wu, C.Y., Yu, J., 2020. The role of gut microbiota in cancer treatment: Friend or foe? *Gut*. 69(10):1867–1876

Chmiela, M., Walczak, N., Rudnicka, K., 2018. Helicobacter pylori outer membrane vesicles involvement in the infection development and Helicobacter pylori-related diseases. *J Biomed Sci* 25, 1–11.

Ciccia, A., Elledge, S.J., 2010. The DNA damage response: making it safe to play with knives. *Mol Cell* 40, 179–204.

Ciorba, M.A., Riehl, T.E., Rao, M.S., Moon, C., Ee, X., Nava, G.M., Walker, M.R., Marinshaw, J.M., Stappenbeck, T.S., Stenson, W.F., 2012. Lactobacillus probiotic protects intestinal epithelium from radiation injury in a TLR-2/cyclo-oxygenase-2-dependent manner. *Gut* 61, 829–838.

Clevers, H., 2006. Wnt/β-catenin signaling in development and disease. *Cell* 127, 469–480.

Cogdill, A.P., Gaudreau, P.O., Arora, R., Gopalakrishnan, V., Wargo, J.A., 2018. The impact of intratumoral and gastrointestinal microbiota on systemic cancer therapy. *Trends Immunol* 39, 900–920.

Coutzac, C., Jouniaux, J.-M., Paci, A., Schmidt, J., Mallardo, D., Seck, A., Asvatourian, V., Cassard, L., Saulnier, P., Lacroix, L., 2020. Systemic short chain fatty acids limit antitumor effect of CTLA-4 blockade in hosts with cancer. *Nat Commun* 11(1):2168.

Dapito, D.H., Mencin, A., Gwak, G.-Y., Pradere, J.-P., Jang, M.-K., Mederacke, I., Caviglia, J.M., Khiabanian, H., Adeyemi, A., Bataller, R., 2012. Promotion of hepatocellular carcinoma by the intestinal microbiota and TLR4. *Cancer Cell* 21, 504–516.

Delia, P., Sansotta, G., Donato, V., Frosina, P., Messina, G., De Renzis, C., Famularo, G., 2007. Use of probiotics for prevention of radiation-induced diarrhea. *World J Gastroenterol: WJG* 13(6):912–915

Derosa, L., Routy, B., Fidelle, M., Iebba, V., Alla, L., Pasolli, E., Segata, N., Desnoyer, A., Pietrantonio, F., Ferrere, G., 2020. Gut bacteria composition drives primary resistance to cancer immunotherapy in renal cell carcinoma patients. *Eur Urol* 78, 195–206.

Dohlman, A.B., Klug, J., Mesko, M., Gao, I.H., Lipkin, S.M., Shen, X., Iliev, I.D., 2022. A pan-cancer mycobiome analysis reveals fungal involvement in gastrointestinal and lung tumors. *Cell* 185, 3807–3822.

Eisenhofer, R., Minich, J.J., Marotz, C., Cooper, A., Knight, R., Weyrich, L.S., 2019. Contamination in low microbial biomass microbiome studies: issues and recommendations. *Trends Microbiol* 27, 105–117.

El Bairi, K., Jabi, R., Trapani, D., Boutallaka, H., Ouled Amar Bencheikh, B., Bouziane, M., Amrani, M., Afqir, S., Maleb, A., 2020. Can the microbiota predict response to systemic cancer therapy, surgical outcomes, and survival? The answer is in the gut. *Expert Rev Clin Pharmacol* 13, 403–421.

Erawijantari, P.P., Mizutani, S., Shiroma, H., Shiba, S., Nakajima, T., Sakamoto, T., Saito, Y., Fukuda, S., Yachida, S., Yamada, T., 2020. Influence of gastrectomy for gastric cancer treatment on faecal microbiome and metabolome profiles. *Gut* 69, 1404–1415.

Fang, J.Y., Richardson, B.C., 2005. The MAPK signalling pathways and colorectal cancer. *Lancet Oncol* 6, 322–327.

Fehrenbacher, L., Spira, A., Ballinger, M., Kowanetz, M., Vansteenkiste, J., Mazieres, J., Park, K., Smith, D., Artal-Cortes, A., Lewanski, C., 2016. Atezolizumab versus docetaxel for patients with previously treated non-small-cell lung cancer (POPLAR): a multicentre, open-label, phase 2 randomised controlled trial. *The Lancet* 387, 1837–1846.

Fu, A., Yao, B., Dong, T., Chen, Y., Yao, J., Liu, Y., Li, H., Bai, H., Liu, X., Zhang, Y., 2022. Tumor-resident intracellular microbiota promotes metastatic colonization in breast cancer. *Cell* 185, 1356–1372.

Gabrilovich, D.I., 2017. Myeloid-derived suppressor cells. *Cancer Immunol Res* 5, 3–8.

Garrett, W.S., 2015. Cancer and the microbiota. *Science (1979)* 348, 80–86.

Gensollen, T., Iyer, S.S., Kasper, D.L., Blumberg, R.S., 2016a. How colonization by microbiota in early life shapes the immune system. *Science (1979)* 352, 539–544.

Gensollen, T., Iyer, S.S., Kasper, D.L., Blumberg, R.S., 2016b. How colonization by microbiota in early life shapes the immune system. *Science (1979)* 352, 539–544.

González, M.F., Díaz, P., Sandoval-Bórquez, A., Herrera, D., Quest, A.F.G., 2021. Helicobacter pylori outer membrane vesicles and extracellular vesicles from Helicobacter pylori-infected cells in gastric disease development. *Int J Mol Sci* 22, 4823.

Gregorieff, A., Clevers, H., 2005. Wnt signaling in the intestinal epithelium: from endoderm to cancer. *Genes Dev* 19, 877–890.

Gunjur, A., 2020. Cancer and the microbiome. *Lancet Oncol* 21, 888.

Guo, Y., Zhang, Y., Gerhard, M., Gao, J.-J., Mejias-Luque, R., Zhang, L., Vieth, M., Ma, J.-L., Bajbouj, M., Suchanek, S., 2020. Effect of Helicobacter pylori on gastrointestinal microbiota: a population-based study in Linqu, a high-risk area of gastric cancer. *Gut* 69, 1598–1607.

Gur, C., Ibrahim, Y., Isaacson, B., Yamin, R., Abed, J., Gamliel, M., Enk, J., Bar-On, Y., Stanietsky-Kaynan, N., Coppenhagen-Glazer, S., 2015. Binding of the Fap2 protein of Fusobacterium nucleatum to human inhibitory receptor TIGIT protects tumors from immune cell attack. *Immunity* 42, 344–355.

Hamada, T., Zhang, X., Mima, K., Bullman, S., Sukawa, Y., Nowak, J.A., Kosumi, K., Masugi, Y., Twombly, T.S., Cao, Y., 2018. Fusobacterium nucleatum in colorectal cancer relates to immune response differentially by tumor microsatellite instability status. *Cancer Immunol Res* 6, 1327–1336.

Harper, J.W., Elledge, S.J., 2007. The DNA damage response: ten years after. *Mol Cell* 28, 739–745.

He, Y., Fu, L., Li, Y., Wang, W., Gong, M., Zhang, J., Dong, X., Huang, J., Wang, Q., Mackay, C.R., 2021. Gut microbial metabolites facilitate anticancer therapy efficacy by modulating cytotoxic CD8+ T cell immunity. *Cell Metab* 33, 988–1000.

Heshiki, Y., Vazquez-Uribe, R., Li, J., Ni, Y., Quainoo, S., Imamovic, L., Li, J., Sørensen, M., Chow, B.K.C., Weiss, G.J., 2020. Predictable modulation of cancer treatment outcomes by the gut microbiota. *Microbiome* 8, 1–14.

Hezaveh, K., Shinde, R.S., Klötgen, A., Halaby, M.J., Lamorte, S., Quevedo, R., Neufeld, L., Liu, Z.Q., Jin, R., Grünwald, B.T., 2022. Tryptophan-derived microbial metabolites activate the aryl hydrocarbon receptor in tumor-associated macrophages to suppress anti-tumor immunity. *Immunity* 55, 324–340.

Holokai, L., Chakrabarti, J., Broda, T., Chang, J., Hawkins, J.A., Sundaram, N., Wroblewski, L.E., Peek Jr, R.M., Wang, J., Helmrath, M., 2019. Increased programmed death-ligand 1 is an early epithelial cell response to Helicobacter pylori infection. *PLoS Pathog* 15, e1007468.

Huang, J., Liu, W., Kang, W., He, Y., Yang, R., Mou, X., Zhao, W., 2022. Effects of microbiota on anticancer drugs: current knowledge and potential applications. *EBioMedicine* 83:104197.

Hui, L., Chen, Y., 2015. Tumor microenvironment: Sanctuary of the devil. *Cancer Lett* 368, 7–13.

Jardim, D.L., Goodman, A., de Melo Gagliato, D., Kurzrock, R., 2021. The challenges of tumor mutational burden as an immunotherapy biomarker. *Cancer Cell* 39, 154–173.

Joyce, J.A., Fearon, D.T., 2015. T cell exclusion, immune privilege, and the tumor microenvironment. *Science (1979)* 348, 74–80.

Kaliannan, K., Donnell, S.O., Murphy, K., Stanton, C., Kang, C., Wang, B., Li, X.-Y., Bhan, A.K., Kang, J.X., 2022. Decreased tissue omega-6/omega-3 fatty acid ratio prevents chemotherapy-induced gastrointestinal toxicity associated with alterations of gut microbiome. *Int J Mol Sci* 23, 5332.

Krajmalnik-Brown R., Ilhan Z.E., Kang D.W., DiBaise J.K., 2012. Effects of gut microbes on nutrient absorption and energy regulation. *Nutr Clin Pract* 27, 201–214.

Kastenhuber, E.R., Lowe, S.W., 2017. Putting p53 in context. *Cell* 170, 1062–1078.

Khan, S., Gerber, D.E., 2020. Autoimmunity, checkpoint inhibitor therapy and immune-related adverse events: a review. In: *Seminars in Cancer Biology*. Elsevier, pp. 93–101.

Knippel, R.J., Drewes, J.L., Sears, C.L., 2021. The cancer microbiome: recent highlights and knowledge gaps. *Cancer Discov* 11, 2378–2395.

Koeppel, M., Garcia-Alcalde, F., Glowinski, F., Schlaermann, P., Meyer, T.F., 2015. Helicobacter pylori infection causes characteristic DNA damage patterns in human cells. *Cell Rep* 11, 1703–1713.

Kominsky, S.L., Vali, M., Korz, D., Gabig, T.G., Weitzman, S.A., Argani, P., Sukumar, S., 2004. Clostridium perfringens enterotoxin elicits rapid and specific cytolysis of breast carcinoma cells mediated through tight junction proteins claudin 3 and 4. *Am J Pathol* 164, 1627–1633.

Kostic, A.D., Chun, E., Robertson, L., Glickman, J.N., Gallini, C.A., Michaud, M., Clancy, T.E., Chung, D.C., Lochhead, P., Hold, G.L., 2013. Fusobacterium nucleatum potentiates intestinal tumorigenesis and modulates the tumor-immune microenvironment. *Cell Host Microbe* 14, 207–215.

LaCourse, K.D., Zepeda-Rivera, M., Kempchinsky, A.G., Baryiames, A., Minot, S.S., Johnston, C.D., Bullman, S., 2022. The cancer chemotherapeutic 5-fluorouracil is a potent Fusobacterium nucleatum inhibitor and its activity is modified by intratumoral microbiota. *Cell Rep* 41(7):111625.

Łaniewski, P., Ilhan, Z.E., Herbst-Kralovetz, M.M., 2020. The microbiome and gynaecological cancer development, prevention and therapy. *Nat Rev Urol* 17, 232–250.

Lavin, M.F., 2007. ATM and the Mre11 complex combine to recognize and signal DNA double-strand breaks. *Oncogene* 26, 7749–7758.

Lee, J.-H., Paull, T.T., 2005. ATM activation by DNA double-strand breaks through the Mre11-Rad50-Nbs1 complex. *Science (1979)* 308, 551–554.

Lee, J.H., Paull, T.T., 2007. Activation and regulation of ATM kinase activity in response to DNA double-strand breaks. *Oncogene* 26, 7741–7748.

Leeming, E.R., Johnson, A.J., Spector, T.D., Le Roy, C.I., 2019. Effect of diet on the gut microbiota: rethinking intervention duration. *Nutrients* 11, 2862.

Li, W., Deng, X., Chen, T., 2021. Exploring the modulatory effects of gut microbiota in anti-cancer therapy. *Front Oncol* 11, 644454.

Li, X., Heyer, W.-D., 2008. Homologous recombination in DNA repair and DNA damage tolerance. *Cell Res* 18, 99–113.

Lim, Y., Tang, K.D., Karpe, A.V, Beale, D.J., Totsika, M., Kenny, L., Morrison, M., Punyadeera, C., 2021. Chemoradiation therapy changes oral microbiome and metabolomic profiles in patients with oral cavity cancer and oropharyngeal cancer. *Head Neck* 43, 1521–1534.

Liou, J.-M., Malfertheiner, P., Lee, Y.-C., Sheu, B.-S., Sugano, K., Cheng, H.-C., Yeoh, K.-G., Hsu, P.-I., Goh, K.-L., Mahachai, V., 2020. Screening and eradication of Helicobacter pylori for gastric cancer prevention: the Taipei global consensus. *Gut* 69, 2093–2112.

Liu, Y., Baba, Y., Ishimoto, T., Tsutsuki, H., Zhang, T., Nomoto, D., Okadome, K., Yamamura, K., Harada, K., Eto, K.,

2021. Fusobacterium nucleatum confers chemoresistance by modulating autophagy in oesophageal squamous cell carcinoma. Br J Cancer 124, 963–974.

Loo, T.M., Kamachi, F., Watanabe, Y., Yoshimoto, S., Kanda, H., Arai, Y., Nakajima-Takagi, Y., Iwama, A., Koga, T., Sugimoto, Y., 2017. Gut microbiota promotes obesity-associated liver cancer through PGE2-mediated suppression of antitumor immunity. Cancer Discov 7, 522–538.

Lou, X., Chen, Z., He, Z., Sun, M., Sun, J., 2021. Bacteria-mediated synergistic cancer therapy: small microbiome has a big hope. Nanomicro Lett 13, 1–26.

Lugano, R., Ramachandran, M., Dimberg, A., 2020. Tumor angiogenesis: causes, consequences, challenges and opportunities. Cell Mol Life Sci 77, 1745–1770.

Ma, C., Han, M., Heinrich, B., Fu, Q., Zhang, Q., Sandhu, M., Agdashian, D., Terabe, M., Berzofsky, J.A., Fako, V., 2018. Gut microbiome-mediated bile acid metabolism regulates liver cancer via NKT cells. Science (1979) 360, eaan5931.

Ma, J., Huang, L., Hu, D., Zeng, S., Han, Y., Shen, H., 2021. The role of the tumor microbe microenvironment in the tumor immune microenvironment: bystander, activator, or inhibitor? J Exp Clin Cancer Res 40, 1–17.

Meisel, M., Hinterleitner, R., Pacis, A., Chen, L., Earley, Z.M., Mayassi, T., Pierre, J.F., Ernest, J.D., Galipeau, H.J., Thuille, N., 2018. Microbial signals drive pre-leukaemic myeloproliferation in a Tet2-deficient host. Nature 557, 580–584.

Milotti, E., Fredrich, T., Chignola, R., Rieger, H., 2020. Oxygen in the tumor microenvironment: mathematical and numerical modeling. Adv Exp Med Biol. 1259:53–76.

Mima, K., Sukawa, Y., Nishihara, R., Qian, Z.R., Yamauchi, M., Inamura, K., Kim, S.A., Masuda, A., Nowak, J.A., Nosho, K., 2015. Fusobacterium nucleatum and T cells in colorectal carcinoma. JAMA Oncol 1, 653–661.

Mimuro, H., Suzuki, T., Nagai, S., Rieder, G., Suzuki, M., Nagai, T., Fujita, Y., Nagamatsu, K., Ishijima, N., Koyasu, S., 2007. Helicobacter pylori dampens gut epithelial self-renewal by inhibiting apoptosis, a bacterial strategy to enhance colonization of the stomach. Cell Host Microbe 2, 250–263.

Mousa, W.K., Chehadeh, F., Husband, S., 2022. Microbial dysbiosis in the gut drives systemic autoimmune diseases. Front Immunol 13, 906258.

Naqash, A.R., Kihn-Alarcón, A.J., Stavraka, C., Kerrigan, K., Vareki, S.M., Pinato, D.J., Puri, S., 2021. The role of gut microbiome in modulating response to immune checkpoint inhibitor therapy in cancer. Ann Transl Med 9(12): 1034.

Narunsky-Haziza, L., Sepich-Poore, G.D., Livyatan, I., Asraf, O., Martino, C., Nejman, D., Gavert, N., Stajich, J.E., Amit, G., González, A., 2022. Pan-cancer analyses reveal cancer-type-specific fungal ecologies and bacteriome interactions. Cell 185, 3789–3806.

Nejman, D., Livyatan, I., Fuks, G., Gavert, N., Zwang, Y., Geller, L.T., Rotter-Maskowitz, A., Weiser, R., Mallel, G., Gigi, E., 2020. The human tumor microbiome is composed of tumor type-specific intracellular bacteria. Science (1979) 368, 973–980.

Oh, B., Boyle, F., Pavlakis, N., Clarke, S., Guminski, A., Eade, T., Lamoury, G., Carroll, S., Morgia, M., Kneebone, A., Hruby, G., Stevens, M., Liu, W., Corless, B., Molloy, M., Libermann, T., Rosenthal, D., Back, M., 2021. Emerging evidence of the gut microbiome in chemotherapy: a clinical review. Front. Oncol. 11:706331.

Oh, B., Eade, T., Lamoury, G., Carroll, S., Morgia, M., Kneebone, A., Hruby, G., Stevens, M., Boyle, F., Clarke, S., 2021. The gut microbiome and gastrointestinal toxicities in pelvic radiation therapy: a clinical review. Cancers (Basel) 13, 2353.

Palamaris, K., Alexandris, D., Stylianou, K., Giatras, I., Stofas, A., Kaitatzoglou, C., Migkou, M., Goutas, D., Psimenou, E., Theodoropoulou, E., 2022. Immune checkpoint inhibitors' associated renal toxicity: a series of 12 cases. J Clin Med 11, 4786.

Panebianco, C., Villani, A., Pisati, F., Orsenigo, F., Ulaszewska, M., Latiano, T.P., Potenza, A., Andolfo, A., Terracciano, F., Tripodo, C., 2022. Butyrate, a postbiotic of intestinal bacteria, affects pancreatic cancer and gemcitabine response in in vitro and in vivo models. Biomed Pharmacother 151, 113163.

Parida, S., Wu, S., Siddharth, S., Wang, G., Muniraj, N., Nagalingam, A., Hum, C., Mistriotis, P., Hao, H., Talbot Jr, C.C., 2021. A procarcinogenic colon microbe promotes breast tumorigenesis and metastatic progression and concomitantly activates notch and β-catenin axes. Cancer Discov 11, 1138–1157.

Parthasarathy, G., Chen, J., Chen, X., Chia, N., O'Connor, H.M., Wolf, P.G., Gaskins, H.R., Bharucha, A.E., 2016. Relationship between microbiota of the colonic mucosa vs feces and symptoms, colonic transit, and methane production in female patients with chronic constipation. Gastroenterology 150, 367–379.

Petroni, G., Cantley, L.C., Santambrogio, L., Formenti, S.C., Galluzzi, L., 2022. Radiotherapy as a tool to elicit clinically actionable signalling pathways in cancer. Nat Rev Clin Oncol 19, 114–131.

Poonacha, K.N.T., Villa, T.G., Notario, V., 2022. The interplay among radiation therapy, antibiotics and the microbiota: impact on cancer treatment outcomes. Antibiotics 11, 331.

Pushalkar, S., Hundeyin, M., Daley, D., Zambirinis, C.P., Kurz, E., Mishra, A., Mohan, N., Aykut, B., Usyk, M., Torres, L.E., 2018. The pancreatic cancer microbiome promotes oncogenesis by induction of innate and adaptive immune suppression. Cancer Discov 8, 403–416.

Rangan, P., Mondino, A., 2022. Microbial short-chain fatty acids: a strategy to tune adoptive T cell therapy. J Immunother Cancer 10.

Rieber, N., Singh, A., Öz, H., Carevic, M., Bouzani, M., Amich, J., Ost, M., Ye, Z., Ballbach, M., Schäfer, I., 2015. Pathogenic fungi regulate immunity by inducing neutrophilic myeloid-derived suppressor cells. Cell Host Microbe 17, 507–514.

Roberts, A.B., Wallace, B.D., Venkatesh, M.K., Mani, S., Redinbo, M.R., 2013. Molecular insights into microbial β-glucuronidase inhibition to abrogate CPT-11 toxicity. Mol Pharmacol 84, 208–217.

Routy, B., Le Chatelier, E., Derosa, L., Duong, C.P.M., Alou, M.T., Daillère, R., Fluckiger, A., Messaoudene, M., Rauber, C., Roberti, M.P., 2018. Gut microbiome influences efficacy of PD-1-based immunotherapy against epithelial tumors. Science (1979) 359, 91–97.

Rubinstein, M.R., Wang, X., Liu, W., Hao, Y., Cai, G., Han, Y.W., 2013. Fusobacterium nucleatum promotes colorectal carcinogenesis by modulating E-cadherin/β-catenin signaling via its FadA adhesin. Cell Host Microbe 14, 195–206.

Sadrekarimi, H., Gardanova, Z.R., Bakhshesh, M., Ebrahimzadeh, F., Yaseri, A.F., Thangavelu, L., Hasanpoor, Z., Zadeh, F.A., Kahrizi, M.S., 2022. Emerging role of human microbiome in cancer development and response to therapy: special focus on intestinal microflora. J Transl Med 20, 1–20.

Sasako, M., Sakuramoto, S., Katai, H., Kinoshita, T., Furukawa, H., Yamaguchi, T., Nashimoto, A., Fujii, M., Nakajima, T., Ohashi, Y., 2011. Five-year outcomes of a randomized phase III trial comparing adjuvant chemotherapy with S-1 versus surgery alone in stage II or III gastric cancer. *J Clin Oncol* 29, 4387–4393.

Sender, R., Fuchs, S., Milo, R., 2016. Are we really vastly outnumbered? Revisiting the ratio of bacterial to host cells in humans. *Cell* 164(3):337–340.

Sharma, P., Hu-Lieskovan, S., Wargo, J.A., Ribas, A., 2017. Primary, adaptive, and acquired resistance to cancer immunotherapy. *Cell* 168, 707–723.

Sharma, P.C., Sharma, D., Sharma, A., Bhagat, M., Ola, M., Thakur, V.K., Bhardwaj, J.K., Goyal, R.K., 2022. Recent advances in microbial toxin-related strategies to combat cancer. In: *Seminars in Cancer Biology*. Elsevier, pp. 753–768.

Shiao, S.L., Kershaw, K.M., Limon, J.J., You, S., Yoon, J., Ko, E.Y., Guarnerio, J., Potdar, A.A., McGovern, D.P.B., Bose, S., 2021. Commensal bacteria and fungi differentially regulate tumor responses to radiation therapy. *Cancer Cell* 39, 1202–1213.

Sikorska, H., Smoragiewicz, W., 2013. Role of probiotics in the prevention and treatment of meticillin-resistant Staphylococcus aureus infections. *Int J Antimicrob Agents* 42, 475–481.

Singh, A., Nayak, N., Rathi, P., Verma, D., Sharma, R., Chaudhary, A., Agarwal, A., Tripathi, Y.B., Garg, N., 2021. Microbiome and host crosstalk: a new paradigm to cancer therapy. In: *Seminars in Cancer Biology*. Elsevier, pp. 71–84.

Sinha, R., Abu-Ali, G., Vogtmann, E., Fodor, A.A., Ren, B., Amir, A., Schwager, E., Crabtree, J., Ma, S., Consortium, M.Q.C.P., 2017. Assessment of variation in microbial community amplicon sequencing by the Microbiome Quality Control (MBQC) project consortium. *Nat Biotechnol* 35, 1077–1086.

Sommer, F., Bäckhed, F., 2013. The gut microbiota-masters of host development and physiology. *Nat Rev Microbiol* 11, 227–238.

Song, X., An, Y., Chen, D., Zhang, W., Wu, X., Li, C., Wang, S., Dong, W., Wang, B., Liu, T., 2022. Microbial metabolite deoxycholic acid promotes vasculogenic mimicry formation in intestinal carcinogenesis. *Cancer Sci* 113, 459–477.

Stearn, E.W., Sturdivant, B.F., Stearn, A.E., 1925. The life history of a micro-parasite isolated from carcinomatous growths. *Proc Natl Acad Sci* 11, 662–669.

Tanoue, T., Morita, S., Plichta, D.R., Skelly, A.N., Suda, W., Sugiura, Y., Narushima, S., Vlamakis, H., Motoo, I., Sugita, K., 2019. A defined commensal consortium elicits CD8 T cells and anti-cancer immunity. *Nature* 565, 600–605.

Tilg, H., Adolph, T.E., Gerner, R.R., Moschen, A.R., 2018. The intestinal microbiota in colorectal cancer. *Cancer Cell* 33, 954–964.

Touchefeu, Y., Montassier, E., Nieman, K., Gastinne, T., Potel, G., Bruley des Varannes, S., Le Vacon, F., de La Cochetière, M., 2014. Systematic review: the role of the gut microbiota in chemotherapy or radiation-induced gastrointestinal mucositis-current evidence and potential clinical applications. *Aliment Pharmacol Ther* 40, 409–421.

Tse, J.W.T., Jenkins, L.J., Chionh, F., Mariadason, J.M., 2017. Aberrant DNA methylation in colorectal cancer: what should we target? *Trends Cancer* 3, 698–712.

Tubbs, A., Nussenzweig, A., 2017. Endogenous DNA damage as a source of genomic instability in cancer. *Cell* 168, 644–656.

van Praagh, J.B., de Goffau, M.C., Bakker, I.S., van Goor, H., Harmsen, H.J.M., Olinga, P., Havenga, K., 2019. Mucus microbiome of anastomotic tissue during surgery has predictive value for colorectal anastomotic leakage. *Ann Surg* 269, 911–916.

Vaupel, P., Harrison, L., 2004. Tumor hypoxia: causative factors, compensatory mechanisms, and cellular response. *Oncologist* 9, 4–9.

Vizcaino, M.I., Crawford, J.M., 2015. The colibactin warhead crosslinks DNA. *Nat Chem* 7, 411–417.

Waldman, A.D., Fritz, J.M., Lenardo, M.J., 2020. A guide to cancer immunotherapy: from T cell basic science to clinical practice. *Nat Rev Immunol* 20, 651–668.

Wang, T., Zheng, N., Luo, Q., Jiang, L., He, B., Yuan, X., Shen, L., 2019. Probiotics Lactobacillus reuteri abrogates immune checkpoint blockade-associated colitis by inhibiting group 3 innate lymphoid cells. *Front Immunol* 10, 1235.

Wang, Y., Wiesnoski, D.H., Helmink, B.A., Gopalakrishnan, V., Choi, K., DuPont, H.L., Jiang, Z.-D., Abu-Sbeih, H., Sanchez, C.A., Chang, C.-C., Parra, E.R., Francisco-Cruz, A., Raju, G.S., Stroehlein, J.R., Campbell, M.T., Gao, J., Subudhi, S.K., Maru, D.M., Blando, J.M., Lazar, A.J., Allison, J.P., Sharma, P., Tetzlaff, M.T., Wargo, J.A., Jenq, R.R., 2018. Fecal microbiota transplantation for refractory immune checkpoint inhibitor-associated colitis. *Nat Med* 24, 1804–1808.

Wei, S.C., Duffy, C.R., Allison, J.P., 2018. Fundamental mechanisms of immune checkpoint blockade therapy. *Cancer Discov* 8, 1069–1086.

Williams, A.B., Schumacher, B., 2016. p53 in the DNA-damage-repair process. *Cold Spring Harb Perspect Med* 6(5): a026070.

Xia, X., Wu, W.K.K., Wong, S.H., Liu, D., Kwong, T.N.Y., Nakatsu, G., Yan, P.S., Chuang, Y.-M., Chan, M.W.-Y., Coker, O.O., 2020. Bacteria pathogens drive host colonic epithelial cell promoter hypermethylation of tumor suppressor genes in colorectal cancer. *Microbiome* 8, 1–13.

Xu, C., Fan, L., Lin, Y., Shen, W., Qi, Y., Zhang, Y., Chen, Z., Wang, L., Long, Y., Hou, T., 2021. Fusobacterium nucleatum promotes colorectal cancer metastasis through miR-1322/CCL20 axis and M2 polarization. *Gut Microbes* 13, 1980347.

Yazbeck, V., Alesi, E., Myers, J., Hackney, M.H., Cuttino, L., Gewirtz, D.A., 2022. An overview of chemotoxicity and radiation toxicity in cancer therapy. *Adv Cancer Res* 155, 1–27.

Yoshimoto, S., Loo, T.M., Atarashi, K., Kanda, H., Sato, S., Oyadomari, S., Iwakura, Y., Oshima, K., Morita, H., Hattori, M., 2013. Obesity-induced gut microbial metabolite promotes liver cancer through senescence secretome. *Nature* 499, 97–101.

Yu, L.-X., Schwabe, R.F., 2017. The gut microbiome and liver cancer: mechanisms and clinical translation. *Nat Rev Gastroenterol Hepatol* 14, 527–539.

Yue, B., Gao, R., Wang, Z., Dou, W., 2021. Microbiota-host-irinotecan axis: a new insight toward irinotecan chemotherapy. *Front Cell Infect Microbiol* 11, 710945.

Zhan, T., Rindtorff, N., Boutros, M., 2017. Wnt signaling in cancer. *Oncogene* 36, 1461–1473.

Zhang, Q., Ma, C., Duan, Y., Heinrich, B., Rosato, U., Diggs, L.P., Ma, L., Roy, S., Fu, Q., Brown, Z.J., 2021. Gut microbiome directs hepatocytes to recruit MDSCs and promote cholangiocarcinoma. *Cancer Discov* 11, 1248–1267.

Zhang, Z., Li, J., Zheng, W., Zhao, G., Zhang, H., Wang, X., Guo, Y., Qin, C., Shi, Y., 2016. Peripheral lymphoid volume expansion and maintenance are controlled by gut microbiota via RALDH+ dendritic cells. *Immunity* 44, 330–342.

Zhao, L.-Y., Mei, J.-X., Yu, G., Lei, L., Zhang, W.-H., Liu, K., Chen, X.-L., Kołat, D., Yang, K., Hu, J.-K., 2023. Role of the gut microbiota in anticancer therapy: from molecular mechanisms to clinical applications. *Signal Transduct Target Ther* 8, 201.

Zhu, R., Lang, T., Yan, W., Zhu, X., Huang, X., Yin, Q., Li, Y., 2021. Gut microbiota: influence on carcinogenesis and modulation strategies by drug delivery systems to improve cancer therapy. *Adv Sci* 8, 2003542.

Zitvogel, L., Ayyoub, M., Routy, B., Kroemer, G., 2016. Microbiome and anticancer immunosurveillance. *Cell* 165, 276–287.

4 Gut Microbiome Modulation for Personalized Cancer Therapies

Lloyd Mabonga, Godfrey Grech, and Zodwa Dlamini

INTRODUCTION

The realization that pathobiont microbial networks play an indispensable function in the initiation and progression of cancer has challenged scientists and prompted therapeutic interrogation on the modulation of the gut microbiome for personalized cancer therapies (Scott et al. 2019). The disappearance of symbiotic microbial communities and their regulating protective mechanisms have been highlighted as the critical players in the initiation and progression of cancers. The preponderance of high-quality biological evidence not only supports the functional role of the gut microbiome in cancer development and progression, but also its role in defining the efficacy and toxicity of chemotherapy and immunotherapy regimens. The gut microbiome communities seem to change concurrently with tumor progression, potentiating metastasis, and therapeutic resistance (Ivleva and Grivennikov, 2022). In this context, the gut microbiome is used to create unique, individualized treatments for the treatment of cancer. The modulation of the gut microbiome towards next-generation oncologic personalized treatments has birthed a new multimodal therapeutic concept that incorporates oncomicrobiome cometabolism of pharmacologicals into cancer care options. The multiparametric functions of the gut microbiome in oncologic pharmacomicrobiomics influence treatment responses and shape oncologic outcomes in cancer (Lee et al. 2021).

Over the years, the management of cancer has solely relied on multimodal therapies, usually including surgery or a mix of cytotoxic and immunologic techniques used throughout extensive and varied patient care courses (Pan et al. 2020). The composition and function of the gut microbiome are incredibly individualized and transient. The microbiome has tremendous functional plasticity when people are healthy. However, changes in food, exposome, xenometabolites, neoadjuvant, and adjuvant medicines that disrupt its structure and function make this less effective throughout cancer treatment (Chrysostomou et al. 2023). This is of pathophysiological significance in cancer patient treatment options because the gut microbiota has a significant role in both the control of the tumor microenvironment and the absorption and breakdown of drugs. It is generally hypothesized that the gut microbiome will have an enormous impact on how well a regimen works and how hazardous it can be. It may also be the key to understanding differential outcomes of oncologic therapeutic interventions (Sánchez-Alcoholado et al. 2020). Thus, gut microbiome modulation remains one of the most critical approaches in leveraging the development of individualized treatment stratifications in cancer therapies.

The curative value of gut microbiota modulation in precision cancer treatments is scientifically proven to be indispensable, however, the modus operandi of the gut microbiome's interactions with the cancer environment remain elusive and yet to be fully characterized (Lee et al. 2021). Over time, knowledge of the relationships between altering gut flora and cancer has grown dramatically, which has contributed to a greater therapeutic comprehension of the gut flora and its direct and indirect implications on individualized medical outcomes. Questions about the relationships between breast cancer subtypes, targeted medicines, and the gut microbiota are becoming clinically important considering increasing evidence of the impact of the gut microbiota on cancer therapy. Modulating the gut microbiota to alleviate the burden of cancer is a novel therapeutic concept. It provides protracted remissions that can be exploited to increase the efficacy and safety of cancer treatment modalities through modulating the central immune mechanism (Lee et al. 2021).

The creation of innovative methods to describe the native gut and target-tissue microbiota, the capacity to understand how its connections with gene networks operate, the progressive understanding of the immune landscape and circulating metabolome, and the successful modulation of the microbiota ecosystem all provide a platform in which the microbiota could be used as a unique tool to enhance personalized therapies in cancer. Multiple strategies—including the use of prebiotics, probiotics, postbiotics, synbiotics, dietary modulations and fecal microbiota transplantation (FMT)—are under investigation to fine-tune the modulation of the gut microbiome towards the development of personalized therapies. Some of the strategies used in modulating the gut microbiome to enhance personalized cancer therapies are discussed below.

STRATEGIES OF GUT MICROBIOTA MODULATION

Diet

The composition of the gut microbiota ecosystem is significantly influenced by diet and previous studies have suggested a strong relationship between diet and the microbiome in cancer progression and treatment response (Chrysostomou et al. 2023). Great emphasis has been made on using diet in modulating the gut microbiome in the etiology of cancer. The modulation of the gut microbiome through dietary intervention consequently orchestrates the broad pathophysiological aspects that include nutritional responses and intestinal and immune system homeostasis in cancer patients (Ting et al. 2022; Rebersek, 2021; McQuade et al. 2019). The diet-microbiota-host interaction drives the impact on the surrounding tissues. Commensal gut bacteria are neither helpful nor bad in and of themselves. Whether our microbiota produces advantageous or harmful metabolites from the food that is digested relies on our diet. Intake of prebiotics (like dietary fiber), a low-fat diet, a plant-based diet, a low or no intake of red and processed meat, or a higher intake of probiotics and postbiotics (like microbial fermentation components, including short-chain fatty acids (SCFAs)) have thus been somewhat linked to suppressive dietary factors in most cancer cases. A diet high in animal fat, protein-based, and low in fiber is thought to increase the risk of developing cancer because it leads to the buildup of bile acids and a reduction in the generation of SCFAs by gut flora (Chrysostomou et al. 2023; Ting et al. 2022; McQuade et al. 2019).

The microbial metagenome contains genes that metabolize a wide range of nutrients, including indigestible carbohydrates like galacto- and fructo-oligosaccharides and host-produced substances like bile acids (Won and Yu, 2019). Research studies on diets high in oligosaccharides, L-leucine, protein (casein and whey), and fish oil provided more evidence of diet-microbiome therapy connections. A dietary SCFA called butyrate has been additionally connected to improved irinotecan activation in various colon cancer cell lines, suggesting that consuming dietary fibers such as fructo-oligosaccharides (FOS), inulin, and isomalto-oligosaccharides lowers the toxicity of irinotecan following increased intestinal butyrate synthesis, as a metabolite of microbiota. Thus, dietary fiber has a tumor-suppressive effect (Chrysostomou et al. 2023; Encarnação et al. 2018). Modulating the gut bacteria performs an essential function in minimizing the risk of carcinogenesis through the digestion and absorption of high-fiber diets and diet-derived SCFAs including butyrate, branched-chain amino acids, and bile acids (Encarnação et al. 2018).

Modulating the gut microbiome through fasting has been recommended as a significant method of reducing irinotecan-related side effects without reducing drug efficacy. A diet that mimics fasting influences the gut microbiome through utilizing the host's systematic and intratumor antitumor immune systems, thereby improving the clinical prognosis and enhancing personalized therapies for cancer patients (Vernieri et al. 2022). A fasting diet reduces peripheral immune-suppressive myeloid cells (CD14$^+$ and CD15$^+$ granulocytes) while increasing the activity of cytotoxic Th1 cells such as cytolytic CD3$^-$CD16$^+$CD56^{dim} natural killer cells and CD8$^+$ T cells. In chronic myeloid leukemia, patients on tyrosine kinase inhibitors observed significantly lower levels of white blood cells, BCR-ABL transcripts and neutrophils after fasting (Yassin et al. 2021). The precise relationship between the modulation of the gut microbiome through fasting and cancer remains elusive. The modulation of the gut microbiome through fasting to enhance the effectiveness of immunotherapy and chemotherapy or to lessen drug toxicity is yet to be fully characterized. Nevertheless, fasting has been recommended as a significant method of reducing irinotecan-related side effects without reducing drug efficacy (Zhuang et al. 2021).

Over-the-counter nutritional supplements which are frequently used by patients as a supplementary to medication have been shown to modulate the gut microbiota for improved clinical effects. The effects of traditional Chinese medicines (TCMs) and dietary changes on the gut microbiome and drug response have also been investigated (Huang et al. 2021). Jujube powder, a fruit extract, enhances CD8 T lymphocytes in colon cancer following CTX therapy, suggesting the supplement's capacity to boost bifidobacterial populations and butyrate production (Zhuang et al. 2021). Ginseng, a common herbal remedy known for its significant anticancer benefits, is also thought to boost the antiproliferative effects of 5-FU in colon cancer cell lines through its modulative effects of the gut microbiome. Ginseng polysaccharides enhance the production of microbially generated valeric acid and decrease L-kynurenine in lung cancer potentiating the anticancer impact of anti-PD-1/L1 immunotherapy. It modulates both microbial composition (e.g., *Bacteroides vulgatus* and *Parabacteroides distasonis*) as well as microbial metabolites (e.g., L-kynurenine and valeric acid). By boosting activated CD8 T cells and reducing Foxp3 regulatory T cells, as well as lowering the kynurenine/tryptophan ratio; combinatorial therapy with ginseng polysaccharides and anti-PD-1 antibody has been shown to improve therapeutic anticancer effects (Huang et al. 2022). Similarly, Gegen Qinlian decoction has been shown to improve the effectiveness of PD-1 inhibitors by altering the gut microbiota and the tumor microenvironment (Lv et al. 2019). The use of nutritional supplements to modulate the gut microbiome's pathophysiological function is an inevitable strategy in personalized cancer therapies. Its capacity to improve anticancer drug efficacy by presiding over microbiota is an interesting phenomenon to investigate.

In colon cancer cell lines, ellagic acid, a dietary derivative of polyphenols, improves chemosensitivity to 5-FU (Kao et al. 2012). Ellagic acid interacts with bacteria in the gut microbiome and produces urolithins (Selma et al. 2017). According to González-Sarrás et al. (2014), urolithin A is one of the ellagic acid's downstream metabolites that may have an antiproliferative effect on colon cancer cells by impeding the cell cycle. Red sage, or dihydrotanshinone I, is a product of *Salvia miltiorrhiza* Bunge extract. Recent research using rats confirms dihydrotanshinone I's positive role in successfully reducing 5-FU and irinotecan-related intestinal toxicity (Wang et al. 2020). There are undoubtedly cues that point to the possibility of exploiting microbiome-diet connections to change the responsiveness of cancer therapies; however, this area of research has not yet been fully investigated through experiments.

The clinical effects of ketogenic diet on cancer patients' ability to respond to personalized cancer therapies observed that the ketogenic diet improved radiotherapy outcomes of tumor growth and overall survival. In hepatocellular carcinoma, the possibility of altering nutrition to enhance therapeutic outcomes showed that changing one's diet and caloric consumption could affect DNA repair, epigenetic gene expression, and genome stability. A phenomenon that extrapolates from the link between hepatocellular carcinoma, obesity, and other metabolic diseases (Oudmaijer et al. 2022). Consumption of red meat and processed animal products is linked to an increased likelihood of cancer. Meat contains heme iron, which is broken down in the gut to form N-nitroso compounds. These compounds have a damaging effect on the cells lining the bowel, which may lead to cancer. Nitrates and nitrites used as preservatives in processed meats are also disintegrated into N-nitroso compounds leading to the same effect (Chrysostomou et al. 2023; Won and Yu, 2019).

Dietary fat affects gut microbial composition and gastrointestinal function. It promotes inflammatory processes and the growth of intestinal tumors by stimulating the hepatic secretion of bile acids to aid in fat emulsification and increasing the enterohepatic circulation of bile acids (Wong and Yu 2019). Pro-carcinogenic and pro-inflammatory advanced glycation end-products (AGEs), which contribute to the production of highly oxidative molecules, are produced because of factors including cooking techniques, especially when AGEs are produced from meals with an animal source. AGEs have been associated with early-onset colorectal cancer (EOCRC), inflammation, and gut dysbiosis. By impairing the function of the mucus barrier, hazardous effects resulting from microbial metabolism such as N-nitroso compounds and hydrogen sulfide cause epithelium hyperproliferation (Rebersek 2021).

Metabolic byproducts can influence the epithelial barrier or the integrity of the gut, inhibit histone deacetylase, reduce or increase inflammation, have tumor-suppressing effects, or change the immune system's response depending on the type of food consumed (McQuade et al. 2019). A diet high in fiber and plant-based foods reduces the likelihood of cancer, cardiovascular diseases, and overall mortality as compared to industrially refined foods (Rebersek, 2021). Such a diet results in gut microbiome metabolites that have a variety of tumor-suppressing and immune-modulating effects, including the maintenance of a healthy epithelial barrier and the integrity of the gut, the induction of T-regulatory cells, the inhibition of histone deacetylase, and the suppression of inflammation. (Wong and Yu 2019).

Obesity, a recognized risk factor for CRC, is directly correlated with diet as well. Adipokines, sex hormones, systemic inflammation, insulin, or insulin-like growth factor 1 signaling, and other factors all play a role in obesity and can lead to the likelihood of CRC (Rebersek 2021). Due to its ability to alter proinflammatory chemicals and oncometabolites produced by microorganisms, the gut microbiota contributes a significant part in these pathways. According to Wong and Yu (2019), obesity is also linked to decreased microbial diversity and changes in the composition of the gut microbiota. Obesity brought on by diet activates numerous signaling pathways that are like those involved in carcinogenesis by increasing histone methylation and acetylation. Due to these connections, controlling one's weight in obese people has the capacity to significantly change the gut microbiota and lower the chance of developing cancer (Rebersek 2021).

A high-salt diet (HSD), which can stimulate NK cells and the gut microbiota (e.g., by increasing the quantity of *Bifidobacterium*), has also been shown to improve anti-PD-1 therapy and tumor retrogression in mice (Rizvi et al. 2021). Future research should further investigate the effects of the microbiome on the synergistic sequels of dietary interventions and anticancer drugs given that several dietary interventions, such as fasting, the ketogenic diet, and histidine supplementation, may sensitize multiple cancer cell types in personalized anticancer therapies (Huang et al. 2022).

PROBIOTICS

Probiotics are live microorganisms that enhance or restore the gut flora to promote health when provided in sufficient proportions (McQuade et al. 2019). They may additionally communicate with the body's immune system, impact the gut metabolome, and change the overall makeup of the gut environment. Probiotics, both natural and genetically modified, have grown in medical importance in relation to chemosensitivity and cancer prevention. They have the potential to be used as live biotherapeutic products (LBPs) to reduce the adverse effects and increase the effectiveness of cancer chemotherapy medications (Huang et al. 2022). A variety of bacterial species may improve the therapeutic efficacy of immune checkpoint inhibitor (ICI) drugs and increase cancer survival (Dizman et al. 2022; Anker et al. 2018), induce interferon producing CD8+ T cells in the gut, and enhance the therapeutic efficacy of ICIs and anticancer drugs.

Probiotics function in three different mechanisms, namely, colonization resistance, modulating immunity, and enhanced gut barrier function, as shown in Figure 4.1. By producing antimicrobial peptides, decreasing luminal pH, and through direct contact with pathogens through competing for resources and space, and forming aggregates with other materials, probiotics prevent the colonization of pathogenic bacteria (Chrysostomou et al. 2023). Depending on the chosen species and strains, probiotics may have distinct immunomodulatory effects that minimize the inflammation of the colon (e.g., activating DCs, increasing Treg expression, lowering Th17, and transforming macrophage to M2 subtype) or improving antitumor immunity (e.g., increasing Th17 while decreasing the expression of Treg at a systemic level, and reducing the expression of tumor CXCR4 and MHC-1) (Huang et al. 2022). Probiotics stimulate tight junction protein expression, mucin synthesis, and epithelial restitution. Probiotic usage in cancer patients has, however,

Gut Microbiome Modulation for Personalized Cancer Therapies

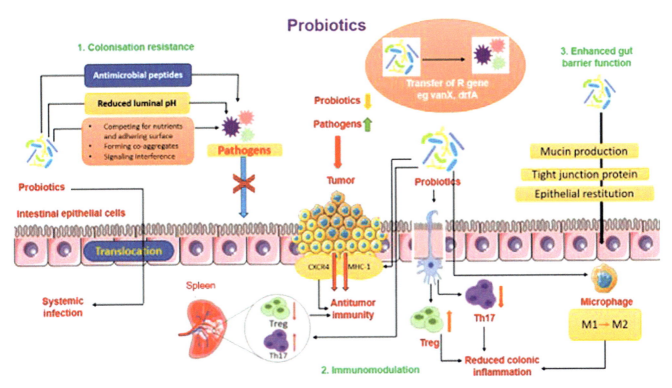

FIGURE 4.1 Probiotics' alleged modes of action and potential risks. Probiotics function in three different mechanisms, namely, colonization resistance, modulating immunity, and enhanced gut barrier function. By producing antimicrobial peptides, decreasing luminal pH, and/or through direct contact with pathogens through vying for resources and space, and forming co-aggregates, probiotics prevent the colonization of pathogenic bacteria (Chrysostomou et al. 2023). Depending on the chosen species and strains, probiotics may have distinct immunomodulatory effects that minimize colonic inflammation (e.g., activating DCs, lowering Th17, increasing Treg expression, and transforming macrophage to M2 subtype) or improving antitumor immunity (e.g., increasing Th17 while decreasing Treg expression at a systemic level, and reducing tumor CXCR4 and MHC-1 expression) (Huang et al. 2022). Probiotics stimulate tight junction protein expression, mucin synthesis, and epithelial restitution. Probiotic usage in cancer patients has, however, also raised certain safety issues, including as the threat of bacterial displacement and systemic encroachment, the potential transmission of resistant genes to local microbiota, and the increase of antimicrobial resistance. Dendritic cells, Th17 T helper cells, MHC-1 major histocompatibility complex class I, CXCR CXC chemokine receptors 4, and Treg T regulatory cells (McQuade et al. 2019).

also raised certain safety issues, including the threat of bacterial displacement and systemic encroachment, the potential transmission of resistant genes to local microbiota, and the increase of antimicrobial resistance (McQuade et al. 2019).

The administration of probiotics can also be used to decrease the negative effects of anticancer drugs. According to Wang et al. (2018), probiotic *Bifidobacterium* strains were given to mice to minimize the immune-related side effects of CTLA-4 inhibitor, such as colitis. Animal models have been used in several research studies that demonstrate probiotics have anticancer properties. Colon cancer development was significantly reduced in mice with tumors treated with *Bifidobacterium infantum* and *bifidum*, *Bacillus polyfermenticus*, and *Lactobacillus acidophilus*, *plantarum*, *rhamnosus*, *casei*, *lactis*, and *salivarius*. Through clinical investigations done in humans, the benefit of probiotics was translated to affect therapeutic results in addition to preventing cancer growth and progression.

Numerous bacteria, including *Lactobacillus* and *Bifidobacterium* spp., have anticancer characteristics, such as the capacity to stop cancer cell development, trigger apoptosis in cancer cells, alter host immunity, neutralize carcinogenic toxins, and produce anticarcinogenic substances like butyrate (McQuade et al. 2019). They are frequently utilized as a dietary supplement by the public. Probiotics serve a variety of purposes, including warding off harmful microbes, preserving intestinal integrity, taking part in metabolic processes within the gut, acting as an anti-inflammatory, triggering an immune response, and modifying the central nervous system's communication with the gut, which in turn promotes anxiolytic, antidepressant, and nociceptive action (Suez et al. 2019).

Several modified microorganisms were created to enhance cancer treatment. An artificial variation of the *E. coli* Nissle 1917 that was created by Canale et al. (2021) boosted intratumorally L-arginine levels, a crucial factor in antitumor activity. This strain's intratumoral injection works in concert with PD-L1 inhibitor to help tumor-bearing mice survive and control their tumors (Canale et al. 2021). The conversion of nutritional glucosinolate from a synthetic drug into the anticancer compound sulforaphane is catalyzed by another modified strain of the *E. coli* Nissle 1917 molecule (Ho et al. 2018). A synchronized lysis circuit (SLC) in a *Salmonella enterica* strain can lyse and release an anticancer toxin at the same time. When this strain and the chemotherapy medication 5-FU were administered together to mice, the antitumor effects were noticeably enhanced compared to either therapy used alone (Huang et al. 2022). The appropriate quantity of probiotics given to patients in the years to come should be determined through clinical and preclinical studies to maximize the functionality of boosting therapeutic efficacy.

It was also investigated how *Lactobacillus fermentum* BR11 may reduce 5-FU-induced intestinal mucositis, indicating that this probiotic could lessen chemotoxicity. Additional studies looking into the positive effects of probiotic mixtures discovered that giving rats VSL#3 probiotic (*Bifidobacterium breve, longum,* and *infantis, Streptococcus thermophiles, Lactobacillus paracasei, delbrueckii* spp. *acidophilus, bulgaricus,* and *plantarum*) along with irinotecan minimized chemotoxicity, as evidenced by decreased diarrhea. By lowering the production of IL-1b, IL-6, and TNF messenger RNAs, *Lactobacillus rhamnosus, casei* and *Bifidobacterium bifidum* have additionally demonstrated defenses against diarrhea brought on by chemotherapy in mice (Rebersek 2021).

Following 5-FU treatment, the DM#1 mixture (*L. acidophilus, Bifidobacterium breve* DM8310, *Streptococcus thermophilus,* and *L. casei*) can reestablish intestinal stability and lessen proinflammatory cytokine activation. The probiotic treatments *L. paracasei, L. rhamnosus, L. acidophilus,* and *Bifidobacterium lactis* in conjunction with 5-FU also produced comparable results. In a sample of 150 patients with colon cancer taking 5-FU, *L. rhamnosus* GG was also demonstrated to have protective effects on anti-PD-1 effectiveness and to be related to decreased diarrhea severity (Quaresma et al. 2020).

Additionally, a recent investigation recommended that *Bifidobacterium infantis* may reduce the harmful effects of chemotherapy (5-FU and oxaliplatin) by reducing Th1 and Th17 activation and boosting cytotoxic regulatory T-cell activity (CD4-CD25-Foxp3 activity) in rats (Rebersek 2021). One of the kinds of bacteria belonging to the *Bifidobacterium* genus that has been hypothesized to offer protection against chemotoxicity is *Bifidobacterium bifidum* G9-1. Co-administration of 5-FU and *Bifidobacterium bifidum* G9-1 resulted in a significant decrease in the intensity of diarrhea as well as a decrease in the levels of pro-inflammatory cytokines and myeloperoxidase (Kato et al. 2017). A protective effect against chemotoxicity is provided by *L. acidophilus*' regulatory effects on the release of proinflammatory cytokines, upregulation of mucin genes, gastrointestinal dysmotility, and myeloperoxidase activity following 5-FU treatment (Oh et al. 2017). After receiving cisplatin therapy, protective properties of *L. acidophilus* were also noted. When *L. acidophilus* and cisplatin were administered together, tumor size was significantly reduced compared to mice not receiving probiotic treatment (Rebersek 2021).

Because some probiotics are created expressly for the treatment of diseases, they can be categorized as LBPs. According to Rebersek (2021), LBPs are living organisms designed to influence the gut environment and alleviate, cure, or forestall diseases in humans. Additionally, techniques that prevent bacterial reproduction in the absence of a certain metabolite (auxotrophy) and restrict the replication of bacterial species to mediate positive pharmacological effects on the host can be incorporated into the design of genetically modified organisms. According to O'Toole et al. (2017), the use of LBPs as a medication has not yet been approved. To assess the effectiveness of a single strain LPB (*Christensenella minuta*) in the treatment of obesity and other metabolic illnesses, first-in-human clinical research has recently been launched. The continuous analysis of this clinical trial will shed light on the advantages of LBPs and, as a result, point the way for adopting LBPs as an alternative therapeutic strategy in clinics (Paquet et al. 2021). Probiotics like *E. coli* Nissle 1917 are frequently utilized to treat a range of digestive issues. To target the tumor itself and stop tumor growth in mice models, *E. coli* Nissle 1917 has been altered to create cytotoxic substances such glidobactin, colibactin, and luminmide (Rebersek 2021).

Probiotics have been recommended for use as a remedy or preventative approach for several other illnesses as well as to ease several health concerns. However, neither preclinical nor clinical studies have proven beneficial for probiotics (Suez et al. 2019). Which bacterial strains should be used for treatment, the ideal strain ratio, the kinds of functions that different strains perform, the physiological effects of probiotics on the body, how they interact with the intestinal microbiome, potential safety concerns associated with their use, and how they affect the host are just a few of the many unanswered questions regarding probiotics that remain (Suez et al. 2019).

PREBIOTICS, POSTBIOTICS, AND SYNBIOTICS

Prebiotics are nondigestible food components that have a favorable effect on the gut microbiota by boosting the proliferation and/or functioning of one or a few specific bacteria in the colon (Wong and Yu 2019). This enhances the host's health. As shown in Figure 4.2 prebiotics purportedly work to promote probiotic growth, encourage selective probiotic fermentation, interact with pathogens to prevent colonization, and act as an anti-inflammatory agent. However, the advantages of prebiotics might not be available to everyone and rely on a person's genetic makeup. In contrast, postbiotics can promote the generation of IgA, demonstrate specific cytotoxicity against tumor cells, and stop healthy epithelial cells from dying (Rebersek 2021).

The probiotics *Bifidobacterium lactis* Bb12 and *Lactobacillus rhamnosus* GG cause changes in the fecal microbiome when combined with a prebiotic like inulin, reducing the number of harmful *Clostridium* strains and increasing the quantity of constructive *Bifidobacterium*

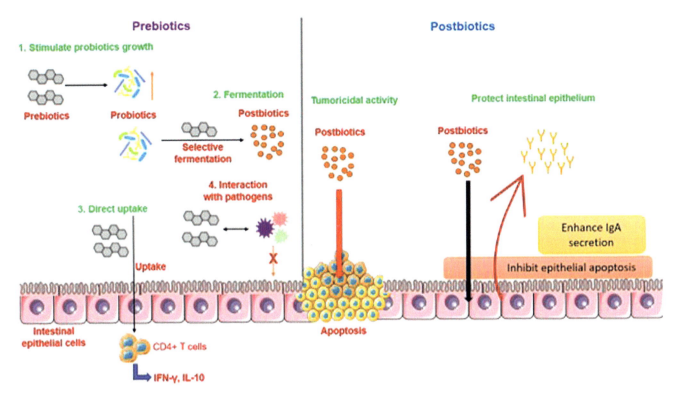

FIGURE 4.2 Potential prebiotic and postbiotic methods of action. Prebiotics purportedly work in the gut by promoting probiotic growth, selective probiotic fermentation, interacting with pathogens to prevent colonization, being absorbed into the intestine, and acting as an anti-inflammatory agent. However, the benefits of prebiotics may not be universal and are dependent on a person's genetic makeup. On the other hand, postbiotics can exhibit selective cytotoxicity towards tumor cells and preventing the death of healthy epithelial cells and promoting IgA production. IFN-γ stands for interferon-γ; IgA stands for immunoglobulin A; IL-10 stands for interleukin-10.

and *Lactobacillus* strains (Rebersek 2021). By promoting the development and performance of commensal microbes like *Bifidobacterium* and *Lactobacillus*, mostly through the generation of SCFAs, prebiotics have a beneficial effect on the gut microbiota. Previous research has suggested that SCFAs can increase the integrity of intestinal epithelium, regulate metabolism, and boost immunity to protect against a variety of disorders. We only have a limited grasp of how prebiotics affect chemotherapy-induced toxicity and chemosensitivity (Samanta et al. 2022). Our understanding of the positive effects of prebiotics is confined to how they demonstrate anticancer effects.

Inulin and oligofructose consumption along with 5-FU in rat models decreased tumor growth and metastasis and improved overall survival. Various chemotherapy drugs, including vincristine, CTX, doxorubicin, methotrexate, and cytarabine, were found to have comparable effects. Additionally, 5-FU and FOS supplements were given to rats to see if they provided any protection against the intestinal mucositis that 5-FU causes. After the administration of FOS, myeloperoxidase activity decreased along with inflammation levels, weight loss was stopped, and intestinal integrity was maintained, pointing to the efficacy of FOS as an adjuvant in preventing intestinal mucositis brought on by 5-FU treatment (Galdino et al. 2018).

Postbiotics are metabolites, functional proteins, extracellular polysaccharides (EPS), SCFAs, peptidoglycan-derived muropeptides, cell lysates, teichoic acid, microbial cell fractions, and pili-type structures that are byproducts of microbial fermentation (Wong and Yu 2019). They are defined as a mixture of micro- and macrocomponents, including dormant microbial cells, cell compartments, cell metabolites, as well and probiotic metabolic byproducts, which, when taken in sufficient quantities, can affect biological functions (Rad et al. 2021a). Postbiotics offer a more secure substitute to probiotics because probiotic bacteria have a challenging time surviving and have positive effects in less-than-ideal growth, distribution, and preservation and preparation settings. Oncomicrobiotics, a mixture of bacteria or bacterial products that enhance the immune response, is one type of postbiotic that may be used to increase the efficacy of prebiotics (Rebersek 2021).

The regulation of gut health and function has undergone a revolution thanks to postbiotics. According to Homayouni Rad et al. (2021), postbiotics may have antihypertensive, anti-inflammatory, immunomodulatory, apoptotic, and antioxidant properties. Numerous in vitro studies have shown that bacterium metabolites from cell-free isolates of *Lactobacillus* strains can control inflammation, cell proliferation, and apoptosis in colorectal cancer (Rad et al.

2021b). Clinical investigations also showed the postbiotics' potential to reduce the risk of colon cancer. A lower concentration of SCFAs and a higher concentration of bile acids are linked to a higher risk of colon cancer, according to research on the metabolomic profiling of individuals with high and insignificant risk of developing colon cancer. Postbiotics may be used as innovative anticancer therapeutics, directly modifying the makeup of the gut microbiota, and indirectly affecting the effectiveness of traditional colorectal cancer treatments by regulating immune activities (Rad et al. 2021b).

It is plausible to suggest that the favorable effects of synbiotic administration are stronger than those of prebiotic or probiotic administration alone (Chrysostomou et al. 2023). Patients with esophageal cancer receiving symbiotic treatment had less severe diarrhea, lymphopenia, and neutropenia brought on by a chemotherapy treatment consisting of docetaxel, cisplatin, and 5-FU when compared to patients receiving only a single strain of *Streptococcus faecalis* as a probiotic (Motoori et al. 2017).

ANTIBIOTICS AND FECAL MICROBIOTA TRANSPLANTATION

Antibiotics and fecal microbiota transplantation as shown in Figure 4.3 are efficient ways to reverse dysbiosis and reestablish equilibrium given that gut dysbiosis frequently contributes to the formation of a range of illnesses. However, because antibiotics also kill commensal microflora, they can also result in dysbiosis in other areas of the body. Antibiotics are exceptionally good at eliminating pathogenic or hazardous bacteria (Huang et al. 2022). Additionally, because commensal microbiota affects how well cancer immunotherapy works to fight cancer, it may be less successful. FMT, on the other hand, involves introducing a new bacterial population to the recipient to treat the existing dysbiosis. However, there is a possibility that the recipient could catch a disease or acquire a pathogen from the donor because the donor's samples include so many unidentified components (Huang et al. 2022).

The prevention of cancer may benefit greatly from the use of selective antibiotics (Wong and Yu 2019). Antibiotics can operate as small molecule inhibitors to lessen side effects from treatment, supplement commensals to enhance cancer therapies, and inhibit cancer-associated bacteria through altering the gut microbiome. One of the particular and selective treatments for cancer-associated *F. nucleatum* is antibiotic therapy. Most B-lactam antibiotics, metronidazole, and clindamycin are efficient at reducing tumor volume in cancer patients and *F. nucleatum* is sensitive to all of them (Ranjbar et al. 2021). Since broad-spectrum antibiotics are known to have a negative effect on immunotherapy responses, it is essential to combine these selective antibiotics with other

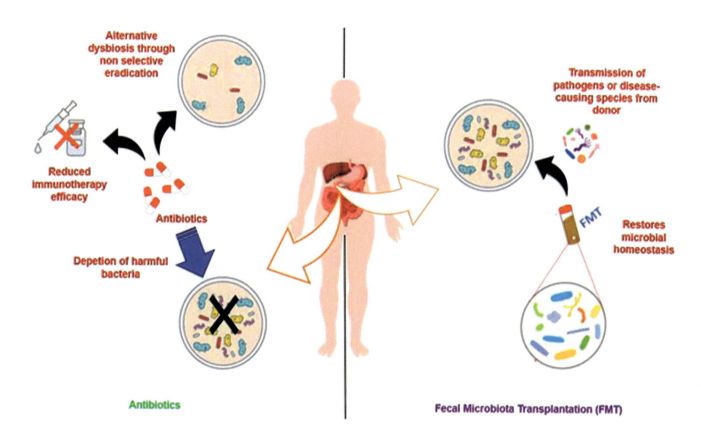

FIGURE 4.3 Potential modes of action for fecal microbiota transplantation (FMT) and antibiotics as well as related safety issues. Antibiotics and fecal microbiota transplantation are efficient ways to reverse dysbiosis and reestablish equilibrium. Antibiotics kill commensal microflora whereas FMT introduces new bacterial population to the recipient (Huang et al. 2022).

gut microbiome-modulating methods, such as diet, prebiotics and probiotics, or fecal microbiota transplantation, for the best results (Wong and Yu 2019).

Antibiotic bacterial ablation reduces the effectiveness of several anticancer medications, such as cyclophosphamide, platinum salts (such as oxaliplatin and cisplatin), anti-CTLA-4, and anti-PD-1/L1 antibodies. This is true even though some members of the gut microbiota are responsible for certain adverse effects of some antitumor drugs (Huang et al. 2022). Because the gut microbiota drives certain immune responses that are essential for the anticancer impact of cyclophosphamide, Viaud et al. (2013) found that treatment with antibiotics caused cyclophosphamide treatment in tumor-bearing animals to fail therapeutically. Additionally, a prospective, multicenter clinical trial showed a link between the usage of broad-spectrum antibiotics and a worse outcome after immune checkpoint inhibitor (ICI) treatment. To achieve the best results from cancer therapy, it is therefore important to limit the use of antibiotics in cancer patients (Huang et al. 2022).

Fecal microbiota transplantation (FMT) is a medical procedure that involves injecting healthy bacteria from a donor into the intestines of patients. FMT is a successful method for reshaping the gut microbiota during cancer treatment. It entails the gut microbiota's most direct modification (Rebersek 2021). FMT preparations can be given directly to patients during a gastroscopy or colonoscopy or by oral administration of lyophilized or frozen capsules. Patients with chronic inflammatory bowel illness, patients who are resistant to conventional medications, and patients suffering from *Clostridium difficile* infection (CDI) have all received treatment with the FMT approach (McQuade et al. 2019).

Rebuilding the gut microbiota and altering the tumor microenvironment are two effects of FMT/anti-PD-1 therapy that also increase CD8+ T cell activation and change gene expression. These encouraging findings point to a potential method for enhancing anti-PD-1 therapy through FMT gut microbiota modulation. Several clinical trials are currently being conducted to evaluate the efficacy and safety of this approach in treating other cancer types (such as lung cancer, gastric cancer, kidney cancer, and prostate cancer), as well as to further evaluate the underlying mode of action of the combined use of FMT and ICIs (Canale et al. 2021; Ho et al. 2018).

The donor selection and screening, donor blood and stool testing, collection, preparation, and storage of feces, as well as the implementation of FMT into clinical practice are all steps that are included in the internationally agreed-upon standards for FMT (Wong and Yu 2019). Establishing a stool bank for freezing excrement is crucial to ensure availability and standardize quality parameters. Other diseases with intestinal dysbiosis are also being treated with FMT, mostly intestinal ailments but also metabolic, neurological, cardiovascular, and rheumatological conditions (Rebersek 2021).

FMT can lessen the negative effects of cancer treatments due to its capacity to restore dysbiosis and reduced variety of the gut microbiota (Huang et al. 2022). The first clinical investigation of ICI-related colitis successfully treated by FMT, together with a changed gut microbiome and a higher percentage of regulatory T cells in the colonic mucosa, was reported by Wang et al. (2018). FMT is also a highly effective and secure treatment for chemotherapy-induced *C. difficile* infection in cancer patients receiving cytotoxic chemotherapy (Dizman et al. 2022; Anker et al. 2018; Viaud et al. 2013). Fecal donor selection and screening provide one of the biggest obstacles in FMT because the effectiveness of this method depends on having accurate inclusion and exclusion criteria for donors.

NANOTECHNOLOGY

Over the past years, nanotechnology regulation of the gut microbiota for cancer therapy has been investigated for cancer treatment, but it is unknown how to use it to modify the gut microbiota to indirectly fight cancer. Recently, some scientists constructed a bacterial outer membrane-coated nanoparticle using a *Helicobacter pylori* membrane that may compete with *H. pylori* to prevent pathogen adherence (Zhang et al. 2019). The study gave us the idea to prepare nanoparticles that might compete with target bacteria to inhibit their attachment and reduce their number in the body, which would enhance anticancer efficacy, even though it did not conclusively show that the suppression of the adhesion of pathogens by such nanoparticles is relevant to cancer therapy. The creation of anticancer nanoformulations employing specific microbial components is another intriguing research field for the treatment of cancer. The immunological environment in cancers and lymph nodes that drain them may be changed by four different-sized nanoformulations synthesized from yeast cell walls, which in turn prevented tumor growth (Xu et al. 2022).

Smaller nanoparticles are more likely to efficiently drain into lymphatic vessels and accumulate in lymph nodes due to their increased mobility and propensity to penetrate tissue barriers. Once in the lymph nodes, they can be readily internalized by immune cells such as dendritic cells, leading to enhanced antigen presentation and activation of T-cell-mediated immune responses against cancer cells (Xu et al. 2022). In contrast, larger nanoparticles may have reduced mobility and penetration into tissue, limiting their ability to reach and accumulate in lymph nodes. Consequently, they may elicit a weaker or delayed immune response compared to smaller nanoparticles (Xu et al. 2022). Hence, the size of nanoformulations plays a significant role in modulating their interaction with the immune system and subsequent anticancer immune responses. By optimizing nanoparticle size to maximize accumulation in tumor-draining lymph nodes, researchers can enhance the efficacy of cancer immunotherapy strategies aimed at harnessing the immune system to target and eradicate tumors (Xu et al. 2022).

BACTERIOPHAGE

According to Zheng et al. (2019), phage-guided manipulation of the gut microbiota can limit bacteria that are associated with chemoresistance and adverse reactions of cancer chemotherapy with great specificity. A phage against *Fusobacterium nucleatum* was isolated by Zheng et al. (2019), who also demonstrated that oral administration of the phage precisely eradicated *F. nucleatum* in mice's gut and *F. nucleatum*-induced chemoresistance to irinotecan. This work highlights bacteriophages as a viable tool for microbiome editing and improving the efficacy of anticancer medications (Zheng et al. 2019), even though both safety and tolerability objectives need to be investigated in the use of phage-drug combinations in the clinic.

Researchers have also suggested employing phages to alter the gut microbiome's composition to treat cancer. Researchers connected azide-modified phages with irinotecan-loaded dextran nanoparticles to prevent *F. nucleatum* from performing a fundamental role in the tumorigenesis of CRC, and it was found that the administration of the combined unit could significantly increase the efficacy of chemotherapy drugs for CRC (Zheng et al. 2019). Bacteriophages can also change the Tumor microenvironment (TME). Researchers placed silver nanoparticles (AgNPs) on the outer surface of the capsid protein of the M13 phage (M13@Ag) because it could preferentially bind to *F. nucleatum* (Dong et al. 2020). The ability of M13@Ag to eradicate *F. nucleatum* in the gut, lessen the growth of immunosuppressive myeloid-derived suppressor cells that *F. nucleatum* causes in tumor locations, and then modify the TME against CRC was further proven (Dong et al. 2020). To further arouse the body's immune system for CRC suppression, the M13 phage may additionally stimulate antigen-presenting cells (Dong et al. 2020).

SPORE-BASED ANTICANCER STRATEGY

A spore is a dormant or reproductive body generated by some microbes, fungi, and plants that can either develop into a new individual on its own or after fusing with another spore. The term "spore" used in this article explicitly refers to the latent body of bacteria and fungi (Zhao et al. 2023; Song et al. 2019). Drug delivery systems are one of the most often used types of spore-based methods. The spores that remain dormant of the probiotic *Bacillus cagulans* can withstand the harsh acidic environment, complex chemicals, and temperature in the gastrointestinal tract, and begin to grow to probiotics under stimulation by some nutrients in the gut (Song et al. 2019). This probiotic is helpful in the management of gut microbial balance and the treatment of intestinal inflammation.

Additionally, the hydrophobic protein covering the spores' surface sheds during germination (Zhao et al. 2023; Aps et al. 2016; Knecht et al. 2011). Song and colleagues created a new oral medication delivery system for cancer therapy based on these physiological characteristics of the spores (Song et al. 2019). The combination can dissolve in the intestinal milieu, which is subsequently followed by the self-assembly of nanoparticles containing chemotherapy medications (Song et al. 2019). More specifically, the spore of *B. coagulans* was remodeled with DCA and loaded with chemotherapeutics. More importantly, this mechanism can safeguard therapeutic agents from the stomach's acidic environment, get past intestinal barriers, and reduce drug degradation in epithelial cells. As a result, the efficiency of tumor inhibition is boosted due to an increase in basolateral medication release into the bloodstream. (Song et al. 2019). The development of an oral drug delivery method for PDAC chemotherapy that could significantly boost intratumorally drug buildup also used *Clostridium butyricum* spores (Han et al. 2022).

Bacterial spores can also be employed to cure cancer. Since *Clostridium* is obligately anaerobic, its spores are solely localized to and emerge in the necrotic/hypoxic portion of solid tumors (Zhao et al. 2023). This has led to extensive research on clostridial spores. As a result, clostridial spores may carry anticancer medications or unique genes that target the TME. Additionally, using clostridial spores helps lessen the negative effects of chemotherapy. Chemotherapy is hazardous mostly because it does not target tumor cells specifically and damages healthy cells. Therefore, when paired with benign prodrug delivery, inoculation of the transgenic bacterial spores can lessen systemic deleterious effects, and genes generating enzymes that convert the safe prodrug into a damaging derivative can be introduced into *Clostridium* (Zhao et al. 2023).

PHYSICAL ACTIVITY

Physical activity (PA) stands out among complementary therapy philosophies as a novel and promising strategy in cancer. According to Villeger et al. (2019), PA appears to have a considerable positive influence on diagnosis, recurrence, mortality, therapeutic efficacy, and side effects associated with cancer and therapy. In numerous observational and experimental research, exercise has been recommended as a practical method to lessen the side effects of cancer and its therapy (Oruç et al. 2019). However, the molecular processes underlying the cancer-preventive effects of exercise are still unknown. There has not been much research done in the literature regarding PA's effects on gut microbiota. According to Oruç et al. (2019), the advantages of exercise may be related to their effects on obesity, oxidative stress, inflammation and/or immunological impairment, mitochondrial dysfunction, and transcriptional misregulation.

Exercise may potentially alter the physiologic microenvironment of tumors and enhance antitumor immunity, according to research investigations. The metabolism and development dynamics of tumors may be positively and persistently impacted by these combined effects of exercise (Zhang et al. 2019). The second hypothesized mechanism that may also highlight the benefits of exercise on cancer is the modulatory effect of PA on colon movement time and on intestinal microbiota. Preclinical research has demonstrated that PA alters the microbiota that is linked with the intestinal mucosa, increases the generation of SCFAs from a variety of sources, and increases microbial metabolic capacity. In severe pathogenic situations like cancer, the effects of PA on the gut microbiota modify the gut microbiota's features more significantly (Villéger et al. 2019).

Considering the potential significance of the "gut microbiota-skeletal muscle" axis, the manipulation of the microbiome by PA may be a ground-breaking concept with broad scientific and societal applications. However, the impact is still not fully understood, particularly in terms of how it can help to lessen the side effects of both cancer and its curative regimens (Zhang et al. 2019). To support the potential interest of PA in gut microbiota regulation for individualized cancer therapy, these interactions need to be further investigated in the context of cancer (Villéger et al. 2019).

OTHER MICROBIOTA-MODULATING AGENTS

Genetic engineering along with surface modification have recently been used to modify bacteria for effective anticancer aims as well as directly boosting the efficacy of anticancer therapy by changing the mix of gut microbes (Zhao et al. 2023). Some researchers have successfully increased the anticancer activity of violacein under hypoxia by transferring the violacein biosynthetic cluster into the *Salmonella* oncolytic strain VNP20009, which serves as a targeted delivery vehicle with tumor-colonizing properties (Zhao et al. 2023; Wu et al. 2022). Another strategy is surface modification, which entails changing several aspects of the bacterial envelope structure to give them new biological characteristics (Sun et al. 2023). Antibodies that disrupt checkpoints and tumor-specific antigens were added to the surface of bacteria, and the modified bacteria successfully inhibited tumor growth in tumor models that overexpressed those antigens (Li et al. 2022).

CASE STUDIES DEMONSTRATING PERSONALIZED THERAPEUTIC APPROACHES

The modulation of the gut microbiome in cancer therapy essentially has two goals: to increase therapeutic efficacy and to lessen toxicity or side effects associated with the medication. A growing number of case studies aiming to achieve clinical translation of microbial therapy are ongoing or have already been completed, and some chosen trials are summarized in Tables 4.1 and 4.2 (Zhao et al. 2023; Juan et al. 2022; Wang et al. 2018). A case study (NCT04116775) in metastatic prostate cancer administered FMT via endoscopy from pembrolizumab-sensitive participants into pembrolizumab-resistant individuals is ongoing with the intention of improving the recipients' antitumor activity and enhancing their tumor sensitivity to ICIs.

TABLE 4.1
Gut microbial modulation associated with anticancer therapeutic efficacy

Intervention	Cancer	Case study	Objective	Outcomes
Primal Defense ULTRA Probiotic Formula	Breast cancer	NCT03358511 (America) Engineering Gut Microbiome to Target Breast Cancer	To assess the efficacy of presurgical antibiotics to influence antitumor immune function	Mean number of cytotoxic T lymphocytes (CD8 + cells)
Probiotic Natural Health Product—RepHresh Pro-B	Breast cancer	NCT03290651 (Canada) Re-setting the Breast Microbiome to Lower Inflammation and Risk of Cancer	To determine if oral antibiotics can change the breast flora	Change in breast microbiota
ProBion Clinica (*Bifidobacterium lactis, L. acidophilus*)	Colon cancer	NCT03072641 (Sweden) Using Probiotics to Reactivate Tumor Suppressor Genes in Colon Cancer	To reactivate the tumor-suppressor genes using probiotics	Changes in microbiota composition after probiotics use
FMT via endoscopy	Prostate cancer	NCT04116775 (America) A phase II Single Arm Study of Fecal Microbiota Transplant (FMT) in Men with Metastatic Castration Resistant Prostate Cancer Whose Cancer Has Not Responded to Enzalutamide + Pembrolizumab	To determine the anticancer effect of fecal microbiota transplant from participants who respond to pembrolizumab into those who have not responded in metastatic castration resistant prostate cancer	Percentage of participants with a PSA decline of ≥50% at any time point on study after FMT
FMT	Melanoma; head and neck squamous cell carcinoma; cutaneous squamous cell carcinoma; clear cell renal cell carcinoma	NCT05286294 (Norway) MITRIC: Microbiota Transplant to Cancer Patients Who Have Failed Immunotherapy Using Feces from Clinical Responders	To turn non-responders to immune checkpoint inhibitors into responders by modulating patients' intestinal microbiota through FMT	Objective tumor response rate, incidence, nature, and severity of FMT-related adverse events

(continued)

TABLE 4.1 (Continued)
Gut microbial modulation associated with anticancer therapeutic efficacy

Intervention	Cancer	Case study	Objective	Outcomes
Investigational FMT capsules	NSCLC, melanoma, and uveal melanoma	NCT04951583 (Canada) Phase II Trial of Fecal Microbial Transplantation in Patients with Advanced Non-Small Cell Lung Cancer and Melanoma Treated with Immune Checkpoint Inhibitors	To assess the impact of FMT on ICI response and survival	Objective response rate in the NSCLC cohort
Probio-M9	Liver cancer	NCT05032014 (China) Probiotics Enhance the Treatment of PD-1 Inhibitors in Patients with Liver Cancer	To assess whether probiotics can improve the efficacy of ICI	Proportion of patients whose tumor volume shrinks to a predetermined value and maintains the minimum time limit
CBM 588 probiotic strain	Renal cell carcinoma	NCT03829111 (America) Pilot Study to Evaluate the Biologic Effect of CBM588 in Combination with Nivolumab/Ipilimumab for Patients with Metastatic Renal Cell Carcinoma	To determine the effect of *clostridium butyricum* CBM 588 probiotic strain (in combination with nivolumab/ipilimumab) on the gut microbiome in patients with metastatic renal cell carcinoma and evaluate the effect of CBM588 on the clinical efficacy of the nivolumab/ipilimumab combination	Change in *Bifidobacterium* composition of stool
Dietary supplement: soluble corn fiber	Colorectal cancer	NCT05516641 (America) Do Prebiotics Change Intestinal Biome in Rectal Cancer Patients Undergoing Neoadjuvant Therapy	To study microbiome modulating treatment could have an impact on CRC outcomes	Gut flora modulation
Behavioral: prolonged nightly fasting	Head and neck cancer	NCT05083416 (America) Effect of Prolonged Nightly Fasting (PNF) on Immunotherapy Treatment Outcomes in Patients with Advanced Head and Neck Cancer (HNSCC)-Role of Gut Microbiome	To evaluate if eating within an 8–10-h window during the day, without any caloric restriction, can lead to better response rates to immunotherapy in head and neck cancer patients	Rates of PNF compliance, change in gut microbiome and microbial metabolites
FMT (donor responder to PD-1 therapy) with pembrolizumab	Melanoma	NCT03341143 (America) Phase II Feasibility Study of Fecal Microbiota Transplant (FMT) in Advanced Melanoma Patients Not Responding to PD-1 Blockade	To study concurrent use of FMT and pembrolizumab in patients with PD-1- resistant melanoma	ORR, change in T cell. composition and function; change in innate and adaptive immune subsets
FMT (colonoscopy and capsules) (donor responder to immunotherapy)	Melanoma	NCT03353402 (Israel) Altering the Gut Microbiota of Melanoma Patients Who Failed Immunotherapy Using Fecal Microbiota Transplantation (FMT) From Responding Patients	To study use of FMT in patients with stage IV metastatic melanoma for whom immunotherapy failed	Incidence of FMT related adverse events, engraftment, changes in composition of immune cell population and activity
Probiotics (La1, BB536)	Colorectal cancer	NCT00936572 (Italy) A Randomized Double-Blind Trial of Perioperative Administration of Probiotics in Colorectal Cancer Patients.	To investigate the effect of probiotics on gut microflora and the immune and inflammatory response	To perform morphological and microbiological evaluation of the colonic microflora, GI function
Saccharomyces boulardii	Colorectal cancer	NCT01609660 (Brazil) Impact of Probiotics on the Intestinal Microbiota and Its Association with Postoperative Outcome After Colorectal Surgery	To assess the impact of probiotics on patients undergoing colorectal resections	To measure mucosal cytokine and SCFA, postoperative complication and hospital LOS

TABLE 4.2
Gut microbial modulation to prevent anticancer therapy-related side effects

Intervention	Cancer	Case study	Objective	Outcomes
Probiotic capsules with *Bifidobacterium longum*, *Lactobacillus acidophilus*, and *Enterococcus faecalis*	Breast cancer	**ChiCTR-INQ-17014181** (China) The Effect of Probiotics on Preventing Patients with Breast Cancer From Cancer-Related Cognitive Impairment and its Mechanism.	To determine the preventive effects of probiotics on CRCI development and underlying mechanisms	Incidence of cancer-related cognitive impairment
Probiotic	Colorectal cancer	**NCT01410955** (Slovakia) Prevention of Irinotecan Induced Diarrhea by Probiotics. A Phase III Study	To determine the effectiveness of the probiotics in the prophylaxis of irinotecan-induced diarrhea due to reduction intestinal beta-D-glucuronidase activity.	Prevention of grade 3–4 diarrhea by probiotics in patients treated with irinotecan-based chemotherapy
Probiotic: Bifilact®	Prostate cancer; gynecologic cancers	**NCT01839721** (Canada) Impact of Probiotic BIFILACT® on Diarrhea in Patients Treated with Pelvic Radiation	To assess probiotic used to prevent or delay radiation induced grade moderate to severe diarrhea with patient treated for pelvic cancer.	The efficacy of probiotic Bifilact®
FMT	Renal cell cancer	**NCT04040712** (Italy) Fecal Microbiota Transplantation to Treat Diarrhea Induced by Tyrosine-kinase Inhibitors in Patients with Metastatic Renal Cell Carcinoma: A Randomized Clinical Trial	To evaluate, through a randomized controlled design, the efficacy of fecal microbiota transplantation (FMT), compared with sham FMT, in treating TKI-induced diarrhea in patients with metastatic renal cell carcinoma.	Rate of patients who experience resolution of diarrhea 4 weeks after the end of treatments
Dietary supplement: oat bran and blueberry husks	Rectal cancer	**NCT03420443** (Sweden) Randomized Clinical Trial of Effects of Synbiotics on Intestinal Microbiota in Patients Undergoing Short-course Preoperative Radiotherapy During Treatment of Rectal Cancer	To investigate how bacteria and fiber interact with the epithelial cells of the gastrointestinal mucosa to reduce inflammation and to diminish tissue damage caused by radiation therapy to patients diagnosed with rectal cancer.	Action of synbiotics on irradiated GI mucosa in rectal cancer treatment
Dietary supplement: inulin, fructo-oligosaccharide and maltodextrine	Endometrial neoplasms	**NCT01549782** (Spain) Effect of a Mixture of Inulin and Fructo-oligosaccharide on Lactobacillus and Bifidobacterium Intestinal Microbiota of Patients Receiving Radiotherapy: A Randomized, Double-blind, Placebo-	To assess the prebiotic effect of a carbohydrate by its capacity to stimulate the proliferation of healthy bacteria (*Bifidobacterium*, *Lactobacillus*) rather than pathogenic bacteria (*Clostridium*, *E. coli*).	Changes in *Lactobacillus* and *Bifidobacterium* populations
FMT via colonoscopy	Malignant genitourinary system neoplasm	**NCT04038619** (America) Fecal Microbiota Transplantation in Treating Immune-Checkpoint Inhibitor Induced-Diarrhea or Colitis in Genitourinary Cancer Patients	To assess the efficacy of FMT for clinical remission/response of immune-related diarrhea/colitis	1. Incidence of FMT-related adverse events 2. Clinical response/remission of immune-related diarrhea/colitis

(continued)

TABLE 4.2 (Continued)
Gut microbial modulation to prevent anticancer therapy-related side effects

Intervention	Cancer	Case study	Objective	Outcomes
FMT capsules	Renal cell carcinoma	NCT04163289 (Canada) Preventing Immune-Related Adverse Events in Renal Cell Carcinoma Patients Treated with Combination Immunotherapy Using Fecal Microbiota Transplantation	To study the safety of FMT combination immunotherapy treatment and reduce occurrence of immune-related toxicities in renal cell carcinoma patients	Occurrence of grade 3 or higher immune-related colitis from the start of treatment with ipilimumab and nivolumab to 120 days after completion of treatment
Probiotic	Pelvic cancer	NCT05032027 (China) A Randomized Controlled Clinical Study of Oral Probiotics on Radiation Enteritis Stage II Induced by Pelvic Concurrent Chemoradiotherapy	To determine if regulating intestinal tract flora will reduce the severity of radiation-induced mucositis in patients receiving pelvic radiotherapy	The incidence of grade 3 enteritis
Dietary intervention: a high-fiber diet rich in polyunsaturated fatty acid	Colorectal cancer	NCT04869956 (Spain) Gut Microbiome Modification Through Dietary Intervention in Patients with Colorectal Cancer: Response to Surgery	To assess the effect of a dietary fiber diet on the prognosis of colorectal cancer patients following surgery	Rate of anastomotic leakage surgical site infection

In another ongoing case study (NCT05032014), probiotics (Probio-49) are being tested to see if they can improve the effectiveness of PD-1 inhibitors for the treatment of liver cancer. Immunotherapy paired with FMT is being used in patients with renal cell carcinoma to lessen immune-related effects. The effectiveness of oral probiotic treatment in preventing radiation injury and associated enteritis is being tested in conjunction with pelvic chemoradiotherapy (NCT05032027) (Zhao et al. 2023). Probiotic supplements are being actively used in another case study to reduce or prevent adverse events that follow chemotherapy to protect breast cancer patients from chemotherapy-related damage. Probiotic supplements help mitigate and stop chemotherapy-related cognitive impairment (CRCI) from happening (Juan et al. 2022).

Additionally, eating a probiotic complex could help thyroid cancer patients who undergo thyroidectomy avoid symptoms connected to thyroid hormone withdrawal, such as dyslipidemia and constipation (Lin et al. 2022). Researchers are interested in the potential outcomes of these studies because they could offer the first-ever convincing proof for applications in medicine involving the gut microbiota, even though more research is still largely needed to identify the more precise and accurate molecular interactions underlying the microbiota and antitumor activity.

LIMITATIONS AND OUTLOOK

There are opportunities and difficulties that need to be recognized and handled in the future of using cancer-associated microorganisms in the clinic. Despite significant attempts to maximize therapeutic efficacy and reduce deleterious toxicities, therapeutic resistance and adverse effects continue to pose the biggest managerial problems in the management of cancer treatment (Chrysostomou et al. 2023). Future personalized cancer strategies must consider the gut microbiome due to its significance for cancer outcomes and the large interindividual variation it exhibits. Consistency in mechanistic understanding of microbial effect on cancer is an indispensable arsenal. It is essential to investigate a holistic strategy that combines microbial modulation treatment in the present cancer management system because of the gut microbiota's significant role and immense potential for the creation of novel anticancer methods (Sun et al. 2023).

Today, the microbiome is a standalone therapeutic target. It is possible to increase illness prognosis and survival by better understanding the direct and indirect roles of gut microbiota, as well as metabolic products and functions produced from it, in cancer (Zhao et al. 2023). Over many years, focused efforts were made to comprehend how the gut microbiome interacted with cytotoxic and immunotherapeutic drugs to enhance therapeutic outcomes. However, many challenges remain for now (Sun et al. 2023). Future investigations must not only use longitudinal sampling procedures, utilizing multi-omic approaches, but also novel large-scale biobanks that consider regional variations in microbiome ecologies if meaningful insights into the therapeutic oncomicrobiome are to be obtained. The most important query, though, is how the microbiome should be modified to enhance patient outcomes from cancer treatment (Zhao et al. 2023).

Thus, the interaction of genetic (genomics), environmental (exposome), and microbial components must be considered in future drug trials. This is difficult since numerous xenobiotics affect both the makeup and functionality of the microbiota. Additional motivation for doing this comes from the possibility that accidental changes to the gut microbiome could harm patients through sepsis, immunological dysfunction, or changed medication metabolism (Zhao et al. 2023). The identification of novel therapeutic targets and the decline in the failure rates of novel treatment candidates are perhaps the two biggest benefits of adding the microbiome into cancer studies. Many microbiome-centered studies have, to date, only provided a single snapshot of the microbiome state before and after disease or treatment and have not considered niche-specific variations or the structural and functional rehabilitation dynamics in the gut microbiome across increasingly long patient journeys (Chrysostomou et al. 2023).

Despite the intriguing findings of microbiome research accumulated over the years, there is still a disconnect between clinical observations and clinical interventions that stratify the microbiome. Although it has been demonstrated that bacteria and medicinal molecules interact strongly, the precise underlying mechanisms are still unknown. The implementation of those solutions also needs to be done with consideration. Due to inconsistent findings across cohorts, the main worry centers on the effectiveness and safety of therapies that modulate the microbiome (Zhao et al. 2023). Additionally, we must carefully consider the fact that interventional investigations are typically carried out in animal models, which offer valuable insights into the interactions between the human microbiome and drugs but do not completely replicate human biology. Therefore, to apply such findings in a therapeutic environment, sizable human-centered research is needed. Future research is required to better understand the fundamental microbiome-drug interactions and find microbiome-derived biomarkers to develop plans for altering the gut microbiome to enhance therapeutic outcomes (Chrysostomou et al. 2023).

The associated clinical therapies targeted at microorganisms have not yet been developed into mature applications for cancer patients, despite mounting evidence shown in human subjects. Individual differences in sensitivity to the same microbial pathogens are one of the immensely complicated factors resulting in this occurrence (Chrysostomou et al. 2023). Can microbe-targeted therapies be added to the current cancer management system to have a more thorough and effective antitumor effect? Since the issue has not yet been solved, more preclinical study and prospective clinical trials are required to identify the difficulties (Zhao et al. 2023). Despite accumulating evidence in human subjects, the accompanying clinical medicines that target microorganisms have not yet been translated into mature applications for cancer patients. One of the incredibly complex elements causing this occurrence is individual variations in sensitivity to the same microbial infections. Can the current cancer management system be supplemented with microbe-targeted medicines to have a more thorough and potent antitumor effect? More preclinical research and prospective clinical trials are needed to discover the issues because the problem has not yet been resolved (Chrysostomou et al. 2023).

Finally, even though there are still many obstacles to overcome, it is imperative to consider a comprehensive strategy that incorporates microbial modulation therapy into the current cancer management system due to the gut microbiota's significant significance and full potential for the development of new anticancer strategies (Chrysostomou et al. 2023). Future research should focus on differentiating microbiota stratification, and the distinct strain found in various hosts might be investigated using a "single microbe" profile, like a single-cell sequence, which can help to accurately capture specific influencing processes. Additionally, specific preclinical models can be employed to test the results in vitro and connect the molecular pathways to applications, such as patient-derived organotypic tumor spheroids in short-term 3D cultures in the same environmental settings (Zhao et al. 2023).

CONCLUSION

It is becoming increasingly obvious that disturbances in the commensal microbiota may contribute to a variety of disease states and their treatment, including cancer, and that they play a significant role in overall health by boosting general immunity (Zhao et al. 2023). Additionally, there is growing evidence that these microbes may increase the risk of developing specific malignancies, either directly by their local presence in the tumor microenvironment or indirectly through the systemic effects of their presence in other parts of the body (such as the gut and the skin). The latter is particularly important since it relates to how gut microbiota can potentially influence the toxicity of immunotherapy as well as conventional chemotherapeutic drugs, thereby altering patient outcomes (Sun et al. 2023). This ecosystem is both peculiarly adaptable and fundamentally adjustable, providing the possibility for practical application of these discoveries. Additionally, outside factors (like diet, antigen exposure, medications, and stress) play a significant role in causing states of health or disease through their interactions with host-specific factors; a significant portion of these influence the microbiota, which raises the possibility that the microbiota may be a common factor (Zhao et al. 2023).

Notably, there are also new, unexpected findings that indicate that we still have a long way to go in understanding the impacts of the human microbiota. For instance, there is a great deal of crosstalk and bidirectional feedback between the gut microbiota and the neurological and endocrine systems. The mechanism of action and the precise bacterial species or group of species that are most crucial in mediating anticancer effects and general health remain unknown because this area is still in its infancy (Zhao et al. 2023). Our understanding of this complex ecosystem can be advanced by collaborative research at every stage, from basic and translational research through clinical investigations and epidemiological analyses. However, it is crucial that we consider all these characteristics going ahead to treat cancer and other diseases, both from a prognosis and a therapeutic standpoint. To achieve the best possible health and to effectively treat disease, multifaceted systems will need to be developed to monitor and modify these elements. Only by using such a strategy can personalized cancer therapies reach their full potential (Chrysostomou et al. 2023).

In this chapter we examined the strategies used in modulating the gut microbiome to enhance personalized cancer therapies. The chapter discussed various strategies that can promote a healthy gut microbial composition and that can be used as potential interventions to manipulate the gut microbiome towards personalized therapeutic approaches in cancer treatment. Studies have been used to find changes in the gut microbiota following treatment and, as a result, to uncover potential bacteria and underlying bacterial functions associated with modulating therapy responses (Zhao et al. 2023). Microbiota unquestionably has significant influence on cancer therapy efficacy and toxicity, even though several research studies provide conclusions with some discrepancies due to interpatient variability and other environmental factors. There is a need for more research on the mechanistic pathways and the functional role of the microbiome in enhancing therapeutic outcomes and reducing toxicity (Chrysostomou et al. 2023).

REFERENCES

Anker, J. F., Naseem, A. F., Mok, H., Schaeffer, A. J., Abdulkadir, S. A. & Thumbikat, P. (2018). Multi-faceted immunomodulatory and tissue-tropic clinical bacterial isolate potentiates prostate cancer immunotherapy. *Nat Commun*, 9(1), 1591:1–14.

Aps, L. R. M. M., Tavares, M. B., Rozenfeld, J. H. K., Lamy, M. T., Ferreira, L. C. S. & Diniz, M. O. (2016). Bacterial spores as particulate carriers for gene gun delivery of plasmid DNA. *J. Biotechnol*, 228, 58–66.

Canale, F. P., Basso, C., Antonini, G., Perotti, M., Li, N., Sokolovska, A., Neumann, J., James, M. J., Geiger, S., Jin, W., Theurillat, J. P., West, K. A., Leventhal, D. S., Lora, J. M., Sallusto, F. & Geiger, R. (2021). Metabolic modulation of tumors with engineered bacteria for immunotherapy. *Nature*, 598(7882), 662–666.

Chrysostomou, D., Roberts, L. A., Marchesi, J. R., & Kinross, J. M. (2023). Gut Microbiota modulation of efficacy and toxicity of cancer chemotherapy and immunotherapy. *Gastroenterology*, 164 (2), 198–213.

Dizman, N., Meza, L., Bergerot, P., Alcantara, M., Dorff, T., Lyou, Y., Frankel, P., Cui, Y., Mira, V., Llamas, M., Hsu, J., Zengin, Z., Salgia, N., Salgia, S., Malhotra, J., Chawla, N., Chehrazi-Raffle, A., Muddasani, R., Gillece, J., Reining, L., Trent, J., Takahashi, M., Oka, K., Higashi, S., Kortylewski, M., Highlander, S. K. & Pal, S. K. (2022). Nivolumab plus ipilimumab with or without live bacterial supplementation in metastatic renal cell carcinoma: a randomized phase 1 trial. *Nat Med*, 28 (4), 704–712.

Dong, X., Pan, P., Zheng, D. W., Bao, P., Zeng, X. & Zhang, X. Z. (2020). Bioinorganic hybrid bacteriophage for modulation of intestinal microbiota to remodel tumor-immune microenvironment against colorectal cancer. *Sci Adv*, 6, eaba1590.

Encarnação, J. C., Pires, A. S., Amaral, R. A., Gonçalves, T. J., Laranjo, M., Casalta-Lopes, J. E., Gonçalves, A. C., Sarmento-Ribeiro, A. B., Abrantes, A. M. & Botelho, M. F. (2018). Butyrate, a dietary fiber derivative that improves irinotecan effect in colon cancer cells. *J Nutr Biochem*, 56, 183–192.

Galdino, F. M. P., Andrade, M. E. R., de Barros, P. A. V., Generosoc, S. V., Alvarez-Leited, J. I., de Almeida-Leitee, C. M., Peluziof, M. C. G., Fernandesb, S. O. A. & Cardosob, V. N. (2018). Pretreatment and treatment with fructo-oligosaccharides attenuate intestinal mucositis induced by 5-FU in mice. *J Funct Foods*, 49, 485–492.

González-Sarrías, A., Giménez-Bastida, J. A., NúñezSánchez, M. Á., Larrosa, M., García-Conesa, M. T., Tomás-Barberán, F. A. & Espín, J. C. (2014). Phase-II metabolism limits the antiproliferative activity of urolithins in human colon cancer cells. *Eur J Nutr*, 53, 853–864.

Han, Z. Y., Chen, Q. W., Fu, Z. J., Cheng, S. X. & Zhang, X. Z. (2022). Probiotic spore-based oral drug delivery system for enhancing pancreatic cancer chemotherapy by gut-pancreas-axis-guided delivery. *Nano Lett*, 22, 8608–8617.

Ho, C. L., Tan, H. Q., Chua, K. J., Kang, A., Lim, K. H., Ling, K. L., Yew, W. S., Lee, Y. S., Thiery, J. P. & Chang, M. W. (2018). Engineered commensal microbes for diet-mediated colorectal-cancer chemoprevention. *Nat Biomed Eng*, 2(1), 27–37.

Homayouni Rad, A., Aghebati-Maleki, L., Samadi-Kafil, H., Abbasi, A. & Khani, N. (2021). Postbiotics as a safe alternative to live probiotic bacteria in the food and pharmaceutical industries. *Sci J Kurdistan Univ Medi Sci*, 26, 132–157.

Huang, J., Liu, D., Wang, Y., Liu, L., Li, J., Yuan, J., Jiang, Z., Jiang, Z., Hsiao, W. W., Liu, H., Khan, I., Xie, Y., Wu, J., Xie, Y., Zhang, Y., Fu, Y., Liao, J., Wang, W., Lai, H., Shi, A., Cai, J., Luo, L., Li, R., Yao, X., Fan, X., Wu, Q., Liu, Z., Yan, P., Lu, J., Yang, M., Wang, L., Cao, Y., Wei, H. & Leung, E. L. (2021). Ginseng polysaccharides alter the gut microbiota and kynurenine/tryptophan ratio, potentiating the antitumor effect of anti-programmed cell death 1/programmed cell death ligand 1 (Anti-PD-1/PD-L1). *Immunotherapy Gut*, 71, 734–745.

Huang, J., Liu, W., Kang, W., He, Y., Yang, R., Mou, X. & Zhao, W. (2022). Effects of microbiota on anticancer drugs: current knowledge and potential applications. *EBio Medicine*, 83, 104197.

Ivleva, E. A. & Grivennikov, S. I. (2022). Microbiota-driven mechanisms at different stages of cancer development. *Neoplasia*, 32, 100829.

Juan, Z., Chen, J., Ding, B., Yongping, L., Liu, K., Wang, L., Le, Y., Liao, Q., Shi, J., Huang, J., Wu, Y., Ma, D., Ouyang, W. & Tong, J. (2022). Probiotic supplements attenuate chemotherapy-related cognitive impairment in patients with breast cancer: a randomised, double-blind, and placebo-controlled trial. *Eur J Cancer*, 161, 10–22.

Kao, T.Y., Chung, Y.C., Hou, Y.C., Tsai, Y. W., Chen, C. H., Chang, H. P., Chou, J. L. & Hsu, C. P. (2012). Effects of ellagic acid on chemosensitivity to 5-fluorouracil in colorectal carcinoma cells. *Anticancer Res*, 32, 4413–4418.

Kato, S., Hamouda, N., Kano, Y., Oikawa, Y., Tanaka, Y., Matsumoto, K. Amagase, K. & Shimakawa, M. (2017). Probiotic bifidobacterium bifidum G9-1 attenuates 5-fluorouracilinduced intestinal mucositis in mice via suppression of dysbiosis-related secondary inflammatory responses. *Clin Exp Pharmacol Physiol*, 44, 1017–1025.

Knecht, L. D., Pasini, P. & Daunert, S. (2011). Bacterial spores as platforms for bioanalytical and biomedical applications. *Anal Bioanal Chem*, 400, 977–989.

Lee, K. A., Luong, M. K., Shaw, H., Nathan, P., Bataille, V. & Spector, T. D. (2021). The gut microbiome: what the oncologist ought to know. *Br J Cancer*, 125(9), 1197–1209.

Li, J., Xia, Q., Guo, H., Fu, Z., Liu, Y., Lin, S. & Liu, J. (2022). Decorating bacteria with triple immune nanoactivators generates tumor-resident living immunotherapeutics. *Angew Chem Int Ed Engl*, 61, e202202409.

Lin, B., Zhao, F., Liu, Y., Wu, X., Feng, J., Jin, X., Yan, W., Guo, X., Shi, S., Li, Z., Liu, L., Chen, H., Wang, H., Wang, S., Lu, Y. & Wei, Y. (2022). Randomized clinical trial: probiotics alleviated oral-gut microbiota dysbiosis and thyroid hormone withdrawal-related complications in thyroid cancer patients before radioiodine therapy following thyroidectomy. *Front Endocrinol. (Lausanne)*, 13, 834674.

Lv, J., Jia, Y., Li, J., Kuai, W., Li, Y., Guo, F., Xu, X., Zhao, Z., Lv, J. & Li, Z. (2019). Gegen qinlian decoction enhances the effect of pd-1 blockade in colorectal cancer with microsatellite stability by remodelling the gut microbiota and the tumour microenvironment. *Cell Death Dis*, 10, 415.

McQuade, J. L., Daniel, C. R., Helmink, B. A. & Wargo, J. A. (2019). Modulating the microbiome to improve therapeutic response in cancer. *Lancet Oncol*, 20(2), e77–e91.

Motoori, M., Yano, M., Miyata, H., Sugimura, K., Saito, T., Omori, T., Fujiwara, Y., Miyoshi, N., Akita, H., Gotoh, K., Takahashi, H., Kobayashi, S., Noura, S., Ohue, M., Asahara, T., Nomoto, K., Ishikawa, O. & Sakon, M. (2017). Randomized study of the effect of synbiotics during neoadjuvant chemotherapy on adverse events in esophageal cancer patients. *Clin Nutr*, 36, 93–99.

O'Toole, P. W., Marchesi, J. R. & Hill, C. (2017). Next-generation probiotics: the spectrum from probiotics to live biotherapeutics. *Nat Microbiol*, 2, 17057.

Oh, N. S., Lee, J. Y., Lee, J. M., Lee, K. W. & Kim, Y. (2017). Mulberry leaf extract fermented with Lactobacillus acidophilus A4 ameliorates 5-fluorouracil-induced intestinal mucositis in rats. *Lett Appl Microbiol*, 64, 459–468.

Oruç, Z. & Kaplan, M. A. (2019). Effect of exercise on colorectal cancer prevention and treatment. *World J. Gastrointest Oncol*, 11, 348–366.

Oudmaijer, C. A. J., Berk, K. A., van der Louw, E. J. T. M., de Man, R., van der Lelij, A. J., Hoeijmakers, J. H. J. & IJzermans, J. (2022). KETO genic diet therapy in patients with HEPatocellular adenoma: study protocol of a matched interventional cohort study. *BMJ Open*, 12, e053559.

Pan, C., Liu, H., Robins, E., Song, W., Liu, D., Li, Z. & Zheng, L. (2020). Next-generation immuno-oncology agents: current momentum shifts in cancer immunotherapy. *J Hematol Oncol*, 13(1), 29.

Paquet, J. C., Claus, S. P., Cordaillat-Simmons, M., Mazier, W., Rawadi, G., Rinaldi, L., Elustondo, F. & Rouanet, A. (2021). Entering first-in-human clinical study with a single-strain live biotherapeutic product: input and feedback gained from the EMA and the FDA. *Front Med (Lausanne)*, 8, 716266.

Quaresma, M., Damasceno, S., Monteiro, C., Lima, F., Mendes, T., Lima, M., Justino, P., Barbosa, A., Souza, M., Souza, E. & Soares, P. (2020). Probiotic mixture containing *Lactobacillus spp.* and *Bifidobacterium spp.* attenuates 5-fluorouracil-induced intestinal mucositis in mice. *Nutr Cancer*, 72, 1355–1365.

Rad, A. H., Aghebati-Maleki, L., Kafil, H. S. & Abbasi A. (2021b). Molecular mechanisms of postbiotics in colorectal cancer prevention and treatment. *Crit Rev Food Sci Nutr*, 61, 1787–1803.

Rad, A. H., Maleki, L. A., Kafil, S. H., Zavoshti F. H. & Abbasi A. (2021a). Postbiotics as promising tools for cancer adjuvant therapy. *Adv Pharm Bull*, 11, 1–5.

Ranjbar, M., Salehi, R., Haghjooy Javanmard, S., Rafiee, L., Faraji, H., Jafarpor, S., Ferns, G. A., Ghayour-Mobarhan, M., Manian, M. & Nedaeinia, R. (2021). The dysbiosis signature of *Fusobacterium nucleatum* in colorectal cancer-cause or consequences? A systematic review. *Cancer Cell Int*, 21, 194.

Rebersek, M. (2021). Gut microbiome and its role in colorectal cancer. *BMC Cancer*, 21, 1325.

Rizvi, Z. A., Dalal. R., Sadhu, S., Kumar, Y., Kumar, S., Gupta, S. K., Tripathy, M. R., Rathore, D. K. & Awasthi, A. (2021). High-salt diet mediates interplay between NK cells and gut microbiota to induce potent tumor immunity. *Sci Adv*, 7, 1–17.

Samanta, S. (2022). Potential impacts of prebiotics and probiotics in cancer prevention. *Anticancer Agents Med Chem*, 22, 605–628.

Sánchez-Alcoholado, L., Ramos-Molina, B., Otero, A., Laborda-Illanes, A., Ordóñez, R., Medina, J. A., Gómez-Millán, J. & Queipo-Ortuño, M. I. (2020). The role of the gut microbiome in colorectal cancer development and therapy response. *Cancers (Basel)*, 12(6), 1406.

Scott, A. J., Alexander, J. L., Merrifield, C. A., Cunningham, D., Jobin, C., Brown, R., Alverdy, J., O'Keefe, S. J., Gaskins, H. R., Teare, J., Yu, J., Hughes, D. J., Verstraelen, H., Burton, J., O'Toole, P. W., Rosenberg, D. W., Marchesi, J. R. & Kinross, J. M. (2019). International cancer microbiome consortium consensus statement on the role of the human microbiome in carcinogenesis. *Gut*, 68 (9), 1624–1632.

Selma, M. V., Beltrán, D., Luna, M. C., Romo-Vaquero, M., García-Villalba, R., Mira, A., Espín. J. C. & Tomás-Barberán, F. A. (2017). Isolation of human intestinal bacteria capable of producing the bioactive metabolite isourolithin a from ellagic acid. *Front Microbiol*, 8, 1521.

Song, Q., Zheng, C., Jia, J., Zhao, H., Feng, Q., Zhang, H., Wang, L., Zhang, Z. & Zhang, Y. A. (2019). A probiotic spore-based oral autonomous nanoparticles generator for cancer therapy. *Adv Mater* 31, e1903793.

Suez, J., Zmora, N., Segal, E. & Elinav, E. (2019). The pros, cons, and many unknowns of probiotics. *Nat Med*, 25(5), 716–729.

Sun, J., Chen, F. & Wu, G. (2023). Potential effects of gut microbiota on host cancers: focus on immunity, DNA damage, cellular pathways, and anticancer therapy. *ISME J*, 17, 1535–1551.

Ting, N. L., Lau, H. C. & Yu, J. (2022). Cancer pharmacomicrobiomics: targeting microbiota to optimize cancer therapy outcomes. *Gut*, 71 (7), 1412–1425.

Vernieri, C., Fucà, G., Ligorio, F., Huber, V., Vingiani, A., Iannelli, F., Raimondi, A., Rinchai, D., Frigè, G., Belfiore, A., Lalli, L., Chiodoni, C., Cancila, V., Zanardi, F., Ajazi, A., Cortellino, S., Vallacchi, V., Squarcina, P., Cova, A., Pesce, S., Frati, P., Mall, R., Corsetto, P. A., Rizzo, A. M,. Ferraris, C., Folli, S., Garassino, M. C., Capri, G., Bianchi, G., Colombo, M. P., Minucci, S., Foiani, M., Longo, V. D., Apolone, G., Torri, V., Pruneri, G., Bedognetti, D., Rivoltini, L. & de Braud, F. (2022). Fasting-mimicking diet is safe and reshapes metabolism and antitumor immunity in patients with cancer. *Cancer Discov*, 12, 90–107.

Viaud, S., Saccheri, F., Mignot, G., Yamazaki, T., Daillère, R., Hannani, D., Enot, D. P., Pfirschke, C., Engblom, C., Pittet, M. J., Schlitzer, A., Ginhoux, F., Apetoh, L., Chachaty, E., Woerther, P. L., Eberl, G., Bérard, M., Ecobichon, C., Clermont, D., Bizet, C., Gaboriau-Routhiau, V., Cerf-Bensussan, N., Opolon, P., Yessaad, N., Vivier, E., Ryffel, B., Elson, C. O., Doré, J., Kroemer, G., Lepage, P., Boneca, I. G., Ghiringhelli,

F. & Zitvogel, L. (2013). The intestinal microbiota modulates the anticancer immune effects of cyclophosphamide. *Science*, 342(6161), 971–976.

Villéger, R., Lopès, A., Carrier, G., Veziant, J., Billard, E., Barnich, N., Gagnière, J., Vazeille, E. & Bonnet, M. (2019). Intestinal microbiota: a novel target to improve anti-tumor treatment? *Int J Mol Sci*, 20(18), 4584.

Wang, Y., Wiesnoski, D. H., Helmink, B. A., Gopalakrishnan, V., Choi, K., DuPont, H. L., Jiang, Z. D., Abu-Sbeih, H., Sanchez, C. A., Chang, C. C., Parra, E. R., Francisco-Cruz, A., Raju, G. S., Stroehlein, J. R., Campbell, M. T., Gao, J., Subudhi, S. K., Maru, D. M., Blando, J. M., Lazar, A. J., Allison, J. P., Sharma, P., Tetzlaff, M. T., Wargo, J. A. & Jenq, R. R. (2018). Fecal microbiota transplantation for refractory immune checkpoint inhibitor-associated colitis. *Nat Med*, 24, 1804–1808.

Wang, L., Wang, R., Wei, G. Y., Wang, S. M. & Du, G. H. (2020). Dihydrotanshinone attenuates chemotherapy-induced intestinal mucositis and alters fecal microbiota in mice. *Biomed Pharmacother*, 128, 110262.

Wong, S. H. & Yu, J. (2019). Gut microbiota in colorectal cancer: mechanisms of action and clinical applications. *Nat Rev Gastroenterol Hepatol*, 16(11), 690–704.

Wu, L., Bao, F., Li, L., Yin, X. & Hua, Z. (2022). Bacterially mediated drug delivery and therapeutics: strategies and advancements. *Adv Drug Deliv Rev*, 187, 114363.

Xu Q., Ni J. J., Han B. X., Yan S. S., Wei X. T., Feng G. J., Zhang H., Zhang L., Li B., Pei Y. F. (2022). Causal relationship between gut microbiota and autoimmune diseases: a two-sample mendelian randomization study. *Front Immunol*, 12, 746998.

Yassin, M. A., Ghasoub, R. S., Aldapt, M. B., Abdulla, M. A., Chandra, P., Shwaylia, H. M., Nashwan, A. J., Kassem, N. A. & Akiki, S. J. (2021). Effects of intermittent fasting on response to tyrosine kinase inhibitors (TKIs) in patients with chronic myeloid leukemia: an outcome of European LeukemiaNet project. *Cancer Control*, 28, 10732748211009256.

Zhang, X., Ashcraft, K. A., Betof Warner, A., Nair, S. K. & Dewhirst, M. W. (2019). Can exercise-induced modulation of the tumor physiologic microenvironment improve antitumor immunity? *Cancer Res*, 79, 2447–2456.

Zhao, L. Y., Mei, J. X., Yu, G., Lei, L., Zhang, W. H., Liu, K., Chen, X. L., Kołat, D., Yang, K. & Hu, J. K. (2023). Role of the gut microbiota in anticancer therapy: from molecular mechanisms to clinical applications. *Sig Transduct Target Ther*, 8, 201.

Zheng, D. W., Dong, X., Pan, P., Chen, K. W., Fan, J. X., Cheng, S. X. & Zhang, X. Z. (2019). Phage-guided modulation of the gut microbiota of mouse models of colorectal cancer augments their responses to chemotherapy. *Nat Biomed Eng*, 3, 717–728.

Zhuang, H., Jing, N., Wang, L., Jiang, G. & Liu, Z. (2021). Jujube powder enhances cyclophosphamide efficiency against murine colon cancer by enriching CD8þ T cells while inhibiting eosinophilia. *Nutrients* 13, 2700.

5 Gut Microbiome and Immunotherapy Resistance

Botle Precious Damane, Lorraine Tshegofatso Maebele, Ramsey Maluleke, Melvin Anyani Ambele, Thanyani Mulaudzi, Jyotsna Batra, and Zodwa Dlamini

INTRODUCTION

The human body comprises about 40 trillion microbes of which most are commensal and contribute to health and disease (Zhao et al., 2023). The diversity of the gut microbiome is affected by lifestyle, drugs, and physiological changes effected by factors such as age or dietary patterns. These alterations in the gut microbiome, referred to as dysbiosis, are correlated with several diseases as evidently indicated by their increased diversity in long-living individuals compared to young adults (Deng et al., 2019). Human beings are constantly exposed to other external microbiota and about 15–20% of cancers are as a result of microbial infections (Bhatt et al., 2017). Attributing cancer initiation and development to microbes is mainly due to the biomolecular chemicals they produce resulting in an epigenetic (Zhao et al., 2023) and immune modulation that is at times species-specific. These include short-chain fatty acids (SCFAs), omega-3 fatty acids, oligo/polysaccharides, and several peptides (Jenab et al., 2020).

The SCFA required as the primary source of energy and related to the integrity of the intestinal epithelial cells is butyrate (Siddiqui and Cresci, 2021). Butyrate assists in regulating inflammatory responses by stimulating the secretion of pro- and anti-inflammatory cytokines such as IFN-γ, TNF-α, IL-6, IL-8 and TGF-β, IL-10, IL-18, respectively. Moreover, butyrate modulates the function of antigen-presenting cells in the gastrointestinal tract (GIT) including dendritic cells (DCs), macrophages, and mast cells (Figure 5.1). Interestingly, SCFA has also been shown to possess biomechanisms that allow them to cross the blood-brain barrier (Siddiqui and Cresci, 2021). The hallmarks of cancer include tumor-induced inflammation and Hanahan suggested that polymorphic microbiomes should also be included. This is based on compelling evidence provided by next-generation sequencing (NGS) which showed the variability and diversity of microbial species amongst individuals and their association with cancer initiation and progression, with the gut microbiome being the most prominent at promoting inflammation, genetic instability, and cancer-favoring cell senescence (Hanahan, 2022).

The gut microbiome-derived metabolites have an impact on the patient's response to cancer immunotherapy and the potential to utilize these metabolites to sensitize patients to immune checkpoint inhibitors (ICIs) is currently being explored (Hersi et al., 2022). This chapter will explore the mechanisms used by the gut microbiome to modulate immune responses and the resultant contribution to immunotherapeutic resistance in cancer.

MICROBIOME TUMOR IMMUNE EVASION AND THE CONCOMITANT BIOMARKERS OF THE DISEASE

Several microbiota have been analyzed and their presence in cancer compared to normal tissue has been suggested as a potential tool for cancer screening. These include microbial metabolites which can be determined non-invasively from liquid biopsies such as stool, urine, saliva, and blood. These include species such as *Desulfovibrio, Faecalibacterium, Oscillospira, Bacteroides fragilis, Escherichia coli, Enterococcus faecalis, Streptococcus gallolyticus,* and *Fusobacterium nucleatum* alone or in combination with each other (Veziant et al., 2021). There are several ways that the gut microbiome utilizes to promote cancer immune evasion. It has been established that chronic inflammation is one of the risk factors of cancer development and cancer itself is known as a chronic inflammatory disease. Thus the gut microbiota can penetrate the epithelial cells and induce inflammatory responses via the induction of related immunosuppressive signaling pathways. The gut microbiota can influence polarization of macrophages into the cancer-favoring M2 phenotype, thus playing a significant role in tumor immune evasion (Figure 5.1). Inflammatory responses can also be induced by activation of tissue factor which then mediates angiogenic processes. Both angiogenesis and chronic inflammatory state can be promoted via the NOD-like receptor-dependent manner by the gut microbiota metabolites (He et al., 2022).

Immune biomarkers for immunotherapy could be evaluated by the assessment of immune responses such as the expression of regulatory cells [macrophages, regulatory T/B cells (T/Bregs), tolerogenic dendritic cells], cytokines, antitumor antigens and circulating tumor DNA (Wang et al., 2022, Iglesias-Escudero et al., 2023). Amongst potential predictive biomarkers of immunotherapeutic response to ICIs, clonal neoantigen burden and tumor mutation burden (TMB) have shown great potential based on their correlation with the effectiveness of ICI treatment in several cancers. However, the former has been shown to be less effective compared to the

DOI: 10.1201/9781032706450-5

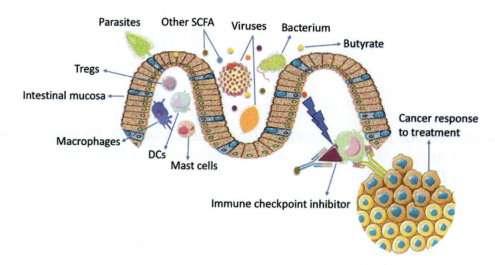

FIGURE 5.1 **The role of microbiota in immune modulation and immunotherapeutic responses.** The presence of different microbiota can induce several immune responses in addition to their secretory molecules such as short-chain fatty acids (SCFAs) with the most studied being butyrate. Conditions brought about by microbiota promote an immunosuppressive environment by inducing the development of regulatory T cells (Tregs) and promoting polarization of the pro-inflammatory M1 macrophages into cancer favoring M2 phenotype. However, butyrate can modulate both pro- and anti-inflammatory responses as well as the function of antigen presenting cells such as macrophages, dendritic, and mast cells making it valuable in immunomodulatory activities and sensitization to immune checkpoint inhibition.

TMB. The expression of programmed cell death ligand (PD-L1) has also shown potential as it is correlated with a positive response rate and overall survival (OS). The expression of PD-L1 in different tissues and sites differs and thus has an association with the response rate (Bai et al., 2020). However, determination of the PD-L1 response rate according to its expression on tumor-infiltrating lymphocytes (TIL) was reported to be more effective as opposed to the assessment of its expression levels on tumor cells (Herbst et al., 2014). The microbiome can modulate these immune parameters and increase ICI efficacy via the induction of cytotoxic lymphocytes, secretion of cytokines, or activation of antigen presentation cells, Figure 5.1 (Araji et al., 2022).

MECHANISMS OF GUT MICROBIOME IMMUNOTHERAPY RESISTANCE

The mechanisms of resistance to cancer immunotherapy are mostly based on the ability to evade the immune system. Immune evasion is mostly by manipulation of the adaptive immune system where T cells end up doing cancer cells' bidding, thus allowing them to survive and thrive. For instance, direct mechanisms of anti-PD/PD-L1 resistance include the downregulation of B7-H1 expression, dysregulation of the interferon signaling pathway, and blocking T cell activities within the tumor microenvironment. The indirect mechanisms could include loss of antigen and presentation abilities (Vesely et al., 2022). The tendency of some microbial species to polarize macrophages into the M2 phenotype contributes to their immunosuppressive effects through the production of cytokines such as IL-10, facilitation of immune checkpoint engagement by the expression of PD-L1, and the elimination of metabolites and production of reactive oxygen species (ROS). Other mechanisms of the M2 phenotype include blocking antitumor activities within the tumor microenvironment via recruitment of regulatory T cells (Tregs) or inhibition of antigen presenting cells such as DCs (DeNardo and Ruffell, 2019).

The tumor associated macrophages (TAMs) which are mainly of the M2 phenotype promote the suppressive tumor microenvironment by expression of immune checkpoint ligands such as PD-L1, PD-L2, and CD155. Attenuation of antitumor immune responses is achieved through binding of these ligands to T cells leading to T cell exhaustion. Although tumor cells express PD-L1, evidence points to TAMs being the most important player in anti-PD/PD-L1 resistance (Sheban, 2023). Anti-PD-1 immunotherapy can lead to the elicitation of T-cell responses to an epitope within the tail length tape measure protein (TMP) of an enterococcal bacteriophage via cross-reactivity with tumor MHC class I–restricted antigens (Fluckiger et al., 2020). It is worth noting that certain bacterial species produce exotoxins capable of destroying host immune cells including macrophages. Adenylate cyclase toxin (ACT) is amongst other species secreted by *Bordetella pertussis*, and has been shown to block macrophages and neutrophils from phagocytosing and destroying the bacterium itself. Anthrax lethal toxin (LT) has also been shown to block the function of macrophages and DCs by inhibiting pro-inflammatory cytokines secretion in both in vitro and in vivo studies (do Vale et al., 2016).

SPECIES-SPECIFIC GUT MICROBIOTA MODULATION OF IMMUNOTHERAPY

BACTEROIDES FRAGILIS

Bacteroides fragilis (*B. fragilis*) is the most abundantly detected, anaerobic Gram-negative bacillus. It is a commensal gut microbiota with the potential to have a negative effect on human health should it invade the intestinal mucosal layer (Cheng et al., 2020). A study conducted on stool samples of patients with colorectal cancer (CRC) found the frequency of *B. fragilis* to be significantly higher at 58.3% compared to healthy controls (26.6%), thus indicating the potential use of fecal enterotoxigenic *B. fragilis* (ETBF) as a diagnostic biomarker of CRC (Haghi et al., 2019). The role of *B. fragilis* in immunotherapeutic responses has long been identified and has been shown to induce sensitivity to cytotoxic T-lymphocyte-associated antigen 4 (CTLA-4) inhibition by favoring the T helper 1 (Th1) immune response, activation of DCs (Lichtenstern and Lamichhane-Khadka, 2023, Vétizou et al., 2015).

Cheng et al. (2020), reviewed *B. fragilis'* role in the development of colon cancer. *B. fragilis* is classified into non-toxigenic *B. fragilis* (NTBF) and ETBF. The distinction between the two is the presence of chronic inflammation inducing and "carcinogenic" *B. fragilis* toxin (BFT). BFT employs several mechanisms to induce CC development. These include the expression of cyclooxygenase (COX)-2 by colonic epithelial cells resulting in the induction of inflammatory responses by prostaglandin E2 (PGE2). Subsequently, PGE2 modulates cell proliferation and activation of oncogenic signaling pathways such as STAT-3 (Figure 5.2) known to have a significant role in cancer development. Furthermore, STAT-3 activation leads to the induction of immunosuppressive signaling involving Tregs which reduces the surrounding IL-2 in favor of Th17, which in turn results in further activation of the STAT-3 pathway.

FUSOBACTERIUM NUCLEATUM

The Gram-negative oral pathobiont, *Fusobacterium nucleatum* (*F. nucleatum*) is associated with several types of cancers. It has a high affinity for adherence with other oral microbial species such as *Streptococcus, Porphyromonas gingivalis, Treponema denticola,* and *Aggregatibacter actinomycetemcomitans*, thus providing structural support and facilitating co-habitation (Alon-Maimon et al., 2022). The detection of the microbiome was performed in CRC tissue and adjacent normal tissue samples using quantitative real-time PCR, and the results were compared with oncogenic mutations including phosphatidylinositol-4,5-bisphosphate 3-kinase (PI3K) CA, *KRAS,* and *BRAF*. Although *B. fragilis* was the most abundant in 66% and 60% of cancerous and normal tissue, respectively, as expected, *F. nucleatum* was identified in 23% of tumors and 13% of normal samples and its levels were higher in the rectum than in the colon. *F. nucleatum* positive tumors had higher frequency of KRAS mutations than their negative counterparts (p-value = 0.02) and BRAF mutation was detected only in 2 (6.6%) *F. nucleatum* positive tumors. However, the *PIK3CA* mutations were not detected (Shariati et al., 2021).

The *F. nucleatum* modulation of immune responses differs in microsatellite instability (MSI) positive CRC tumors. An enhanced response to PD-1/PD-L1 inhibitors was observed in mismatch repair-deficient (dMMR) CRC, with a rate of 75%, compared to mismatch repair-proficient (pMMR) CRC, which had a rate of 11.8%. This difference was attributed to the higher abundance of *F. nucleatum* in the former CRC tissues. This was confirmed by co-treatment of mouse models xenografts with *F. nucleatum* and PD-1/PD-L1 inhibitors resulting in a significant reduction in tumor growth. Furthermore, *F. nucleatum* facilitated the expression of PD-L1 via the activation of the stimulator of interferon genes (STING) signaling pathway which upregulated the levels of interferon-gamma (IFN-γ) and CD8+ tumor-infiltrating lymphocytes (TILs), thus enhancing tumor sensitivity to PD-L1 inhibition, Figure 5.2 (Gao et al., 2021). Contradictory to these findings, Kim et al. (2023) noted a reduced disease-free survival and OS in patients with stage III CRC infected with *F. nucleatum*. This was due to the apparent upregulation of immunosuppressive Tregs resulting in depletion of cytotoxic T cells and promotion of exhausted CD8+ T cells thus reducing adaptive antitumor immunity in CRC (Kim et al., 2023). Borowsky et al. (2021) also indicated the association of *F. nucleatum* with reduced stromal memory helper T cells required for sustained antitumor immune responses. Thus more studies are required to further understand the role of *F. nucleatum* as an immune modulator and how its immunomodulatory properties affect patients' responses to ICIs.

AKKERMANSIA MUCINIPHILA

Akkermansia muciniphila (*Akk*) is a Gram-negative anaerobic bacterium that colonizes the intestinal mucosa. This bacterium is capable of degrading the intestinal mucosa. Degradation of mucin results in the production of acetate and propionate, which further act as substrates for other bacteria (Rodrigues et al., 2022). Macrophages infected with *Akk* were shown to have the propensity to polarize into the tumor-favoring M2 phenotype. Treatment of gliadin-stimulated macrophages (M1 phenotype) with *Akk*-induced M2 phenotype which was confirmed by gene and protein expression analysis that showed increased anti-inflammatory cytokines; IL-10 and TGF-β from pro-inflammatory IL-6 and TNF-alpha expressed by macrophages treated with gliadin alone (Molaaghaee-Rouzbahani et al., 2023). Modulation of inflammatory responses by reducing the frequency of CD16/CD32+ macrophages and activation of antitumor cytotoxic T cells with reduction of PD-1 to hinder colitis-associated colorectal cancer (CAC) progression was also reported (Wang et al., 2020).

Moreover, *Akk* increased sensitivity to PD-1 inhibition by upregulation of CCR9+CXCR3+CD4+ T lymphocytes into mouse tumor beds (Routy et al., 2018). Studies show that *Akk* contributes to ICIs response in several cancers including non-small cell lung cancer (NSCLC). Treatment of NSCLC with PD-1/PD-L1 has been successful but only in a fraction (35%) of patients. However, most of these patients develop resistance and rapid progression of the disease. Treatment is mostly given to patients with PD-L1 positive tumors and in some cases, combination with chemotherapy will be administered to patients with PD-L1 negative tumors. The difference in objective response rates (ORR) between *Akk*+ and *Akk*− patients was 28% and 18%, respectively. Mouse models treated with fecal microbiota

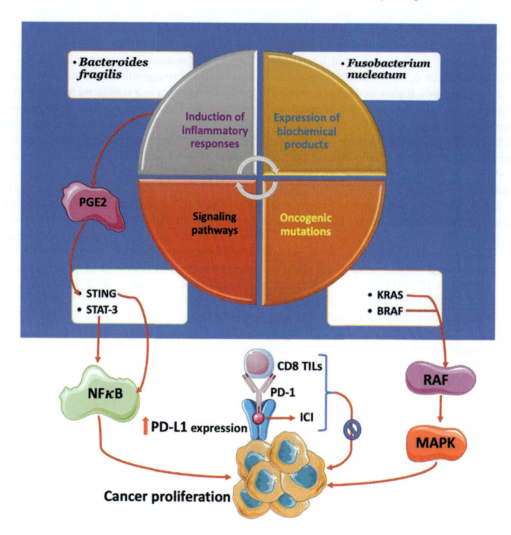

FIGURE 5.2 *Fusobacterium nucleatum* and *Bacteroides fragilis* involvement in the induction of cancer favoring mechanisms. Both species modulate immune response by regulating inflammatory responses, and the expression of biochemical products which further contribute to immunotherapeutic responses by inducing specific cancer-related signaling pathways. *B. fragilis* induces inflammation via prostaglandin E2 (PGE2) resulting in activation of the oncogenic Signal transducer and activator of transcription 3 (STAT-3) signaling pathway which modulates cancer cell proliferation. *F. nucleatum*-positive tumors have an abundance of KRAS mutations and a smaller percentage of BRAF mutations. These mutations are linked to the activation of the MAPK signaling pathway associated with cancer proliferation. *F. nucleatum* halts cancer progression by promoting increased expression of PD-L1 by tumors and therefore increasing their sensitivity to immunotherapy. Protein kinase B (Akt), Mitogen-activated protein kinase (MAPK), Kirsten rat sarcoma viral oncogene homolog (KRAS), Immune checkpoint Inhibitor (ICI).

transplantation (FMT) from responder NSCLC patients were also positive for *Akk* regardless of PD-L1 expression compared to non-responder FMT (Derosa et al., 2022).

Ruminococcaceae

Ruminococcaceae are a group of anaerobic commensal Gram-positive gut microbiota residing in the colonic mucosal biofilm. The species is responsible for the maintenance of gut health and is associated with modulation of immunotherapy responses in several solid cancers including pancreatic ductal adenocarcinoma (PDAC) and metastatic melanoma mouse model (Qi et al., 2022). Ruminococcaceae (p = 0.03) was amongst bacterium such as Barnesiellaceae (p = 0.02), and Tannerellaceae (p = 0.03) with higher percentages and lower levels of Clostridiaceae (p = 0.03) in NSCLC patients with disease control during first-line immunotherapy. However, the risk of mortality increased with the abundance of Ruminococcaceae family (p < 0.0001) and low abundance of Clostridaceae (p = 0.005) (Grenda et al., 2022).

The role of polyphenols in overcoming resistance to oncotherapies is described in detail elsewhere (Maleki Dana et al., 2022). Castalagin is the active compound in the polyphenol-rich berry camu-camu (*Myrciaria dubia*). Castalagin was shown to have a preference for binding to the cellular envelope of *Ruminococcus*. Syngeneic C57BL/6 mice were implanted subcutaneously with MCA-205 Sarcoma and E0771 Breast Cancer cells FMT from different non-responding NSCLC patients and later treated with αPD-1 or isotype control with or without Castalagin or water. Castalagin-induced abundance of Ruminococcaceae and *Alistipes* associated with the efficacy of anti-PD-1 therapy by suppressing the expression/recruitment of Tregs in the tumor microenvironment. Additionally, obesity is known as one of the risk factors for cancer initiation and progression. Castalagin contributed to the enhancement of metabolic activity through the upregulation of taurine-conjugated bile acids. The study provided evidence that supplementation of castalagin followed by FMT from ICI-refractory patients could enhance anti-PD-1 activity thus suggesting castalagin as a prebiotic to assist in resistance to anti-PD-1 inhibition (Messaoudene et al., 2022).

HPV-RELATED IMMUNOTHERAPEUTIC RESISTANCE

Human Papillomavirus (HPV)

HPV is responsible for 26% of new gastrointestinal tract incidences globally with the highest prevalence in colon cancer. HPV is associated with the occurrence of oral, pharyngeal, and anal cancers, and is a provocative risk factor for esophageal, gastric, liver, and colorectal cancers. HPV infects the cutaneous or the basal epithelial cells of the mucosa by entering their nucleus through the attachment of their L1 and L2 capsid proteins to epithelial cell receptors (Baj et al., 2022). The HPV high-risk types—HPV 16, 18, 31, 33, and 45—are associated with the occurrence of genital, anal, laryngeal, oral, esophageal, and probably gastric cancers (Fakhraei et al., 2016). The presence of HPV oncoproteins E6 and E7 facilitates the epithelial cell cycle which increases viral replication (Lin et al., 2020). The HPV status is of great prognostic significance in head and neck squamous cell carcinoma (HNSCC). However, despite advancements in research, the contribution of HPV in the pathogenesis of HNSCC as well as other cancers is underutilized for the modification of treatment guidelines or successful development of immunotherapy targeting HPV cancers. (Wang et al., 2019).

A significant increase in tumor-infiltrating T cells (TILs), activation of immune effector cells, and T-cell receptors diversity was observed in HPV-positive (HPV+) HNSCC indicating constant/chronic inflammatory responses associated with HPV infection (Wang et al., 2019). An increase in TILs and PD-L1 overexpression in HPV+ oropharyngeal squamous cell carcinomas (OSCC) compared to HPV-negative (HPV-) OSCC distinguished the immunologically hot and cold status of HPV+ and HPV- tumors, respectively (Tosi et al., 2022). The immunologically hot tumors create a favorable environment for immunotherapy, especially the ICIs. In the presence of high levels of TILs, ICIs disrupt the immune checkpoint axis as a result suppressing immune evasion and promoting antitumor immunity. The ICIs monotherapy is more effective in hot tumors as compared to cold tumors (Wang et al., 2023). Another study reported the increased expression of PD-1, lymphocyte activation gene-3 (LAG-3), T cell immunoglobulin mucin-3 (TIM-3), and T cell immunoglobulin and ITIM domain (TIGIT) in HPV+ HNSCC than in HPV- HNSCC, which could generate a therapeutic benefit as ICIs target these molecules (Gameiro et al., 2018).

The HNSCC patients who are HPV+ demonstrated an improved response rate and OS. This was indicated by a meta-analysis study that showed that HPV+ cancer patients have greater chances of responding to immunotherapy as compared to HPV- patients with a risk ratio of 1.29. The study reported an OS of 11.5 months in HPV+ patients which was greater than the 6.3 months OS of HPV- patients (Galvis et al., 2020). These clinical outcomes were also shown to be associated with PD-L1 expression levels (Galvis et al., 2020, Seiwert et al., 2016). However, the association of immunotherapy response with the presence of HPV remains controversial as it was also stated that immunotherapy can improve clinical outcomes regardless of HPV status (Julian et al., 2021). Nevertheless, this is a promising indication that patients with HPV-associated malignancies may benefit from ICIs. The presence of these controversies warrants the need for more research to improve the availability of data and to provide further clarification and understanding (Pharaon et al., 2021).

A phase Ib/II clinical trial evaluating MEDI0457 (DNA immunotherapy targeting HPV16/18 E6/E7 with IL-12 encoding plasmids) immunotherapy in 22 patients with advanced p16+ HNSCC reported that 18 patients showed high IFNγ levels suggesting an increase in antigen-specific T-cell activity (Aggarwal et al., 2019). Furthermore, MEDI0457 was found to induce HPV-specific CD8+ T cells with a shift of CD8+/FoxP3+ ratio in four of five tumor samples post immunotherapy. An induction in HPV16-specific PD-1+ CD8+ T cells was observed in a metastatic disease treated with anti-PD-1 therapy (Aggarwal et al., 2019). This shows immunotherapy targeting HPV such as MEDI0457 can generate strong HPV antigen-specific immune responses with the potential to improve clinical outcomes in HPV-associated HNSCC. Another study investigating the predictive value of HPV status for ICIs treatment reported more benefit from PD-1/PD-L1 inhibitors in HPV+ than HPV- patients with an objective response rate of 21.9% and 14.1%, respectively, with odds ratio of 1.79, p = 0.01 (Wang et al., 2019). This demonstrates the beneficial effect of HPV status in predicting the effectiveness of PD-1 inhibitors in HNSCC.

The use of engineered T cell receptor (TCR) T cells to target HPV+ cancers in an effort to improve clinical outcomes of HPV+ cancer patients is being evaluated, including in clinical trials with some still ongoing. A genetically engineered T cell containing the dominant E6-reactive TCR clonotype sequence from PBMCs of HPV16+ anal cancer patients showed specific recognition and killing of HPV-16+ cervical, head, and neck cancer cell lines (Draper et al., 2015). This may pave the way for the development of possible novel immunotherapy that is specific to HPV16+ cancers in different anatomical sites. Another genetically engineered T cell expressing HPV-16

E7-specific HLA-A*02:01-restricted TCR from cervical cancer was shown to kill HPV-16+ cervical and oropharyngeal cancer cell lines regressed tumors in a mouse model of HPV16+ human cervical cancer (Jin et al., 2018). This finding has led to a phase I/II trial of TCR gene therapy targeting HPV-16 E7 for HPV-associated cancers (NCT02858310), which is still ongoing.

Also, the diversity and relative abundance of TCR repertoire genes was investigated in women with HPV16+ cervical cancer of grade 3 or higher (CIN3+) compared to women who cleared an incident HPV16 infection without developing precancer/cancer using NGS technology (Lang Kuhs et al., 2018). Interestingly, the findings showed differences in TCR repertoire were greater in women with CIN3+ as compared to disease-free women who cleared the incidental HPV16 infection, thus suggesting a significantly different TCR repertoire in the two cohorts (Lang Kuhs et al., 2018). In summary, HPV+ cancers pose a great challenge to immunotherapy due to its complex nature in modifying the tumor microenvironment through immune effector cells, and therefore it is important to consider a combination of different immunotherapeutic approaches in treating cancers based on their HPV status.

CLINICAL APPLICATIONS AND STRATEGIES TO OVERCOME RESISTANCE

FMT is suggested as one of the potential therapies that can be utilized to overcome ICIs resistance. FMT in combination with anti-PD1 proved safe for the treatment of patients with pancreatic cancer (Unknown, 2023). Donor feces are manipulated to correct microbial dysbiosis in the recipient for health benefits. The efficacy of ICI responder-derived FMT was tested in preclinical germ-free mouse models (Matson et al., 2018). Following this, human studies have interrogated whether this is species-specific and have shown that every cancer has a specific microbial taxon that affects the response to anti-PD-1 immunotherapy. Thus several clinical trials (Table 5.1) have been conducted to evaluate the effect of gut microbiome modulation on cases such as anti-PD-1 refractory melanoma (NCT03341143). Sero-matched patients with primary refractory melanoma were treated with responder-derived FMT along with Pembrolizumab. Patients experienced no unusual toxicity. The response to therapy was directly proportional to the abundance of microbial taxa associated with a positive response rate and an increase in anticancer immune response via the activation of CD8+ T cells and reduced IL-8 expressing myeloid cells (Davar et al., 2021).

Microbial Ecosystem Therapeutics (MET) is a newly developed alternative treatment of FMT. Its advantage over FMT is the ability to scale up the production of microbiota. Thus a 30-species microbial consortium (Microbial Ecosystem Therapeutic 4, MET4) was administered in combination with ICIs in an early-phase clinical trial to assess safety, tolerability, and ecological responses. The efficacy of this combination therapy is to be interrogated in phase II clinical trials in other solid cancers. What was noticed in this study was the abundance of microbial taxa varied amongst patients and this correlated with response to ICI therapy (Spreafico et al., 2023).

CHALLENGES AND LIMITATIONS

Several studies have indicated the contribution of microbiota in promoting immunosuppression linked to cancer progression. The positive immunotherapeutic response is shown to be directly proportional to microbial dysbiosis which in turn influences the expression of some immune checkpoints markers (Aghamajidi and Maleki Vareki, 2022). For instance, equal frequencies of *Clostridium* species and *B. fragilis* was shown to promote intestinal induced Tregs (iTregs). The production of SCFAs including butyrate by the former was shown to be responsible for the induction of iTregs. With regards to *B. fragilis*, only polysaccharide A (PSA)-expressing strains could induce iTregs formation through the activation of toll-like receptor 2. Correlating this to immunotherapeutic responses, PD-L1 in particular induces iTregs differentiation via the expression of Foxp3 and inhibition of the PI3K/protein kinase B (Akt)/mTOR signaling cascade and upregulates phosphatase and tensin homolog (PTEN) to promote the transformation of iTregs (Dai et al., 2020).

A specific set of microbial signatures that are associated with immune modulation and therapeutic response to ICIs have not been fully established. There is a high discrepancy in microbiota taxa within the same cancers and at times in the same study cohorts. In an attempt to resolve this discrepancy, a study generated a common signature from their study cohort (MELRESIST) and three other studies, and reported that the signature they identified had strong evidence of predicting ICIs response with 91% accuracy compared to the other three studies (Villemin et al., 2023). Therefore, treatment with microbiota to sensitize patients to immunotherapy might be species specific depending on the cancer type. These might not be the only challenge as treatment by FMT is mostly invasive and administered via the gastrointestinal tract using esophagogastroduodenoscopy (EGD), colonoscopy, feeding tubes, or rectal enemas. The choice of EGD requires the practitioner to be cautious when administering FMT in patients with a history of gastrointestinal surgery as these patients might develop adverse events including aspiration (Dai et al., 2020). There are other safety concerns associated with FMT, such as the potential transfer of pathogens as a patient has previously died from this procedure. The long-term effects of FMT are not known as gut microbiota is unique for each patient and FMT effects vary (Xu et al., 2022).

FUTURE DIRECTIONS

The gut microbiome is a crucial modulator of tumor development, progression and therapy response (Pandey and Khan, 2023). These microorganisms induce T cell responses (Duarte Mendes et al., 2022) or utilize certain

TABLE 5.1
Clinical trials assessing safety and efficacy of microbial transplantation in immunotherapy resistant cancers

Cancer	ICI	Treatment plan	Outcome measures	Trial ID
Melanoma	Pembrolizumab or Nivolumab	Patients received FMT a week prior to treatment with ICIs.	Assessment of treatment effect on antitumor activity, on commensal gut microbiome, on CD4 /CD8 T cells levels and on ICIs (PD-1, PD-L1, TIM-3, LAG-3, TIGIT and BTLA) on CD8 T cells and the expression of HLA-DR CD38, and CD28.	NCT03772899
Advanced solid tumors	Any approved immunotherapy for the specific solid cancer	The study is a proof-of-concept trial recruiting patients already on immunotherapy and those who will be placed on immunotherapy.	The ultimate objective is to develop microbiome biomarkers for cancer immunotherapy. Overall response rate will be evaluated by assessing tumor progression every 4–8 weeks for up to 6 months	NCT04264975
Stage III / IV resected melanoma	Any approved PD-1/ PD-L1 inhibitors	MET-4 was administered with anti-PD1 alone or in combination with anti-CTLA-4 for 1 week, and maximum of 2 weeks prior ICIs treatment until unacceptable toxicity, confirmed PD or completion of 1 year ICIs. treatment.	The study assessed the safety, tolerability, and engraftment of MET-4 strains when given in combination with ICIs.	NCT03686202
Melanoma	Pembrolizumab Anti-PD-1 treatment	Patients will receive FMT from an ICI responding donor.	Tumor immune infiltration, abundance of gut microbiome and CD8 + PD1+ T cells will be measured and ORR, PFS, and OS assessed.	NCT03341143 NCT05251389
Not specified	Not specified	Non-responding stage IV cancer patients will receive a single-dose FMT after at least full cycle of ICI therapy.	Change in the intestinal microbiome community, response rate to microbial change and frequency of circulating tumor infiltrating and intestinal immune cells.	NCT05273255
Melanoma, NSCLC, CSCC, HNSCC, renal clear cell carcinoma, or MSI+ solid cancer	PD1/PD-L1 and/or CTLA-4 and/or LAG-3 inhibitors, or combinations thereof.	FMT treatment plan not outlined.	Safety assessed as a measure of incidence, nature, and severity of adverse events and response measured by OS, ORR, and PFS. Assessment of immunological markers and microbial composition will be performed.	NCT05286294
Genitourinary, melanoma, lung, ovarian, uterine, cervical, and breast cancers	Any ICI	FMT will be administered via colonoscopy.	This study is unique in that it focuses on assessing safety and the efficacy of FMT in ICI induced diarrhea or colitis in cancer. Frequency of immune cells such as CD4 and CD8 T cells, Tregs cells, macrophages and cytokine levels will be measured in tissue/blood/stool samples.	NCT04038619
Lung cancer	PD-L1 in combination with chemotherapy	Oral administration of 10 FMT capsules in the morning and afternoon when starting chemo-immunotherapy cycle then every 3 weeks.	Quantification of serum antibody levels and lymphocyte levels will be performed.	NCT05502913

Immune checkpoint inhibitor (ICI), Overall survival (OS), objective tumor response rate (ORR), progression-free survival (PFS), B and T lymphocyte attenuator (BTLA), and human leucocyte antigens (HLA).

metabolites that modulate immunological pathways leading to an improved immunotherapeutic response or resistance. The ability of microbiota to improve immunotherapeutic response or resistance is attributed to its composition (Hersi et al., 2022). Modulating the gut microbiota may improve ICIs response (Duarte Mendes et al., 2022) and FMT is one of the methods of manipulating the gut microbiome to improve immunotherapeutic response (Li et al., 2022). However, FMT is associated with safety concerns such as transferring pathogens from donor to recipient as well as the uncertainty of its long-term effects. This can be resolved by screening donor microbiota using FDA-approved guidelines before transferring into patients (Xu et al., 2022). The existing data indicate that the role of HPV in the modulation of immunotherapy remains controversial and this requires more research to address the effect of HPV on immunotherapy response (Pharaon et al., 2021). The gut microbiota is not well characterized, and therefore future research should focus on improving knowledge by characterizing gut microbiota and their mechanism of action in immunotherapy response (Sampsell et al., 2020).

CONCLUSION

Immunotherapy has demonstrated a therapeutic advantage in medical oncology; however, resistance is still a bottleneck in its application. The gut microbiome composition and diversity have an integral role in cancer immunotherapy resistance or response. Thus understanding the various mechanisms of the gut microbiota in modulating immune responses and ultimate therapeutic responses can assist in developing therapeutic strategies for circumventing immunotherapy resistance. Preclinical mouse model studies have demonstrated that modulation of immunotherapy response via administration of FMT has beneficial effects in overcoming immunotherapy resistance in several cancers. Several studies have also indicated that different cancers have different species of microbiota. Current clinical trial studies isolating microbiota from patients responding positively to immunotherapy have also shown that the composition of the microbiome can be cancer specific. Thus FMT could be a promising future targeted therapy that could mainly be utilized to decipher immunotherapy resistance. However, there are concerns associated with FMT therapy such as safety concerns which can be resolved through screening of the donor microbiota, improved methods of stool processing and analysis, and lastly by tailoring FMT therapy for specific types of cancers in alignment or consideration of the individual's own microbial composition. Diet and lifestyle supporting the growth and activity of the desired microbiota can be incorporated to enhance immunotherapeutic effects (Figure 5.3).

REFERENCES

AGGARWAL, C., COHEN, R. B., MORROW, M. P., KRAYNYAK, K. A., SYLVESTER, A. J., KNOBLOCK, D. M., BAUML, J. M., WEINSTEIN, G. S., LIN, A., BOYER, J., SAKATA, L., TAN, S., ANTON, A., DICKERSON, K., MANGROLIA, D., VANG, R., DALLAS, M., OYOLA, S., DUFF, S., ESSER, M., KUMAR, R., WEINER, D., CSIKI, I. & BAGARAZZI, M. L. 2019. Immunotherapy targeting HPV16/18 generates potent immune responses in HPV-associated head and neck cancer. *Clin Cancer Res*, 25, 110–124.

AGHAMAJIDI, A. & MALEKI VAREKI, S. 2022. The effect of the Gut microbiota on systemic and anti-tumor immunity and response to systemic therapy against cancer. *Cancers (Basel)*, 14(15):3563.

ALON-MAIMON, T., MANDELBOIM, O. & BACHRACH, G. 2022. Fusobacterium nucleatum and cancer. *Periodontology 2000*, 89, 166–180.

ARAJI, G., MAAMARI, J., AHMAD, F. A., ZAREEF, R., CHAFTARI, P. & YEUNG, S. J. 2022. The emerging role of the Gut microbiome in the cancer response to immune checkpoint inhibitors: a narrative review. *J Immunother Precis Oncol*, 5, 13–25.

BAI, R., LV, Z., XU, D. & CUI, J. 2020. Predictive biomarkers for cancer immunotherapy with immune checkpoint inhibitors. *Biomark Res*, 8, 34.

BAJ, J., FORMA, A., DUDEK, I., CHILIMONIUK, Z., DOBOSZ, M., DOBRZYŃSKI, M., TERESIŃSKI, G., BUSZEWICZ, G., FLIEGER, J. & PORTINCASA, P. 2022. The involvement of human Papilloma Virus in gastrointestinal cancers. *Cancers (Basel)*, 14(11):2607.

BHATT, A. P., REDINBO, M. R. & BULTMAN, S. J. 2017. The role of the microbiome in cancer development and therapy. *CA Cancer J Clin*, 67, 326–344.

BOROWSKY, J., HARUKI, K., LAU, M. C., DIAS COSTA, A., VÄYRYNEN, J. P., UGAI, T., ARIMA, K., DA SILVA, A., FELT, K. D., ZHAO, M., GURJAO, C., TWOMBLY, T. S., FUJIYOSHI, K., VÄYRYNEN, S. A., HAMADA, T., MIMA, K., BULLMAN, S., HARRISON, T. A., PHIPPS, A. I., PETERS, U., NG, K., MEYERHARDT, J. A., SONG, M., GIOVANNUCCI, E. L., WU, K., ZHANG, X., FREEMAN, G. J., HUTTENHOWER, C., GARRETT, W. S., CHAN, A. T., LEGGETT, B. A., WHITEHALL, V. L. J., WALKER, N., BROWN, I., BETTINGTON, M., NISHIHARA, R., FUCHS, C. S., LENNERZ, J. K., GIANNAKIS, M., NOWAK, J. A. & OGINO, S. 2021. Association of Fusobacterium nucleatum with specific T-cell subsets in the colorectal carcinoma microenvironment. *Clin Cancer Res*, 27, 2816–2826.

CHENG, W. T., KANTILAL, H. K. & DAVAMANI, F. 2020. The mechanism of bacteroides fragilis toxin contributes to colon cancer formation. *Malays J Med Sci*, 27, 9–21.

DAI, Z., ZHANG, J., WU, Q., FANG, H., SHI, C., LI, Z., LIN, C., TANG, D. & WANG, D. 2020. Intestinal microbiota: a new force in cancer immunotherapy. *Cell Commun Signal*, 18, 90.

DAVAR, D., DZUTSEV, A., MCCULLOCH, J. A., RODRIGUES, R. R., CHAUVIN, J.-M., MORRISON, R. M., DEBLASIO, R. N., MENNA, C., DING, Q., PAGLIANO, O., ZIDI, B., ZHANG, S., BADGER, J. H., VETIZOU, M., COLE, A. M., FERNANDES, M. R., PRESCOTT, S., COSTA, R. G., BALAJI, A. K., MORGUN, A., VUJKOVIC-CVIJIN, I., WANG, H., BORHANI, A. A., SCHWARTZ, M. B., DUBNER, H. M., ERNST, S. J., ROSE, A., NAJJAR, Y. G., BELKAID, Y., KIRKWOOD, J. M., TRINCHIERI, G. & ZAROUR, H. M. 2021. Abstract LB062: efficacy of Responder-derived Fecal Microbiota Transplant (R-FMT) and pembrolizumab in anti-PD-1 refractory patients with advanced melanoma. *Cancer Res*, 81, LB062–LB062.

DENARDO, D. G. & RUFFELL, B. 2019. Macrophages as regulators of tumour immunity and immunotherapy. *Nat Rev Immunol*, 19, 369–382.

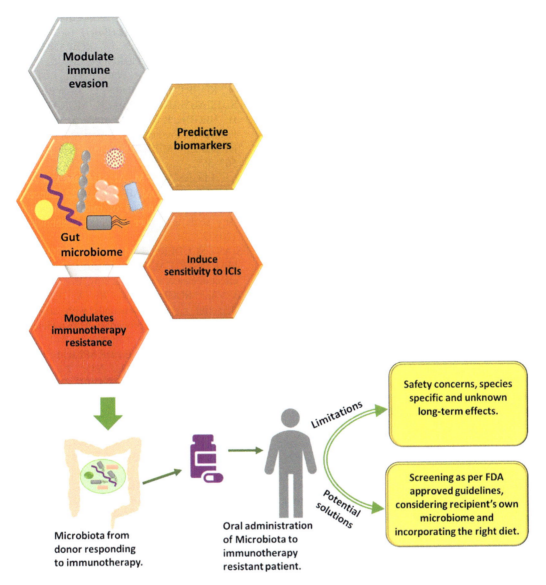

FIGURE 5.3 **Summary of the modulation of gut microbiome as a potential tool to circumvent anti-ICI resistance in cancers.** The gut microbiome is involved in the modulation of the immune system and concomitant immunotherapy resistance. Moreover, specific sets of microbes can be utilized as potential predictive biomarkers as well as therapeutic strategies to improve sensitivity to immune checkpoint inhibitor (ICI) therapy. Strategies to improve patients' response to immunotherapy include the administration of fecal microbial transplantation (FMT) whereby stools from patients responding to immunotherapy are processed and administered to patients with resistant cancers. However, the use of FMT is limited by the concerns around safety, the diverse composition of microbiota which has shown that cancers are species-specific, and unknown long-term effects. Attempts to resolve these challenges might include standardization of vigorous screening methods of donor samples to isolate specific microbes that can benefit a specific individual (considering the recipient's own microbial composition) with a specific type of cancer and incorporating the right diet and lifestyle to support the survival of the desired microbiota.

DENG, F., LI, Y. & ZHAO, J. 2019. The gut microbiome of healthy long-living people. *Aging (Albany NY),* 11, 289–290.

DEROSA, L., ROUTY, B., THOMAS, A. M., IEBBA, V., ZALCMAN, G., FRIARD, S., MAZIERES, J., AUDIGIER-VALETTE, C., MORO-SIBILOT, D., GOLDWASSER, F., SILVA, C. A. C., TERRISSE, S., BONVALET, M., SCHERPEREEL, A., PEGLIASCO, H., RICHARD, C., GHIRINGHELLI, F., ELKRIEF, A., DESILETS, A., BLANC-DURAND, F., CUMBO, F., BLANCO, A., BOIDOT, R., CHEVRIER, S., DAILLÈRE, R., KROEMER, G., ALLA, L., PONS, N., LE CHATELIER, E., GALLERON, N., ROUME, H., DUBUISSON, A., BOUCHARD, N., MESSAOUDENE, M., DRUBAY, D., DEUTSCH, E., BARLESI, F., PLANCHARD, D., SEGATA, N., MARTINEZ, S., ZITVOGEL, L., SORIA, J. C. & BESSE, B. 2022. Intestinal Akkermansia muciniphila predicts clinical response to PD-1 blockade in patients with advanced non-small-cell lung cancer. *Nat Med,* 28, 315–324.

DO VALE, A., CABANES, D. & SOUSA, S. 2016. Bacterial toxins as pathogen weapons against phagocytes. *Front Microbiol,* 7, 42.

DRAPER, L. M., KWONG, M. L., GROS, A., STEVANOVIĆ, S., TRAN, E., KERKAR, S., RAFFELD, M., ROSENBERG, S. A. & HINRICHS, C. S. 2015. Targeting of HPV-16+ epithelial cancer cells by TCR gene engineered T cells directed against E6. *Clin Cancer Res*, 21, 4431–4439.

DUARTE MENDES, A., VICENTE, R., VITORINO, M., SILVA, M. & ALPUIM COSTA, D. 2022. Modulation of tumor environment in colorectal cancer – could gut microbiota be a key player? *Front Gastroenterol*, 1.

FAKHRAEI, F., HAGHSHENAS, M. R., HOSSEINI, V., RAFIEI, A., NAGHSHVAR, F. & ALIZADEH-NAVAEI, R. 2016. Detection of human papillomavirus DNA in gastric carcinoma specimens in a high-risk region of Iran. *Biomed Rep*, 5, 371–375.

FLUCKIGER, A., DAILLÈRE, R., SASSI, M., SIXT, B. S., LIU, P., LOOS, F., RICHARD, C., RABU, C., ALOU, M. T., GOUBET, A. G., LEMAITRE, F., FERRERE, G., DEROSA, L., DUONG, C. P. M., MESSAOUDENE, M., GAGNÉ, A., JOUBERT, P., DE SORDI, L., DEBARBIEUX, L., SIMON, S., SCARLATA, C. M., AYYOUB, M., PALERMO, B., FACCIOLO, F., BOIDOT, R., WHEELER, R., BONECA, I. G., SZTUPINSZKI, Z., PAPP, K., CSABAI, I., PASOLLI, E., SEGATA, N., LOPEZ-OTIN, C., SZALLASI, Z., ANDRE, F., IEBBA, V., QUINIOU, V., KLATZMANN, D., BOUKHALIL, J., KHELAIFIA, S., RAOULT, D., ALBIGES, L., ESCUDIER, B., EGGERMONT, A., MAMI-CHOUAIB, F., NISTICO, P., GHIRINGHELLI, F., ROUTY, B., LABARRIÈRE, N., CATTOIR, V., KROEMER, G. & ZITVOGEL, L. 2020. Cross-reactivity between tumor MHC class I-restricted antigens and an enterococcal bacteriophage. *Science*, 369, 936–942.

GALVIS, M. M., BORGES, G. A., OLIVEIRA, T. B. D., TOLEDO, I. P. D., CASTILHO, R. M., GUERRA, E. N. S., KOWALSKI, L. P. & SQUARIZE, C. H. 2020. Immunotherapy improves efficacy and safety of patients with HPV positive and negative head and neck cancer: a systematic review and meta-analysis. *Crit Rev Oncol/Hematol*, 150, 102966.

GAMEIRO, S. F., GHASEMI, F., BARRETT, J. W., KOROPATNICK, J., NICHOLS, A. C., MYMRYK, J. S. & MALEKI VAREKI, S. 2018. Treatment-naïve HPV+ head and neck cancers display a T-cell-inflamed phenotype distinct from their HPV- counterparts that has implications for immunotherapy. *Oncoimmunology*, 7, e1498439.

GAO, Y., BI, D., XIE, R., LI, M., GUO, J., LIU, H., GUO, X., FANG, J., DING, T., ZHU, H., CAO, Y., XING, M., ZHENG, J., XU, Q., XU, Q., WEI, Q. & QIN, H. 2021. Fusobacterium nucleatum enhances the efficacy of PD-L1 blockade in colorectal cancer. *Signal Transduct Target Ther*, 6, 398.

GRENDA, A., IWAN, E., KRAWCZYK, P., FRĄK, M., CHMIELEWSKA, I., BOMBA, A., GIZA, A., ROLSKA-KOPIŃSKA, A., SZCZYREK, M., KIESZKO, R., KUCHARCZYK, T., JAROSZ, B., WASYL, D. & MILANOWSKI, J. 2022. Attempting to identify bacterial allies in immunotherapy of NSCLC patients. *Cancers (Basel)*, 14(24):6250.

HAGHI, F., GOLI, E., MIRZAEI, B. & ZEIGHAMI, H. 2019. The association between fecal enterotoxigenic B. fragilis with colorectal cancer. *BMC Cancer*, 19, 879.

HANAHAN, D. 2022. Hallmarks of cancer: new dimensions. *Cancer Discovery*, 12, 31–46.

HE, Y., HUANG, J., LI, Q., XIA, W., ZHANG, C., LIU, Z., XIAO, J., YI, Z., DENG, H., XIAO, Z., HU, J., LI, H., ZU, X., QUAN, C. & CHEN, J. 2022. Gut microbiota and tumor immune escape: a new perspective for improving tumor immunotherapy. *Cancers (Basel)*, 14(21):5317.

HERBST, R. S., SORIA, J. C., KOWANETZ, M., FINE, G. D., HAMID, O., GORDON, M. S., SOSMAN, J. A., MCDERMOTT, D. F., POWDERLY, J. D., GETTINGER, S. N., KOHRT, H. E., HORN, L., LAWRENCE, D. P., ROST, S., LEABMAN, M., XIAO, Y., MOKATRIN, A., KOEPPEN, H., HEGDE, P. S., MELLMAN, I., CHEN, D. S. & HODI, F. S. 2014. Predictive correlates of response to the anti-PD-L1 antibody MPDL3280A in cancer patients. *Nature*, 515, 563–567.

HERSI, F., ELGENDY, S. M., AL SHAMMA, S. A., ALTELL, R. T., SADIEK, O. & OMAR, H. A. 2022. Cancer immunotherapy resistance: The impact of microbiome-derived short-chain fatty acids and other emerging metabolites. *Life Sci*, 300, 120573.

IGLESIAS-ESCUDERO, M., ARIAS-GONZÁLEZ, N. & MARTÍNEZ-CÁCERES, E. 2023. Regulatory cells and the effect of cancer immunotherapy. *Mol Cancer*, 22, 26.

JENAB, A., ROGHANIAN, R. & EMTIAZI, G. 2020. Bacterial natural compounds with anti-inflammatory and immunomodulatory properties (Mini review). *Drug Des Devel Ther*, 14, 3787–3801.

JIN, B. Y., CAMPBELL, T. E., DRAPER, L. M., STEVANOVIĆ, S., WEISSBRICH, B., YU, Z., RESTIFO, N. P., ROSENBERG, S. A., TRIMBLE, C. L. & HINRICHS, C. S. 2018. Engineered T cells targeting E7 mediate regression of human papillomavirus cancers in a murine model. *JCI Insight*, 3.

JULIAN, R., SAVANI, M. & BAUMAN, J. E. 2021. Immunotherapy approaches in HPV-associated head and neck cancer. *Cancers (Basel)*, 13(23):5889.

KIM, H. S., KIM, C. G., KIM, W. K., KIM, K.-A., YOO, J., MIN, B. S., PAIK, S., SHIN, S. J., LEE, H., LEE, K., KIM, H., SHIN, E.-C., KIM, T.-M. & AHN, J. B. 2023. Fusobacterium nucleatum induces a tumor microenvironment with diminished adaptive immunity against colorectal cancers. *Front Cell Infect Microbiol*, 13.

LANG KUHS, K. A., LIN, S. W., HUA, X., SCHIFFMAN, M., BURK, R. D., RODRIGUEZ, A. C., HERRERO, R., ABNET, C. C., FREEDMAN, N. D., PINTO, L. A., HAMM, D., ROBINS, H., HILDESHEIM, A., SHI, J. & SAFAEIAN, M. 2018. T cell receptor repertoire among women who cleared and failed to clear cervical human papillomavirus infection: an exploratory proof-of-principle study. *PLoS One*, 13, e0178167.

LI, X., ZHANG, S., GUO, G., HAN, J. & YU, J. 2022. Gut microbiome in modulating immune checkpoint inhibitors. *EBio Med*, 82, 104163.

LICHTENSTERN, C. R. & LAMICHHANE-KHADKA, R. 2023. A tale of two bacteria – Bacteroides fragilis, Escherichia coli, and colorectal cancer. *FrontBacteriol*, 2.

LIN, D., KOUZY, R., ABI JAOUDE, J., NOTICEWALA, S. S., DELGADO MEDRANO, A. Y., KLOPP, A. H., TANIGUCHI, C. M. & COLBERT, L. E. 2020. Microbiome factors in HPV-driven carcinogenesis and cancers. *PLoS Pathog*, 16, e1008524.

MALEKI DANA, P., SADOUGHI, F., ASEMI, Z. & YOUSEFI, B. 2022. The role of polyphenols in overcoming cancer drug resistance: a comprehensive review. *Cell Mol Biol Lett*, 27, 1.

MATSON, V., FESSLER, J., BAO, R., CHONGSUWAT, T., ZHA, Y., ALEGRE, M. L., LUKE, J. J. & GAJEWSKI, T. F. 2018. The commensal microbiome is associated with anti-PD-1 efficacy in metastatic melanoma patients. *Science*, 359, 104–108.

MESSAOUDENE, M., PIDGEON, R., RICHARD, C., PONCE, M., DIOP, K., BENLAIFAOUI, M., NOLIN-LAPALME, A., CAUCHOIS, F., MALO, J., BELKAID, W., ISNARD, S., FRADET, Y., DRIDI, L., VELIN, D., OSTER, P., RAOULT, D., GHIRINGHELLI, F., BOIDOT, R., CHEVRIER, S., KYSELA, D. T., BRUN, Y. V., FALCONE, E. L., PILON, G., OÑATE, F. P., GITTON-QUENT, O., LE CHATELIER, E., DURAND, S., KROEMER, G., ELKRIEF, A., MARETTE, A., CASTAGNER, B. & ROUTY, B. 2022. A natural polyphenol exerts antitumor activity and circumvents anti–PD-1 resistance through effects on the Gut microbiota. *Cancer Discov*, 12, 1070–1087.

MOLAAGHAEE-ROUZBAHANI, S., ASRI, N., SAPONE, A., BAGHAEI, K., YADEGAR, A., AMANI, D. & ROSTAMI-NEJAD, M. 2023. Akkermansia muciniphila exerts immunomodulatory and anti-inflammatory effects on gliadin-stimulated THP-1 derived macrophages. *Sci Rep*, 13, 3237.

PANDEY, P. & KHAN, F. 2023. Gut microbiome in cancer immunotherapy: current trends, translational challenges and future possibilities. *Biochim Biophys Acta (BBA) – Gen Subj*, 1867, 130401.

PHARAON, R. R., XING, Y., AGULNIK, M. & VILLAFLOR, V. M. 2021. The role of immunotherapy to overcome resistance in viral-associated head and neck cancer. *Front Oncol*, 11, 649963.

QI, X., LIU, Y., HUSSEIN, S., CHOI, G., KIMCHI, E. T., STAVELEY-O'CARROLL, K. F. & LI, G. 2022. The species of Gut bacteria associated with antitumor immunity in cancer therapy. *Cells*, 11, 3684.

RODRIGUES, V. F., ELIAS-OLIVEIRA, J., PEREIRA Í, S., PEREIRA, J. A., BARBOSA, S. C., MACHADO, M. S. G. & CARLOS, D. 2022. Akkermansia muciniphila and Gut immune system: a good friendship that attenuates inflammatory Bowel disease, obesity, and diabetes. *Front Immunol*, 13, 934695.

ROUTY, B., LE CHATELIER, E., DEROSA, L., DUONG, C. P. M., ALOU, M. T., DAILLÈRE, R., FLUCKIGER, A., MESSAOUDENE, M., RAUBER, C., ROBERTI, M. P., FIDELLE, M., FLAMENT, C., POIRIER-COLAME, V., OPOLON, P., KLEIN, C., IRIBARREN, K., MONDRAGÓN, L., JACQUELOT, N., QU, B., FERRERE, G., CLÉMENSON, C., MEZQUITA, L., MASIP, J. R., NALTET, C., BROSSEAU, S., KADERBHAI, C., RICHARD, C., RIZVI, H., LEVENEZ, F., GALLERON, N., QUINQUIS, B., PONS, N., RYFFEL, B., MINARD-COLIN, V., GONIN, P., SORIA, J.-C., DEUTSCH, E., LORIOT, Y., GHIRINGHELLI, F., ZALCMAN, G., GOLDWASSER, F., ESCUDIER, B., HELLMANN, M. D., EGGERMONT, A., RAOULT, D., ALBIGES, L., KROEMER, G. & ZITVOGEL, L. 2018. Gut microbiome influences efficacy of PD-1–based immunotherapy against epithelial tumors. *Science*, 359, 91–97.

SAMPSELL, K., HAO, D. & REIMER, R. A. 2020. The Gut microbiota: a potential gateway to improved health outcomes in breast cancer treatment and survivorship. *Int J Mol Sci*, 21(23):9239.

SEIWERT, T. Y., BURTNESS, B., MEHRA, R., WEISS, J., BERGER, R., EDER, J. P., HEATH, K., MCCLANAHAN, T., LUNCEFORD, J., GAUSE, C., CHENG, J. D. & CHOW, L. Q. 2016. Safety and clinical activity of pembrolizumab for treatment of recurrent or metastatic squamous cell carcinoma of the head and neck (KEYNOTE-012): an open-label, multicentre, phase 1b trial. *Lancet Oncol*, 17, 956–965.

SHARIATI, A., RAZAVI, S., GHAZNAVI-RAD, E., JAHANBIN, B., AKBARI, A., NORZAEE, S. & DARBAN-SAROKHALIL, D. 2021. Association between colorectal cancer and Fusobacterium nucleatum and Bacteroides fragilis bacteria in Iranian patients: a preliminary study. *Infect Agents Cancer*, 16, 41.

SHEBAN, F. 2023. It takes two to tango: the role of tumor-associated macrophages in T cell-directed immune checkpoint blockade therapy. *Front Immunol*, 14.

SIDDIQUI, M. T. & CRESCI, G. A. M. 2021. The immunomodulatory functions of butyrate. *J Inflamm Res*, 14, 6025–6041.

SPREAFICO, A., HEIRALI, A. A., ARAUJO, D. V., TAN, T. J., OLIVA, M., SCHNEEBERGER, P. H. H., CHEN, B., WONG, M. K., STAYNER, L. A., HANSEN, A. R., SAIBIL, S. D., WANG, B. X., COCHRANE, K., SHERRIFF, K., ALLEN-VERCOE, E., XU, W., SIU, L. L. & COBURN, B. 2023. First-in-class Microbial Ecosystem Therapeutic 4 (MET4) in combination with immune checkpoint inhibitors in patients with advanced solid tumors (MET4-IO trial). *Ann Oncol*, 34, 520–530.

TOSI, A., PARISATTO, B., MENEGALDO, A., SPINATO, G., GUIDO, M., DEL MISTRO, A., BUSSANI, R., ZANCONATI, F., TOFANELLI, M., TIRELLI, G., BOSCOLO-RIZZO, P. & ROSATO, A. 2022. The immune microenvironment of HPV-positive and HPV-negative oropharyngeal squamous cell carcinoma: a multiparametric quantitative and spatial analysis unveils a rationale to target treatment-naïve tumors with immune checkpoint inhibitors. *J Exp Clin Cancer Res*, 41, 279.

UNKNOWN. 2023. Fecal microbiota transplantation plus anti-PD-1 is safe in a first-line setting. *Cancer Discov*, 13, 1957.

VESELY, M. D., ZHANG, T. & CHEN, L. 2022. Resistance mechanisms to anti-PD cancer immunotherapy. *Annu Rev Immunol*, 40, 45–74.

VÉTIZOU, M., PITT, J. M., DAILLÈRE, R., LEPAGE, P., WALDSCHMITT, N., FLAMENT, C., RUSAKIEWICZ, S., ROUTY, B., ROBERTI, M. P., DUONG, C. P., POIRIER-COLAME, V., ROUX, A., BECHAREF, S., FORMENTI, S., GOLDEN, E., CORDING, S., EBERL, G., SCHLITZER, A., GINHOUX, F., MANI, S., YAMAZAKI, T., JACQUELOT, N., ENOT, D. P., BÉRARD, M., NIGOU, J., OPOLON, P., EGGERMONT, A., WOERTHER, P. L., CHACHATY, E., CHAPUT, N., ROBERT, C., MATEUS, C., KROEMER, G., RAOULT, D., BONECA, I. G., CARBONNEL, F., CHAMAILLARD, M. & ZITVOGEL, L. 2015. Anticancer immunotherapy by CTLA-4 blockade relies on the gut microbiota. *Science*, 350, 1079–1084.

VEZIANT, J., VILLÉGER, R., BARNICH, N. & BONNET, M. 2021. Gut microbiota as potential biomarker and/or therapeutic target to improve the management of cancer: focus on colibactin-producing Escherichia coli in colorectal cancer. *Cancers (Basel)*, 13(9):2215.

VILLEMIN, C., SIX, A., NEVILLE, B. A., LAWLEY, T. D., ROBINSON, M. J. & BAKDASH, G. 2023. The heightened importance of the microbiome in cancer immunotherapy. *Trends Immunol*, 44, 44–59.

WANG, D.-R., WU, X.-L. & SUN, Y.-L. 2022. Therapeutic targets and biomarkers of tumor immunotherapy: response versus non-response. *Signal Transduct Target Ther*, 7, 331.

WANG, J., SUN, H., ZENG, Q., GUO, X.-J., WANG, H., LIU, H.-H. & DONG, Z.-Y. 2019. HPV-positive status associated with inflamed immune microenvironment and improved response to anti-PD-1 therapy in head and neck squamous cell carcinoma. *Sci Rep,* 9, 13404.

WANG, L., GENG, H., LIU, Y., LIU, L., CHEN, Y., WU, F., LIU, Z., LING, S., WANG, Y. & ZHOU, L. 2023. Hot and cold tumors: immunological features and the therapeutic strategies. *Med Commun (2020),* 4, e343.

WANG, L., TANG, L., FENG, Y., ZHAO, S., HAN, M., ZHANG, C., YUAN, G., ZHU, J., CAO, S., WU, Q., LI, L. & ZHANG, Z. 2020. A purified membrane protein from *Akkermansia muciniphila* or the pasteurised bacterium blunts colitis associated tumourigenesis by modulation of CD8+ T cells in mice. *Gut,* 69, 1988–1997.

XU, H., CAO, C., REN, Y., WENG, S., LIU, L., GUO, C., WANG, L., HAN, X., REN, J. & LIU, Z. 2022. Antitumor effects of fecal microbiota transplantation: Implications for microbiome modulation in cancer treatment. *Front Immunol,* 13:949490.

ZHAO, L.-Y., MEI, J.-X., YU, G., LEI, L., ZHANG, W.-H., LIU, K., CHEN, X.-L., KOŁAT, D., YANG, K. & HU, J.-K. 2023. Role of the gut microbiota in anticancer therapy: from molecular mechanisms to clinical applications. *Signal Transduct Target Ther,* 8, 201.

6 Gut Microbiome and Chemotherapy Resistance

Sikhumbuzo Z. Mbatha, Botle Precious Damane, Kevin Gaston, and Zodwa Dlamini

INTRODUCTION

Cancer poses a major health burden worldwide. The cancer incidence rate was estimated at more than 19.3 million new patients with approximately 10 million deaths annually according to GLOBOCAN 2020 (Sung et al., 2021; Chhikara and Parang, 2023). Cancer is a heterogeneous set of diseases affecting multiple pathways in the body. Cancer development is linked to a number of risk factors including genetic abnormalities, lifestyle factors (i.e., obesity, smoking, and diet), as well as environmental factors and infectious agents. Over and above these factors certain human microbiome niches were noted recently to be significant contributing factors to oncogenesis and tumor advancement (Doocey et al., 2022). The human microbiome consists of approximately 100 trillion communities of different microorganisms occupying the various epithelial surfaces of the human being, with the largest grouping found in the intestines (Garajová et al., 2021). It is now established that the gut microbiome is heterogeneous, exhibiting temporo-spatial fluctuation, and that it significantly influences a range of human illnesses, including cancer. Research has demonstrated that the intestinal microorganisms significantly affect oncogenesis, tumor progression, and management of malignancies, the effect may either be detrimental or beneficial to the patient, depending on the patient's intestinal microbe composition and the prevailing species (Vivarelli et al., 2019). For example, *Helicobacter pylori* and *Fusobacterium nucleatum* promote cancer development and progression of gastric adenocarcinoma and colorectal cancer respectively, whereas *Streptococcus thermophilus* and *Lactobacillus gallinarum* suppress carcinogenesis. Numerous studies have revealed that the gut microbiome does not only affect the pathogenesis of cancers of the gastro-intestinal tract (GIT) system but is also linked to other cancers occurring outside the gut including cancers of the ovary, lung, prostate, and breast (Oh et al., 2021). Moreover, the microenvironment around the tumor plays a pivotal role in chemoresistance.

The TME is a dynamic entity made up of multiple cell types (including malignant cells, cells of the endothelium, mesenchymal stem cells (MSCs), fibroblasts, cancer stem cells (CSC) and cells obtained from bone marrow), oxygen, nutrients, and extracellular matrix (ECM) (Senthebane et al., 2017). The gut microbiota uses a variety of processes, such as microbial enzymatic degradation, drug metabolism, and modulation of immunity, to influence the body's reaction to anticancer treatments. Current cancer treatment protocols include cytotoxic chemotherapy, monoclonal antibodies, and immune checkpoint inhibitors, with cytotoxic chemotherapeutic agents usually constituting the first-line regimens and the most commonly used agents (Huang et al., 2022). Despite progress in the past decades with the introduction of immunotherapy and targeted therapies, the main treatment modalities still remain chemotherapy and radiotherapy with or without surgery (Wei et al., 2021). Research shows that the gut microbiome does not only impact tumor pathogenesis but also chemotherapy-induced toxicities and modulates treatment response to immunotherapy. Other previous research indicates that the makeup and variety of the gut microbiome, as well as its changes prior to, during, and/or following chemotherapy treatment, impact the frequency of unfavorable events and the effectiveness of the treatment (Oh et al., 2021). The natural microbiome in most instances provides a protective microenvironment, and its disturbance or dysbiosis may lead to enhanced tumor progression and chemoresistance (Chambers et al., 2022). Progress in sequencing technologies over the past three decades has generated data illustrating that the constituent organisms of the healthy gut microbiome are predominantly the bacterial phyla Bacteroidetes, Firmicutes, and Proteobacteria, with the other non-bacterial microorganisms contributing more towards the balance and variety of the human gut microbiome (Sevcikova et al., 2022). The advent of sequencing technologies and especially sequencing of microbial small-subunit ribosomal RNA genes (16S ribosomal DNA) has significantly increased the armamentarium available to researchers for characterization of intestinal microbial communities from patient's fecal samples, at different time points (Eckburg et al., 2005).

THE HUMAN GUT MICROBIOTA AND CHEMOTHERAPY

The intestinal microbiome consists of trillions of microorganisms including bacteria, archaebacteria, viruses, and fungi, together with their overall genetic material (Shreiner et al., 2015). The human gut microbiome is acquired from the mother and evolves with the host throughout the course of the host's life, and its constitution is determined by various factors such as the host's genetic make-up, dietary habits, environmental exposures and lifestyle. This evolution in turn influences the metabolic constitution of the host, affects the inflammatory and immune pathways, and modulates the interplay between host anticancer mechanisms and host carcinogenic metabolism (Nicholson et al., 2012). The gut microbiota of humans is constituted of approximately 380 billion microorganisms, with dominant phyla being the Fusobacteria, Bacteroidetes, Proteobacteria, Firmicutes, Actinobacteria, and Verrucomicrobia (Eckburg et al., 2005; Wei et al., 2021).

Available research indicates that gut microbiota may directly or indirectly modify the toxicity and efficacy of chemotherapeutic agents by altering a broad range of chemical signaling pathways, thereby affecting the efficiency of almost all classes of chemotherapeutic agents. A review by Alexander et al. suggested that the intestinal microbes influence chemotherapy via a structured mechanism they named "TIMER," which includes the **T**ranslocation of bacteria from bowel to systemic circulation, **I**mmunomodulation with gut bacteria regulating immune response to cancer drugs, **M**etabolism affected by the side effect of gastrointestinal toxicity causing mucositis diarrhea, **E**nzyme microbial degradation, and **R**educed diversity and ecological variation in intestinal microbes, caused by the chemotherapy agents themselves (Alexander et al., 2017).

Chemotherapy-Induced Changes on the Gut Microbiome

The administration of chemotherapy during the management of various cancers induces significant and impactful changes to the constituent organisms and diversification of the gastrointestinal microbiota (Stringer et al., 2009; van Vliet et al., 2009). A major complication related to chemotherapy is the induction of severe intestinal mucositis with resultant diarrhea, nausea, vomiting, malnutrition, and increased risk of infections leading to treatment disruptions or premature cessation of chemotherapy and eventual development of resistance (Van Vliet et al., 2010). Table 6.1 lists some of the examples of this chemotherapy-induced modulation.

An understanding of pretreatment microbiome composition is crucial to identifying patients who are at high risk of developing chemotherapy-related infections, leading to increased morbidity, increased chances of treatment failure, and increased mortality during treatment, especially in hematological malignancies (Rusu et al., 2018; Wardill et al., 2021). Therefore, accurate characterization of the microbiome prior to treatment could potentially serve as a biomarker and present an opportunity to modulate or support the microbiome with antibiotics, probiotics, synbiotics, etc. (Scott et al., 2018; Oh et al., 2021; Galloway-Peña et al., 2020).

CHEMOTHERAPY RESISTANCE

Cancer chemoresistance is a known scenario where the cancer develops drug tolerance with a resultant diminished response to the pharmaceutical treatment. Chemoresistance develops as a result of complicated genetic and environmental interactions within the patient. It is induced by a wide range of elements, such as the TME, genetic alterations, epigenetic variations, changes in drug transportation and efflux, epithelial-mesenchymal transition (EMT), and other mechanisms (Ramos et al., 2021; Du and Shim, 2016). Up to 90% of cancer-related deaths can be attributed to chemoresistance and the resultant decline in the efficacy and effectiveness of chemotherapy. Chemotherapy resistance is classified into two distinct forms: intrinsic or acquired. This distinction is based on the period when it occurs and these two forms may occur independently or sometimes overlap. Intrinsic resistance is resistance that existed prior to initiation of treatment, whereas acquired resistance develops sometime after initiation of treatment. The rate of drug resistance is evenly distributed between the two classes, affecting about 50% of patients per each class (Wang et al., 2019; Yu et al., 2017).

MECHANISMS OF CHEMORESISTANCE

Resistance to chemotherapy develops through a variety of pathways that ultimately lead to inactivation of chemotherapy agents, these include autophagy and suppression of apoptosis, epigenetic variations, altered gene amplification, and DNA double-strand breaks repair (Sevcikova et al., 2022). A considerable contribution towards chemoresistance may be due to changes in trans-cellular chemical transportation mechanisms and increased outflow of anticancer drugs resulting in decreased intracellular drug accumulation (Wang et al., 2019).

Alterations in drug transportation

Translocation of bodily substrates such as amino acids, lipids, peptides, ions, sugars, and xenobiotic components through cell membranes may be facilitated by an ATP-dependent group of proteins which belong to the transport superfamily called ATP-binding cassette (ABC) transporter proteins. These ABC transporters are structurally composed of at least two transmembrane domains and two nucleotide-binding domains. The common forms of these transporter molecules include the P-glycoprotein (P-gp), ABCG2, and major vault protein (MVP) (Altenberg, 2004). Increased expression of transporter proteins has been positively related to the evolution of chemoresistance. For example, overexpression of ABCG 2, alternatively called the breast cancer resistance protein (BCRP), or placenta-specific ABC protein (ABCP), or mitoxantrone resistance protein (MXR1), may be seen in a number of malignant cells that are drug resistant as well as in normal tissues that have barrier functions (including the placenta, bowel, liver) promoting the efflux of cytotoxic drugs (Lu and Shervington, 2008). In normal barrier organs like the placenta, prostate, small intestine, brain, colon, liver, mammary glands, and kidney ABCG2 is endogenously expressed to protect tissues against toxic chemicals. In a study by Chang et al. ABCG2 demonstrated increased expression in the mitoxantrone (MX)-resistant MCF-7/

TABLE 6.1
Chemotherapy induced gut microbiome modulation

Cancer	Chemotherapy regimen	Microbiome changes after chemotherapy — Increased abundances	Decreased microbes	Reference
Colorectal cancer	FOLFIRI	*Faecalibacterium, Clostridiales, phascolarctobacterium, Humicola,* and *Rhodotorula*	*Saccharomycetales Candida Tremellomycetes Magnusiomyces, Dipodascaceae, Malassezia,* and *Lentinula*	(Shuwen et al., 2020)
Non-hodgkins lymphoma	*Aracytine Etoposide, Carmustine* and *Melphalan*	Proteobacteria	*Bifidobacterium, Actinobacteria, Clostridium, Firmicutes, Oscillospira, Anaerostipes, Lachnospira, Blautia, Ruminococcus, Roseburia, Dorea, Adlercreutzia, Coprococcus, Collinsella*	(Montassier et al., 2015)
Pediatric acute myeloid leukemia	High-Dose Etoposide Cytarabine Daunorubicine	Enterococci	*Bacteroides* species, *Faecalibacterium, Prausnitzii, Clostridium,* Cluster Xiva, *Bifidobacterium*	(van Vliet et al., 2009)
Adult acute myeloid leukemia (AML)	AML Induction Chemotherapies: High-intensity regimens with-fludarabine and non-fludarabine regimens. Regimen based on Hypomethylating agent Low-dose cytarabine	*Staphylococcus*	Shannon Diversity In stool: *Blautia* & *Clostridiales* Oral swab: *Gemella* & *Viellonellaceae,* Prevotellaceae	(Galloway-Peña et al., 2020, Wei et al., 2021)
Advanced esophageal cancer	Docetaxel, cisplatin, and 5-fluorouracil (5-FU) (DCF therapy)	*Enterococcus, Staphylococcus, C. difficile* and methicillin-sensitive coagulase-negative *Staphylococcus aureus*	*Bifidobacterium* and *Lactobacillus*	(Motoori et al., 2017)
Acute lymphoblastic leukemia (ALL)	Induction chemotherapy, consolidation chemotherapy, and maintenance therapy	*Parabacteroides Lachnospiraceae,* UCG-005 and *Lachnoclostridium Ruminococcus gnavus Ruminococcus torques*	Bacteroidetes (*Alistipes*)	(Rajagopala et al., 2020)
Ovarian cancer	Carboplatin/ cisplatin, and paclitaxel	*Firmicutes, Bacteroides, Faecalibacterium, Coprococcus, Bilophila, Collinsella,* and *Blautia*	Proteobacteria Enterobacteriaceae, *Klebsiella, Enterobacter*	(Tong et al., 2020)

MX cell line in relation to the normal MCF 7 parental cell line. They also noted that estrogen seemed to upregulate the tolerance of MCF-7 cancer cells to mitoxantrone by generating the expression of ABCG2 after the estrogen receptor α (ERα) had been inhibited. They concluded that estrogen prompted ABCG2 expression via ERα mechanism, and this overexpression of ABCG2 led to MCF-7 acquiring more tolerance towards MX (Chang et al., 2017).

MVP or Lung Resistance-Related Protein (LRP) is a transporter of cytotoxic DNA targeting drugs that is overexpressed in non-small cell lung carcinoma (NSCLC), B-cell lymphoma, and gliomas. It can also potentially be utilized as an independent biomarker of chemoresistance in patients with cancer of the ovaries and acute leukemia. It facilitates primary chemoresistance by modifying the nucleocytoplasmic transportation of hormones, ribosomes, mRNA, and drugs (Zheng, 2017).

Epithelial-mesenchymal transition (EMT) is a physiological, temporo-spatially well-defined process that follows a specific stepwise and sequential set of events whose final outcome is the mutation of epithelial cells into mesenchymal cells or tissue. The process is active during the embryonic developmental stage as well as after birth, however post-natally it is a common feature of tumorigenesis where it is inappropriately activated and the normal processes disrupted (Nisticò et al., 2012). EMT is now recognized as an aggravating factor of chemoresistance in a broad range of malignancies. One of its main mechanisms is the overexpression of ABC transporter proteins observed in cancer cells that have been through the EMT process which causes uncontrolled drug efflux leading to chemoresistance (Du and Shim, 2016).

Gene repair and gene amplification

Chemotherapeutic agents destroy cancer cells by direct or indirect disruption of DNA in the nucleus and/or mitochondria. For instance, 5-fluorouracil (5-FU) and cisplatin are frequently used drugs that damage DNA. Cancer cells have the ability to activate the DNA repair pathway, which enables the cell to identify and correct damage to DNA molecules and eliminate DNA lesions brought on by chemotherapy resulting in chemoresistance and enhanced cancer cell survival. These DNA lesions include double-strand breaks (DSBs), single-strand breaks (SSBs), chemical modifications of the bases or sugars, mismatches, and inter-strand or intra-strand crosslinks (Li et al., 2021). The two main types of DNA repair mechanisms that cause chemoresistance to DNA-targeting drugs are nucleotide excision repair and base excision repair (Zheng, 2017). Approximately 10% of human cancers develop chemoresistance through the mechanism of gene amplification occurring in malignant cells which is associated with the overexpression of proteins involved in a particular drug's mechanism of action and poor prognosis (Albertson, 2006). For example, acute leukemia may develop resistance to methotrexate as a result of amplification of gene coding for dihydrofolate reductase enzyme, whose activity is increased in resistant cells (Gorlick et al., 1996).

Epigenetic changes

The role of epigenetic modifications in the development of chemoresistance is becoming more widely acknowledged. Epigenetic alterations include DNA methylation, modulation of histones, chromatin remodeling, and changes related to actions of non-coding RNA (Easwaran et al., 2014).

DNA demethylation occurring in the promoter region of a tumor promoter gene will lead to the upregulation of that gene which may induce drug resistance. An investigation into the mechanisms underlying the acquisition of acquired chemoresistance to antiangiogenic therapy in hepatocellular carcinoma showed that an expression of G-actin monomer binding protein thymosin β4 (Tβ4) was enhanced by the demethylation of DNA and active modulation of histone H3 at the promoter region in the resistant hepatocellular carcinoma (HCC) cell line. The HCC cell line developed stem cell-like capabilities as a result of this Tβ4 overexpression, which also caused *in vivo* Sorafenib resistance. Sorafenib acts by inhibition of the vascular endothelial growth factor (VEGF) receptor (Ohata et al., 2017).

In some instances, the development of drug resistance is facilitated by long non-coding RNAs (lncRNAs) and microRNAs (miRNAs). They act by regulating the expression of proteins that promote resistance to anticancer drugs, control autophagy and apoptosis, and modulate metabolism of chemo drugs, altering drug targets and influencing DNA repair mechanisms. For example, lncRNA urothelial cancer-associated 1 (UCA1) was found to be upregulated in cisplatin-resistant bladder cancer cells in comparison to responsive cells, whereas the overexpression of miR-134, miR-487b, and miR-655 was shown to enhance transforming growth factor beta (TGF-β)-induced epithelial-mesenchymal transition and drug resistance to Gefitinib in non-small cell lung cancer (Wang et al., 2019).

Tumor microenvironment

The TME is a dynamic entity defined by the presence of multiple cell types, oxygen, nutrients, and extracellular matrix (ECM) (Senthebane et al., 2017). All the components of the TME contribute towards tumor metabolism. The components of the TME have a specific metabolic landscape that facilitates cancer cells' adaptation and therefore influences tumor progression (Elia and Haigis, 2021). The metabolites of the gut microbiome are key factors that modulate the TME, thereby promoting cancer progression and inducing chemoresistance. Microbiota-derived metabolites regulate several cancer promoting signaling pathways and the differentiation of immune cells such as regulatory T cells. These metabolites have the ability to control inflammatory reactions by causing macrophages to express pro-inflammatory cytokines (Yang et al., 2023).

A critical part of tumor cellular growth is the close cooperation between cells and their respective microenvironments. Cellular and non-cellular components of the TME interact closely with each other to promote cancer heterogeneity that is commonly observed in solid tumors, and this heterogeneity promotes the development of chemoresistance. The ECM forms thick fibers within the tumor creating a mechanical boundary blocking the free transfer of chemotherapeutic drugs. Levels of oxygenation impact cellular growth. For example, cells in oxygen poor environments tend to divide slowly, causing them to respond poorly to chemotherapeutic agents whilst at the same time the hypoxic environment may activate genes that promote neovascularization and cell survival. Low pH or acidic conditions in TME can hamper the activation of various chemotherapeutic drugs, thereby decreasing their cytotoxicity towards cancer cells. Intra- and extracellular variations in pH both within and around the malignant cells can have a sustained impact on the efficacy of anticancer drugs (Senthebane et al., 2017).

Autophagy

The complex cellular process of autophagy is an intricate process that causes intracellular and cellular structures to self-degrade during times of cellular stress, cell nutrient variations, and cellular development. Its main purpose is the restoration of cellular energy balance during these critical periods. It uses various signaling pathways to promote or prevent cell death. Autophagy can be classified into three forms, namely micro- or macroautophagy and chaperone-mediated autophagy (Pu et al., 2022; Lu et al., 2020). Autophagy can be seen as a survival mechanism of characterized degradation of cytosolic components by the lysosomal system in order to remove damaged misfolded proteins, clearance of damaged organelles including mitochondria, removal of intracellular pathogens and other cytoplasmic components (Glick et al., 2010). Figure 6.1 below summarizes the mechanism of autophagy that develops in cellular stress conditions, such as those induced in cancer cells.

It is now well accepted that autophagy may play a complex role in the emergence of drug resistance in a variety of cancer cells, including those found in certain solid and non-solid tumors (i.e., acute myeloid leukemia). Autophagy is controlled by a group of highly conserved genes called autophagy-related genes (ATGs). It can be activated by stress-inducing factors like hypoglycemic states, hypoxia, AMP/ATP, amino acids, and growth factors. The ATGs participate, amongst other processes, in apoptosis, necrosis, and regulation of drug resistance via autophagy. The initiation of autophagy is facilitated by a large complex named ULK1-FIP200-ATG13 complex, which is constituted by the Unc-51-like autophagy activating kinase 1 (ULK1), the autophagy-related gene 13 (ATG13) and the FAK family kinase-interacting protein of 200 KDa (FIP200) (Li et al., 2019). Autophagy can promote cell survival or lead to cell death. Because of this duality, it frequently promotes significant resistance to chemotherapy when autophagy protects cancer cells against apoptosis induced by chemotherapy (Pu et al., 2022).

Numerous relevant research has demonstrated that autophagy may provide cancer cells with a defense mechanism that enhances chemoresistance. Autophagy promotes tumor cell survival by a variety of mechanisms and molecules during treatment with anticancer drugs, including EGFR signaling, PI3K/AKT/ mTOR pathways, p53, VEGF, MAPK14/p38α signaling, and microRNAs (Sui et al., 2013).

MICROBIOME-INDUCED CHEMORESISTANCE

CHEMOTHERAPY AGENTS

Platinum-based therapies (oxaliplatin and cisplatin)

Platinum-based chemotherapeutics (oxaliplatin and cisplatin) induce tumor cell death by causing intra-chain crosslinking-mediated DNA damage which activates pro-apoptotic pathways. Furthermore, research indicates that an increased output of reactive oxygen species (ROS) promotes oxaliplatin (OXA)-induced DNA damage. Oxaliplatin may cause intestinal dysbiosis that encourages the onset of chemotherapy-induced mechanical hyperalgesia which is characterized by debilitating neuropathic pain that leads to premature abrupt treatment disruption and eventual failure to complete treatment regimens (Liu et al., 2022).

Chambers et al conducted a study on mouse models looking at the consequences of disrupting the gut microbiome by administration of antibiotics. They assessed tumor growth and response to cisplatin-based chemotherapy on epithelial ovarian cancer (EOC). They collected C57BL/6J female mice at 6 weeks of age and gave them either a placebo of plain water or antibiotic-containing water (ampicillin, neomycin,

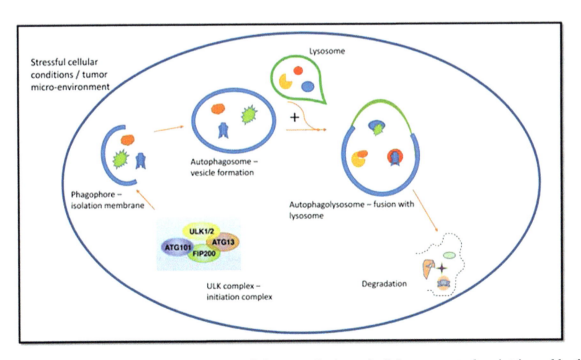

FIGURE 6.1 Mechanism of autophagy in response to cellular stress: In times of cellular stress *autophagy* is triggered by the ULK complex. In TME, initiating factors include hypoxia, low glucose, AMP/ATP, amino acids, and growth factors. The phagophore is an isolation membrane that originates from endoplasmic reticulum, plasma or mitochondrial membranes. Its lengthening is facilitated by the ATG5-ATG12-ATG16 axis. Whereas the development of autophagosomes is catalyzed by LC3-ATG3-ATG4-ATG7. The amalgamation of the autophagosome and the lysosome involves Syntaxin 17 and SNARE. Autophagy directly affects the proliferation, invasiveness, and metastatic potential of malignant cells, and can mediate chemoresistance induced by the TME (Li et al., 2019).

metronidazole, and vancomycin). After being given antibiotic (ABS) containing water for 2 weeks, the mice were injected intraperitoneally with murine EOC cell lines ID8 or ID8-VEGF, and than subsequently 2 weeks after cancer cell line injection the mice were injected intraperitoneally with cisplatin on a weekly basis for the rest of the study period. Whilst at the same time, tumor growth was assessed on a weekly basis starting from the time of injection with the cell lines. They noted that ID8 and ID8-VEGF EOC tumor growth was significantly increased in the ABS-treated mice, the efficacy of cisplatin therapy was attenuated and there was development of cisplatin resistance in antibiotics-treated mice compared with control-treated mice. Their experiments highlighted the fact that antibiotics caused significant alterations to the gut microbiome and microbial metabolites, which in turn impacted on ovarian cancer growth and diminished response to chemotherapy. The ABS-mediated microbiome disruption led to chemoresistance and poor overall survival (Chambers et al., 2022).

Cyclophosphamide

Cyclophosphamide (CTX) is an alkylating agent that inhibits tumor growth by prompting the host's immune system to kill immunogenic cancer cells. CTX undermines the immunosuppressive T cells and enhances the action of CD4+ T helper 1 (Th1) and T helper (Th17) cells that modulate cancer growth (Sistigu et al., 2011). Gut microbiotas affect the immune response that is induced by cyclophosphamide. Cyclophosphamide damages the mucosal barrier of the bowel resulting in translocation of gut bacteria into lymphatic tissues or organs. These bacteria stimulate the host's immune response by promoting the manufacture of pathogenic T helper cell 17 (pTh17) and memory Th1 cells, thereby improving the antitumor effect of CTX. Antibiotics can destroy the Gram-positive bacteria which decreases the production of pTh17 and thus the efficacy of CTX is also decreased. Two bacteria species that have been shown to be translocated from gut to lymphoid organs during cyclophosphamide therapy are *Enterococcus hirae* and *Barnesiella*, causing a rise in the intratumoral CD8/Treg ratio (Liu et al., 2022; Viaud et al., 2013).

Viaud et al. treated naïve mice with non-myeloablative doses of cyclophosphamide or doxorubicin, and found that chemotherapy gave rise to crucial structural alterations in the intestinal mucosa that are closely linked to the disruption of normal intestinal barrier functions. These changes included a rise in the number of Paneth and goblet cells in the intestinal villi and crypts, small bowel villi shortening, rifts in the mucosal barrier, interstitial edema, and focal aggregation of mononuclear cells in the lamina propria. The intestinal barrier disruption was associated with the translocation of a select group of microbes from the bowel to mesenteric lymph nodes and spleen in more than half of the CTX-treated mice. The translocated organisms included *Enterococcus hirae*, *Lactobacillus johnsonii*, and *Lactobacillus murinus*. When they assessed the microbiota composition in the intestinal mucosa of mice with subcutaneous cancers, they identified a significant microbial deviation that was however only realized a week after administration of cyclophosphamide. This dysbiosis was characterized by the reduction in Firmicutes phylum distributed within four genera and groups (*Coprococcus*, *Roseburia*, unclassified *Lachnospiraceae*, and *Clostridium* cluster XIVa) and reduction in the abundance of lactobacilli and enterococci (Viaud et al., 2013).

The administration of antibiotics, particularly vancomycin, has been shown to decrease the potency of cyclophosphamide, inducing resistance in MCA205 induced mice. *Barnesiella intestini hominis* impacts tumor immune response by promoting the production and accumulation of cytotoxic CD8+ T cells, increasing the response of Th1 cells, and promoting infiltration of IFN-γ–producing T cells in the tumor microenvironment after CTX treatment. Therefore, the reduction in *Barnesiella intestini hominis* and *Enterococcus hirae* promotes chemoresistance to CTX (Chrysostomou et al., 2023; Daillère et al., 2016).

Fluoropyrimidine analogs

One of the most used drugs in cancer treatment is 5-fluorouracil (5-FU). 5-FU is utilized in the management of several malignancies, including colorectal cancer, breast cancer, and gastric cancer. 5-FU is a fluorinated analog of uracil. Its mechanism of action involves the inhibition of thymidylate synthase, resulting in DNA breaks formation, disturbances in DNA replication with cell cycle arrest, disturbances in RNA synthesis and resultant cellular death (Huang et al., 2022).

5-FU works by promoting neutrophil infiltration and abnormal inflammatory processes, and also causing upregulation of TNF-α, IL-1β, and other secondary inflammatory agents. Treatment with 5-FU, even of short duration, has a profound and direct impact on the bacteria that are resident in the gastrointestinal tract. For example, after 2–3 days of treatment the *Staphylococcus*, *Escherichia coli*, and *Clostridium* numbers were diminished in the stomach whilst in the jejunum *Clostridium* and *Lactobacillus* were diminished, however intestinal *E. coli* was enriched.

The 5-FU-induced disruption of the gut microbiota and mucin secretion may lead to severe mucositis. Severe mucositis leads to severe diarrhea which negatively impacts the efficacy and treatment compliance. 5-FU also causes quantitative decline in intestinal goblet cells (Liu et al., 2022). Yuan et al. in their study of mice injected with colorectal cancer cells and then treated with 5-FU found that in the 5-FU treated mice there was decreased alpha diversity and significant change in the microbial composition, the relative abundance of genera *Bacteroides*, *Rikenella*, *Blautia*, *Mucispirillum*, *Escherichia-Shigella*, *Alloprevotella*, *Enterobacter*, Lachnospiraceae_NK4 A136_group, and *Mycoplasma* were increased while that of unidentified Lachnospiraceae, *Rikenella*, *Lactobacillus*, and *Alistipes* decreased in the FU group compared to control group. The administration of both antibiotics and 5-FU caused significant dysbiosis which was associated with decreased effectiveness of anticancer therapy resulting in a higher tumor/body weight ratio in the group that was treated with ABS-5

FU in comparison to the 5-FU only treatment group (Yuan et al., 2018). Zhang et al. demonstrated that high numbers of *Fusobacterium nucleatum* in colorectal cancer correlated with a 12-fold increase in the expression of BIRC3 gene and protein. BIRC3 inhibits the caspase cascades, thereby inhibiting apoptosis. Their result showed that 5-FU efficacy was significantly attenuated by *Fusobacterium* leading to chemoresistance (Zhang et al., 2019).

Gemcitabine

Gemcitabine is a deoxycytidine nucleoside derivative with anti-proliferative properties that depends on the inhibition of several pathways related to DNA synthesis and arrest of cell cycle progression at the G1/S-phase. Gemcitabine is used to treat pancreatic ductal adenocarcinoma (PDAC), cholangiocarcinomas, advanced breast cancers, carcinoma of the bladder, and non-small cell lung cancer (Toschi et al., 2005; Valle et al., 2014). It is transported into the cells by several human nucleoside transporters wherein it undergoes intracellular phosphorylation to gemcitabine diphosphate (dFdCDP) by pyrimidine nucleoside monophosphate kinase. dFdCTP eventually gets incorporated into DNA during replication where it blocks the elongation of the DNA chain causing cell death by apoptosis (Amrutkar and Gladhaug, 2017).

Gammaproteobacteria induces cancer chemoresistance to Gemcitabine by breaking it down into its inactive form 2',2'-difuorodeoxyuridine. The long subtype of bacterial cytidine deaminase (CDDL), primarily produced by Gammaproteobacteria, is essential for the metabolism of bacteria. Research shows that bacteria are a crucial component of the PDAC microenvironment and mediate chemoresistance by lowering the concentration of chemo-drugs inside the tumor (Sayin et al., 2023). Geller et al. conducted a mouse model study where they subcutaneously transplanted *Mycoplasma hyorhinis*-positive or -negative MC-26 mouse colon carcinoma cells into the flanks of BALB/c mice and found that the *Mycoplasma hyorhinis*-infected carcinoma cells were resistant to gemcitabine. They also analyzed fresh human PDAC tissue specimens and discovered that 51.7% were infected with *Gammaproteobacteria*. They cultured bacteria from 15 samples of human PDAC tissues and found that 93% rendered the RKO and HCT116 human colon carcinoma cell lines fully resistant to gemcitabine (Geller et al., 2017).

Irinotecan

Irinotecan, also called CPT- 111, is a DNA topoisomerase I (Top1) inhibitor that is often utilized in the management of solid tumors. It is predominantly used in the treatment of colorectal cancer and pancreatic cancer but also in the management of ovarian cancer, lung cancer, and other solid tumors (Reyhanoglu and Smith, 2023). Irinotecan's mechanism of action primarily involves the arrest of cell replication leading to cell death. DNA topoisomerase I facilitates DNA replication and transcription by reducing the supercoiling and twisting of the double-stranded DNA helix during essential cellular processes such as transcription, repair recombination, and replication. Irinotecan inhibits this action of topoisomerases; their interaction leads to the formation of irinotecan-Top1-DNA complexes that collide with advancing replication forks forming double-stranded DNA breaks leading to irreversible cessation of cellular replication and cell death (Xu and Villalona-Calero, 2002). Treatment with irinotecan is associated with physiological and intestinal disturbances and constituent alterations in gut microbiota, imbalances in the tumor microenvironment, which further increases the effects of harmful bacteria. This disharmony is called "microbial–host–irinotecan axis imbalance." These changes attenuate drug efficacy and increase the toxicity of chemotherapy (Liu et al., 2022). The severe toxicities induced by irinotecan include myelosuppression, peripheral neuropathy, nausea, vomiting, and diarrhea, all leading to interruption or premature termination of treatment, reduced quality of life, negative impact on prognosis, and increased risk of treatment-related deaths (Eng, 2009; Bailly, 2019).

β-Glucorinodase is a microbiome-encoded enzyme mainly produced by four microbial "phyla," namely Bacteroides, Firmicutes, Verrucomicrobia, and Proteobacteria. It is involved in the metabolism of exogenous compounds in the intestinal tract and begets drug-related intestinal toxicities, including CPT11 toxicities where the CPT11 active metabolite SN38G (which is metabolized and then inactivated in the liver) is reactivated by β-glucorinodase to toxic SN38 in the intestinal lumen leading to dose-limiting toxicities and reducing drug efficacy (Parvez et al., 2021, Yue et al., 2021). Additionally, studies show that the dysbiosis caused by CPT11-induced suppression of the release of microbial metabolites, such as short-chain fatty acids (SCFA), exacerbates the toxicity of CPT11. CPT11 treatment also causes augmentation in the number of pathogenic microbes leading to disruption of the host's immunological state and impairment of chemotherapeutic outcomes. For example, *Eschericia* spp., *Shigella* spp., *Clostridium difficile*, *Parasutteralla*, *Lactococcus*, *Streptococcus*, and *Staphylococcus* spark acute inflammatory response including the release of pro-inflammatory cytokines IL-6, IL-1β, and IL-18, activation of caspase-1, and activation of NF-ƙB pathway (Yue et al., 2021).

BACTERIA

Fusobacterium nucleatum

Fusobacterium nucleatum is a Gram-negative, non-sporulating anaerobic species that is one of the constituents of the gut microbiota. It is found throughout the gastrointestinal system including the oral cavity. It is not only linked to the emergence of benign dental diseases such as periodontitis and gingivitis but is also implicated in the pathogenesis of malignant conditions of the gastrointestinal system, including esophageal and colorectal cancer. Evidence suggests that its abundance confers aggressive tumor biology that is associated with poor prognosis and metastatic disease. A recent study analyzed 120 resected ESCC specimens from patients who had preoperative chemotherapy and 30 pre-treatment biopsies looking at the *F. nucleatum* burden on tumor and correlated it to tumor's response to chemotherapy, their results illustrated that patients with high intra-tumoral quantities of *F. nucleatum* appear to have greater resistance to anticancer drug therapy (cisplatin, 5-fluorouracil, and docetaxel). This study demonstrated, using multiplexed visualization methods such as transmission electron microscopy (TEM) and laser scanning confocal microscopy (LSCM), that *F. nucleatum* has a propensity for cell adhesion and invasiveness allowing it to thrive as an intracellular pathogen, which explains its enrichment in ESCC cells. The evidence suggests that the mechanism of action leading to chemoresistance is due to the modulation of cell autophagy by *F. nucleatum* (Liu et al., 2021).

Another study by Yu and colleagues looked at the interconnection between *F. nucleatum*, recurrence, and chemoresistance in colorectal cancer. They analyzed their previous data comparing it with pyro-sequenced data using a Roche 454 GS FLX in 16 CRC tissues from patients with recurrence versus 15 CRC tissues from patients who did not have recurrence. They then applied the LEfSe algorithm to identify any possible differences in the composition of the bacteria. The LEfSe algorithm being described as linear discriminant analysis Effect Size algorithm which is a computational statistical analysis tool useful in metagenomics and understanding of different microbial communities (Segata et al., 2011). They found that *Prevotella*, *Fusobacterium*, *Anaerosporobacter*, *Parvimonas*, and *Peptostreptococcus* were enriched in recurrent CRC tissues compared to non-recurrent CRC tissues, with *Fusobacterium* being the most abundant. They subsequently evaluated the abundance rates of *F. nucleatum* in 48 CRC tissues from patients who did not develop any recurrence and 44 CRC tissues from patients who developed recurrence and established that the quantity of *F. nucleatum* was higher in CRC tissues of patients with recurrence. Subsequent analysis showed that *F. nucleatum* infection enhanced CRC resistance to 5-FU and oxaliplatin via coordinating the autophagy network of ULK1/ATG7, TLR4-MYD88, miR18a*, and miR4802 to biologically regulate CRC chemoresistance. Data showed that the recurrence-free survival was significantly shorter in the *F. nucleatum*-high group when compared to the *F. nucleatum*-low group (Yu et al., 2017). Figure 6.2 below summarizes the *F. nucleatum*-induced chemoresistance via autophagy in colorectal cancer (CRC) cells.

Bacteroides

Laura et al., in their study assessing how gut microbiota might influence the success of neoadjuvant chemotherapy in urothelial carcinoma, examined the gut microbiome of 29 bladder cancer patients undergoing neoadjuvant chemotherapy and compared them with 26 healthy controls and also conducted murine studies in C57BL/6 female and male mice. Their research found that compared to complete

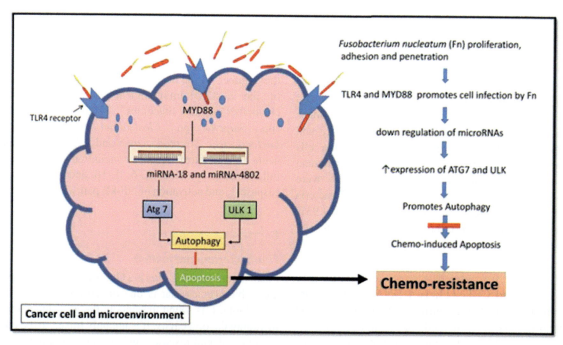

FIGURE 6.2 **Mechanism of chemoresistance conferred by *F. nucleatum* in colorectal cancer.** *Fusobacterium nucleatum (Fn)* activates the autophagy pathway in CRC cells and induces chemoresistance by protecting CRC cells from chemotherapy induced apoptosis. *Fn* enrichment is associated with CRC recurrence and poorer outcomes. *Fusobacterium* was the most dominant phylotype in CRC (colorectal cancer) tissues and the most enriched bacteria in recurrent CRC tissues (Yu et al., 2017). The TLR4 and MYD88 innate immune signaling pathway is triggered when there is enrichment of *Fn*. The *Fn*–mediated chemoresistance is dependent on the TLR4 and MYD88 pathway initiating autophagy. TLR4 and MYD88 cause a selective loss and significant downregulation of miR-18a* and miR-4802. MiRNAs downregulation leads to increased ULK1 and ATG7 expression which promotes autophagy and thus prevents chemotherapy induced apoptosis (Yu et al., 2017).

responders, non-responders were more likely to experience a statistically significant sustained increase or high abundance of *Bacteroides* throughout chemotherapy compared to complete responders (p<0.001). This quantitative elevation of *Bacteroides* during neoadjuvant chemotherapy correlated with the finding of residual disease during the radical cystectomy regardless of the chemotherapy regimen given (Laura et al., 2023).

B. fragilis and *B. thetaiotaomicron*

Pancreatic adenocarcinoma has been shown to be usually infected with intestinal bacteria that translocates from the gut, particularly duodenum, into the tumor and these bacteria modulate the activation of antitumor immune response. A recent study of 30 patients with metastatic PDAC, 23 of whom had not received any antibiotic treatment, analyzed the constituent organisms of gut microbiota before the initiation of chemotherapy. The cohort was separated into responders and non-responders, mainly based on radiological response or progression-free survival (PFS) and a decrease in serum tumor markers. They found that the microbiota was distinct between the two groups, with responders showing enrichment with *B. fragilis* and *B. thetaiotaomicron*. To assess for a potential cause-and-effect relationship between the microbiota and the response to chemotherapy, they introduced microbiota from selected responders and non-responders into gnotobiotic mice and then injected them with pancreatic cancer cells orthotopically. Using 16S rRNA sequencing they detected intra-tumoral bacteria in only 2 out of 12 tumors and deduced that response to chemotherapy was rather indirectly influenced by the circulating microbiota-derived metabolites. Further analysis demonstrated that the microbiota-derived tryptophan metabolite 3-IAA (indole-3-acetic acid (3-IAA) was elevated in the serum of mice and humans that responded

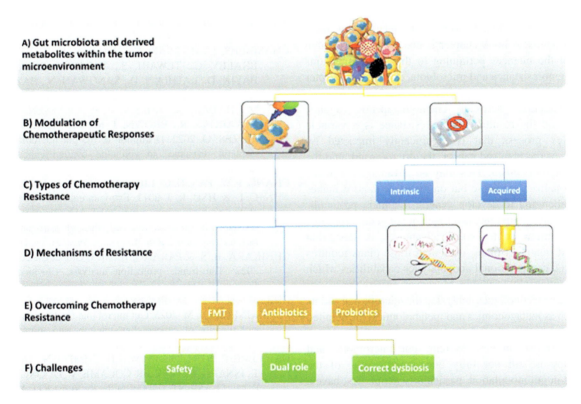

FIGURE 6.3 **Modulation of the tumor microenvironment by the gut microbiota and chemotherapy resistance.** (A) Contribution of the tumor microenvironment and several types of tumor-infiltrating immune cells and microbial species to chemoresistance. (B) The gut microbiota can modulate chemotherapy resistance by induction of cellular and molecular signaling pathways. These can lead to sensitivity to chemotherapeutic treatment resulting in cancer cell death or resistance to chemotherapy. (C) Chemotherapeutic resistance can either be intrinsic or acquired. (D) Intrinsic resistance is due to mechanisms induced by the gut microbiota such as modulation of gene expression or DNA breaks repair mechanisms. Adaptive is due to the introduction of chemotherapeutic drugs which can also result in alteration of genetic mechanisms. (E) The composition and diversity of the gut microbiota are the major determinants of therapeutic responses. Thus, gut-microbiome-related resistance to therapy can be overcome by fecal microbial transplantation (FMT) of positive responders to cancer patients who have developed resistance to therapy. Probiotics have also been shown to improve response to therapy by correcting the patient's microbial composition. Antibiotics also assist to a certain extent to clear microbes known to be responses to suppressing therapeutic responses. (F) However, the challenge with FMT is the concern for its safety, methods of preparation, and scaling up prior to administration. Antibiotics on the other hand serve as a double-edged sword by their inability to eradicate only unneeded microbiota resulting in therapeutic resistance. The effectiveness of probiotics in correcting dysbiosis to improve therapeutic response is also questionable as the same probiotics are not effective in all cancers and should be patient specific.

to chemotherapy. The study confirmed that *Bacteroides fragilis* and *Bacteroides thetaiotaomicron* are able to produce significant amounts of the 3-IAA metabolite and that they were abundant in the microbiota of responders (Tintelnot et al., 2023).

GUT MICROBIOTA MODULATION

Gut microbiota can be modulated using various strategies to counter the chemoresistance conferred by microbial organisms. These strategies include dietary modification, fecal microbial transplantation, prescription of antibiotics, probiotics, prebiotics, and synbiotics (Motoori et al., 2017; Scott et al., 2018). Figure 6.3 summarizes the modulation techniques available.

Limitations

Both the microbiome and cancer are diverse entities whose ultimate form and composition are determined by a number of variables, including genetic factors, environmental exposures, and dietary habits. A book chapter is not exhaustive enough to cover all the nuances pertaining to the interconnections between chemoresistance and microbiota, as such our chapter attempts to provide a summary of a vast topic.

The interaction between chemotherapeutic agents, microbiota and the resultant chemoresistance is a variable and complex process that is significantly impacted by specificities of the involved cancer, the drug(s) used, and the dominant microorganism. This may be advantageous in the era of personalized medicine but on the other hand it makes it more challenging to develop generic treatment protocols. Although the inter-individual heterogeneity of gut microbiome and cancer might confer some advantages in designing personalized treatment plans, designing those plans requires high-powered computational and analytics capabilities which are not yet universally available. Moreover, despite the advent of new research technologies analyzing the microbiome and its actions, such as metagenomics and metabolomics, the detailed molecular mechanism that controls the complex interactions between intestinal immune system, gut microbiota, and chemotherapy is still not fully understood. Some of the agents used in gut modulation, particularly antibiotics, have a diametrically opposed impact on the drug efficacy depending on the prevailing microorganism and insulting cancer. They may promote cancer cell survival or cancer cell death.

CONCLUSION

The different chemotherapeutic agents interact closely with the gut microbiota inducing alterations in the microbial composition and microbial abundances, especially of bacteria. The microbial disturbances can induce the emergence of chemoresistance in several cancers or may even on occasion lead to improved chemosensitivity. The final outcome being determined by the predominant microbial organism. Chemotherapy-induced dysbiosis can be seen either early after initiation of treatment or later on, with effects lasting for months after termination of therapy. Modulation of microbiota seems to have a significant impact on chemoresistance by eliminating protective microbes or it can improve chemosensitivity and reduce complications by eliminating harmful bacteria.

REFERENCES

ALBERTSON, D. G. 2006. Gene amplification in cancer. *Trends in Genetics*, 22, 447–455.

ALEXANDER, J. L., WILSON, I. D., TEARE, J., MARCHESI, J. R., NICHOLSON, J. K. & KINROSS, J. M. 2017. Gut microbiota modulation of chemotherapy efficacy and toxicity. *Nature Reviews Gastroenterology & Hepatology*, 14, 356–365.

ALTENBERG, G. A. 2004. Structure of multidrug-resistance proteins of the ATP-binding cassette (ABC) superfamily. *Current Medicinal Chemistry - Anti-Cancer Agents*, 4, 53–62.

AMRUTKAR, M. & GLADHAUG, I. P. 2017. Pancreatic cancer chemoresistance to gemcitabine. *Cancers*, 9, 157.

BAILLY, C. 2019. Irinotecan: 25 years of cancer treatment. *Pharmacological Research*, 148, 104398.

CHAMBERS, L. M., ESAKOV RHOADES, E. L., BHARTI, R., BRALEY, C., TEWARI, S., TRESTAN, L., ALALI, Z., BAYIK, D., LATHIA, J. D., SANGWAN, N., BAZELEY, P., JOEHLIN-PRICE, A. S., WANG, Z., DUTTA, S., DWIDAR, M., HAJJAR, A., AHERN, P. P., CLAESEN, J., ROSE, P., VARGAS, R., BROWN, J. M., MICHENER, C. M. & REIZES, O. 2022. Disruption of the gut microbiota confers cisplatin resistance in epithelial ovarian cancer. *Cancer Research*, 82, 4654–4669.

CHANG, F. W., FAN, H. C., LIU, J. M., FAN, T. P., JING, J., YANG, C. L. & HSU, R. J. 2017. Estrogen enhances the expression of the multidrug transporter gene ABCG2-increasing drug resistance of breast cancer cells through estrogen receptors. *International Journal of Molecular Sciences*, 18, 163.

CHHIKARA, B. S. & PARANG, K. 2023. Global Cancer Statistics 2022: The trends projection analysis. *Chemical Biology Letters*, 10, 451.

CHRYSOSTOMOU, D., ROBERTS, L. A., MARCHESI, J. R. & KINROSS, J. M. 2023. Gut microbiota modulation of efficacy and toxicity of cancer chemotherapy and immunotherapy. *Gastroenterology*, 164, 198–213.

DAILLÈRE, R., VÉTIZOU, M., WALDSCHMITT, N., YAMAZAKI, T., ISNARD, C., POIRIER-COLAME, V., DUONG, CONNIE P. M., FLAMENT, C., LEPAGE, P., ROBERTI, MARIA P., ROUTY, B., JACQUELOT, N., APETOH, L., BECHAREF, S., RUSAKIEWICZ, S., LANGELLA, P., SOKOL, H., KROEMER, G., ENOT, D., ROUX, A., EGGERMONT, A., TARTOUR, E., JOHANNES, L., WOERTHER, P.-L., CHACHATY, E., SORIA, J.-C., GOLDEN, E., FORMENTI, S., PLEBANSKI, M., MADONDO, M., ROSENSTIEL, P., RAOULT, D., CATTOIR, V., BONECA, IVO G., CHAMAILLARD, M. & ZITVOGEL, L. 2016. *Enterococcus hirae* and *Barnesiella intestinihominis* facilitate cyclophosphamide-induced therapeutic immunomodulatory effects. *Immunity*, 45, 931–943.

DOOCEY, C. M., FINN, K., MURPHY, C. & GUINANE, C. M. 2022. The impact of the human microbiome in tumorigenesis, cancer progression, and biotherapeutic development. *BMC Microbiology*, 22, 53.

DU, B. & SHIM, J. S. 2016. Targeting Epithelial-Mesenchymal Transition (EMT) to overcome drug resistance in cancer. *Molecules*, 21, 965.

EASWARAN, H., TSAI, H. C. & BAYLIN, S. B. 2014. Cancer epigenetics: Tumor heterogeneity, plasticity of stem-like states, and drug resistance. *Molecular Cell*, 54, 716–727.

ECKBURG, P. B., BIK, E. M., BERNSTEIN, C. N., PURDOM, E., DETHLEFSEN, L., SARGENT, M., GILL, S. R., NELSON, K. E. & RELMAN, D. A. 2005. Diversity of the human intestinal microbial flora. *Science*, 308, 1635–1638.

ELIA, I. & HAIGIS, M. C. 2021. Metabolites and the tumour microenvironment: From cellular mechanisms to systemic metabolism. *Nature Metabolism*, 3, 21–32.

ENG, C. 2009. Toxic effects and their management: Daily clinical challenges in the treatment of colorectal cancer. *Nature Reviews Clinical Oncology*, 6, 207–218.

GALLOWAY-PEÑA, J. R., SHI, Y., PETERSON, C. B., SAHASRABHOJANE, P., GOPALAKRISHNAN, V., BRUMLOW, C. E., DAVER, N. G., ALFAYEZ, M., BODDU, P. C., KHAN, M. A. W., WARGO, J. A., DO, K. A., JENQ, R. R., KONTOYIANNIS, D. P. & SHELBURNE, S. A. 2020. Gut microbiome signatures are predictive of infectious risk following induction therapy for acute myeloid leukemia. *Clinical Infectious Diseases*, 71, 63–71.

GARAJOVÁ, I., BALSANO, R., WANG, H., LEONARDI, F., GIOVANNETTI, E., DENG, D. & PETERS, G. J. 2021. The role of the microbiome in drug resistance in gastrointestinal cancers. *Expert Review of Anticancer Therapy*, 21, 165–176.

GELLER, L. T., BARZILY-ROKNI, M., DANINO, T., JONAS, O. H., SHENTAL, N., NEJMAN, D., GAVERT, N., ZWANG, Y., COOPER, Z. A., SHEE, K., THAISS, C. A., REUBEN, A., LIVNY, J., AVRAHAM, R., FREDERICK, D. T., LIGORIO, M., CHATMAN, K., JOHNSTON, S. E., MOSHER, C. M., BRANDIS, A., FUKS, G., GURBATRI, C., GOPALAKRISHNAN, V., KIM, M., HURD, M. W., KATZ, M., FLEMING, J., MAITRA, A., SMITH, D. A., SKALAK, M., BU, J., MICHAUD, M., TRAUGER, S. A., BARSHACK, I., GOLAN, T., SANDBANK, J., FLAHERTY, K. T., MANDINOVA, A., GARRETT, W. S., THAYER, S. P., FERRONE, C. R., HUTTENHOWER, C., BHATIA, S. N., GEVERS, D., WARGO, J. A., GOLUB, T. R. & STRAUSSMAN, R. 2017. Potential role of intratumor bacteria in mediating tumor resistance to the chemotherapeutic drug gemcitabine. *Science*, 357, 1156–1160.

GLICK, D., BARTH, S. & MACLEOD, K. F. 2010. Autophagy: Cellular and molecular mechanisms. *The Journal of Pathology*, 221, 3–12.

GORLICK, R., GOKER, E., TRIPPETT, T., WALTHAM, M., BANERJEE, D. & BERTINO, J. R. 1996. Intrinsic and acquired resistance to methotrexate in acute leukemia. *New England Journal of Medicine*, 335, 1041–1048.

HUANG, J., LIU, W., KANG, W., HE, Y., YANG, R., MOU, X. & ZHAO, W. 2022. Effects of microbiota on anticancer drugs: Current knowledge and potential applications. *EBioMedicine*, 83, 104197.

LAURA, B., RASHIDA, G., MOHIT, S., MEGAN, P., DANIEL, G., GHATALIA, P., HENKEL, V., ADAM, C., JASON, R. B., ANDRES, C., KIRTISHRI, M., RAYMOND, P., ELIZABETH, P., ALEXANDER, K., MAHMOUD, G., MOHAMMED, E., MAURICIO, R., ROBERT, U., LEE, P. & PHILIP, H. A. 2023. Role of gut microbiome in neoadjuvant chemotherapy response in urothelial carcinoma: A multi-institutional prospective cohort evaluation. *bioRxiv*, 2023.01.21.525021.

LI, L.-Y., GUAN, Y.-D., CHEN, X.-S., YANG, J.-M. & CHENG, Y. 2021. DNA repair pathways in cancer therapy and resistance. *Frontiers in Pharmacology*, 11, 629266.

LI, X., ZHOU, Y., LI, Y., YANG, L., MA, Y., PENG, X., YANG, S., LIU, J. & LI, H. 2019. Autophagy: A novel mechanism of chemoresistance in cancers. *Biomedicine & Pharmacotherapy*, 119, 109415.

LIU, L., BAI, Y., XIANG, L., QI, W., GAO, L., LI, X., LI, H., WANG, B. & CHEN, H. 2022. Interaction between gut microbiota and tumour chemotherapy. *Clinical and Translational Oncology*, 24, 2330–2341.

LIU, Y., BABA, Y., ISHIMOTO, T., TSUTSUKI, H., ZHANG, T., NOMOTO, D., OKADOME, K., YAMAMURA, K., HARADA, K., ETO, K., HIYOSHI, Y., IWATSUKI, M., NAGAI, Y., IWAGAMI, S., MIYAMOTO, Y., YOSHIDA, N., KOMOHARA, Y., OHMURAYA, M., WANG, X., AJANI, J. A., SAWA, T. & BABA, H. 2021. Fusobacterium nucleatum confers chemoresistance by modulating autophagy in oesophageal squamous cell carcinoma. *British Journal of Cancer*, 124, 963–974.

LU, C. & SHERVINGTON, A. 2008. Chemoresistance in gliomas. *Molecular and Cellular Biochemistry*, 312, 71–80.

LU, K. H., LU, E. W., LIN, C. W., YANG, J. S. & YANG, S. F. 2020. New insights into molecular and cellular mechanisms of zoledronate in human osteosarcoma. *Pharmacology & Therapeutics*, 214, 107611.

MONTASSIER, E., GASTINNE, T., VANGAY, P., AL-GHALITH, G. A., BRULEY DES VARANNES, S., MASSART, S., MOREAU, P., POTEL, G., DE LA COCHETIÈRE, M. F., BATARD, E. & KNIGHTS, D. 2015. Chemotherapy-driven dysbiosis in the intestinal microbiome. *Alimentary Pharmacology & Therapeutics*, 42, 515–528.

MOTOORI, M., YANO, M., MIYATA, H., SUGIMURA, K., SAITO, T., OMORI, T., FUJIWARA, Y., MIYOSHI, N., AKITA, H., GOTOH, K., TAKAHASHI, H., KOBAYASHI, S., NOURA, S., OHUE, M., ASAHARA, T., NOMOTO, K., ISHIKAWA, O. & SAKON, M. 2017. Randomized study of the effect of synbiotics during neoadjuvant chemotherapy on adverse events in esophageal cancer patients. *Clinical Nutrition*, 36, 93–99.

NICHOLSON, J. K., HOLMES, E., KINROSS, J., BURCELIN, R., GIBSON, G., JIA, W. & PETTERSSON, S. 2012. Host-gut microbiota metabolic interactions. *Science*, 336, 1262–1267.

NISTICÒ, P., BISSELL, M. J. & RADISKY, D. C. 2012. Epithelial-mesenchymal transition: General principles and pathological relevance with special emphasis on the role of matrix metalloproteinases. *Cold Spring Harbor Perspectives in Biology*, 4, a011908.

OH, B., BOYLE, F., PAVLAKIS, N., CLARKE, S., GUMINSKI, A., EADE, T., LAMOURY, G., CARROLL, S., MORGIA, M., KNEEBONE, A., HRUBY, G., STEVENS, M., LIU, W., CORLESS, B., MOLLOY, M., LIBERMANN, T., ROSENTHAL, D. & BACK, M. 2021. Emerging evidence of the gut microbiome in chemotherapy: A clinical review. *Frontiers in Oncology*, 11, 706331.

OHATA, Y., SHIMADA, S., AKIYAMA, Y., MOGUSHI, K., NAKAO, K., MATSUMURA, S., AIHARA, A., MITSUNORI, Y., BAN, D., OCHIAI, T., KUDO, A., ARII, S., TANABE, M. & TANAKA, S. 2017. Acquired resistance with epigenetic alterations under long-term antiangiogenic therapy for hepatocellular carcinoma. *Molecular Cancer Therapeutics,* 16, 1155–1165.

PARVEZ, M. M., BASIT, A., JARIWALA, P. B., GÁBORIK, Z., KIS, E., HEYWARD, S., REDINBO, M. R. & PRASAD, B. 2021. Quantitative investigation of irinotecan metabolism, transport, and gut microbiome activation. *Drug Metabolism and Disposition,* 49, 683–693.

PU, Y., WANG, J. & WANG, S. 2022. Role of autophagy in drug resistance and regulation of osteosarcoma (Review). *Molecular and Clinical Oncology,* 16, 72.

RAJAGOPALA, S. V., SINGH, H., YU, Y., ZABOKRTSKY, K. B., TORRALBA, M. G., MONCERA, K. J., FRANK, B., PIEPER, R., SENDER, L. & NELSON, K. E. 2020. Persistent gut microbial dysbiosis in children with Acute Lymphoblastic Leukemia (ALL) during chemotherapy. *Microbial Ecology,* 79, 1034–1043.

RAMOS, A., SADEGHI, S. & TABATABAEIAN, H. 2021. Battling chemoresistance in cancer: Root causes and strategies to uproot them. *International Journal of Molecular Sciences,* 22, 9451.

REYHANOGLU, G. & SMITH, T. 2023. *Irinotecan.* StatPearls. Treasure Island (FL): StatPearls Publishing Copyright © 2023, StatPearls Publishing LLC.

RUSU, R.-A., SÎRBU, D., CURȘEU, D., NĂSUI, B., SAVA, M., VESA, Ș. C., BOJAN, A., LISENCU, C. & POPA, M. 2018. Chemotherapy-related infectious complications in patients with Hematologic malignancies. *Journal of Research in Medical Sciences,* 23, 68.

SAYIN, S., ROSENER, B., LI, C. G., HO, B., PONOMAROVA, O., WARD, D. V., WALHOUT, A. J. M. & MITCHELL, A. 2023. Evolved bacterial resistance to the chemotherapy gemcitabine modulates its efficacy in co-cultured cancer cells. *eLife,* 12, e83140.

SCOTT, A. J., MERRIFIELD, C. A., YOUNES, J. A. & PEKELHARING, E. P. 2018. Pre-, pro- and synbiotics in cancer prevention and treatment – A review of basic and clinical research. *Ecancermedicalscience,* 12, 869.

SEGATA, N., IZARD, J., WALDRON, L., GEVERS, D., MIROPOLSKY, L., GARRETT, W. S. & HUTTENHOWER, C. 2011. Metagenomic biomarker discovery and explanation. *Genome Biology,* 12, R60.

SENTHEBANE, D. A., ROWE, A., THOMFORD, N. E., SHIPANGA, H., MUNRO, D., MAZEEDI, M., ALMAZYADI, H. A. M., KALLMEYER, K., DANDARA, C., PEPPER, M. S., PARKER, M. I. & DZOBO, K. 2017. The role of tumor microenvironment in chemoresistance: To survive, keep your enemies closer. *International Journal of Molecular Sciences,* 18, 1586.

SEVCIKOVA, A., IZOLDOVA, N., STEVURKOVA, V., KASPEROVA, B., CHOVANEC, M., CIERNIKOVA, S. & MEGO, M. 2022. The impact of the microbiome on resistance to cancer treatment with chemotherapeutic agents and immunotherapy. *International Journal of Molecular Sciences,* 23, 488.

SHREINER, A. B., KAO, J. Y. & YOUNG, V. B. 2015. The gut microbiome in health and in disease. *Current Opinion in Gastroenterology,* 31, 69–75.

SHUWEN, H., XI, Y., YUEFEN, P., JIAMIN, X., QUAN, Q., HAIHONG, L., YIZHEN, J. & WEI, W. 2020. Effects of postoperative adjuvant chemotherapy and palliative chemotherapy on the gut microbiome in colorectal cancer. *Microbial Pathogenesis,* 149, 104343.

SISTIGU, A., VIAUD, S., CHAPUT, N., BRACCI, L., PROIETTI, E. & ZITVOGEL, L. 2011. Immunomodulatory effects of cyclophosphamide and implementations for vaccine design. *Seminars in Immunopathology,* 33, 369–383.

STRINGER, A. M., GIBSON, R. J., BOWEN, J. M., LOGAN, R. M., ASHTON, K., YEOH, A. S., AL-DASOOQI, N. & KEEFE, D. M. 2009. Irinotecan-induced mucositis manifesting as diarrhoea corresponds with an amended intestinal flora and mucin profile. *International Journal of Experimental Pathology,* 90, 489–499.

SUI, X., CHEN, R., WANG, Z., HUANG, Z., KONG, N., ZHANG, M., HAN, W., LOU, F., YANG, J., ZHANG, Q., WANG, X., HE, C. & PAN, H. 2013. Autophagy and chemotherapy resistance: A promising therapeutic target for cancer treatment. *Cell Death & Disease,* 4, e838.

SUNG, H., FERLAY, J., SIEGEL, R. L., LAVERSANNE, M., SOERJOMATARAM, I., JEMAL, A. & BRAY, F. 2021. Global Cancer Statistics 2020: GLOBOCAN estimates of incidence and mortality worldwide for 36 cancers in 185 countries. *CA Cancer J Clin,* 71, 209–249.

TINTELNOT, J., XU, Y., LESKER, T. R., SCHÖNLEIN, M., KONCZALLA, L., GIANNOU, A. D., PELCZAR, P., KYLIES, D., PUELLES, V. G., BIELECKA, A. A., PESCHKA, M., CORTESI, F., RIECKEN, K., JUNG, M., AMEND, L., BRÖRING, T. S., TRAJKOVIC-ARSIC, M., SIVEKE, J. T., RENNÉ, T., ZHANG, D., BOECK, S., STROWIG, T., UZUNOGLU, F. G., GÜNGÖR, C., STEIN, A., IZBICKI, J. R., BOKEMEYER, C., SINN, M., KIMMELMAN, A. C., HUBER, S. & GAGLIANI, N. 2023. Microbiota-derived 3-IAA influences chemotherapy efficacy in pancreatic cancer. *Nature,* 615, 168–174.

TONG, J., ZHANG, X., FAN, Y., CHEN, L., MA, X., YU, H., LI, J., GUAN, X., ZHAO, P. & YANG, J. 2020. Changes of intestinal microbiota in ovarian cancer patients treated with surgery and chemotherapy. *Cancer Management and Research,* 12, 8125–8135.

TOSCHI, L., FINOCCHIARO, G., BARTOLINI, S., GIOIA, V. & CAPPUZZO, F. 2005. Role of gemcitabine in cancer therapy. *Future Oncology,* 1, 7–17.

VALLE, J. W., FURUSE, J., JITLAL, M., BEARE, S., MIZUNO, N., WASAN, H., BRIDGEWATER, J. & OKUSAKA, T. 2014. Cisplatin and gemcitabine for advanced biliary tract cancer: A meta-analysis of two randomised trials. *Annals of Oncology,* 25, 391–398.

VAN VLIET, M. J., HARMSEN, H. J., DE BONT, E. S. & TISSING, W. J. 2010. The role of intestinal microbiota in the development and severity of chemotherapy-induced mucositis. *PLOS Pathogens,* 6, e1000879.

VAN VLIET, M. J., TISSING, W. J., DUN, C. A., MEESSEN, N. E., KAMPS, W. A., DE BONT, E. S. & HARMSEN, H. J. 2009. Chemotherapy treatment in pediatric patients with acute myeloid leukemia receiving antimicrobial prophylaxis leads to a relative increase of colonization with potentially pathogenic bacteria in the gut. *Clinical Infectious Diseases,* 49, 262–270.

VIAUD, S., SACCHERI, F., MIGNOT, G., YAMAZAKI, T., DAILLÈRE, R., HANNANI, D., ENOT, D. P., PFIRSCHKE, C., ENGBLOM, C., PITTET, M. J., SCHLITZER, A., GINHOUX, F., APETOH, L., CHACHATY, E., WOERTHER, P. L., EBERL, G., BÉRARD, M., ECOBICHON, C., CLERMONT, D., BIZET, C., GABORIAU-ROUTHIAU, V., CERF-BENSUSSAN, N., OPOLON, P., YESSAAD, N., VIVIER, E., RYFFEL, B., ELSON, C. O., DORÉ,

J., KROEMER, G., LEPAGE, P., BONECA, I. G., GHIRINGHELLI, F. & ZITVOGEL, L. 2013. The intestinal microbiota modulates the anticancer immune effects of cyclophosphamide. *Science,* 342, 971–976.

VIVARELLI, S., SALEMI, R., CANDIDO, S., FALZONE, L., SANTAGATI, M., STEFANI, S., TORINO, F., BANNA, G. L., TONINI, G. & LIBRA, M. 2019. Gut microbiota and cancer: From pathogenesis to therapy. *Cancers (Basel),* 11, 38.

WANG, X., ZHANG, H. & CHEN, X. 2019. Drug resistance and combating drug resistance in cancer. *Cancer Drug Resistance,* 2, 141–160.

WARDILL, H. R., VAN DER AA, S. A. R., DA SILVA FERREIRA, A. R., HAVINGA, R., TISSING, W. J. E. & HARMSEN, H. J. M. 2021. Antibiotic-induced disruption of the microbiome exacerbates chemotherapy-induced diarrhoea and can be mitigated with autologous faecal microbiota transplantation. *European Journal of Cancer,* 153, 27–39.

WEI, L., WEN, X. S. & XIAN, C. J. 2021. Chemotherapy-induced intestinal microbiota dysbiosis impairs mucosal homeostasis by modulating toll-like receptor signaling pathways. *International Journal of Molecular Sciences,* 22, 9474.

XU, Y. & VILLALONA-CALERO, M. A. 2002. Irinotecan: Mechanisms of tumor resistance and novel strategies for modulating its activity. *Annals of Oncology,* 13, 1841–1851.

YANG, Q., WANG, B., ZHENG, Q., LI, H., MENG, X., ZHOU, F. & ZHANG, L. 2023. A review of gut microbiota-derived metabolites in tumor progression and cancer therapy. *Advanced Science,* 10, 2207366.

YU, T., GUO, F., YU, Y., SUN, T., MA, D., HAN, J., QIAN, Y., KRYCZEK, I., SUN, D., NAGARSHETH, N., CHEN, Y., CHEN, H., HONG, J., ZOU, W. & FANG, J.-Y. 2017. Fusobacterium nucleatum promotes chemoresistance to colorectal cancer by modulating autophagy. *Cell,* 170, 548–563.e16.

YUAN, L., ZHANG, S., LI, H., YANG, F., MUSHTAQ, N., ULLAH, S., SHI, Y., AN, C. & XU, J. 2018. The influence of gut microbiota dysbiosis to the efficacy of 5-Fluorouracil treatment on colorectal cancer. *Biomedicine & Pharmacotherapy,* 108, 184–193.

YUE, B., GAO, R., WANG, Z. & DOU, W. 2021. Microbiota-host-irinotecan axis: A new insight toward irinotecan chemotherapy. *Frontiers in Cellular and Infection Microbiology,* 11, 710945.

ZHANG, S., YANG, Y., WENG, W., GUO, B., CAI, G., MA, Y. & CAI, S. 2019. Fusobacterium nucleatum promotes chemoresistance to 5-fluorouracil by upregulation of BIRC3 expression in colorectal cancer. *Journal of Experimental & Clinical Cancer Research,* 38, 14.

ZHENG, H.-C. 2017. The molecular mechanisms of chemoresistance in cancers. *Oncotarget,* 8, 59950–59964.

7 Gut Microbiome Biomarkers for Colorectal Cancer Diagnosis and Prognosis

Rahaba Marima, Afra Basera, Patrick T. Dumakude, Olalekan Fadebi, Linomtha Gabada, Amahle Nyalambisa, Lydia Mphahlele, Egnesious Sambo, Kamal S. Saini, and Zodwa Dlamini

INTRODUCTION

The gut microbiome is an exciting frontier in cancer research and management. There are approximately 100 trillion microbial cells present in a human body, most of which are found in the gut (Mármol et al., 2017). This microbial community is termed the microbiome and includes a plethora of microbes, such as, archaea, fungi, viruses, and anaerobic bacteria (Scarpellini et al., 2015). However, more studies gravitate towards bacteria as they are most abundant. These microbial populations play significant roles in maintaining body homeostasis. Some of their roles in the host include modulating the human immune system, preventing colonization by enteropathogenic bacteria and helping extract energy from indigestible carbohydrates such as pectin (Geuking et al., 2014). Research shows that changes in normal flora may result in disease. Dysbiosis is a condition whereby the interaction between the host and the gut flora is altered and may lead to inflammatory bowel disease or colorectal cancer (CRC) (Quaglio et al., 2022). Furthermore, the gut microbiome can also influence distant organs through microorganism-associated molecular patterns (MAMPs) and other bacterial metabolites (Tao et al., 2015, Yu and Schwabe, 2017). Modifications in the intestinal microbiome can be attributed to intrinsic and extrinsic factors, and present with significant inter-human gut microbiome variability. While the human genome is about 99.9% identical to each other, the human gut microbiome is about 85% distinct from each other (Usell et al., 2012, Anipindi and Bitetto, 2022). This distinct gap may render potency towards the gut microbiome use in early cancer diagnosis.

Microbial signatures can be developed by using modifications in microbiota constitution from antibiotics, probiotics, and anticancer therapies (Bhatt et al., 2017). Although more research is warranted, research demonstrating unique microbial signatures in various malignancies including CRC could aid in the development of specific biomarkers correlating with prognosis. For example, in murine-based models, it has been demonstrated that fecal microbial transplantation with unique microbial signatures decreases DNA damage from radiation. Thus the identification of these microbial signatures may aid in the identification of cancer patient's radiosensitivity (Anipindi and Bitetto, 2022). The complex mechanisms of the gut microbiota cognate with tumor development and progression are multifaceted and remain to be understood. This chapter aims to discuss the utility of the gut microbiome biomarkers in CRC by deciphering role of gut microbiome biomarkers in CRC development and progression, in CRC signaling pathways and highlighting their role in non-invasive CRC "biopsies."

GUT MICROBIOME BIOMARKERS IN CRC DEVELOPMENT AND PROGRESSION

The gut microbiome has been linked to the development and progression of CRC and is partially responsible for the initial inflammatory response and changes to various cancer signaling pathways (Maisonneuve et al., 2018, Montalban-Arques and Scharl, 2019, Gopalakrishnan et al., 2018). The presence of specific bacterial strains, as well as altered composition and fungal strains in colorectal adenomas, has been shown to be associated with the advancement of CRC (Rebersek, 2021, Allen and Sears, 2019). An interwoven connection exists among the gut, tumor microbiomes, and the immune system during cancer progression (Inamura, 2018, Scott et al., 2019). Eubiosis is a condition of health in which the intestinal microbiome is observed to be healthy, with an uncompromised mucosal barrier and mucus layer as well as an equilibrium between immune cells and IgA secretion, proinflammation, and anti-inflammatory cytokines. On the other hand, these traits are not in equilibrium in dysbiosis. In contrast to a healthy gut microbiome, the CRC microbiota contains a distinct make-up of bacterial species, including those linked to the disease such as *Escherichia coli, Bacteroides fragilis, Streptococcus gallolyticus,* and *Enterococcus faecalis.* Recently found strains of bacteria associated with CRC are *Porphyromonas, Fusobacterium nucleatum, Peptostreptococcus, Parvimonas,* and *Prevotella* (Rebersek, 2021). The presence of these strains of bacteria in detectable amounts in the tumor and fecal specimen of patients can serve as CRC biomarkers (Wong and Yu, 2019, Grenham et al., 2011). The gut microbiota influences CRC growth through several pathways, including immune response control, inflammatory, and changed metabolism of food components, which can result in the synthesis of hazardous microbiological byproducts like metabolites or genotoxin (Ternes et al., 2020, Schwabe and Jobin, 2013, Montalban-Arques and Scharl, 2019).

Chronic inflammation in the colorectal epithelium is influenced by gut microbes. Typhoid toxins secreted by *Salmonella* and colibactin secreted by *Escherichia coli* result in the generation of pro-inflammatory cytokines and bacterial adhesion (Kim and Lee, 2021, André et al., 2020). Chronic inflammation and elevated reactive oxygen species (ROS) are key factors associated with CRC, while DNA damage of epithelial cells is also a crucial factor in CRC development by gut microbiota (Kim and Lee, 2021).

The bacterium *Streptococcus bovis* which is typically found in the gastrointestinal tract (GIT), is established to induce endocarditis or bacteremia and is a precursor of colon cancer (Gupta et al., 2010). Via an inflammation-based series of tumor formation or integration of interleukin (IL)-1, cyclooxygenase-2 (COX-2), and IL-8 (Biarc et al., 2004, Rebersek, 2021), *S. bovis* actively contributes to the development of CRC. Additionally, an established strain for the development of CRC is *Fusobacterium nucleatum* (Castellarin et al., 2012). Commensal *Fusobacterium* spp. have been linked to CRC in humans, however, it is uncertain whether they are directly or indirectly pro-carcinogenic based on a metagenomic study (Rebersek, 2021). Bacteria can cause cancer either directly (in the case of a driver) or indirectly (in the case of a passenger). In the tumor microenvironment, passenger bacteria multiply as opportunistic bacteria (Wong and Yu, 2019, Saus et al., 2019, Rebersek, 2021). *Fusobacterium nucleatum* is reported to produce Fusobacterium adhesin A (FadA), a distinct protein, which promotes the initiation of the β-catenin signaling pathway following binding to E-cadherin, known to be a strong inducer of cancer (Rebersek, 2021). Furthermore, superoxides are naturally produced in the gut by commensal *Enterococcus faecalis*. Infection with *Enterococcus faecalis* promotes DNA damage to the intestinal epithelial cells by producing larger quantities of the superoxide. The *Enterococcus faecalis* strain was reported to be present in significantly higher numbers in CRC patients than in healthy individuals (Wang et al., 2012). Studies reported that *Enterococcus faecalis* is capable of producing hydroxyl radicals (Huycke et al., 2001, Huycke and Moore, 2002). These potent mutagens may result in DNA cleavage, point mutations, and protein-DNA crosslinking, which may lead to genomic instability and raise the probability of CRC (Evans et al., 2004). Previous study has revealed an association between the gut microbiome and colorectal adenomas, which are precursors to CRC (Wong and Yu, 2019). Furthermore, research found that *Fusobacterium nucleatum* created a pro-inflammatory milieu in the adenomatous polyposis coli (APC) +/- murine CRC model, causing neoplasia progression in intestinal epithelial cells (Kim and Lee, 2021, Li et al., 2019). Figure 7.1 illustrates the role of different bacterial strains on cellular processes in promoting CRC.

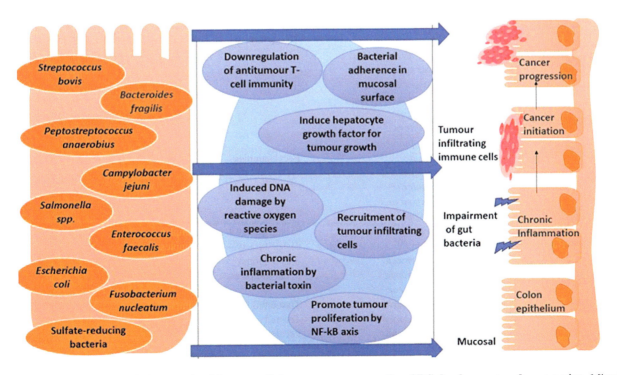

FIGURE 7.1 **The influence of the gut microbiota on cellular processes, promoting CRC development and progression.** Microbial toxins induce chronic inflammation, DNA damage, and the downregulation of antitumor cells, resulting in CRC.

GUT MICROBIOME BIOMARKERS IN CRC DIAGNOSIS: EXPLORING TISSUE AND FECAL BIOPSIES

According to recent research, the interplay between immune control and anticancer immunotherapies could be affected by the gut microbiota (Asseri et al., 2023). The evaluation of molecular pathology is essential for neoplasia therapy since tumor grade and the likelihood of metastasis affect the therapeutic approach and chance of success thereof. The availability of tumor biopsies and their limited breadth of sampling (i.e., only one tiny slice of a big, diverse, or metastatic tumor) place restrictions on tissue-based analysis using tumor biopsies (Newsome and Jobin, 2021, Zhang et al., 2021). Non-tissue or liquid biopsies-based technologies have received widespread attention. Cell-free tumor's DNA (ctDNA) and ctRNA, which are found in bodily fluids such as blood plasma, urine, and spinal fluid are used to screen for tumor type and grade. One key benefit of liquid biopsies is that several samples can be collected in a minimally invasive manner, and that the ctDNA is indicative of both nearby tumors and distant locations of metastases. However, these tests necessitate extensive processing, have large false positive or negative rates, and are mainly useful for tumor types with a significant burden of mutations. These liquid samples can be analyzed for early cancer identification, supplementary staging, prognosis evaluation, medication resistance monitoring, and minimal residual disease (MRD) monitoring. Moreover, recent microbiome research suggests that the microbial composition and metabolites in feces can predict the development of CRC and response to chemotherapy or immunotherapy (Newman et al., 2019, Neish, 2009, Zhang et al., 2021, David et al., 2023, Ding et al., 2020).

Invasive procedures are still employable for diagnosis of CRC, this includes endoscopy and surgical method to access bowel tissues. However, because it is more pertinent to the pathological mechanisms involved in CRC development, tissue microbiome continues to have significant scientific relevance. The multifariousness of the tissue microbiome can be detected in various CRC stages and also in the microbiomes of tumor tissues from various intestinal sites, which is significant to bolster their possible contribution to the early diagnosis of CRC. This is in line with the findings of fecal and blood microbiomes in the early detection of CRC (Zhou et al., 2022).

In order to improve the effectiveness of therapies, such as immunotherapy, the gut microbiota has become a novel prognostic biomarker and possible therapeutic target (Rahman et al., 2022, Sillo et al., 2023). Few biomarkers have been successfully used to diagnose CRC as of yet. Therefore, tumor heterogeneity may be one rationale for such biomarker-directed immunotherapy. The primary characteristic of carcinogenesis is tumor heterogeneity, which is associated with unsuccessful drug therapy (Ao et al., 2021). Table 7.1 shows CRC-enriched gut microbiota from tissue and fecal biopsies.

TABLE 7.1

Gut microbiome CRC potential biomarkers

Taxonomy	Bacterial species	Source	Reference
Firmicutes	Streptococcus bovis	Tissue biopsy	(Liu et al., 2023)
	Streptococcus thermophilus		
	Streptococcus spp.		
	Peptostreptococcus stomatis		
	Peptostreptococcus anerobius		
	Parvimonas micra		
	Gemella merbilorum		
	Selenomonas sputigena		
	Staphylococceae	Fecal samples	
	Enterococcus faecalis		
	Parvimonas micra		
	Solobacterium moorei		
	Clostridium symbiosum		
Fusobacteria	Fusobacterium nucleatum	Tissue biopsy + fecal samples	
Bacteroidetes	BFT-producing Bacteroides fragilis	Tissue biopsy + fecal samples	
	Prevotella intermedia	Tissue biopsy	
	Prevotella nigrescencs	Fecal samples	
	Porhyromonadaceae		
Proteobacteria	Colibactin Escherichia coli	Tissue biopsy + fecal samples	
	Campylobacter gracilis	Tissue biopsy	
	Campylobacter rectus	Fecal samples	
	Shigella spp.		
Actinobacteria	Coriobateriaceae	Tissue biopsy + fecal samples	
	Actinomyces odontolyticus	Tissue biopsy	
	Atopobium parvulum		

GUT MICROBIOME BIOMARKERS IN CRC SIGNALING PATHWAYS

The development of spontaneous CRC is an organized chain of events known as the adenoma-carcinoma sequence (ACS), which denotes the change of the typical epithelium of the colon to an adenomatous intermediary, eventually leading to adenocarcinoma (Bennedsen et al., 2022). The gut microbiome induces tumorigenesis by regulating various signaling pathways in the host. Pathogenic bacteria's proteins, enzymes, and toxins adhere to host cells, altering their regular function and encouraging different tumors and malignancies (Vivarelli et al., 2019, Akbar et al., 2022). Metabolites and enzymes released due to dysbiosis result in the host's DNA breaks (Halazonetis, 2004, Frisan, 2016), altered DNA damage response and repair (Lara-Tejero and Galán, 2000), and disruption of intercellular junctions (Murata-Kamiya et al., 2007, Wu et al., 2007), which promote cancer initiation, development, and progression (Yao and Dai, 2014). Advances in sequencing have shown how certain bacteria can influence cancer signaling pathways, including the Wnt, TGF-β, PI3K, MAPK, AKT, and EGFR/MPK1 pathways (Bennedsen et al., 2022, Lee et al., 2021, Ramanan et al., 2012). Bacteria inculpated in these signaling pathways can function as biomarkers for prognosis and diagnosis in CRC (Wirbel et al., 2019, Dai et al., 2018). There is accumulating evidence that the microbiome modulates antitumor immune regulation. Short-chain fatty acids, including sodium butyrate, that result from microbiota promote the formation of memory T cells and modulate the activity of regulatory T cells (Czajka-Francuz et al., 2023).

THE INFLUENCE OF THE GUT MICROBIOME ON THE WNT PATHWAY

The Wnt signaling pathway is a conserved mechanism that regulates essential elements of the fate of cells (Komiya and Habas, 2008). The attachment of the Wnt protein to its receptor disassembles APC, a tumor-suppressor, and the complex (GSK3-β and β-catenin), elevating the quantity of β-catenin in the cytoplasm, causing it to translocate into the nucleus thus increasing transcription (Li and Lai, 2009, Novellasdemunt et al., 2015, Humphries and Wright, 2008). However, abnormal Wnt signaling activity has been linked to several biological events associated with malignancies and tumor progression (Zhao et al., 2023, Zhan et al., 2017). Multiple bacterial virulence components which target the Wnt/b-catenin pathway have lately been discovered, leading to inflammatory reactions (Wang et al., 2018). One instance is *Fusobacterium nucleatum*, whose involvement in CRC has been widely documented (Villar-Ortega et al., 2022, Gethings-Behncke et al., 2020). *Fusobacterium nucleatum* stimulates the Wnt/β-catenin pathway by upregulating cyclin-dependent kinase 5 (Cdk5), thus encouraging cell growth and migration (Li et al., 2021, Mima et al., 2016). Other studies show that *Fusobacterium nucleatum* induced β-catenin-modulated transcription and elevated the quantities of transcription factors and transforming genes (c-Myc and Cyclin D1) through the binding of its adhesion molecule FadA to E-cadherin (Rubinstein et al., 2013). Moreover, the attachment of FadA to E-cadherin increases levels of Annexin A1, thus impacting the signaling pathway (Rubinstein et al., 2019). Li et al. used a mouse model with an adenomatous polyposis coli (Apc) gene mutation through fecal microbiota transplantation (FMT) to study the impact of gut microbiota in the development of intestinal adenoma. The findings showed intestinal adenoma-adenocarcinoma in $Apc^{min/+}$ mice increased by the gut microbiota of CRC patients. In addition, there was a disturbance of the gastrointestinal barrier, persistent mild inflammation, Wnt signaling pathway activation, and a disruption in the balance in the gut microbiome (Li et al., 2019). A virulence factor known as BFT, released by Enterotoxigenic *Bacteroides fragilis* (ETBF), can stimulate Wnt signaling by cleaving E-cadherin (Wu et al., 2003).

THE INFLUENCE OF THE GUT MICROBIOME ON THE PI3K/AKT PATHWAY

The PI3K/AKT/mTOR signaling pathway regulates the cell cycle (Terracciano et al., 2019). This is observed when KRAS, a monomeric guanosine triphosphatase (GTPase) relays information from the epidermal growth factor receptor (EGFR) when EGF binds to the EGFR. The activation of KRAS by the binding of guanosine triphosphate (GTP) causes the activation of phosphatidylinositol 3-kinase (PI3K), which then induces the phosphorylation of the serine/threonine kinase AKT via the mammalian kinase target of rapamycin (mTOR). The phosphorylation of AKT causes its movement into the nucleus, wherein it modulates the transcription of genes concerned with cell viability (Goel et al., 2015, Testa et al., 2018, Long et al., 2019). Although additional studies are warranted, a study by Long et al. (2019) elucidated the influence of microbes on the PI3K/AKT pathway in CRC. *Peptostreptococcus anaerobius* was reported to upregulate the expression of the PI3K and AKT proteins. This study revealed an increase in cell growth via the PI3K/AKT pathway, as the levels of proliferating cell nuclear antigen (a cell growth marker) were elevated in the presence of *Peptostreptococcus anaerobius* (Long et al., 2019). Similarly, an investigation has documented the tumorigenic effect of microbes in relation to EGFR. Exposure of CRC cells to *Listeria monocytogenes* medium revealed increased expression of ErbB2 and ErbB3, which promotes cell invasion (Oliveira et al., 2005). While the cancer signaling pathways mechanisms have been documented in CRC, the specific mechanisms of the association of the intestinal microbiome and these signaling pathways are yet to be clarified.

THE INFLUENCE OF THE GUT MICROBIOME ON THE MAPK PATHWAY

Apart from signaling via the PI3K/AKT system, KRAS signals via the mitogen-activated protein kinase (MAPK) module. RAS, a GTPase protein, initially stimulates the RAF kinase, triggering MEK-activating MAPKs, including ERK (Saini et al., 2013). The aforementioned MAPK proteins activate transcription factors, causing their translocation into the nucleus and regulating the transcription of targeted genes associated with migratory and differentiation activities (Guo et al., 2020). *Porphyromonas gingivalis*, previously associated with periodontitis and later discovered to be abundant in excremental and mucosal specimens from individuals with CRC, increased CRC growth by activating the MAPK and PI3K/AKT pathways (Mu et al., 2020).

THE INFLUENCE OF THE GUT MICROBIOME ON THE TGF-β SIGNALING PATHWAY

Transforming growth factors (TGFs) are multifaceted cytokines that play significant roles in a myriad of biological phenomenon, including growth, differentiation, and immune modulation; despite that, it is uncertain how these mechanisms have a role in colon tumor suppression (Daniel et al., 2017). In CRC, the transforming growth factor-β (TGF-β) type II receptor gene is mutated, resulting in the loss of transforming growth factor receptor 2 (TGFR2) expression, consequently affecting TGF-β signaling. Mutations in mothers against decapentaplegic (SMAD) genes impair TGF-β signaling at rates of 3.4% (SMAD2), 4.3% (SMAD3), and 8.6% (SMAD4) in spontaneous CRC tumors (Fleming et al., 2013). SMAD2/3 forms a transcriptional complex with SMAD4 (co-SMAD). SMAD3 alterations can inhibit SMAD3 transcription (Monteleone et al., 2001). Increased synthesis of SMAD7 in diseased gut mucosa specimens from individuals with active ulcerative colitis and Crohn's disease inhibits TGFR1 kinase-modulated phosphorylation of SMAD3 protein and impairs TGF-β signaling (Hayashi et al., 1997). TGFBR2 alterations, SMAD2/3/4 alterations, and high SMAD7 concentrations, when combined, impair TGF-β signaling and promote CRC development (Svrcek et al., 2007, Yashiro, 2014).

Because TGF-β signaling has been established as a key regulator of immunological tolerance and T-cell homeostasis, its deficiency is shown to worsen inflammation in the mouse colon (Daniel et al., 2017). An induced deficiency of SMAD3 (SMAD3$^{-/-}$) in a mouse model revealed that exposure to *Helicobacter pylori* resulted in a prolonged inflammatory condition. Furthermore, the presence of *Helicobacter pylori* in the colon alters the transcripts of *c-myc*, tumor necrosis factor-α, and interleukins 1α (IL-1α), IL-1β, IL-6, IFN-γ, which form part of the TGF-β pathway, suggesting that bacteria may be pivotal in triggering CRC through the TGF-β (Maggio-Price et al., 2006).

Additionally, deficiencies in SMAD3 reportedly cause microbial alterations to bacterial functions. An instance is the cutback of RNA counts of Butyrate Kinase (Buk), a crucial butyrate gene, responsible for maintaining the colon epithelium by *Lachnospiraceae* bacterium A4 potentially causing tumor development. Furthermore, *Mucispirillum schaedleri* was demonstrated to promote lipopolysaccharide production, which is linked to an inflammatory reaction (Daniel et al., 2017). Figure 7.2 demonstrates CRC signaling pathways associated with gut bacteria.

GUT MICROBIOME BIOMARKERS AS PROGNOSTICATORS IN CRC

The gut microbiota's potential to influence responses to cancer treatment, including chemotherapy and radiotherapy, has

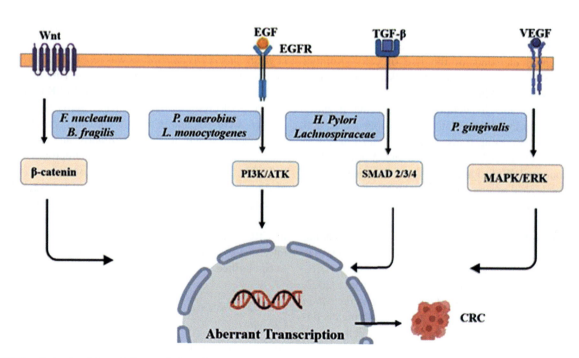

FIGURE 7.2 **Gut microbiome influenced signaling pathways involved in CRC.** Several bacteria affect the Wnt, PI3K/ATK, TGF-β and MAPK signaling pathways, promoting the tumorigenic processes in CRC.

been extensively investigated. Alexander et al. introduced the "TIMER" framework—Translocation, Immunomodulation, Metabolism, Enzymatic degradation, and Reduced diversity and ecological variation—in elucidating how intestinal bacteria impact chemotherapy efficacy (Alexander et al., 2017). Preclinical studies have demonstrated the gut microbiome's involvement in the efficacy of various chemotherapies including cyclophosphamide, oxaliplatin, or gemcitabine in CRC and other malignancies (Viaud et al., 2013, Geller et al., 2017, Iida et al., 2013). Chemotherapy has the effect of increasing the diversity of the microbiomes and decreasing the quantity of species linked to poor prognoses (Csendes et al., 2022). Thirty-one individuals in a breast cancer randomized controlled experiment collating metronomic capecitabine to a standard dose revealed that the chemotherapy dose changed the microbiome profile (Guan et al., 2020). Recent research in lung cancer patients identified specific gut bacteria, such as *Streptococcus mutans* and *Enterococcus casseliflavus*, associated with improved chemotherapy outcomes (Iida et al., 2013).

Despite promising preclinical evidence, clinical research on gut microbial biomarkers for predicting chemotherapy responses is limited. Two Asian cohort studies in 2020 evaluated the intestinal microbiome's ability to predict rectal cancer patients undergoing preoperative concurrent chemoradiation (Jang et al., 2020, Yi et al., 2021). These studies identified potential microbial biomarkers for response prediction, focusing on butyrate-producing bacteria and microbial compositions associated with responders (Yi et al., 2021, Jang et al., 2020). Although gut dysbiosis has been investigated as a prognostic biomarker for radiotherapy-induced mucositis, its direct impact on patient responses to radiotherapy remains underexplored. Recent research in mice has suggested the potential of microbiota-associated markers to predict radiation injury (Guo et al., 2021). However, additional clinical research is necessary to determine the bacterial communities responsible for radioresistance. Cyclophosphamide treatment was reported to assist Gram-positive bacteria translocation into secondary lymphoid organs, increasing the development of "pathogenic" T helper 17 cells and memory Th1 immune responses in mice models. Meanwhile, resistance to cyclophosphamide in secondary lymphoid organs, where it increased the formation of "pathogenic" T helper 17 cells, was observed in mice with lower T helper 17 responses when germ-free or treated with memory Th1 immune responses. Antimicrobial resistance to cyclophosphamide has been observed in mice. This was validated by another investigation in which two bacteria, *Enterococcus hirae* and *Barnesiella intestinihominis* facilitated the anticancer impact of cyclophosphamide in lung and ovarian malignancies by elevating the intratumoral CD8/Treg ratio in secondary lymphoid organs, and by infiltrating IFN-producing T cells into tumor lesions and resected cancers. In another study, IFN-producing T cells were infiltrated into cancer lesions by raising the intratumoral CD8/Treg ratio in secondary lymphoid organs and by elevating the intratumoral CD8/Treg ratio in secondary lymphoid organs (Temraz et al., 2019).

Anastomotic leaks (AL) represent a critical postoperative complication in CRC surgery, despite surgical advancements and perioperative care (Stormark et al., 2020). Animal models have linked specific microorganisms, including *Enterococcus faecalis* and *Pseudomonas aeruginosa*, with the development of AL due to their collagenolytic properties and matrix metalloproteinase (MMP-9) activation (Shogan et al., 2015). Clinical evidence supports these findings, with *Enterococcus faecalis* colonization in individuals with colorectal AL suggesting its potential as a means of screening (Komen et al., 2014). Mucosa-associated microbiota composition has also been explored, indicating associations between microbial diversity and specific bacteria with AL risk (van Praagh et al., 2016, Palmisano et al., 2020). Surgical site infections (SSI) and postoperative ileus (POI) are issues that arise after colorectal surgery. Clinical studies have connected specific bacteria, such as *Faecalibacterium*, *Staphylococcus aureus*, *Pseudomonas aeruginosa*, and *Enterococcus* spp., with these complications (Jin et al., 2020, Ohigashi et al., 2013). However, additional clinical studies are needed to identify microbial signatures associated with postoperative issues in colorectal surgery, with ongoing prospective studies aiming to shed more light on this subject (Veziant et al., 2020).

GUT MICROBIOME GENETIC ENGINEERING IN ADVANCING CRC PROGNOSIS

Recent advances in genetically engineering the gut microbiome in CRC prognosis have been reported (Chung et al., 2021, Hamidi Nia and Claesen, 2022, Arnold et al., 2023). For example, various types of microbes can be engineered to serve either as diagnostic, prognostic markers, or therapeutic targets for CRC, through synthetic biology. *Acinetobacter baylyi* is one of the bacteria that has been engineered for CRC prognosis. This bacterium is used for its ability to invade the GIT and acquire environmental DNA from lysed cells and incorporate it into its genome via the process of DNA-DNA hybridization, and is a preferred use for its non-pathogenicity properties to humans. Since these bacteria can reside within the mice's gut but are generally foreign in the human gut, scientists delivered *Acinetobacter baylyi* bacteria rectally in a CRC mouse model. Furthermore, mutated KRAS oncogene and KanR gene (which provides bacterial resistance to the antibacterial agent kanamycin) were co-inserted using CRISPR-Cas-9. Then the highly competent *Acinetobacter baylyi* took up tumor DNA shed into the colorectal lumen and integrated it into its genome through homologous recombination (via homologous arms possessed both by KRAS and engineered bacteria). As a result, the KanR gene was activated in a process, with the acquired kanamycin resistance by bacteria serving as the output signal (Cooper et al., 2017, Cooper et al., 2023, Rajagopala et al., 2017). The engineered bacteria demonstrated that a living biosensor is capable of detecting mammalian DNA shed from CRC in vivo in the gut (Cooper et al., 2023).

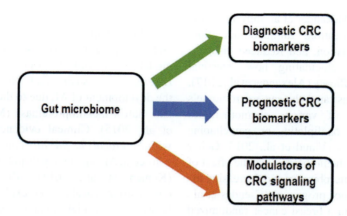

FIGURE 7.3 Summary of gut microbiome potential use as CRC biomarkers. The gut has been demonstrated to be a distinct feature between healthy individuals and CRC patients, and this is accompanied by its high inter-human variability. With improved evidence and better comprehension of the CRC signaling pathways, the gut microbiome has great potential in CRC diagnosis and prognosis.

CHALLENGES AND OUTLOOK OF GUT MICROBIOME BIOMARKERS IN CRC DIAGNOSIS AND PROGNOSIS

The research paradigm in understanding mechanisms of gut microbiome's role in CRC is shifting and this is in part attributable to advances in sequencing technologies, including long and short sequencing reads. However, the mechanisms are still not fully understood. While the mere presence or absence of microbial species in the gut provides limited information, advances in NGS and computational biology play a significant role in providing a clue into the mechanisms involved in the association between CRC and the gut microbiome. Although the bacteriome forms a large part of the intestinal microbiome and its association to CRC, altered fungal microbiota and viromes have also been implicated in interacting with gut bacteria to alter patients' response to CRC treatment. A significant amount of research has been invested in the gut bacteriome, while many more efforts are necessary to decipher the complex mechanisms of bacterial, viral, fungal, and other microbial interactions in addressing the existing research gap. Next, the gut microbiome also interacts with a plethora of host factors, further complicating the understanding of this microbe-host association. Additionally, variances in the intestinal tract physiology, genetics and the dietary patterns between gnotobiotic animal models and humans have been reported. These differences restrict how these models are used to examine the human gut microbiome in CRC, despite preclinical advances made in these models. Thus such generated data are to be interpreted with caution, necessitating a transdisciplinary research team approach. The gut microbiome interacts with cellular, molecular, and physiologic elements of the host and other extrinsic factors. Understanding the integrated complexity of these mechanisms holds great potential in unlocking gut microbiome diagnostic and prognostic potential in CRC.

CONCLUSIONS

The human gut microbiome has been reported as a CRC risk factor, associated with the initiation, development, and progression of CRC. While research has established the association between CRC and the gut microbiome, precise mechanisms of this relationship remain to be fully investigated. Although the mere presence or absence of microbes in the gut confers inadequate information, unique microbial signatures are key in the probable utilization of the intestinal microbiome as diagnostic and prognostic markers. While NGS sequencing techniques have made significant strides in gut microbiome CRC translational research, data inconsistency and inaccuracy has been reported with short read NGS approaches, thereby preferring long-read sequencers for greater accuracy. The parallel similarity of the gut microbiome across various types of cancer also limits its clinical applicability. Next, differential microbiome dysbiosis patterns across various studies have been reported, and these may be attributed to external and intrinsic factors, thus impeding with the translational utility of gut microbiome biomarkers in CRC. As such key variables have been identified in addressing these gaps. Thus improved knowledge on the precise gut microbiome mechanisms in CRC will be made clearer, and this will pave way into the gut microbiome diagnostic and prognostic translational use. Figure 7.3 summarizes the potential diagnostic and prognostic values of the gut microbiome in CRC.

REFERENCES

AKBAR, N., KHAN, N. A., MUHAMMAD, J. S. & SIDDIQUI, R. 2022. The role of gut microbiome in cancer genesis and cancer prevention. *Health Sci Rev,* 2, 100010.

ALEXANDER, J. L., WILSON, I. D., TEARE, J., MARCHESI, J. R., NICHOLSON, J. K. & KINROSS, J. M. 2017. Gut microbiota modulation of chemotherapy efficacy and toxicity. *Nat Rev Gastroenterol Hepatol,* 14, 356–365.

ALLEN, J. & SEARS, C. L. 2019. Impact of the gut microbiome on the genome and epigenome of colon epithelial cells: contributions to colorectal cancer development. *Genome Med,* 11, 1–18.

ANDRÉ, T., SHIU, K.-K., KIM, T. W., JENSEN, B. V., JENSEN, L. H., PUNT, C., SMITH, D., GARCIA-CARBONERO, R., BENAVIDES, M. & GIBBS, P. 2020. Pembrolizumab in microsatellite-instability–high advanced colorectal cancer. *N Engl J Med,* 383, 2207–2218.

ANIPINDI, M. & BITETTO, D. 2022. Diagnostic and therapeutic uses of the microbiome in the field of oncology. *Cureus*, 14, 1–13.

AO, H., XIN, Z. & JIAN, Z. 2021. Liquid biopsy to identify biomarkers for immunotherapy in hepatocellular carcinoma. *Biomark Res*, 9, 1–9.

ARNOLD, J., GLAZIER, J. & MIMEE, M. 2023. Genetic engineering of resident bacteria in the Gut microbiome. *J Bacteriol*, 205, e0012723.

ASSERI, A.H., BAKHSH, T., ABUZAHRAH, S.S., ALI, S. & RATHER, I.A., 2023. The gut dysbiosis-cancer axis: Illuminating novel insights and implications for clinical practice. *Frontiers in Pharmacology*, 14, 1–12.

BENNEDSEN, A. L., FURBO, S., BJARNSHOLT, T., RASKOV, H., GÖGENUR, I. & KVICH, L. 2022. The gut microbiota can orchestrate the signaling pathways in colorectal cancer. *Apmis*, 130, 121–139.

BHATT, A. P., REDINBO, M. R. & BULTMAN, S. J. 2017. The role of the microbiome in cancer development and therapy. *CA: A Cancer J Clin*, 67, 326–344.

BIARC, J., NGUYEN, I. S., PINI, A., GOSSE, F., RICHERT, S., THIERSE, D., VAN DORSSELAER, A., LEIZE-WAGNER, E., RAUL, F. & KLEIN, J.-P. 2004. Carcinogenic properties of proteins with pro-inflammatory activity from Streptococcus infantarius (formerly S. bovis). *Carcinogenesis*, 25, 1477–1484.

CASTELLARIN, M., WARREN, R. L., FREEMAN, J. D., DREOLINI, L., KRZYWINSKI, M., STRAUSS, J., BARNES, R., WATSON, P., ALLEN-VERCOE, E. & MOORE, R. A. 2012. Fusobacterium nucleatum infection is prevalent in human colorectal carcinoma. *Genome Res*, 22, 299–306.

CHUNG, Y., RYU, Y., AN, B. C., YOON, Y.-S., CHOI, O., KIM, T. Y., YOON, J., AHN, J. Y., PARK, H. J., KWON, S.-K., KIM, J. F. & CHUNG, M. J. 2021. A synthetic probiotic engineered for colorectal cancer therapy modulates gut microbiota. *Microbiome*, 9, 122.

COOPER, R. M., TSIMRING, L. & HASTY, J. 2017. Inter-species population dynamics enhance microbial horizontal gene transfer and spread of antibiotic resistance. *Elife*, 6, e25950.

COOPER, R. M., WRIGHT, J. A., NG, J. Q., GOYNE, J. M., SUZUKI, N., LEE, Y. K., ICHINOSE, M., RADFORD, G., RYAN, F. J. & KUMAR, S. 2023. Engineered bacteria detect tumor DNA. *Science*, 381, 682–686.

CSENDES, D., GUTLAPALLI, S. D., PRAKASH, K., SWARNAKARI, K. M., BAI, M., MANOHARAN, M. P., RAJA, R., JAMIL, A., DESAI, A., DESAI, D. M. & KHAN, S. 2022. Gastrointestinal microbiota and breast cancer chemotherapy interactions: a systematic review. *Cureus*, 14, e31648.

CZAJKA-FRANCUZ, P., PRENDES, M. J., MANKAN, A., QUINTANA, Á., PABLA, S., RAMKISSOON, S., JENSEN, T. J., PEIRÓ, S., SEVERSON, E. A., ACHYUT, B. R., VIDAL, L., POELMAN, M. & SAINI, K. S. 2023. Mechanisms of immune modulation in the tumor microenvironment and implications for targeted therapy. *Front Oncol*, 13, 1200646.

DAI, Z., COKER, O. O., NAKATSU, G., WU, W. K., ZHAO, L., CHEN, Z., CHAN, F. K., KRISTIANSEN, K., SUNG, J. J. & WONG, S. H. 2018. Multi-cohort analysis of colorectal cancer metagenome identified altered bacteria across populations and universal bacterial markers. *Microbiome*, 6, 1–12.

DANIEL, S. G., BALL, C. L., BESSELSEN, D. G., DOETSCHMAN, T. & HURWITZ, B. L. 2017. Functional changes in the gut microbiome contribute to transforming growth factor β-deficient colon cancer. *Msystems*, 2, e00065–17.

DAVID, P., MITTELSTÄDT, A., KOUHESTANI, D., ANTHUBER, A., KAHLERT, C., SOHN, K. & WEBER, G. F. 2023. Current applications of liquid biopsy in gastrointestinal cancer disease—from early cancer detection to individualized cancer treatment. *Cancers*, 15, 1924.

DING, Y., LI, W., WANG, K., XU, C., HAO, M. & DING, L. 2020. Perspectives of the application of liquid biopsy in colorectal cancer. *BioMed Res Int*, 2020, 1–13.

EVANS, M. D., DIZDAROGLU, M. & COOKE, M. S. 2004. Oxidative DNA damage and disease: induction, repair and significance. *Mutat Res Rev Mutat Res*, 567, 1–61.

FLEMING, N. I., JORISSEN, R. N., MOURADOV, D., CHRISTIE, M., SAKTHIANANDESWAREN, A., PALMIERI, M., DAY, F., LI, S., TSUI, C. & LIPTON, L. 2013. SMAD2, SMAD3 and SMAD4 mutations in colorectal cancer. *Cancer Res*, 73, 725–735.

FRISAN, T. 2016. Bacterial genotoxins: the long journey to the nucleus of mammalian cells. *Biochim Biophys Acta (BBA) Biomembr*, 1858, 567–575.

GELLER, L. T., BARZILY-ROKNI, M., DANINO, T., JONAS, O. H., SHENTAL, N., NEJMAN, D., GAVERT, N., ZWANG, Y., COOPER, Z. A. & SHEE, K. 2017. Potential role of intratumor bacteria in mediating tumor resistance to the chemotherapeutic drug gemcitabine. *Science*, 357, 1156–1160.

GETHINGS-BEHNCKE, C., COLEMAN, H. G., JORDAO, H. W., LONGLEY, D. B., CRAWFORD, N., MURRAY, L. J. & KUNZMANN, A. T. 2020. Fusobacterium nucleatum in the colorectum and its association with cancer risk and survival: a systematic review and meta-analysis. *Cancer Epidemiol Biomark Prev*, 29, 539–548.

GEUKING, M. B., KÖLLER, Y., RUPP, S. & MCCOY, K. D. 2014. The interplay between the gut microbiota and the immune system. *Gut Microbes*, 5, 411–418.

GOEL, S., HUANG, J. & KLAMPFER, L. 2015. K-Ras, intestinal homeostasis and colon cancer. *Curr Clin Pharmacol*, 10, 73–81.

GOPALAKRISHNAN, V., HELMINK, B. A., SPENCER, C. N., REUBEN, A. & WARGO, J. A. 2018. The influence of the gut microbiome on cancer, immunity, and cancer immunotherapy. *Cancer Cell*, 33, 570–580.

GRENHAM, S., CLARKE, G., CRYAN, J. F. & DINAN, T. G. 2011. Brain–gut–microbe communication in health and disease. *Front Physiol*, 2, 94.

GUAN, X., MA, F., SUN, X., LI, C., LI, L., LIANG, F., LI, S., YI, Z., LIU, B. & XU, B. 2020. Gut microbiota profiling in patients with HER2-negative metastatic breast cancer receiving metronomic chemotherapy of capecitabine compared to those under conventional dosage. *Front Oncol*, 10, 902.

GUO, H., CHOU, W.-C., LAI, Y., LIANG, K., TAM, J., BRICKEY, W., CHEN, L., MONTGOMERY, N. D., LI, X. & BOHANNON, L. M. 2021. Multi-omics analyses of radiation survivors identify radioprotective microbes and metabolites. *J Immunol*, 206, 99.02.

GUO, Y. J., PAN, W. W., LIU, S. B., SHEN, Z. F., XU, Y. & HU, L. L. 2020. ERK/MAPK signalling pathway and tumorigenesis. *Exp Ther Med*, 19, 1997–2007.

GUPTA, A., MADANI, R. & MUKHTAR, H. 2010. Streptococcus bovis endocarditis, a silent sign for colonic tumour. *Colorectal Dis*, 12, 164–171.

HALAZONETIS, T. D. 2004. Constitutively active DNA damage checkpoint pathways as the driving force for the high frequency of p53 mutations in human cancer. *DNA Repair,* 3, 1057–1062.

HAMIDI NIA, L. & CLAESEN, J. 2022. Engineered cancer targeting microbes and encapsulation devices for human gut microbiome applications. *Biochemistry,* 61, 2841–2848.

HAYASHI, H., ABDOLLAH, S., QIU, Y., CAI, J., XU, Y.-Y., GRINNELL, B. W., RICHARDSON, M. A., TOPPER, J. N., GIMBRONE, M. A. & WRANA, J. L. 1997. The MAD-related protein Smad7 associates with the TGFβ receptor and functions as an antagonist of TGFβ signaling. *Cell,* 89, 1165–1173.

HUMPHRIES, A. & WRIGHT, N. A. 2008. Colonic crypt organization and tumorigenesis. *Nat Rev Cancer,* 8, 415–424.

HUYCKE, M. M., MOORE, D., JOYCE, W., WISE, P., SHEPARD, L., KOTAKE, Y. & GILMORE, M. S. 2001. Extracellular superoxide production by Enterococcus faecalis requires demethylmenaquinone and is attenuated by functional terminal quinol oxidases. *Mol Microbiol,* 42, 729–740.

HUYCKE, M. M. & MOORE, D. R. 2002. In vivo production of hydroxyl radical by Enterococcus faecalis colonizing the intestinal tract using aromatic hydroxylation. *Free Rad Biol Med,* 33, 818–826.

IIDA, N., DZUTSEV, A., STEWART, C. A., SMITH, L., BOULADOUX, N., WEINGARTEN, R. A., MOLINA, D. A., SALCEDO, R., BACK, T. & CRAMER, S. 2013. Commensal bacteria control cancer response to therapy by modulating the tumor microenvironment. *Science,* 342, 967–970.

INAMURA, K. 2018. Colorectal cancers: an update on their molecular pathology. *Cancers,* 10, 26.

JANG, B.-S., CHANG, J. H., CHIE, E. K., KIM, K., PARK, J. W., KIM, M. J., SONG, E.-J., NAM, Y.-D., KANG, S. W. & JEONG, S.-Y. 2020. Gut microbiome composition is associated with a pathologic response after preoperative chemoradiation in patients with rectal cancer. *Int J Rad Oncol Biol Phys,* 107, 736–746.

JIN, Y., GENG, R., LIU, Y., LIU, L., JIN, X., ZHAO, F., FENG, J. & WEI, Y. 2020. Prediction of postoperative ileus in patients with colorectal cancer by preoperative gut microbiota. *Front Oncol,* 10, 526009.

KIM, J. & LEE, H. K. 2021. Potential role of the gut microbiome in colorectal cancer progression. *Front Immunol,* 12, 807648.

KOMEN, N., SLIEKER, J., WILLEMSEN, P., MANNAERTS, G., PATTYN, P., KARSTEN, T., DE WILT, H., VAN DER HARST, E., VAN LEEUWEN, W. & DECAESTECKER, C. 2014. Polymerase chain reaction for Enterococcus faecalis in drain fluid: the first screening test for symptomatic colorectal anastomotic leakage. The appeal-study: analysis of parameters predictive for evident anastomotic leakage. *Int J Colorectal Disease,* 29, 15–21.

KOMIYA, Y. & HABAS, R. 2008. Wnt signal transduction pathways. *Organogenesis,* 4, 68–75.

LARA-TEJERO, M. & GALÁN, J. E. 2000. A bacterial toxin that controls cell cycle progression as a deoxyribonuclease I-like protein. *Science,* 290, 354–357.

LEE, C. S., SONG, I. H., LEE, A., KANG, J., LEE, Y. S., LEE, I. K., SONG, Y. S. & LEE, S. H. 2021. Enhancing the landscape of colorectal cancer using targeted deep sequencing. *Sci Rep,* 11, 8154.

LI, F.-Y. & LAI, M.-D. 2009. Colorectal cancer, one entity or three. *J Zhejiang Univ Sci B,* 10, 219–229.

LI, L., LI, X., ZHONG, W., YANG, M., XU, M., SUN, Y., MA, J., LIU, T., SONG, X. & DONG, W. 2019. Gut microbiota from colorectal cancer patients enhances the progression of intestinal adenoma in Apcmin/+ mice. *EBio Med,* 48, 301–315.

LI, X., HUANG, J., YU, T., FANG, X., LOU, L., XIN, S., JI, L., JIANG, F. & LOU, Y. 2021. Fusobacterium nucleatum promotes the progression of colorectal cancer through Cdk5-activated Wnt/β-catenin signaling. *Front Microbiol,* 11, 545251.

LIU, Y., LAU, H. C.-H., CHENG, W. Y. & YU, J. 2023. Gut microbiome in colorectal cancer: clinical diagnosis and treatment. *Genomics Proteomics Bioinformatics,* 21, 84–96.

LONG, X., WONG, C. C., TONG, L., CHU, E. S., HO SZETO, C., GO, M. Y., COKER, O. O., CHAN, A. W., CHAN, F. K. & SUNG, J. J. 2019. Peptostreptococcus anaerobius promotes colorectal carcinogenesis and modulates tumour immunity. *Nat Microbiol,* 4, 2319–2330.

MAGGIO-PRICE, L., TREUTING, P., ZENG, W., TSANG, M., BIELEFELDT-OHMANN, H. & IRITANI, B. M. 2006. Helicobacter infection is required for inflammation and colon cancer in SMAD3-deficient mice. *Cancer Res,* 66, 828–838.

MAISONNEUVE, C., IRRAZABAL, T., MARTIN, A., GIRARDIN, S. E. & PHILPOTT, D. J. 2018. The impact of the gut microbiome on colorectal cancer. *Annu Rev Cancer Biol,* 2, 229–249.

MÁRMOL, I., SÁNCHEZ-DE-DIEGO, C., PRADILLA DIESTE, A., CERRADA, E. & RODRIGUEZ YOLDI, M. J. 2017. Colorectal carcinoma: a general overview and future perspectives in colorectal cancer. *Int J Mol Sci,* 18, 197.

MIMA, K., NISHIHARA, R., QIAN, Z. R., CAO, Y., SUKAWA, Y., NOWAK, J. A., YANG, J., DOU, R., MASUGI, Y. & SONG, M. 2016. Fusobacterium nucleatum in colorectal carcinoma tissue and patient prognosis. *Gut,* 65, 1973–1980.

MONTALBAN-ARQUES, A. & SCHARL, M. 2019. Intestinal microbiota and colorectal carcinoma: Implications for pathogenesis, diagnosis, and therapy. *EBio Med,* 48, 648–655.

MONTELEONE, G., KUMBEROVA, A., CROFT, N. M., MCKENZIE, C., STEER, H. W. & MACDONALD, T. T. 2001. Blocking Smad7 restores TGF-β1 signaling in chronic inflammatory bowel disease. *J Clin Invest,* 108, 601–609.

MU, W., JIA, Y., CHEN, X., LI, H., WANG, Z. & CHENG, B. 2020. Intracellular Porphyromonas gingivalis promotes the proliferation of colorectal cancer cells via the MAPK/ERK signaling pathway. *Front Cell Infect Microbiol,* 10, 584798.

MURATA-KAMIYA, N., KURASHIMA, Y., TEISHIKATA, Y., YAMAHASHI, Y., SAITO, Y., HIGASHI, H., ABURATANI, H., AKIYAMA, T., PEEK, R. & AZUMA, T. 2007. Helicobacter pylori CagA interacts with E-cadherin and deregulates the β-catenin signal that promotes intestinal transdifferentiation in gastric epithelial cells. *Oncogene,* 26, 4617–4626.

NEISH, A. S. 2009. Microbes in gastrointestinal health and disease. *Gastroenterology,* 136, 65–80.

NEWMAN, T. M., VITOLINS, M. Z. & COOK, K. L. 2019. From the table to the tumor: the role of mediterranean and Western dietary patterns in shifting microbial-mediated signaling to impact breast cancer risk. *Nutrients,* 11, 2565.

NEWSOME, R. C. & JOBIN, C. 2021. Microbiome-derived liquid biopsy: new hope for cancer screening? *Clin Chem,* 67, 463–465.

NOVELLASDEMUNT, L., ANTAS, P. & LI, V. S. 2015. Targeting Wnt signaling in colorectal cancer. a review in the theme: cell signaling: proteins, pathways and mechanisms. *Am J Physiol Cell Physiol,* 309, C511-C521.

OHIGASHI, S., SUDO, K., KOBAYASHI, D., TAKAHASHI, T., NOMOTO, K. & ONODERA, H. 2013. Significant changes in the intestinal environment after surgery in patients with colorectal cancer. *J Gastrointest Surg,* 17, 1657–1664.

OLIVEIRA, M. J., LAUWAET, T., DE BRUYNE, G., MAREEL, M. & LEROY, A. 2005. Listeria monocytogenes produces a pro-invasive factor that signals via ErbB2/ErbB3 heterodimers. *J Cancer Res Clin Oncol,* 131, 49–59.

PALMISANO, S., CAMPISCIANO, G., IACUZZO, C., BONADIO, L., ZUCCA, A., COSOLA, D., COMAR, M. & DE MANZINI, N. 2020. Role of preoperative gut microbiota on colorectal anastomotic leakage: preliminary results. *Updates Surg,* 72, 1013–1022.

QUAGLIO, A. E. V., GRILLO, T. G., DE OLIVEIRA, E. C. S., DI STASI, L. C. & SASSAKI, L. Y. 2022. Gut microbiota, inflammatory bowel disease and colorectal cancer. *World J Gastroenterol,* 28, 4053–4060.

RAHMAN, M. M., ISLAM, M. R., SHOHAG, S., AHASAN, M. T., SARKAR, N., KHAN, H., HASAN, A. M., CAVALU, S. & RAUF, A. 2022. Microbiome in cancer: Role in carcinogenesis and impact in therapeutic strategies. *Biomed Pharmacother,* 149, 112898.

RAJAGOPALA, S. V., VASHEE, S., OLDFIELD, L. M., SUZUKI, Y., VENTER, J. C., TELENTI, A. & NELSON, K. E. 2017. The human microbiome and cancer. *Cancer Prev Res,* 10, 226–234.

RAMANAN, V. K., SHEN, L., MOORE, J. H. & SAYKIN, A. J. 2012. Pathway analysis of genomic data: concepts, methods, and prospects for future development. *Trends Genet,* 28, 323–332.

REBERSEK, M. 2021. Gut microbiome and its role in colorectal cancer. *BMC Cancer,* 21, 1325.

RUBINSTEIN, M. R., BAIK, J. E., LAGANA, S. M., HAN, R. P., RAAB, W. J., SAHOO, D., DALERBA, P., WANG, T. C. & HAN, Y. W. 2019. Fusobacterium nucleatum promotes colorectal cancer by inducing Wnt/β-catenin modulator Annexin A1. *EMBO Rep,* 20, e47638.

RUBINSTEIN, M. R., WANG, X., LIU, W., HAO, Y., CAI, G. & HAN, Y. W. 2013. Fusobacterium nucleatum promotes colorectal carcinogenesis by modulating E-cadherin/β-catenin signaling via its FadA adhesin. *Cell Host & Microbe,* 14, 195–206.

SAINI, K. S., LOI, S., DE AZAMBUJA, E., METZGER-FILHO, O., SAINI, M. L., IGNATIADIS, M., DANCEY, J. E. & PICCART-GEBHART, M. J. 2013. Targeting the PI3K/AKT/mTOR and Raf/MEK/ERK pathways in the treatment of breast cancer. *Cancer Treat Rev,* 39, 935–946.

SAUS, E., IRAOLA-GUZMÁN, S., WILLIS, J. R., BRUNET-VEGA, A. & GABALDÓN, T. 2019. Microbiome and colorectal cancer: roles in carcinogenesis and clinical potential. *Mol Aspects Med,* 69, 93–106.

SCARPELLINI, E., IANIRO, G., ATTILI, F., BASSANELLI, C., DE SANTIS, A. & GASBARRINI, A. 2015. The human gut microbiota and virome: potential therapeutic implications. *Digest Liver Dis,* 47, 1007–1012.

SCHWABE, R. F. & JOBIN, C. 2013. The microbiome and cancer. *Nat Rev Cancer,* 13, 800–812.

SCOTT, A. J., ALEXANDER, J. L., MERRIFIELD, C. A., CUNNINGHAM, D., JOBIN, C., BROWN, R., ALVERDY, J., O'KEEFE, S. J., GASKINS, H. R. & TEARE, J. 2019. International Cancer Microbiome Consortium consensus statement on the role of the human microbiome in carcinogenesis. *Gut,* 68, 1624–1632.

SHOGAN, B. D., BELOGORTSEVA, N., LUONG, P. M., ZABORIN, A., LAX, S., BETHEL, C., WARD, M., MULDOON, J. P., SINGER, M. & AN, G. 2015. Collagen degradation and MMP9 activation by Enterococcus faecalis contribute to intestinal anastomotic leak. *Sci Translat Med,* 7, 286ra68.

SILLO, T. O., BEGGS, A. D., MIDDLETON, G. & AKINGBOYE, A. 2023. The Gut microbiome, microsatellite status and the response to immunotherapy in colorectal cancer. *Int J Mol Sci,* 24, 1–15.

STORMARK, K., KRARUP, P. M., SJÖVALL, A., SØREIDE, K., KVALØY, J. T., NORDHOLM-CARSTENSEN, A., NEDREBØ, B. & KØRNER, H. 2020. Anastomotic leak after surgery for colon cancer and effect on long-term survival. *Colorectal Dis,* 22, 1108–1118.

SVRCEK, M., EL-BCHIRI, J., CHALASTANIS, A., CAPEL, E., DUMONT, S., BUHARD, O., OLIVEIRA, C., SERUCA, R., BOSSARD, C. & MOSNIER, J.-F. 2007. Specific clinical and biological features characterize inflammatory bowel disease–associated colorectal cancers showing microsatellite instability. *J Clin Oncol,* 25, 4231–4238.

TAO, X., WANG, N. & QIN, W. 2015. Gut microbiota and hepatocellular carcinoma. *Gastrointest Tumors,* 2, 33–40.

TEMRAZ, S., NASSAR, F., NASR, R., CHARAFEDDINE, M., MUKHERJI, D. & SHAMSEDDINE, A. 2019. Gut microbiome: a promising biomarker for immunotherapy in colorectal cancer. *Int J Mol Sci,* 20, 4155.

TERNES, D., KARTA, J., TSENKOVA, M., WILMES, P., HAAN, S. & LETELLIER, E. 2020. Microbiome in colorectal cancer: how to get from meta-omics to mechanism? *Trends Microbiol,* 28, 401–423.

TERRACCIANO, L. M., PISCUOGLIO, S. & NG, C. K. Y. 2019. Hepatocellular carcinoma: pathology and genetics. *In:* BOFFETTA, P. & HAINAUT, P. (eds.) *Encyclopedia of cancer* (3rd ed.). Oxford: Academic Press.

TESTA, U., PELOSI, E. & CASTELLI, G. 2018. Colorectal cancer: genetic abnormalities, tumor progression, tumor heterogeneity, clonal evolution and tumor-initiating cells. *Med Sci,* 6, 31.

USELL, L., METCALF, J., PARFREY, L. & KNICGHT, R. 2012. Defining the human microbiome. *Nutr Rev,* 70, S38–S44.

VAN PRAAGH, J. B., DE GOFFAU, M. C., BAKKER, I. S., HARMSEN, H. J., OLINGA, P. & HAVENGA, K. 2016. Intestinal microbiota and anastomotic leakage of stapled colorectal anastomoses: a Pilot study. *Surg Endoscopy,* 30, 2259–2265.

VEZIANT, J., POIROT, K., CHEVARIN, C., CASSAGNES, L., SAUVANET, P., CHASSAING, B., ROBIN, F., GODFRAIND, C., BARNICH, N. & PEZET, D. 2020. Prognostic value of a combination of innovative factors (gut microbiota, sarcopenia, obesity, metabolic syndrome) to predict surgical/oncologic outcomes following surgery for sporadic colorectal cancer: a prospective cohort study protocol (METABIOTE). *BMJ Open,* 10, e031472.

VIAUD, S., SACCHERI, F., MIGNOT, G., YAMAZAKI, T., DAILLÈRE, R., HANNANI, D., ENOT, D. P., PFIRSCHKE, C., ENGBLOM, C. & PITTET, M. J. 2013. The intestinal microbiota modulates the anticancer immune effects of cyclophosphamide. *Science,* 342, 971–976.

VILLAR-ORTEGA, P., EXPÓSITO-RUIZ, M., GUTIÉRREZ-SOTO, M., JIMÉNEZ, M. R.-C., NAVARRO-MARÍ, J. M. & GUTIÉRREZ-FERNÁNDEZ, J. 2022. The association between Fusobacterium nucleatum and cancer colorectal: a systematic review and meta-analysis. *Enferm Infecc Microbiol Clinica (English Ed.)*, 40, 224–234.

VIVARELLI, S., SALEMI, R., CANDIDO, S., FALZONE, L., SANTAGATI, M., STEFANI, S., TORINO, F., BANNA, G. L., TONINI, G. & LIBRA, M. 2019. Gut microbiota and cancer: from pathogenesis to therapy. *Cancers (Basel)*, 11, 38.

WANG, J., LU, R., FU, X., DAN, Z., ZHANG, Y.-G., CHANG, X., LIU, Q., XIA, Y., LIU, X. & SUN, J. 2018. Novel regulatory roles of Wnt1 in infection-associated colorectal cancer. *Neoplasia*, 20, 499–509.

WANG, T., CAI, G., QIU, Y., FEI, N., ZHANG, M., PANG, X., JIA, W., CAI, S. & ZHAO, L. 2012. Structural segregation of gut microbiota between colorectal cancer patients and healthy volunteers. *The ISME J*, 6, 320–329.

WIRBEL, J., PYL, P. T., KARTAL, E., ZYCH, K., KASHANI, A., MILANESE, A., FLECK, J. S., VOIGT, A. Y., PALLEJA, A., PONNUDURAI, R., SUNAGAWA, S., COELHO, L. P., SCHROTZ-KING, P., VOGTMANN, E., HABERMANN, N., NIMÉUS, E., THOMAS, A. M., MANGHI, P., GANDINI, S., SERRANO, D., MIZUTANI, S., SHIROMA, H., SHIBA, S., SHIBATA, T., YACHIDA, S., YAMADA, T., WALDRON, L., NACCARATI, A., SEGATA, N., SINHA, R., ULRICH, C. M., BRENNER, H., ARUMUGAM, M., BORK, P. & ZELLER, G. 2019. Meta-analysis of fecal metagenomes reveals global microbial signatures that are specific for colorectal cancer. *Nat Med*, 25, 679–689.

WONG, S. H. & YU, J. 2019. Gut microbiota in colorectal cancer: mechanisms of action and clinical applications. *Nat Rev Gastroenterol Hepatol*, 16, 690–704.

WU, S., MORIN, P. J., MAOUYO, D. & SEARS, C. L. 2003. Bacteroides fragilis enterotoxin induces c-Myc expression and cellular proliferation. *Gastroenterology*, 124, 392–400.

WU, S., RHEE, K.-J., ZHANG, M., FRANCO, A. & SEARS, C. L. 2007. Bacteroides fragilis toxin stimulates intestinal epithelial cell shedding and γ-secretase-dependent E-cadherin cleavage. *J Cell Sci*, 120, 1944–1952.

YAO, Y. & DAI, W. 2014. Genomic Instability and Cancer. *J Carcinogenesis Mutagenesis*, 5, 1–16.

YASHIRO, M. 2014. Ulcerative colitis-associated colorectal cancer. *World J Gastroenterol: WJG*, 20, 16389.

YI, Y., SHEN, L., SHI, W., XIA, F., ZHANG, H., WANG, Y., ZHANG, J., WANG, Y., SUN, X. & ZHANG, Z. 2021. Gut microbiome components predict response to neoadjuvant chemoradiotherapy in patients with locally advanced rectal cancer: a prospective, longitudinal study. *Clin Cancer Res*, 27, 1329–1340.

YU, L.-X. & SCHWABE, R. F. 2017. The gut microbiome and liver cancer: mechanisms and clinical translation. *Nat Rev Gastroenterol Hepatol*, 14, 527–539.

ZHAN, T., RINDTORFF, N. & BOUTROS, M. 2017. Wnt signaling in cancer. *Oncogene*, 36, 1461–1473.

ZHANG, F., FERRERO, M., DONG, N., D'AURIA, G., REYES-PRIETO, M., HERREROS-POMARES, A., CALABUIG-FARINAS, S., DURENDEZ, E., APARISI, F. & BLASCO, A. 2021. Analysis of the gut microbiota: an emerging source of biomarkers for immune checkpoint blockade therapy in non-small cell lung cancer. *Cancers*, 13, 2514.

ZHAO, L.-Y., MEI, J.-X., YU, G., LEI, L., ZHANG, W.-H., LIU, K., CHEN, X.-L., KOŁAT, D., YANG, K. & HU, J.-K. 2023. Role of the gut microbiota in anticancer therapy: from molecular mechanisms to clinical applications. *Signal Transduct Target Ther*, 8, 201.

ZHOU, P., YANG, D., SUN, D. & ZHOU, Y. 2022. Gut microbiome: new biomarkers in early screening of colorectal cancer. *J Clin Lab Anal*, 36, e24359.

8 Microbial Metabolites and Cancer

Benny Mosoane, Masibulele Nonxuba, Jessica McIntyre, Meshack Bida, Tsholofelo Kungoane, and Zodwa Dlamini

INTRODUCTION

The microbial-derived metabolites are key hubs that connect the gut microbiome to cancer progression, remodeling of the tumor microenvironment, and regulation of key signaling pathways in cancer cells as well as immune cells. The broad roles of microbial metabolites in cancer make them target points for investigating novel cancer therapies which may ineluctably benefit many cancer patients. There is therefore a need for more relevant data in this field.

Microbial metabolites have both carcinogenic effects and anticancer effects. The gut *Lactobacillus reuterin*-derived metabolite, reuterin is an example of a metabolite that exert anticancer effects by effecting protein oxidation and preventing ribosomal biogenesis to inhibit colorectal cancer (CRC) (Bell et al., 2022). Another protective metabolite derived from the gut microorganisms is butyrate which increases RNA expression of claudins to effectively protect the intestinal epithelia cells from damage, thereby preventing colon cancer development (Mathewson et al., 2016, Encarnação et al., 2018). When butyrate has accumulated, it operates as a histone deacetylase (HDAC) inhibitor where it terminates progression of cell cycle via altered expression of genes to enhance chemotherapy response (Mathebela et al., 2022). Many microbial metabolites inhibit the survival and proliferation of tumor cells through the induction of apoptosis (Figure 8.1) (Jaye et al., 2022).

The concentration scale of the metabolites derived from the gut microorganisms may show paradoxical carcinogenic effects. Short-chain fatty acids (SCFAs) can inhibit the progression of CRC when their levels are within ordinary physiologic span. SCFAs have been found to be raised in hepatocellular carcinoma (HCC) that is associated with non-alcoholic fatty liver disease (Yang et al., 2023, Encarnação et al., 2018, Mathewson et al., 2016). The secondary bile acids products of bacterial metabolism of chenodeoxycholic acid, lithocholic acid (LCA), and deoxycholic acid (DCA) SHOW varied carcinogenic effects in different body organs. LCA suppresses breast cancer (BC) by inducing apoptosis of cancer cells (Luu et al., 2018) and DCA inhibits tumor invasion and migration in gastric cancer (Pyo et al., 2015). Secondary bile acids in higher concentration have been associated with colon cancer (Ou et al., 2012).

Accumulation of gut bacteria-derived metabolites within the tumor microenvironment (TME) can behave as ligands for particular active protein receptors and regulators. These metabolites modulate signaling pathways and affect various gene expression in the cells. In addition, they affect the concentration of various other cytokines in the TME. One example of microbial metabolite reshaping TME and influencing tumor progression is in cervical cancer. Microbe produced lactate binds to the surface of cervical squamous epithelial cells (GPR81 receptor) to activate the wingless-related integration site (Wnt)/β-catenin signal pathway. Activation of the Wnt pathway is responsible for enhancing the *Fut8* expression which encodes α-1,6 fucosyltransferase that increases cellular fucosylation levels of the vaginal epithelium, effectively preventing the progression of cervical cancer (Fan et al., 2021).

To improve the effectiveness of anticancer treatment, priority should include reducing drug side effects, refining the drugs' ability to destroy tumors, and reducing the emergence of drug resistance. With increased understanding of the role of microbial metabolites in cancer progression, their rational use with standard cancer treatments (chemotherapy, radiotherapy, and immunotherapy) affords an advancement for research in trying to find more efficient cancer treatments. Research shows that the use of gut microbiota-derived metabolites, such as kynurenic acid (KYNA), propionate, and indole-3-caboxaldehyde, in patients receiving radiotherapy protect from radiotherapy side effects, thus improving survival rates (Alexander et al., 2017). SCFAs that are generally linked to anticancer properties can incapacitate the efficacy of radiation therapy. When SCFAs producing bacteria are depleted using vancomycin in mice gut, the antitumor properties of radiotherapy become enhanced (Shiao et al., 2021, Guo et al., 2020).

Microbial metabolites impede the effectiveness and safety of the conventional cancer therapies, namely radiotherapy, chemotherapy, and immunotherapy. Microorganisms participate in the metabolism of a large number of chemotherapeutic agents resulting in thye formation of microbial metabolites which are different from the parent drug with regards to potency, anticancer effectiveness, and toxicity (Alexander et al., 2017, Yang et al., 2023). A search for compounds which can strengthen the effectiveness of chemotherapeutic agents has turned into a popular research focus and metabolites derived from the gut microbiota seem to be such compounds.

This chapter focuses on the role of bioactive gut microbiota-derived metabolites in the development, progression, and modulation of cancer. This chapter will also explore the

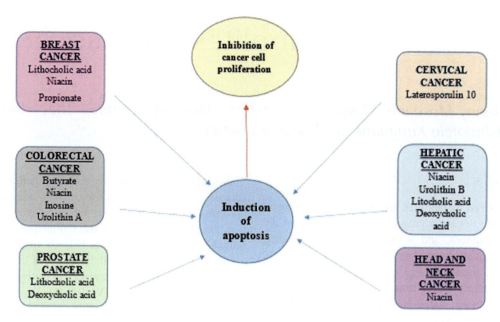

FIGURE 8.1 **Inhibitory effects of gut microbial metabolites on breast, prostate, liver, head and neck, colon and cervical cancer are achieved via induction of apoptosis.** These metabolites then inhibit proliferation and survival of the cancer cells.

potential personalized therapeutic strategies targeting microbial metabolites. Lastly, the chapter highlights some ideas for future scientific research.

BIOACTIVE METABOLITES PRODUCED BY GUT BACTERIA

Metabolites derived from microbiota regulate signaling pathways that influence the health of the host. These metabolites may have only carcinogenic effects or anticarcinogenic effects, although some exhibit paradoxical functions. Whether a metabolite is carcinogenic or anticarcinogenic, one needs to be aware of the condition under which a metabolite functions. An example of a metabolite that is influenced by the condition under which it functions is inosine which is a known inhibitor of Th1 differentiation but may promote differentiation of Th1 when exposed to an exogenous IFN-γ (He et al., 2017). The concentration level of metabolites plays a critical role in influencing their function. The nature of the tumor and tumor heterogeneity are some of the factors that can influence functions of the microbial metabolite. The biological functions of gut-derived microbial metabolites on the progression of tumor and tumor treatment are summarized in Table 8.1. The table also draws attention to the metabolites with known paradoxical functions in cancer.

The paradoxical functions of bioactive metabolites produced by gut bacteria are an engrossing area that warrant further attention in the field of cancer. Taking a look at SCFAs that have proven to have powerful anticarcinogenic effects, SCFAs have however been noted to contribute to the progression of cancer under certain circumstances. SCFAs promote the differentiation of immune cells, downregulate immune mediators that promote inflammation, inhibit angiogenesis in tumors, modulate pH in the intestines, and sustain basement membrane integrity (Gomes et al., 2023). Given these properties, it becomes logical that increased production of SCFAs can constitute an important therapeutic strategy, particularly in CRC patients that lower SCFAs concentrations compared to healthy subjects.

The patients with non-alcoholic fatty liver disease-associated HCC have showed a significant elevation of SCFAs. These SCFAs act as immunosuppressive agents by increasing T-regulator cells and cripple the function of CD8+ T-cells. Alongside regulation of the intracellular activity of β-catenin, butyrate, an example of SCFAs, promotes the transformation of APC$^{Min/+}$MSH2$^{-/-}$ mice colonocytes into cancer cells.

DCA activates vascular growth factor 2 and promotes vasculogenic mimicry to induce CRC (Song et al., 2022). LCA restricts the growth of CRC by promoting secretion of IL-8 through ERK1/2 activation and inhibition of PTEN by inducing miR21. DCA induces the expression of E-cadherin and mucin 2 in gastric cancer cell lines MKN45 and SNU-216 to epithelial mesenchymal transition. This is achieved by decreasing the expression of matrix metalloproteinase and Snail (Huang et al., 2015, Kozak et al., 2020).

Trimethylamine N-oxide (TMAO), a metabolic product of dietary choline and L-carnitine produced by intestinal microbiota, is thought to participate in the progression of cancer. The mechanism of TMAO in cancer progression is not yet fully elucidated, however it is believed that TMAO induces inflammation and oxide damage to promote cancer progression. TMAO aggravates colitis and occurrence of CRC via the inhibition of autophagy that is mediated by AFT16L1 within the epithelial cells of the colon (Salem et al., 2015). By activation of NLRP3 inflammasome, TMAO is able to regulate

TABLE 8.1
Selected examples of gut-derived microbial metabolites with their associated microorganisms and the biologic functions of the metabolites and their role in cancer

Metabolites	Microorganisms	Biological functions	References
Short chain fatty acids (SCFAs)	• *Fecalibacterium prausnitzii* • *Lactobacillus pentosus* • *Clostridium butyricum*	• Suppress the proliferation and induce apoptosis of colon cancer cells by activating G-protein coupled receptors • Induces aberrant proliferation and transformation of colon epithelial cells by regulating activity of B-catenin	(Sun et al., 2017, Zhang et al., 2020)
Reuterin	• *Lactobacillus reuteri*	• Induces oxidative distress and inhibit protein translation	(Bell et al., 2022)
Lithocholic acid (LCA)	• *Lactobacillus* • *Clostridium* • *Bacteriodes*	• Restricts colon cancer growth by secreting IL-8 through ERK1/2 • Induces apoptosis in breast cancer and nephroblastoma	(Nguyen et al., 2017, Luu et al., 2018)
Deoxycholic acid (DCA)	• *Bacteroides* • *Clostridium*	• Promotes epithelial mesenchymal transition and the formation of vasculogenic mimicry in colon cancer cells	(Song et al., 2022)
Inosine	• *Bifidobacterium pseudolongum*	• Promotes T-helper 1 differentiation in the presence of exogenous interferon gamma • Inhibits differentiation of T-helper 1 and 2 cells in the absence of interferon gamma	(Mager et al., 2020)
Lipopolysacharride (LPS)	• Gram negative bacteria	• Promotes cancer progression by activating Toll-like receptor 4 signaling which induces inflammation	(Zhu et al., 2016)
Taurine	• *Deltaproteobacteria*	• Maintains intestinal microbial homeostasis and mitigates inflammation	(Levy et al., 2015)
Kynurenic acid (KYNA)	• *Lichnospiraceae* • *Enterococcaceae*	• Inhibits MAPK and PI3K-Akt signaling pathway to block colon cancer cells proliferation	(Guo et al., 2020)
Manumycin A	• Streptomycin	• Inhibits Ras farnesylation and secretion of exosome to present cancer progression	(Cho et al., 2015)
Urolithin A	• *Enterococcus fecium*	• Regulates many signaling pathways that control inflammation	(Totiger et al., 2019)
Urolithin B	• Unknown	• Inactivates Wnt/B-catenin signaling to inhibit proliferation of hepatocellular carcinoma cells	(Lv et al., 2019)
Trimethylamine N-oxide (TMAO)	• *Lactobacillus*	• Promotes the proliferation of HCT116 cells	(Yang et al., 2022)
Ursodeoxycholic acid (UDCA)	• *Clostridium*	• Inhibits NF-kB activity and suppress upregulation of Cox-2 to prevent progression of colon cancer cells • In high concentration, it promotes neoplasia in patient with ulcerative colitis and primary sclerosing cholangitis	(Yang et al., 2022, Liu et al., 2022, Weingarden et al., 2016)
γ-Aminobutyric acid (GABA)	• *Lactobacillus* • *Parabacterium* • *Bifidobacterium*	• Modulates gut–brain axis	(Liao et al., 2022)
Hippurate	• *Bifidobacterium*	• Activates natural killer cells to kill tumor cells in the presence of high levels of interferon gamma	(Rizvi et al., 2021, Huang et al., 2020)
Niacin	• *Bacteroides*	• Induces cell killing effects on cancer stem cell in low concentration • May promote cancer stem cell proliferation in high concentration	(Sen et al., 2017)
s-equol	*Lactococcus garviae*	• Upregulates mi-R10A-5p to prevent proliferation of human breast cancer MCF-7 Cells	(Zhang et al., 2019)

Note: Metabolites with known paradoxical functions are in bold letters.

AGT16L proteins that tightly control autophagy (Wang et al., 2022a, Yue et al., 2017).

TMAO has shown the ability to induce the secretion of vascular endothelial growth factor receptor A (VEGA) to promote angiogenesis and the proliferation of the HCT116 colon cancer stem cells (Jalandra et al., 2022). TMAO induces reactive oxygen species (ROS), which at higher concentration often correlate with DNA damage (Yue et al., 2017). Antithetical to the promotion of tumor progression, TMOA activates the immune system in cancer patients, augmenting the effects of immunotherapy. The combination of immune check point inhibitors and TMOA has shown significant reduction of tumor burden in pancreatic ductal adenocarcinoma (PDAC) mouse models (Mirji et al., 2022).

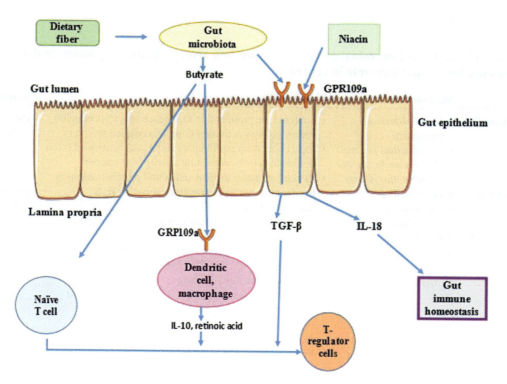

FIGURE 8.2 **The interaction of gut microbiota butyrate and niacin in the protection of the colon epithelial cells.** Niacin and butyrate act on G-protein-coupled receptor 109a (Grp109a) receptor to trigger production of interleukin-18 (IL-18) and transforming growth factor-β (TGF-β). Grp receptors are also present on the macrophages and dendritic cells which produce IL-10 and retinoic acid when activated by butyrate. Butyrate facilitate differentiation of naïve CD4 lymphocytes into T regulator cells.

Another important bioactive metabolite produced by gut microbiota (*Lactobacillus* and *Bacteroides* species) is the vitamin niacin. Low concentration of niacin has been found to kill colon cancer stem cells, however in higher concentration niacin can promote proliferation of CRC stem cells (Sen et al., 2017). Interaction of butyrate and niacin, both acting on Grp109a receptor, is cytoprotective of the colon epithelial cells and maintains immune homeostasis (Figure 8.2) (Lee and Hase, 2014). This interaction results in the production of IL-18, IL-10, and retinoic acids to activate T-regulator cells. At the epigenetic regulatory regions of FoxP3, butyrate upregulates acetylation histone H3 to facilitate differentiation of naïve CD4 lymphocytes into T regulator cells (Lal et al., 2009, Wang et al., 2015).

Ursodeoxycholic acid (UDCA), another secondary bile acid produced by gut microbiota, exerts diametrical functions in CRC. This metabolite suppresses upregulation of cyclooxygenase-2 and inhibits nuclear factor kappa B (NFκB) signaling to prevent the progression of CRC (Liu et al., 2022). By unclear mechanisms, UDCA exhibits cancer-promoting effects in ulcerative colitis and primary sclerosing cholangitis (Eaton et al., 2011).

IMPACT OF BIOACTIVE METABOLITES IN CANCER DEVELOPMENT AND PROGRESSION

For a tumor to progress, tumor cells employ manifold approaches that adjust the signaling pathways intrinsically and extrinsically, particularly in the surrounding cells to create a TME that promotes proliferation and metastasis. Reprogramming of TME and alteration of the signaling pathways are continuous processes that in turn affect the progression of tumor. Autocrine stimulation that activates the signaling of mitogen-activated protein kinase (MAPK) through the secretion of hepatocyte growth factor (HGF) studied in SNU-484 cells is a perfect example of the promotion and progression of gastric cancer (Park et al., 2005). The presence of gut microbial-derived metabolites in the TME modulate signaling pathways and affect gene expression of tumor cells. Multiple cytokines in the TME can be affected by the accumulation of bioactive bacterial metabolites. Microbial-derived metabolites therefore affect the progression of the tumor by modulating cellular signaling pathways and altering the TME.

The complex network of signaling pathways in tumor progression control cell proliferation, apoptosis, and epithelial mesenchymal transition (EMT). Several of the signaling pathways are activated or inhibited by gut microbiota-derived metabolites and these include critical pathways such as MAPK, phosphatidylinositol-3-kinase (PI3K)/serine/threonine protein kinase (Akt) (Figure 8.3), NFκB signaling, Wnt/β-catenin, and janus kinase (JAK)/signal transducer and activator of transcription 3 (STAT3) signaling pathways. The secondary bile acid products of bacterial metabolism, such as LCA, also activate ERK1/2 in CRC cells and trigger secretion of IL-8 to accelerate carcinogenesis (Liu et al., 2022).

Microbial Metabolites and Cancer

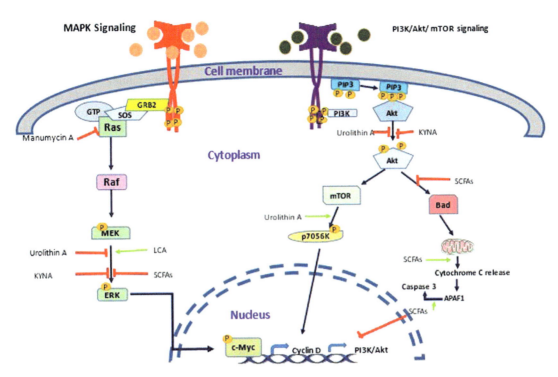

FIGURE 8.3 The gut microbiota-derived metabolites involved in the regulation of mitogen-activated protein kinase (MAPK) and phosphatidylinositol-3-kinase (PI3K)/ a serine/threonine protein kinase (Akt) signaling pathway in tumor cells. Manumycin A inhibits Ras activation to reduce extracellular signal-regulated kinase (ERK) phosphorylation. Kynurenic acid (KYNA), Urolithin A (UA), and short-chain fatty acids (SCFAs) inhibit the phosphorylation of ERK. Lithocholic acid (LCA) facilitates phosphorylation of ERK. Phosphorylated ERK (p-ERK) translocate into the nucleus and phosphorylates c-Myc which regulates the expression of Cyclin D affecting cancer progression. PI3K-Akt signaling inhibits apoptosis partially by suppressing the release of cytochrome c from mitochondria, thus reducing the activity of caspases, especially caspase 3. UA inhibits the activity of p70 ribosomal S6 protein kinase (p70S6K) which is a downstream effector of mTOR and impairs the overall translational capacity of cancer cells.

MAPK Signaling Pathway

Activated MAPK phosphorylates cytoplasmic proteins and translocates into the nucleus to phosphorylate nuclear transcription factors and regulate expression of cancer-related genes such as *C-myc, Oct4*, and *Sox2*. The four signaling pathways of MAPK in eukaryote cells are extracellular signal-regulated kinase (ERK1/2), ERK5, c-jun N-terminal kinase (JNK), and p38 MAPK. Microbial metabolites that regulate MAPK signaling include a tryptophan-derived metabolite, KYNA, which interferes with the proliferation of CRC by decreasing the activity of p38 and ERK1/2 kinases (Walczak et al., 2020). *Streptomyces*, an environmental microbe that is commonly found in the soil, can hide in the human body acting as part of the microbiota. Manumycin A is a secondary metabolite of *Streptomyces* which inhibits Ras farnesylation and prevents anchoring of RAS to the cell membrane (Cuozzo et al., 2023, Tisi et al., 2020). By inhibition of the Ras/Raf/Erk1/2 signaling pathway, manumycin A averts biosynthesis and secretion of exosomes in castration resistance prostate cancer cells (Datta et al., 2017).

Short-chain fatty acids bind to free fatty acid receptor 3 (FFAR3) to inhibit MAPK signaling in BC cells driving them towards non-invasive phenotype (Thirunavukkarasan et al., 2017). Urolithin A (UA), a metabolite product of *Enterococcus faecium* regulates MAPK signaling and prevents development of multiple cancers by controlling inflammation. UA prevents tumor progression by blunting activation of MAPK signaling by interfering with JNK and p38 kinases phosphorylation, thereby decreasing the release of pro-inflammatory factors (Abdelazeem et al., 2021). In the CRC, butyrate activates the MAPK signaling pathway but does not lead to cancer progression, instead this results in activation of apoptosis. Butyrate upregulates the expression of toll like receptor-4 (TLR4) and activates the natural immune system against tumor cells (Xiao et al., 2018).

PI3k/Akt Signaling Pathway

The PI3K/Akt signaling pathway activates mammalian target of rapamycin (mTOR) to regulate cell growth and protein synthesis in the presence of growth signals. In the presence of survival signals, the PI3K/Akt pathway is inhibited and the cell activates apoptosis-related proteins (Meng et al., 2017). Amongst the gut-derived microbial metabolites that inhibit PI3K/Akt signaling is the SCFAs which reduce the signaling pathway activity in CRC cells contributing to cellular apoptosis. In CRC cells, SCFAs decrease phosphorylation of BCL2-associated agonist of cell death (Bad) to enhance pro-apoptotic functions of Bad. When Bad is activated, it increases efflux of cytochrome c from the mitochondria to produce additional cleaved caspase 3, bringing about apoptosis (Ma et al., 2019).

In CRC cells, KYNA blocks cell proliferation by reducing phosphorylation of Akt to inhibit PI3K-Akt-mTOR signaling (Walczak et al., 2020). UA exerts anticancer effects in PDAC by inhibiting PI3K-Akt-mTOR signaling. UA inhibits Akt and p70 ribosomal S6 protein kinase (p70A6K) phosphorylation (Totiger et al., 2019). S-equol is another bacterial metabolite from the daidzein isoflavone which prevents the proliferation of MCF-7 human BC cells. S-equol upregulates miR-10a-5p which binds directly to 3' untranslated region of PI3K3CA to repress PI3K-Akt signaling (Zhang et al., 2019).

Nuclear Factor Kappa B Signaling (NFκB)

NFκB signaling plays a crucial role in inflammation than can lead to cancer. NFκB regulates natural immunity against tumors, preventing tumor progression. In the cytoplasm, NFκB-related proteins exist as latent transcription regulators because they couple with the inhibitor of NFκB (IκB). The phosphorylation of IκB by IκB kinase β (IKKβ) uncouples NFκB from IκB to allow translocation of NFκB into the nucleus to regulate the expression of target genes.

Gut-derived microbial metabolites can meddle with the NFκB signaling pathway. UA can inhibit the expression of TLR4 and phosphorylation of IκB to block NFκB to reduce the transcription of pro-inflammatory cells in lipopolysaccharide (LPS)-induced macrophages derived from the bone marrow (Abdelazeem et al., 2021). Butyrate on the other side enhances TLR4-mediated NFκB signaling in CRC cells to potentiate antitumor natural immunity (Xiao et al., 2018). Therefore, both UA and butyrate show CRC antitumor effects acting on NFκB signaling in different cell types. The combination of butyrate and UA will have more therapeutic benefits in the treatment of CRC.

Wnt/β-Catenin Signaling Pathway

The Wnt signaling dysfunction has been implicated in several cancers. Activated Wnt signaling molecules bind to Frizzled class of cell surface receptors to turn off the destruction of β-catenin that translocates into the nucleus. In the nucleus, β-catenin binds to T cell factor 4 (TCF-4) and lymphoid enhancer binding factor 1 (LEF-1) to coactivate expression of target genes. In HCC, Urolithin B (UB) inactivates the Wnt/β-catenin signaling pathway to induce cell cycle arrest and apoptosis in cancer cells (Garavaglia et al., 2022). In CRC cells harboring mutation in adenoma polyposis coli (APC) or β-catenin, butyrate induces autophagy that disrupts Wnt signaling (Garavaglia et al., 2022). A soil-dwelling bacterial *Myxcoccus fulvus* produces n-butane, a metabolite that inhibits the Wnt/β-catenin signaling pathway and induces apoptosis in the cells of BC (Park et al., 2021).

The JAK/STAT3 Signaling Pathway

The JAK/STAT3 cascade is a crucial cancer-promoting inflammatory signaling pathway. Metabolites derived from *Fecalibacterium* genus inhibit IL-6/STAT3 signaling in BC cells to inhibit tumor growth (Ma et al., 2020). Some studies show that STAT3 signaling can have pro-cancer and anticancer effects (Pencik et al., 2015, Nguyen et al., 2021). LCA suppresses STAT3 activity to promote carcinogenesis (Nguyen et al., 2017).

Other Signaling Pathways

The Ras-related C3 botulinum toxin substrate 1 (Rac1)/p21 protein-activated kinase 1 (PAK1) is another signaling system that is associated with many cancers. The Rac1/Pak1 signaling controls polymerization of actin, a process linked to cell proliferation and mobility. The activity of Rac1 and polymerization of PAK1 are reduced by UA to inhibit proliferation and migration of cancer cells (Alauddin et al., 2020).

The nuclear factor erythroid 2-related factor 2 (Nrf2) signaling pathway regulates cellular antioxidant activity. Nrf2 activity is regulated by UA in the intestine and liver to decrease oxidative stress-induced inflammatory damage and prevent progression of CRC and HCC (Djedjibegovic et al., 2020, Xiao et al., 2022).

Another signaling pathway that promotes progression of cancer is Hippo/yes-associated protein (YAP) signaling. Binding of SCFAs to FFAR2 on the surface of BC cells inhibits Hippo/YAP signaling, resulting in the increased expression of E-cadherin, which prevents the formation of invasive phenotype BC cells (Thirunavukkarasan et al., 2017).

MICROBIAL METABOLITES MODULATION

Immune Responses

Emerging research has uncovered the involvement of microbial-derived metabolites and their receptors in orchestrating the host immune response by controlling the immune system development, differentiation, and activity. Currently, a wide range of microbial-derived metabolites are significantly known for their influential role in stimulating immune response towards pathogens and suppressing immune responses towards food antigens. Similarly, these metabolites have been recognized for preventing chronic inflammation that may potentially lead to the development of carcinogenesis. In other words, gut microbials often produce widely diverse metabolites through microbials providing co-stimulatory signals that may produce pro-inflammatory cytokines to induce an immune response.

SCFAs, such as butyrate, acetate, and propionate, are gut microbial-derived metabolites through anaerobic fermentation of dietary fiber (Zhou et al., 2022). These metabolites are rapidly absorbed through the apical membrane of intestinal epithelial cells where they bind to a class of G-protein coupled receptors for the activation of various signaling processes that are associated with anti-inflammatory effects and immune homeostasis in health while they drive the expression of immune and inflammatory mediators' pathology (Duan et al., 2023, Kim et al., 2014).

As the main energy source for colon epithelial cells, butyrate also activates anti-inflammation signaling cascades that support the regulation of immune response. This includes the induction of T-cell (Tregs) differentiation which suppresses excessive immune activation and affects the function of macrophages and dendritic cells. This metabolite also aids its anti-inflammatory function by increasing the levels of IL18, an anti-inflammatory cytokine, while decreasing pro-inflammatory cytokines (IL6, IL12, IL17) secreted by macrophages. In addition, butyrate inhibits NF-kB activity, a transcriptional factor that upregulates pro-inflammatory-associated genes, by preventing it from translocating to the nucleus and binding to the DNA, which may result from the inhibition of histone deacetylases (Canani et al., 2011). In human colonocytes, the inhibition of NF-kB by butyrate is also achieved through the increase of the transcription and activity of peroxisome proliferator-activated receptor gamma (Hodgkinson et al., 2023).

Gut bacteria metabolize dietary proteins and produce various amino acid-derived metabolites, including tryptophan metabolites like indole derivatives. These metabolites can regulate the function of immune cells, such as T lymphocytes and antigen-presenting cells, and participate in maintaining immune tolerance.

The gut microbiota can modify bile acids through deconjugation and dehydroxylation, producing secondary bile acid metabolites. These metabolites can impact immune responses through binding to specific receptors like farnesoid X receptor and G protein-coupled bile acid receptor 1, which are expressed on immune cells and regulate inflammatory processes (Larabi et al., 2023).

TUMOR GROWTH

While the interaction between the environmental and genetic factors of the host has been widely acknowledged for their essential contribution to the evolution and progression of tumor, the effects of intratumoral microbial population in cancer biology is a newly raised concept. Previously, it was assumed that the microbes that were habiting tumor isolates were merely contaminants instead of tumor associates (Robinson et al., 2017). However, developing results from a comprehensive study that included more than 1,500 tumor samples suggested that the human tumor microbes are mostly intracellular and constitute tumor-site-specific properties (Nejman et al., 2020). Even though the exact mechanism that associates these microbes with cancer is not thoroughly investigated, the interaction between the two is highly attributed to the compromised balance between the host and the microbial, causing the dynamic of this relationship to change, triggering favorable conditions for cancer development.

The TME is a compounded and constantly evolving structure that is composed of various compositions, depending on the tumor type, to ensure the growth, invasion, and metastasis of the tumor (Baghban et al., 2020). The induction of inflammatory mediators and the recruitment of immune cells by the gut microbial-derived metabolites influence the alteration of the TME, by influencing the neoplastic process and fostering the growth, invasion, and metastases of cancer cells (Zhou et al., 2022). Based on this crosstalk, signaling pathways that regulate cellular proliferation, cell apoptosis, epithelial-mesenchymal transition, as well as other physiological activities in various cell types of cancer are either activated or inhibited by the gut microbiota-derived metabolites to influence the development of cancer.

Depending on a particular condition and cancer type, SCFAs have been reported to possess tumor-promoting or tumor-suppressing effects which allow them to perform as a double-edged sword in tumor development. Previous studies have shown that SCFA, mainly butyrate, inhibits tumor invasion and migration through the inhibition of histone deacetylase activity (Son and Cho, 2023). Furthermore, the upregulation of SCFA in CRC has been associated with apoptosis and cell stress response (Fung et al., 2011), downregulating adhesion protein $\alpha_2\beta_1$ integrin (Buda et al., 2003), and upregulating proapoptotic protein BAK (Chirakkal et al., 2006). In prostate cancer, SCFA was found to promote cell proliferation by increasing the levels of IGF1 (Matsushita et al., 2021).

The secondary bile acid metabolites have long been heavily implicated in carcinogenesis, causing ROS production increase and the reduction of pro-apoptotic effects. Studies have shown that LCA regulates Th17 and Treg cells (Hang et al., 2019), inhibits HLA class I genes (Arvind et al., 1994), and induces endoplasmic reticulum stress and mitochondrial dysfunction in human prostate cancer cells (Gafar et al., 2016). Deoxycholic acid can cause DNA DSBs and apoptosis (Powolny et al., 2001), and is thought to have a link to oncogenic mutations of proto-oncogene KRAS (Narahara et al., 2000).

Another double-edged sword metabolite whose effects have been associated with tumor progression and suppression is polyamines, metabolites from arginine. They have been shown to inhibit prostate cancer growth (Kee et al., 2004), protect cells from ROS (Khan et al., 1992), and downregulate estrogen receptor alpha (ER-α) in BC cells (Huang et al., 2006). Moreover, polyamines increase skin cancer risks in mouse models (Wang et al., 2007) and cause DNA damage and apoptosis of the immune cells in gastric cancer as the result of the *H. pylori* downstream effect (Xu et al., 2004).

TUMOR ANGIOGENESIS

Tumor angiogenesis is a multistep process that encompasses complex multifactorial components and cell types. In contrast to vasculogenesis, a process by which blood vessels are produced *de novo* via cell determination of endothelial cell precursors, angioblasts, angiogenesis involves the development of new blood vessels from the pre-existing vessels (Dudley and Griffioen, 2023). While this process is firmly tuned by the balance between pro-angiogenic and anti-angiogenic molecular factors and occurs transiently in physiology, upon disturbance in pathological tissues, including cancer, pro-angiogenic factors are often secreted in abundance compared to anti-angiogenic factors, defined as an angiogenic switch (Lugano et al., 2020).

Angiogenesis remains a hallmark in cancer pathology, playing a vital part in tumor progression and metastasis. When the tumor has grown beyond the diameter of approximately 1–2 millimeters in size, a delivery network that provides oxygen, nutrients, and waste disposal to the growing tumor cell is initiated, involving the activation of endothelial cells (EC) in response to hypoxia by angiogenic stimuli and the breakdown of the perivascular extracellular matrix and the basement membrane by the proteolytic enzymes to ensure EC invasion and tube formation. Apart from tumor growth, angiogenesis also facilitates the dissemination of tumor cells to distal sites, promoting metastases (Saman et al., 2020).

Inside the TME, several pro-angiogenic molecules are produced by the tumor cells, owing to their expression on the tumor and EC to induce angiogenesis. These molecules include vascular endothelial growth factor, platelet-derived growth factor, fibroblast growth factor, and many more (Lugano et al., 2020). While the involvement of these molecules in tumor growth and metastasis has been intensively studied *in vitro* and *in vivo*, a growing body of evidence has highlighted the induction of tumor angiogenesis by gut microbiota.

Drug Metabolism

The necessity to break boundaries in cancer therapy and eradicate tumor cells has long been the driving force in anticancer research. Due to the drawbacks that cancer treatments are known to have, the need to develop new drug treatments remains a desperate need. Currently, chemotherapy is one of the most administered treatments for cancer. Even though it has been shown to improve the survival outcome of patients, chemotherapy does not have the ability to target specific cells, and it damages healthy cells, including those of the immune system. As a result, patients often experience intolerable adverse events and become drug-resistant (Mills et al., 2022). Immunotherapy on the other hand is a new modality in cancer therapy. Since its initial approval for the treatment of melanoma, it has become a standard care treatment for various other malignancies including prostate cancer (Slaney and Kershaw, 2020). It has demonstrated a remarkable impact on clinical outcomes even though these effective results have only been witnessed in a small subset of malignancies and a handful of patients with those diseases.

Given the wide roles of microbes in cancer, the reasonable usage of their metabolites in combination with the abovementioned standard therapies has been shown by numerous studies to be a potential breakthrough for innovative cancer therapy. However, more relevant results associated with this relationship are needed (Yang et al., 2023).

Most recently, research has shown that the therapeutic effects of oxaliplatin have been enhanced by butyrate through the inhibition of HDAC and the induction of the DNA binding 2 (ID2) inhibitors. In this regard, E2A is inhibited by ID2, and the levels of IL-12 receptors are induced on the CD8+ T cell surface to improve anticancer effects (He et al., 2021). Pentanoate and butyrate are the key metabolites that regulate the effects of immunotherapy through HDAC inhibition and the enhancement of mTOR activity in T cells. Accordingly, TNF-α and IFN-γ are secreted by the T cells to enhance the antitumor efficacy of chimeric antigen receptor T cells and CTLAs (Smith et al., 2023).

THE POTENTIAL OF TARGETING SPECIFIC MICROBIAL METABOLITES AS THERAPEUTIC APPROACHES FOR PERSONALIZED CANCER THERAPIES

Novel therapeutic strategies explored based on the understanding of microbiota are summarized in Figure 8.4. The potential approaches include diet, use of phages, manipulation of the microbiota-gut-brain axis, genetic engineering, design of new therapeutic agents, and transplantation of fecal matter.

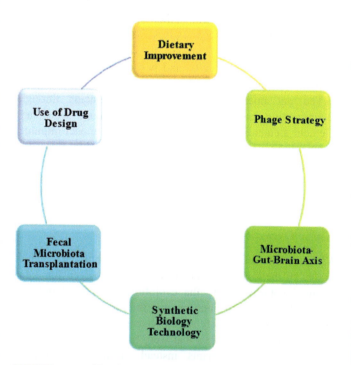

FIGURE 8.4 Novel strategies for cancer treatment by modulating microbiota-derived metabolites. Dietary improvements like increased fiber intake can provide sufficient substrate for microorganisms which results in increased generation of short-chain fatty acids. The use of phages to eliminate certain microorganisms that secrete metabolites that render cancer therapy ineffective has been one effective strategy. Fecal microbiota transplantation and microbiota-gut-brain axis can effectively manipulate microbial species and metabolites. Microbial metabolites affect the mental status by regulating functions of multiple immune cells. Synthetic biology techniques can be used to edit and regulate microbial metabolites systems at the genetic level.

Improving dietary habits can shape the types of microbial metabolites produced by the gut microbiota. Despite carrying known adverse health effects, such as high blood pressure, promotion of renal cell carcinoma, and spurring of Alzheimer's disease, a high-salt diet has been found to thwart cancer progression and refine antitumor immunity (Deckers et al., 2014, He et al., 2020). Increased hippurate-producing *Bifidobacterium* has been associated with a high-salt diet. Higher concentrations of the microbial metabolite hippurate and NF-kB enhances the aptness of natural killer T (NKT) cells to kill tumor cells and boosts the efficiency of PD-1 antibodies (Rizvi et al., 2021).

Controlling dietary fat and cholesterol can help reduce incidences of HCC which can result from upregulation of senescent associated secretory phenotype (SASP) and cyclooxygenase 2 through toll-like receptor-2 (TLR2). Upregulation of SASP results from the alliance of obesity-induced lipoteichoic acid and DCA (microbial metabolite) (Coppé et al., 2010, Zhang et al., 2021).

Deoxynivalenol, a metabolite which is present in many contaminated foods, has been found to increase the production of reactive oxygen species and induce apoptosis in human prostate cancer cells. In addition, deoxynivalenol regulates PI3K/Akt signaling in non-neoplastic prostate epithelial cells to induce apoptosis and autophagy (Kowalska et al., 2022).

Phages are viruses that target bacteria and replicate in the bacteria. The utility of phages to regulate gut microbiota and microbial metabolites is another tool explored in cancer therapy. Delivery of irinotecan via phages that targets *Fusobacterium nucleatum* can reduce these tumor-promoting bacteria in CRC (Wang et al., 2022b).

Chronic mental stress, depression, and anxiety have been associated with cancer progression and effects of treatment manipulation of microbiota-gut-brain axis is one measure of therapeutic approaches in cancer (Clapp et al., 2017). This is in part impelled by the fact that gut bacteria are able to produce neurotransmitters such as dopamine and γ-aminobutyric acid (GABA). GABA affects the state of anxiety and depression and modulates immune functioning (Jin et al., 2013). Microbial metabolite 4-ethylphenyl sulfate fine-tunes brain activity in anxious mice. SCFA modulates neuronal activity, and disturbance of SCFA metabolism can result in depression-like behavior (Liu et al., 2023, Jameson et al., 2020).

The level of microbial metabolites can be adjusted by genetic engineering through modulation of inducible promoters of commensal bacteria. Increased concentration of L-arginine in tumors is known to amplify the potency of immunotherapy. Through genetic engineering, the deletion of the arginine inhibitory gene ArgR and incorporation of ArgA^{fbr} into the *Escherichia coli* genome increases the concentration of L-arginine (Nie et al., 2023, Canale et al., 2021). Another strategy used to enhance the effectiveness of anti-PD-1 is to make usage of genetically engineered *Enterococcus faecalis* whereby *sagA* is inserted (Griffin et al., 2021).

Designing drugs that inhibit or allow production, release, and delivery of microbial metabolites is a strategy that enables scientists to focus not only on metabolites produced by commensal gut microbiota. Designing chemotherapeutic agents based on the structure of the metabolites will help harness more from beneficial metabolites.

Fecal microbiota transplantation (FMT) from a healthy donor into a patient with gut microbiota dysbiosis can help regulate their dysregulated microbiota (Gupta et al., 2016). Dysregulation can result from a variety of chemotherapeutics. FMT has improved chemotherapy response in non-responders and enhanced drug efficacy in the setting of resistance (Biazzo and Deidda, 2022, Zhang et al., 2022).

LIMITATIONS

Despite major strides made, there are several unknown mechanisms through which gut microbiota-derived metabolites influence the progression of cancer. Current research is focused on the relationship between certain metabolites and cancer treatment, however limited attention is given to the causal mechanisms. The microbiome produces enormous amounts of metabolites, and the current knowledge is based on a handful of these metabolites, thus there is a need to expand further. This knowledge needs to expand beyond the gut to other organs of the body. Moreover, fungi-derived metabolites are also known to influence cancer progression and are effective in cancer treatment, however there is limited exploration in this terrain.

CONCLUSIONS

Cancer remains a concern for human health and a largely complex disease to treat. This chapter explored the association of gut microbiota-derived metabolites and cancer, focusing on cancer progression and harnessing this knowledge to exploit novel treatment strategies. Microbial metabolites regulate cancer progression by remodeling of TME, modulating the immune function, and influencing signaling pathways. Paradoxical functions of certain microbial metabolites and the context in which they employ their functions are illustrated. Based on the understanding of the gut microbiota-derived metabolites, therapeutic approaches for cancer treatment by modulating microbial metabolites have also been explored.

REFERENCES

ABDELAZEEM, K. N. M., KALO, M. Z., BEER-HAMMER, S. & LANG, F. 2021. The gut microbiota metabolite urolithin A inhibits NF-κB activation in LPS stimulated BMDMs. *Sci Rep,* 11, 7117.

ALAUDDIN, M., OKUMURA, T., RAJAXAVIER, J., KHOZOOEI, S., PÖSCHEL, S., TAKEDA, S., SINGH, Y., BRUCKER, S. Y., WALLWIENER, D., KOCH, A. & SALKER, M. S. 2020. Gut bacterial metabolite Urolithin A decreases actin polymerization and migration in cancer cells. *Mol Nutr Food Res,* 64, e1900390.

ALEXANDER, J. L., WILSON, I. D., TEARE, J., MARCHESI, J. R., NICHOLSON, J. K. & KINROSS, J. M. 2017. Gut microbiota modulation of chemotherapy efficacy and toxicity. *Nat Rev Gastroenterol Hepatol,* 14, 356–65.

ARVIND, P., PAPAVASSILIOU, E. D., TSIOULIAS, G. J., DUCEMAN, B. W., LOVELACE, C. I., GENG, W., STAIANO-COICO, L. & RIGAS, B. 1994. Lithocholic acid inhibits the expression of HLA class I genes in colon adenocarcinoma cells. Differential effect on HLA-A, -B and -C loci. *Mol Immunol,* 31, 607–14.

BAGHBAN, R., ROSHANGAR, L., JAHANBAN-ESFAHLAN, R., SEIDI, K., EBRAHIMI-KALAN, A., JAYMAND, M., KOLAHIAN, S., JAVAHERI, T. & ZARE, P. 2020. Tumor microenvironment complexity and therapeutic implications at a glance. *Cell Commun Signal,* 18, 59.

BELL, H. N., REBERNICK, R. J., GOYERT, J., SINGHAL, R., KULJANIN, M., KERK, S. A., HUANG, W., DAS, N. K., ANDREN, A., SOLANKI, S., MILLER, S. L., TODD, P. K., FEARON, E. R., LYSSIOTIS, C. A., GYGI, S. P., MANCIAS, J. D. & SHAH, Y. M. 2022. Reuterin in the healthy gut microbiome suppresses colorectal cancer growth through altering redox balance. *Cancer Cell,* 40, 185–200.e6.

BIAZZO, M. & DEIDDA, G. 2022. Fecal microbiota transplantation as new therapeutic avenue for human diseases. *J Clin Med,* 11, 4119.

BUDA, A., QUALTROUGH, D., JEPSON, M. A., MARTINES, D., PARASKEVA, C. & PIGNATELLI, M. 2003. Butyrate downregulates alpha2beta1 integrin: A possible role in the induction of apoptosis in colorectal cancer cell lines. *Gut,* 52, 729–34.

CANALE, F. P., BASSO, C., ANTONINI, G., PEROTTI, M., LI, N., SOKOLOVSKA, A., NEUMANN, J., JAMES, M. J., GEIGER, S., JIN, W., THEURILLAT, J. P., WEST, K. A., LEVENTHAL, D. S., LORA, J. M., SALLUSTO, F. & GEIGER, R. 2021. Metabolic modulation of tumours with engineered bacteria for immunotherapy. *Nature,* 598, 662–6.

CANANI, R. B., COSTANZO, M. D., LEONE, L., PEDATA, M., MELI, R. & CALIGNANO, A. 2011. Potential beneficial effects of butyrate in intestinal and extraintestinal diseases. *World J Gastroenterol,* 17, 1519–28.

CHIRAKKAL, H., LEECH, S. H., BROOKES, K. E., PRAIS, A. L., WABY, J. S. & CORFE, B. M. 2006. Upregulation of BAK by butyrate in the colon is associated with increased Sp3 binding. *Oncogene,* 25, 7192–200.

CHO, J. J., CHAE, J. I., KIM, K. H., CHO, J. H., JEON, Y. J., OH, H. N., YOON, G., YOON, D. Y., CHO, Y. S., CHO, S. S. & SHIM, J. H. 2015. Manumycin A from a new Streptomyces strain induces endoplasmic reticulum stress-mediated cell death through specificity protein 1 signaling in human oral squamous cell carcinoma. *Int J Oncol,* 47, 1954–62.

CLAPP, M., AURORA, N., HERRERA, L., BHATIA, M., WILEN, E. & WAKEFIELD, S. 2017. Gut microbiota's effect on mental health: The gut-brain axis. *Clin Pract,* 7, 987.

COPPÉ, J. P., DESPREZ, P. Y., KRTOLICA, A. & CAMPISI, J. 2010. The senescence-associated secretory phenotype: The dark side of tumor suppression. *Annu Rev Pathol,* 5, 99–118.

CUOZZO, S., DE MORENO DE LEBLANC, A., LEBLANC, J. G., HOFFMANN, N. & TORTELLA, G. R. 2023. Streptomyces genus as a source of probiotics and its potential for its use in health. *Microbiol Res,* 266, 127248.

DATTA, A., KIM, H., LAL, M., MCGEE, L., JOHNSON, A., MOUSTAFA, A. A., JONES, J. C., MONDAL, D., FERRER, M. & ABDEL-MAGEED, A. B. 2017. Manumycin A suppresses exosome biogenesis and secretion via targeted inhibition of Ras/Raf/ERK1/2 signaling and hnRNP H1 in castration-resistant prostate cancer cells. *Cancer Lett,* 408, 73–81.

DECKERS, I. A., VAN DEN BRANDT, P. A., VAN ENGELAND, M., SOETEKOUW, P. M., BALDEWIJNS, M. M., GOLDBOHM, R. A. & SCHOUTEN, L. J. 2014. Long-term dietary sodium, potassium and fluid intake; exploring potential novel risk factors for renal cell cancer in the Netherlands Cohort Study on diet and cancer. *Br J Cancer,* 110, 797–801.

DJEDJIBEGOVIC, J., MARJANOVIC, A., PANIERI, E. & SASO, L. 2020. Ellagic acid-derived urolithins as modulators of oxidative stress. *Oxid Med Cell Longev,* 2020, 5194508.

DUAN, H., WANG, L., HUANGFU, M. & LI, H. 2023. The impact of microbiota-derived short-chain fatty acids on macrophage activities in disease: Mechanisms and therapeutic potentials. *Biomed Pharmacother,* 165, 115276.

DUDLEY, A. C. & GRIFFIOEN, A. W. 2023. Pathological angiogenesis: Mechanisms and therapeutic strategies. *Angiogenesis,* 26, 313–47.

EATON, J. E., SILVEIRA, M. G., PARDI, D. S., SINAKOS, E., KOWDLEY, K. V., LUKETIC, V. A., HARRISON, M. E., MCCASHLAND, T., BEFELER, A. S., HARNOIS, D., JORGENSEN, R., PETZ, J. & LINDOR, K. D. 2011. High-dose ursodeoxycholic acid is associated with the development of colorectal neoplasia in patients with ulcerative colitis and primary sclerosing cholangitis. *Am J Gastroenterol,* 106, 1638–45.

ENCARNAÇÃO, J. C., PIRES, A. S., AMARAL, R. A., GONÇALVES, T. J., LARANJO, M., CASALTA-LOPES, J. E., GONÇALVES, A. C., SARMENTO-RIBEIRO, A. B., ABRANTES, A. M. & BOTELHO, M. F. 2018. Butyrate, a dietary fiber derivative that improves irinotecan effect in colon cancer cells. *J Nutr Biochem,* 56, 183–92.

FAN, Q., WU, Y., LI, M., AN, F., YAO, L., WANG, M., WANG, X., YUAN, J., JIANG, K., LI, W. & LI, M. 2021. Lactobacillus spp. create a protective micro-ecological environment through regulating the core fucosylation of vaginal epithelial cells against cervical cancer. *Cell Death Dis,* 12, 1094.

FUNG, K. Y., BRIERLEY, G. V., HENDERSON, S., HOFFMANN, P., MCCOLL, S. R., LOCKETT, T., HEAD, R. & COSGROVE, L. 2011. Butyrate-induced apoptosis in HCT116 colorectal cancer cells includes induction of a cell stress response. *J Proteome Res,* 10, 1860–9.

GAFAR, A. A., DRAZ, H. M., GOLDBERG, A. A., BASHANDY, M. A., BAKRY, S., KHALIFA, M. A., ABUSHAIR, W., TITORENKO, V. I. & SANDERSON, J. T. 2016. Lithocholic acid induces endoplasmic reticulum stress, autophagy and mitochondrial dysfunction in human prostate cancer cells. *PeerJ,* 4, e2445.

GARAVAGLIA, B., VALLINO, L., FERRARESI, A., ESPOSITO, A., SALWA, A., VIDONI, C., GENTILLI, S. & ISIDORO, C. 2022. Butyrate inhibits colorectal cancer cell proliferation through autophagy degradation of β-catenin regardless of APC and β-catenin mutational status. *Biomedicines,* 10, 1131.

GOMES, S., RODRIGUES, A. C., PAZIENZA, V. & PRETO, A. 2023. Modulation of the tumor microenvironment by microbiota-derived short-chain fatty acids: Impact in colorectal cancer therapy. *Int J Mol Sci,* 24, 5069.

GRIFFIN, M. E., ESPINOSA, J., BECKER, J. L., LUO, J. D., CARROLL, T. S., JHA, J. K., FANGER, G. R. & HANG, H. C. 2021. Enterococcus peptidoglycan remodeling promotes checkpoint inhibitor cancer immunotherapy. *Science,* 373, 1040–6.

GUO, H., CHOU, W. C., LAI, Y., LIANG, K., TAM, J. W., BRICKEY, W. J., CHEN, L., MONTGOMERY, N. D., LI, X., BOHANNON, L. M., SUNG, A. D., CHAO, N. J., PELED, J. U., GOMES, A. L. C., VAN DEN BRINK, M. R. M., FRENCH, M. J., MACINTYRE, A. N., SEMPOWSKI, G. D., TAN, X., SARTOR, R. B., LU, K. & TING, J. P. Y. 2020. Multi-omics analyses of radiation survivors identify radioprotective microbes and metabolites. *Science,* 370, eaay9097.

GUPTA, S., ALLEN-VERCOE, E. & PETROF, E. O. 2016. Fecal microbiota transplantation: In perspective. *Therap Adv Gastroenterol,* 9, 229–39.

HANG, S., PAIK, D., YAO, L., KIM, E., TRINATH, J., LU, J., HA, S., NELSON, B. N., KELLY, S. P., WU, L., ZHENG, Y., LONGMAN, R. S., RASTINEJAD, F., DEVLIN, A. S., KROUT, M. R., FISCHBACH, M. A., LITTMAN, D. R. & HUH, J. R. 2019. Bile acid metabolites control T(H)17 and T(reg) cell differentiation. *Nature,* 576, 143–8.

HE, B., HOANG, T. K., WANG, T., FERRIS, M., TAYLOR, C. M., TIAN, X., LUO, M., TRAN, D. Q., ZHOU, J., TATEVIAN, N., LUO, F., MOLINA, J. G., BLACKBURN, M. R., GOMEZ, T. H., ROOS, S., RHOADS, J. M. & LIU, Y. 2017. Resetting microbiota by Lactobacillus reuteri inhibits T reg deficiency-induced autoimmunity via adenosine A2A receptors. *J Exp Med,* 214, 107–23.

HE, W., XU, J., MU, R., LI, Q., LV, D. L., HUANG, Z., ZHANG, J., WANG, C. & DONG, L. 2020. High-salt diet inhibits tumour growth in mice via regulating myeloid-derived suppressor cell differentiation. *Nat Commun,* 11, 1732.

HE, Y., FU, L., LI, Y., WANG, W., GONG, M., ZHANG, J., DONG, X., HUANG, J., WANG, Q., MACKAY, C. R., FU, Y. X., CHEN, Y. & GUO, X. 2021. Gut microbial metabolites facilitate anticancer therapy efficacy by modulating cytotoxic CD8(+) T cell immunity. *Cell Metab,* 33, 988–1000.e7.

HODGKINSON, K., EL ABBAR, F., DOBRANOWSKI, P., MANOOGIAN, J., BUTCHER, J., FIGEYS, D., MACK, D. & STINTZI, A. 2023. Butyrate's role in human health and the current progress towards its clinical application to treat gastrointestinal disease. *Clin Nutr,* 42, 61–75.

HUANG, L., WU, R. L. & XU, A. M. 2015. Epithelial-mesenchymal transition in gastric cancer. *Am J Transl Res,* 7, 2141–58.

HUANG, Y. W., LIN, C. W., PAN, P., SHAN, T., ECHEVESTE, C. E., MO, Y. Y., WANG, H. T., ALDAKKAK, M., TSAI, S., OSHIMA, K., YEARSLEY, M., XIAO, J., CAO, H., SUN, C., DU, M., BAI, W., YU, J. & WANG, L. S. 2020. Black raspberries suppress colorectal cancer by enhancing Smad4 expression in colonic epithelium and natural killer cells. *Front Immunol,* 11, 570683.

HUANG, Y., KEEN, J. C., PLEDGIE, A., MARTON, L. J., ZHU, T., SUKUMAR, S., PARK, B. H., BLAIR, B., BRENNER, K., CASERO, R. A., JR. & DAVIDSON, N. E. 2006. Polyamine analogues down-regulate estrogen receptor alpha expression in human breast cancer cells. *J Biol Chem,* 281, 19055–63.

JALANDRA, R., MAKHARIA, G. K., SHARMA, M. & KUMAR, A. 2022. Inflammatory and deleterious role of gut microbiota-derived trimethylamine on colon cells. *Front Immunol,* 13, 1101429.

JAMESON, K. G., OLSON, C. A., KAZMI, S. A. & HSIAO, E. Y. 2020. toward understanding microbiome-neuronal signaling. *Mol Cell,* 78, 577–83.

JAYE, K., LI, C. G., CHANG, D. & BHUYAN, D. J. 2022. The role of key gut microbial metabolites in the development and treatment of cancer. *Gut Microbes,* 14, 2038865.

JIN, Z., MENDU, S. K. & BIRNIR, B. 2013. GABA is an effective immunomodulatory molecule. *Amino Acids,* 45, 87–94.

KEE, K., FOSTER, B. A., MERALI, S., KRAMER, D. L., HENSEN, M. L., DIEGELMAN, P., KISIEL, N., VUJCIC, S., MAZURCHUK, R. V. & PORTER, C. W. 2004. Activated polyamine catabolism depletes acetyl-CoA pools and suppresses prostate tumor growth in TRAMP mice. *J Biol Chem,* 279, 40076–83.

KHAN, A. U., MEI, Y. H. & WILSON, T. 1992. A proposed function for spermine and spermidine: Protection of replicating DNA against damage by singlet oxygen. *Proc Natl Acad Sci U S A,* 89, 11426–7.

KIM, C. H., PARK, J. & KIM, M. 2014. Gut microbiota-derived short-chain Fatty acids, T cells, and inflammation. *Immune Netw,* 14, 277–88.

KOWALSKA, K., KOZIEŁ, M. J., HABROWSKA-GÓRCZYŃSKA, D. E., URBANEK, K. A., DOMIŃSKA, K. & PIASTOWSKA-CIESIELSKA, A. W. 2022. Deoxynivalenol induces apoptosis and autophagy in human prostate epithelial cells via PI3K/Akt signaling pathway. *Arch Toxicol,* 96, 231–41.

KOZAK, J., FORMA, A., CZECZELEWSKI, M., KOZYRA, P., SITARZ, E., RADZIKOWSKA-BÜCHNER, E., SITARZ, M. & BAJ, J. 2020. Inhibition or reversal of the epithelial-mesenchymal transition in gastric cancer: Pharmacological approaches. *Int J Mol Sci,* 22, 277.

LAL, G., ZHANG, N., VAN DER TOUW, W., DING, Y., JU, W., BOTTINGER, E. P., REID, S. P., LEVY, D. E. & BROMBERG, J. S. 2009. Epigenetic regulation of Foxp3 expression in regulatory T cells by DNA methylation. *J Immunol,* 182, 259–73.

LARABI, A. B., MASSON, H. L. P. & BÄUMLER, A. J. 2023. Bile acids as modulators of gut microbiota composition and function. *Gut Microbes,* 15, 2172671.

LEE, W.-J. & HASE, K. 2014. Gut microbiota-generated metabolites in animal health and disease. *Nature Chemical Biology,* 10, 416–24.

LEVY, M., THAISS, C. A., ZEEVI, D., DOHNALOVÁ, L., ZILBERMAN-SCHAPIRA, G., MAHDI, J. A., DAVID, E., SAVIDOR, A., KOREM, T., HERZIG, Y., PEVSNER-FISCHER, M., SHAPIRO, H., CHRIST, A., HARMELIN, A., HALPERN, Z., LATZ, E., FLAVELL, R. A., AMIT, I., SEGAL, E. & ELINAV, E. 2015. Microbiota-modulated metabolites shape the intestinal microenvironment by regulating NLRP6 inflammasome signaling. *Cell,* 163, 1428–43.

LIAO, Y., FAN, L., BIN, P., ZHU, C., CHEN, Q., CAI, Y., DUAN, J., CAI, Q., HAN, W., DING, S., HU, X., ZHANG, Y., YIN, Y. & REN, W. 2022. GABA signaling enforces intestinal germinal center B cell differentiation. *Proc Natl Acad Sci U S A,* 119, e2215921119.

LIU, L., WANG, H., CHEN, X., ZHANG, Y., ZHANG, H. & XIE, P. 2023. Gut microbiota and its metabolites in depression: From pathogenesis to treatment. *EBioMedicine,* 90, 104527.

LIU, Y., ZHANG, S., ZHOU, W., HU, D., XU, H. & JI, G. 2022. Secondary bile acids and tumorigenesis in colorectal cancer. *Front Oncol,* 12, 813745.

LUGANO, R., RAMACHANDRAN, M. & DIMBERG, A. 2020. Tumor angiogenesis: Causes, consequences, challenges and opportunities. *Cell Mol Life Sci*, 77, 1745–70.

LUU, T. H., BARD, J. M., CARBONNELLE, D., CHAILLOU, C., HUVELIN, J. M., BOBIN-DUBIGEON, C. & NAZIH, H. 2018. Lithocholic bile acid inhibits lipogenesis and induces apoptosis in breast cancer cells. *Cell Oncol (Dordr)*, 41, 13–24.

LV, M. Y., SHI, C. J., PAN, F. F., SHAO, J., FENG, L., CHEN, G., OU, C., ZHANG, J. F. & FU, W. M. 2019. Urolithin B suppresses tumor growth in hepatocellular carcinoma through inducing the inactivation of Wnt/β-catenin signaling. *J Cell Biochem*, 120, 17273–82.

MA, H., YU, Y., WANG, M., LI, Z., XU, H., TIAN, C., ZHANG, J., YE, X. & LI, X. 2019. Correlation between microbes and colorectal cancer: Tumor apoptosis is induced by sitosterols through promoting gut microbiota to produce short-chain fatty acids. *Apoptosis*, 24, 168–83.

MA, J., SUN, L., LIU, Y., REN, H., SHEN, Y., BI, F., ZHANG, T. & WANG, X. 2020. Alter between gut bacteria and blood metabolites and the anti-tumor effects of Faecalibacterium prausnitzii in breast cancer. *BMC Microbiol*, 20, 82.

MAGER, L. F., BURKHARD, R., PETT, N., COOKE, N. C. A., BROWN, K., RAMAY, H., PAIK, S., STAGG, J., GROVES, R. A., GALLO, M., LEWIS, I. A., GEUKING, M. B. & MCCOY, K. D. 2020. Microbiome-derived inosine modulates response to checkpoint inhibitor immunotherapy. *Science*, 369, 1481–9.

MATHEBELA, P., DAMANE, B. P., MULAUDZI, T. V., MKHIZE-KHWITSHANA, Z. L., GAUDJI, G. R. & DLAMINI, Z. 2022. Influence of the microbiome metagenomics and epigenomics on gastric cancer. *Int J Mol Sci*, 23, 13750.

MATHEWSON, N. D., JENQ, R., MATHEW, A. V., KOENIGSKNECHT, M., HANASH, A., TOUBAI, T., ORAVECZ-WILSON, K., WU, S. R., SUN, Y., ROSSI, C., FUJIWARA, H., BYUN, J., SHONO, Y., LINDEMANS, C., CALAFIORE, M., SCHMIDT, T. M., HONDA, K., YOUNG, V. B., PENNATHUR, S., VAN DEN BRINK, M. & REDDY, P. 2016. Gut microbiome-derived metabolites modulate intestinal epithelial cell damage and mitigate graft-versus-host disease. *Nat Immunol*, 17, 505–13.

MATSUSHITA, M., FUJITA, K., HAYASHI, T., KAYAMA, H., MOTOOKA, D., HASE, H., JINGUSHI, K., YAMAMICHI, G., YUMIBA, S., TOMIYAMA, E., KOH, Y., HAYASHI, Y., NAKANO, K., WANG, C., ISHIZUYA, Y., KATO, T., HATANO, K., KAWASHIMA, A., UJIKE, T., UEMURA, M., IMAMURA, R., RODRIGUEZ PENA, M. D. C., GORDETSKY, J. B., NETTO, G. J., TSUJIKAWA, K., NAKAMURA, S., TAKEDA, K. & NONOMURA, N. 2021. Gut microbiota-derived short-chain fatty acids promote prostate cancer growth via IGF1 signaling. *Cancer Res*, 81, 4014–26.

MENG, Y., WANG, W., KANG, J., WANG, X. & SUN, L. 2017. Role of the PI3K/AKT signalling pathway in apoptotic cell death in the cerebral cortex of streptozotocin-induced diabetic rats. *Exp Ther Med*, 13, 2417–22.

MILLS, H., ACQUAH, R., TANG, N., CHEUNG, L., KLENK, S., GLASSEN, R., PIRSON, M., ALBERT, A., HOANG, D. T. & VAN, T. N. 2022. The use of bacteria in cancer treatment: A review from the perspective of cellular microbiology. *Emerg Med Int*, 2022, 8127137.

MIRJI, G., WORTH, A., BHAT, S. A., EL SAYED, M., KANNAN, T., GOLDMAN, A. R., TANG, H. Y., LIU, Q., AUSLANDER, N., DANG, C. V., ABDEL-MOHSEN, M., KOSSENKOV, A., STANGER, B. Z. & SHINDE, R. S. 2022. The microbiome-derived metabolite TMAO drives immune activation and boosts responses to immune checkpoint blockade in pancreatic cancer. *Sci Immunol*, 7, eabn0704.

NARAHARA, H., TATSUTA, M., IISHI, H., BABA, M., UEDO, N., SAKAI, N., YANO, H. & ISHIGURO, S. 2000. K-ras point mutation is associated with enhancement by deoxycholic acid of colon carcinogenesis induced by azoxymethane, but not with its attenuation by all-trans-retinoic acid. *Int J Cancer*, 88, 157–61.

NEJMAN, D., LIVYATAN, I., FUKS, G., GAVERT, N., ZWANG, Y., GELLER, L. T., ROTTER-MASKOWITZ, A., WEISER, R., MALLEL, G., GIGI, E., MELTSER, A., DOUGLAS, G. M., KAMER, I., GOPALAKRISHNAN, V., DADOSH, T., LEVIN-ZAIDMAN, S., AVNET, S., ATLAN, T., COOPER, Z. A., ARORA, R., COGDILL, A. P., KHAN, M. A. W., OLOGUN, G., BUSSI, Y., WEINBERGER, A., LOTAN-POMPAN, M., GOLANI, O., PERRY, G., ROKAH, M., BAHAR-SHANY, K., ROZEMAN, E. A., BLANK, C. U., RONAI, A., SHAOUL, R., AMIT, A., DORFMAN, T., KREMER, R., COHEN, Z. R., HARNOF, S., SIEGAL, T., YEHUDA-SHNAIDMAN, E., GAL-YAM, E. N., SHAPIRA, H., BALDINI, N., LANGILLE, M. G. I., BEN-NUN, A., KAUFMAN, B., NISSAN, A., GOLAN, T., DADIANI, M., LEVANON, K., BAR, J., YUST-KATZ, S., BARSHACK, I., PEEPER, D. S., RAZ, D. J., SEGAL, E., WARGO, J. A., SANDBANK, J., SHENTAL, N. & STRAUSSMAN, R. 2020. The human tumor microbiome is composed of tumor type-specific intracellular bacteria. *Science*, 368, 973–80.

NGUYEN, T. T., LIAN, S., UNG, T. T., XIA, Y., HAN, J. Y. & JUNG, Y. D. 2017. Lithocholic acid stimulates IL-8 expression in human colorectal cancer cells via activation of Erk1/2 MAPK and suppression of STAT3 activity. *J Cell Biochem*, 118, 2958–67.

NGUYEN, T. T., UNG, T. T., LI, S., SAH, D. K., PARK, S. Y., LIAN, S. & JUNG, Y. D. 2021. Lithocholic acid induces miR21, promoting PTEN inhibition via STAT3 and ERK-1/2 signaling in colorectal cancer cells. *Int J Mol Sci*, 22, 10209.

NIE, M., WANG, J. & ZHANG, K. 2023. A novel strategy for L-arginine production in engineered Escherichia coli. *Microb Cell Fact*, 22, 138.

OU, J., DELANY, J. P., ZHANG, M., SHARMA, S. & O'KEEFE, S. J. 2012. Association between low colonic short-chain fatty acids and high bile acids in high colon cancer risk populations. *Nutr Cancer*, 64, 34–40.

PARK, J., YOO, H. J., YU, A. R., KIM, H. O., PARK, S. C., JANG, Y. P., LEE, C., CHOE, W., KIM, S. S., KANG, I. & YOON, K. S. 2021. Non-polar myxococcus fulvus KYC4048 metabolites exert anti-proliferative effects via inhibition of Wnt/β-catenin signaling in MCF-7 breast cancer cells. *J Microbiol Biotechnol*, 31, 540–9.

PARK, M., PARK, H., KIM, W. H., CHO, H. & LEE, J. H. 2005. Presence of autocrine hepatocyte growth factor-Met signaling and its role in proliferation and migration of SNU-484 gastric cancer cell line. *Exp Mol Med*, 37, 213–9.

PENCIK, J., SCHLEDERER, M., GRUBER, W., UNGER, C., WALKER, S. M., CHALARIS, A., MARIÉ, I. J., HASSLER, M. R., JAVAHERI, T., AKSOY, O., BLAYNEY, J. K., PRUTSCH, N., SKUCHA, A., HERAC, M., KRÄMER, O. H., MAZAL, P., GREBIEN, F., EGGER, G., POLI, V., MIKULITS, W., EFERL, R., ESTERBAUER, H., KENNEDY, R., FEND, F., SCHARPF, M., BRAUN, M., PERNER, S.,

LEVY, D. E., MALCOLM, T., TURNER, S. D., HAITEL, A., SUSANI, M., MOAZZAMI, A., ROSE-JOHN, S., ABERGER, F., MERKEL, O., MORIGGL, R., CULIG, Z., DOLZNIG, H. & KENNER, L. 2015. STAT3 regulated ARF expression suppresses prostate cancer metastasis. *Nat Commun,* 6, 7736.

POWOLNY, A., XU, J. & LOO, G. 2001. Deoxycholate induces DNA damage and apoptosis in human colon epithelial cells expressing either mutant or wild-type p53. *Int J Biochem Cell Biol,* 33, 193–203.

PYO, J. S., KO, Y. S., KANG, G., KIM, D. H., KIM, W. H., LEE, B. L. & SOHN, J. H. 2015. Bile acid induces MUC2 expression and inhibits tumor invasion in gastric carcinomas. *J Cancer Res Clin Oncol,* 141, 1181–8.

RIZVI, Z. A., DALAL, R., SADHU, S., KUMAR, Y., KUMAR, S., GUPTA, S. K., TRIPATHY, M. R., RATHORE, D. K. & AWASTHI, A. 2021. High-salt diet mediates interplay between NK cells and gut microbiota to induce potent tumor immunity. *Sci Adv,* 7, eabg5016.

ROBINSON, K. M., CRABTREE, J., MATTICK, J. S., ANDERSON, K. E. & DUNNING HOTOPP, J. C. 2017. Distinguishing potential bacteria-tumor associations from contamination in a secondary data analysis of public cancer genome sequence data. *Microbiome,* 5, 9.

SALEM, M., AMMITZBOELL, M., NYS, K., SEIDELIN, J. B. & NIELSEN, O. H. 2015. ATG16L1: A multifunctional susceptibility factor in Crohn disease. *Autophagy,* 11, 585–94.

SAMAN, H., RAZA, S. S., UDDIN, S. & RASUL, K. 2020. Inducing angiogenesis, a key step in cancer vascularization, and treatment approaches. *Cancers (Basel),* 12, 1172.

SEN, U., SHENOY, P. S. & BOSE, B. 2017. Opposing effects of low versus high concentrations of water soluble vitamins/dietary ingredients Vitamin C and niacin on colon cancer stem cells (CSCs). *Cell Biol Int,* 41, 1127–45.

SHIAO, S. L., KERSHAW, K. M., LIMON, J. J., YOU, S., YOON, J., KO, E. Y., GUARNERIO, J., POTDAR, A. A., MCGOVERN, D. P. B., BOSE, S., DAR, T. B., NOE, P., LEE, J., KUBOTA, Y., MAYMI, V. I., DAVIS, M. J., HENSON, R. M., CHOI, R. Y., YANG, W., TANG, J., GARGUS, M., PRINCE, A. D., ZUMSTEG, Z. S. & UNDERHILL, D. M. 2021. Commensal bacteria and fungi differentially regulate tumor responses to radiation therapy. *Cancer Cell,* 39, 1202–13.e6.

SLANEY, C. Y. & KERSHAW, M. H. 2020. Challenges and opportunities for effective cancer immunotherapies. *Cancers (Basel),* 12, 3164.

SMITH, E. J., BEAUMONT, R. E., MCCLELLAN, A., SZE, C., PALOMINO LAGO, E., HAZELGROVE, L., DUDHIA, J., SMITH, R. K. W. & GUEST, D. J. 2023. Tumour necrosis factor alpha, interleukin 1 beta and interferon gamma have detrimental effects on equine tenocytes that cannot be rescued by IL-1RA or mesenchymal stromal cell-derived factors. *Cell Tissue Res,* 391, 523–44.

SON, M. Y. & CHO, H. S. 2023. Anticancer effects of gut microbiota-derived short-chain fatty acids in cancers. *J Microbiol Biotechnol,* 33, 849–56.

SONG, X., AN, Y., CHEN, D., ZHANG, W., WU, X., LI, C., WANG, S., DONG, W., WANG, B., LIU, T., ZHONG, W., SUN, T. & CAO, H. 2022. Microbial metabolite deoxycholic acid promotes vasculogenic mimicry formation in intestinal carcinogenesis. *Cancer Sci,* 113, 459–77.

SUN, M., WU, W., LIU, Z. & CONG, Y. 2017. Microbiota metabolite short chain fatty acids, GPCR, and inflammatory bowel diseases. *J Gastroenterol,* 52, 1–8.

THIRUNAVUKKARASAN, M., WANG, C., RAO, A., HIND, T., TEO, Y. R., SIDDIQUEE, A. A., GOGHARI, M. A. I., KUMAR, A. P. & HERR, D. R. 2017. Short-chain fatty acid receptors inhibit invasive phenotypes in breast cancer cells. *PLoS One,* 12, e0186334.

TISI, R., GAPONENKO, V., VANONI, M. & SACCO, E. 2020. Natural products attenuating biosynthesis, processing, and activity of ras oncoproteins: State of the art and future perspectives. *Biomolecules,* 10, 1535.

TOTIGER, T. M., SRINIVASAN, S., JALA, V. R., LAMICHHANE, P., DOSCH, A. R., GAIDARSKI, A. A., 3RD, JOSHI, C., RANGAPPA, S., CASTELLANOS, J., VEMULA, P. K., CHEN, X., KWON, D., KASHIKAR, N., VANSAUN, M., MERCHANT, N. B. & NAGATHIHALLI, N. S. 2019. Urolithin A, a novel natural compound to target PI3K/AKT/mTOR pathway in pancreatic cancer. *Mol Cancer Ther,* 18, 301–11.

WALCZAK, K., WNOROWSKI, A., TURSKI, W. A. & PLECH, T. 2020. Kynurenic acid and cancer: Facts and controversies. *Cell Mol Life Sci,* 77, 1531–50.

WANG, D., YUAN, T., LIU, J., WEN, Z., SHEN, Y., TANG, J., WANG, Z. & WU, X. 2022a. ATG16L2 inhibits NLRP3 inflammasome activation through promoting ATG5-12-16L1 complex assembly and autophagy. *Eur J Immunol,* 52, 1321–34.

WANG, L., LIU, Y., HAN, R., BEIER, U., BHATTI, T., AKIMOVA, T., GREENE, M., HIEBERT, S. & HANCOCK, W. 2015. FOXP3+ regulatory T cell development and function require histone/protein deacetylase 3. *The Journal of Clinical Investigation,* 125, 1111–23.

WANG, X., FEITH, D. J., WELSH, P., COLEMAN, C. S., LOPEZ, C., WOSTER, P. M., O'BRIEN, T. G. & PEGG, A. E. 2007. Studies of the mechanism by which increased spermidine/spermine N1-acetyltransferase activity increases susceptibility to skin carcinogenesis. *Carcinogenesis,* 28, 2404–11.

WANG, Y., LIU, Z., CHEN, Q., YI, L., XU, Z., CAI, M., QIN, J., ZHANG, Y., DU, G., HONG, J., GUO, X. & LIU, C. 2022b. Isolation and characterization of novel Fusobacterium nucleatum bacteriophages. *Front Microbiol,* 13, 945315.

WEINGARDEN, A. R., CHEN, C., ZHANG, N., GRAIZIGER, C. T., DOSA, P. I., STEER, C. J., SHAUGHNESSY, M. K., JOHNSON, J. R., SADOWSKY, M. J. & KHORUTS, A. 2016. Ursodeoxycholic acid inhibits clostridium difficile spore germination and vegetative growth, and prevents the recurrence of Ileal Pouchitis associated with the infection. *J Clin Gastroenterol,* 50, 624–30.

XIAO, T., WU, S., YAN, C., ZHAO, C., JIN, H., YAN, N., XU, J., WU, Y., LI, C., SHAO, Q. & XIA, S. 2018. Butyrate upregulates the TLR4 expression and the phosphorylation of MAPKs and NK-κB in colon cancer cell in vitro. *Oncol Lett,* 16, 4439–47.

XIAO, Y., HUANG, R., WANG, N., DENG, Y., TAN, B., YIN, Y., QI, M. & WANG, J. 2022. Ellagic acid alleviates oxidative stress by mediating Nrf2 signaling pathways and protects against paraquat-induced intestinal injury in piglets. *Antioxidants (Basel),* 11, 252.

XU, H., CHATURVEDI, R., CHENG, Y., BUSSIERE, F. I., ASIM, M., YAO, M. D., POTOSKY, D., MELTZER, S. J., RHEE, J. G., KIM, S. S., MOSS, S. F., HACKER, A., WANG, Y., CASERO, R. A., JR. & WILSON, K. T. 2004. Spermine oxidation induced by Helicobacter pylori results in apoptosis and DNA damage: Implications for gastric carcinogenesis. *Cancer Res,* 64, 8521–5.

YANG, Q., WANG, B., ZHENG, Q., LI, H., MENG, X., ZHOU, F. & ZHANG, L. 2023. A review of gut microbiota-derived metabolites in tumor progression and cancer therapy. *Adv Sci (Weinh),* 10, e2207366.

YANG, S., DAI, H., LU, Y., LI, R., GAO, C. & PAN, S. 2022. Trimethylamine N-oxide promotes cell proliferation and angiogenesis in colorectal cancer. *J Immunol Res,* 2022, 7043856.

YUE, C., YANG, X., LI, J., CHEN, X., ZHAO, X., CHEN, Y. & WEN, Y. 2017. Trimethylamine N-oxide prime NLRP3 inflammasome via inhibiting ATG16L1-induced autophagy in colonic epithelial cells. *Biochem Biophys Res Commun,* 490, 541–51.

ZHANG, J., REN, L., YU, M., LIU, X., MA, W., HUANG, L., LI, X. & YE, X. 2019. S-equol inhibits proliferation and promotes apoptosis of human breast cancer MCF-7 cells via regulating miR-10a-5p and PI3K/AKT pathway. *Arch Biochem Biophys,* 672, 108064.

ZHANG, J., WU, K., SHI, C. & LI, G. 2022. Cancer immunotherapy: Fecal microbiota transplantation brings light. *Curr Treat Options Oncol,* 23, 1777–92.

ZHANG, S., DOGAN, B., GUO, C., HERLEKAR, D., STEWART, K., SCHERL, E. J. & SIMPSON, K. W. 2020. Short chain fatty acids modulate the growth and virulence of pathosymbiont escherichia coli and host response. *Antibiotics (Basel),* 9, 462.

ZHANG, X., COKER, O. O., CHU, E. S., FU, K., LAU, H. C. H., WANG, Y. X., CHAN, A. W. H., WEI, H., YANG, X., SUNG, J. J. Y. & YU, J. 2021. Dietary cholesterol drives fatty liver-associated liver cancer by modulating gut microbiota and metabolites. *Gut,* 70, 761–74.

ZHOU, X., KANDALAI, S., HOSSAIN, F. & ZHENG, Q. 2022. Tumor microbiome metabolism: A game changer in cancer development and therapy. *Front Oncol,* 12, 933407.

ZHU, G., HUANG, Q., HUANG, Y., ZHENG, W., HUA, J., YANG, S., ZHUANG, J., WANG, J. & YE, J. 2016. Lipopolysaccharide increases the release of VEGF-C that enhances cell motility and promotes lymphangiogenesis and lymphatic metastasis through the TLR4- NF-κB/JNK pathways in colorectal cancer. *Oncotarget,* 7, 73711–24.

9 Gut–Brain Axis and Cancer: Delving into the Intricate Connection Between the Gut and the Brain

Rodney Hull, Georgios Lolas, and Zodwa Dlamini

INTRODUCTION

Over the last 15 years, it has become evident that there is a strong association between changes in the microbiota composition (dysbiosis), various host diseases (Bäckhed et al., 2005; Sommer and Bäckhed, 2013; Clarke et al., 2013), and numerous physiological processes within the host (Bäckhed et al., 2005; Lloyd-Price et al., 2016; Sommer and Bäckhed, 2013; Uchimura et al., 2018). In normal healthy conditions where the composition of the gut microbiota is not altered the interaction between the gut microbiota and various tissues assists in protection against pathogens, nutrient digestion and absorption, development, and education of the immune system (Bäckhed et al., 2005; Lloyd-Price et al., 2016; Sommer and Bäckhed, 2013, Uchimura et al., 2018). The gut microbiota has the potential to impact tissues and organs beyond its immediate vicinity (Duvallet et al., 2017; Gil-Cruz et al., 2019) including the central nervous system (CNS) (Clarke et al., 2013, Sudo et al., 2004). The interaction between gut microbiota and CNS is referred to as the gut–brain axis (GBA), which has been extensively studied in recent years. This axis can be defined as the communication between the CNS, the intestine, and the microbiota (Sudo et al., 2004; Yano et al., 2015; Skonieczna-Żydecka et al., 2018). This communication between the gut and brain is bidirectional, involving both direct and indirect pathways. These pathways include the endocrine axis, hypothalamic-pituitary-adrenal axis (HPA), immune chemokines and cytokines, autonomic nervous system (ANS), enteric nervous system, and microbiota (Duvallet et al., 2017; Burberry et al., 2020, Blacher et al., 2019). The gut-microbiota-brain axis is influenced by signaling initiated by the microbiota, through neurotransmitters (Yano et al., 2015; O'Keefe, 2016) and microbial metabolites (Skonieczna-Żydecka et al., 2018; Ellwardt et al., 2016; O'Keefe, 2016).

It is likely that the various ways microbes can interact with the nervous system may be mechanistically connected, explaining how this interaction can promote either good health or diseases such as cancer following dysbiosis. The relationship between bacterial infection and cancer was demonstrated by the work of William Coley, who infected cancer patients with live or heat-killed *Streptococcus* and *Serratia* species, which commonly resulted in the cancer going into remission. Previously, the treatment was not further investigated due to its tendency to cause infection and patient mortality (Coley, 1891). This is now beginning to change as fecal transfers, microbe metabolites, and probiotics are being explored as likely cancer treatments (Xavier et al., 2020; Sepich-Poore et al., 2021). This treatment was and is successful most likely due to the ability of these bacteria or their metabolites to induce inflammation and an immune reaction (Bickels et al., 2002; Starnes, 1992). The CNS is an immune-privileged organ, with the blood-brain barrier (BBB) regulating the entry of molecules, ions, and cells into the brain (Engelhardt and Liebner, 2014), and providing the brain with protection from pathogens and unwanted immune reactions (Daneman and Prat, 2015). However, active immune cells can cross the BBB and can also enter the brain via the choroid plexus, and the lymphatic vessels (Inserra et al., 2018). Certain bacterial metabolites have also been shown to be able to cross the BBB (Uchimura et al., 2018; Buffington et al., 2016).

Apart from the necessity of angiogenesis and the development of the lymphatic system for cancer progression and metastasis, it is now accepted that neo neurogenesis, the formation of new nerve tissue (Figure 9.1) provides cancer cells with pathways for migration and invasion into different tissues throughout the body (Zahalka and Frenette, 2020). Moreover, these newly formed nerve fibers serve as communication channels between tumor cells and various cells and tissues via chemokines and neurotransmitters. The presence of numerous receptors for these molecules on cancer cells suggests their significance in facilitating interactions, further supported by the ability of cancer cells to produce and release them themselves (Zahalka and Frenette, 2020).

This chapter will review the interaction between the gut microbiome and the nervous system. And the role this interaction may have on the development and progression of various cancers due to gut microbiome dysbiosis.

GUT–BRAIN AXIS

The first hints of the existence of a gut–brain axis, was the ability of an individual's emotional state on digestion (Heym

DOI: 10.1201/9781032706450-9

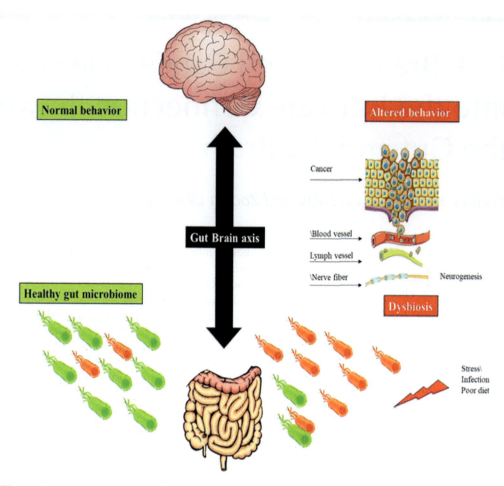

FIGURE 9.1 **The gut–brain axis and its role in the development and progression of cancer.** Dysbiosis caused by various factors, including poor diet, infection, and stress, results in changes in the composition of the gut microbiome. This can result in changes in the process of neurogenesis. This can lead to increased cancer cell migration along these new nerve fibers in the same way cancer cells can migrate along blood and lymph vessels. These new nerve fibers also provide cancer cells with new signals that can promote survival, growth, and migration.

et al., 2019; Rhee et al., 2009). By utilizing germ-free (GF) animal models, researchers have been able to demonstrate that changes in the microbiome result in altered cognitive function (Diaz Heijtz et al., 2011; Gareau et al., 2011). Furthermore, studies have shown that supplementation of specific strains of bacteria through probiotics can influence human (Pinto-Sanchez et al., 2017) and animal (Savignac et al., 2014) behavior. Multiple tissues and cell types are involved in this multifaceted microbiota-gut-brain axis, including the gut, the brain, various glands, immune cells, and gastrointestinal microbiota (Figure 9.2) (Cryan and Dinan, 2012).

Communication between the brain and gut occurs through both the central (Ma et al., 2019) and enteric nervous (Kuwahara et al., 2020) systems. Multiple tissues and cell types are involved in this multifaceted microbiota-gut-brain axis (Carabotti et al., 2015; Sherman et al., 2015). The interaction between the brain and the gut can be influenced by changes in the microbiome that impact immune system functioning (Kamada et al., 2013). Dysbiosis resulting from a weakened immune response may contribute to cancer development and progression (Mangani et al., 2017).

The bacteria in the human gut can be classified into three enterotypes, depending on the dominant genus present. These three most common genera are *Bacteroides, Prevotella*, and *Ruminococcus* (Arumugam et al., 2011). By altering the make-up of the microbiota, through for instance antibiotic treatment, can impact the gut–brain axis, especially the interaction between the microbe-enteric nervous system and the brain (O'Mahony et al., 2014). Cancer treatments like radiotherapy can also affect the makeup of the microbial community (Jones et al., 2020). Dysbiosis of the gut microbiome was initially only associated with the development of colon cancer. However, it is now understood that alterations in microbial composition and the presence of non-native microbes can play a role in the development of various types of cancer, such as prostate, pancreatic (Riquelme et al., 2019), leukemia (Meisel et al., 2018), and brain cancers (Subramaniam et al., 2020).

The components of the GBA include the microbes and their secreted signaling factors, the vagus nerve, and the BBB. Microorganisms produce and secrete metabolites as a result of their regular cellular processes. These metabolites play an important role in the ability of the microbiome to influence the nervous system and the resulting contribution of the gut–brain axis to the development and progression of cancer. For instance the chances of developing colon cancer

Gut–Brain Axis and Cancer

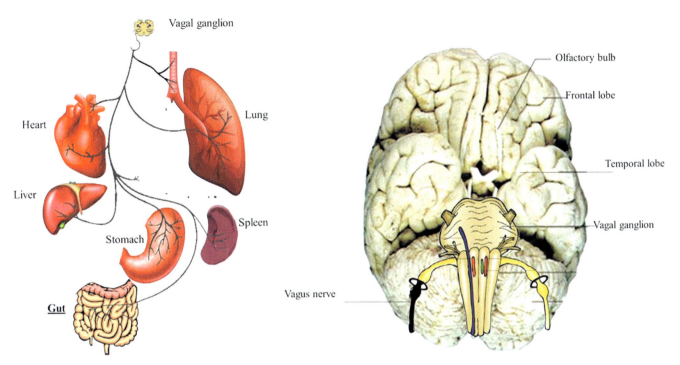

FIGURE 9.2 **The vagus nerve.** (A) The path of the vagus nerve throughout the body as it connects the gut to the brain. It also connects the stomach, spleen, liver, heart, and lungs. (B) The position of the vagal ganglion and vagus nerve in the brain.

are increased through the activity of commensal gut bacteria that secrete metabolites that contribute to DNA damage and chromosomal instability (Chu et al., 2004). Short-chain fatty acids (SCFAs) are produced by anaerobic commensal bacteria fermenting non-digestible carbohydrates. SCFAs include butyrate, acetate, propionate, and ketone bodies (Stilling et al., 2016). Butyrate has the ability to affect the nervous system, especially at high concentrations. It is able to indirectly regulate the activity of various cells including immune cells and nerve cells within the vagus nerve (Stilling et al., 2016). Butyrate and other SCFAs bind to various receptors, including MCT1/SLC16A1; SMCT1/SLC5A8; GPR43/FFAR2; GPR41/FFAR3, and GPR109a/HCAR2 (Stilling et al., 2016). Butyrate acts as an anticancer agent by inhibiting the activity of histone deacetylases (HDACs) (Stilling et al., 2016), decreasing the expression of proteins involved in survival, apoptosis resistance, and proliferation (Donohoe et al., 2014). This was demonstrated through the discovery that individuals with colon cancer had lower amounts of butyrate-producing bacteria in their stool and consequently lower levels of butyrate (Singh et al., 2014).

The vagus nerve emerges from the brain and connects the heart, lungs, and digestive system to the parasympathetic nervous system (Prescott and Liberles, 2022) (Figure 9.2). This means that the vagus nerve conveys signals between the gut and the CNS (Forsythe et al., 2014). Cancer progression and metastasis is associated with increased vagus nerve activity (De Couck et al., 2018). Communication between the vagus nerve and the gut occurs through neurotransmitters. These neurotransmitters are released in response to changes in the gut, such as dysbiosis, environmental changes, infection by pathogens, and the presence of cancer cells in the gut (Browning et al., 2006). The increase or decrease in the release of these neurotransmitters in response to these various changes can lead to aberrant digestion, gastric motility, or signal transmission along the GBA (Travagli and Anselmi, 2016). These neurotransmitters along with other factors are secreted by the enteroendocrine cells lining the gut during the digestion and processing of ingested food. These factors allow these cells to communicate with the neurons and the microbiota (Gribble and Reimann, 2016). The aforementioned bacterial metabolites secreted by the microbes in the gut are also able to bind to receptors on the enteroendocrine cells. These cells also produce hormones such as serotonin or 5-hydroxytryptamine (5-HT), cholecystokinin (CCK), and peptide YY (PYY) (Palazzo et al., 2007).

The BBB is composed of the endothelial cells forming the capillaries of the brain. These cells attach to each other tightly with various physical barriers. These cells are held together by tight and adherens junctions, as well as multiple layers of membranes (Banks, 2009). The selectivity of the BBB ensures that only a specific sub-set of molecules (signaling molecules, nutrients, and minerals) and cells can gain access to the brain. Signaling molecules conveying messages from the gut are among those that can cross the BBB (Banks, 2009). The ability of the BBB to prevent the free movement of cells also helps to prevent brain metastasis for most cancers. However, in addition to this protective role, the BBB also interferes with the treatment of brain cancers as it also excludes many chemotherapeutic agents/drugs, while many of the drugs that do cross the BBB also weaken it, thereby facilitating metastasis (Blecharz et al., 2015). Many gut microbiome metabolites share characteristics with molecules that do cross the BBB and as such they are also able to cross the BBB (Banks, 2009). Various experiments using germ-free mice have demonstrated that the microbiota is also able to influence the integrity of the BBB. This is achieved through molecules secreted by the microbes in the gut assisting in the expression of molecules required in the formation of tight junctions. Consequently, these germ-free mice had a more permeable BBB due to the absence of these molecules that are normally secreted by the gut microbes. *Clostridium tyrobutyricum* is a bacterium that is known to produce high levels of butyrate and inoculating these mice with *C. tyrobutyricum* leads to the restoration of BBB integrity (Braniste et al., 2014). The selective communication between the immune and nervous system ensured by the BBB means that only certain immune cells and factors associated with immunity can cross the BBB (Banks, 2015).

THE MICROBIOTA AND THE IMMUNE SYSTEM IN NERVE-RELATED CANCER

The immune system plays an important role in the GBA, and the development of cancer is related to interactions with the nervous system. The immune system will respond differently to different populations of gut microbiota, with dysbiosis altering the immune response. This activation of the immune response occurs in different ways through different signaling pathways and molecules. The lymphatic system is involved in many of these immune responses to various microbes. It is only in the last decade that a lymphatic system was determined to exist in the brain. Previously, it was believed that the brain did not possess a lymphatic system or anything that could function as one. However, the discovery of the glymphatic system, a lymphatic drainage system, is immunologically significant (Dissing-Olesen et al., 2015). The glymphatic system facilitates bidirectional communication between the peripheral lymphatic and central nervous systems and may play a role in neuroinflammation (Erickson et al., 2012).

The innate immune system has evolved to recognize patterns associated with pathogens, such as their molecules and recognition receptors otherwise known as pathogen-associated molecular patterns (PAMPs). This triggers the activation of the inflammasome, leading to a pro-apoptotic response and the release of IL-1β and IL-18 proteins (Cui et al., 2014). The innate immune system is able to differentiate between different populations of gut microbiota and selectively activate the inflammasome, with the intensity of the response varying depending on the microbes present. In mouse models, inflammasome activation has been shown to induce cognitive and behavioral changes, illustrating that inflammation can impact neuronal function (Kaufmann et al., 2017). Pro-inflammatory molecules such as IL1β, IL6, IL8, IL12, GM-CSF, and TNFα are known to be involved in the development and progression of brain cancer (Braganhol et al., 2015). These pro-inflammatory cytokines are secreted by pro-oncogenic immune cells such as T-helper-17 (Th17) cells. The development of these cells can be instigated by dendritic cells, responding to certain commensal gut bacteria (Bene et al., 2017; Grivennikov et al., 2012). As a result, studies have shown that germ-free mice exhibit lower levels of pro-inflammatory cytokines due to decreased inflammatory response (Atarashi et al., 2008).

The activity of the immune system can be regulated by gut microbes through substances they secrete. These microbial substances are often metabolic byproducts that result from the normal functioning of these organisms. These microbial metabolites can have varying effects on the immune system's response to cancer cells, either promoting or inhibiting. These metabolites are secreted into the gut where they enter the circulatory or lymphatic systems (Sharon et al., 2014).

The bacteria *Fusobacterium nucleatum* can dampen the immune response towards tumor cells by expressing the adhesion protein Fap2. This particular protein possesses the ability to inhibit the tumor killing functions of cytotoxic immune cells. Moreover, it inhibits the immune response even further by activating T-cell immunoreceptor tyrosine-based inhibitory motif domains (TIGIT), which are receptor proteins found on the surface of T cells and serve to restrict their activity (Gur et al., 2015). Consequently, an increase in the abundance of *F. nucleatum* is linked to an immune reaction characterized by a rise in tumor-associated macrophages, which suppresses antitumor T-cell responses (Kostic et al., 2013).

The microbiota is also able to initiate an anticancer immune response. For example, intestinal bacteria of the genus *Bifidobacterium* result in an increase in the ability of cytotoxic T cells via the dendritic cells (Sivan et al., 2015). *Bacteroides fragilis* secretes polysaccharides, such as polysaccharide A (PSA), which enhance antitumour immune function by increasing Toll-like receptor 4 (TLR4) and IL-12-dependent TH1 responses (Vétizou et al., 2015). These bacteria seem to increase the immune response by inhibiting cytotoxic T-lymphocyte-associated protein 4 (CTLA4). Inhibition of this protein using anti-CTLA4 antibodies is a common treatment for many cancers as this protein is a negative regulator of the T cell responses. This is demonstrated by the fact that the effectiveness of these antibodies depends on the presence of these anti-tumor immune-stimulating bacteria in the gut (Vétizou et al., 2015).

These metabolites secreted by microbes can also include various neurotransmitters and neuromodulators with activity in the CNS (Wikoff et al., 2009). These include SCFAs that are able to decrease the release of pro-inflammatory cytokines. These cytokines affect the number of Th1 cells. SCFAs promote the development of Tregs, which release IL10. IL-10 impairs anticancer immune cell activity, leading to cancer development (Sun et al., 2017). Since SCFAs are secreted by *Bacteroides fragilis*, high levels of this bacteria lead to the formation of more Tregs and higher levels of IL-10 (Coyte et al., 2015).

Gut microbe dysbiosis can affect the CNS through NF-κB signaling via activation of the immune system. *Campylobacter jejuni* is a microbe whose metabolites activate cytokines which in turn activate NF-κB (Masanta et al., 2013). NF-κB signaling has been observed to induce inflammation in the CNS of mice. This NF-κB signaling was also associated with decreased expression of brain-derived neurotrophic factor (BDNF) (Jang et al., 2018). The formation of new nervous tissue and fibers requires BDNF and promotes the development and progression of cancer as new nerve fibers provide a pathway for the expansion and migration of tumors (Kumar et al., 2007). The NFκB pathway also activates signal transducer and activator of transcription 3 (STAT3) signaling. In brain cancers STAT3 signaling is associated with an aggressive disease that progresses rapidly and can be used as a biomarker for a poor prognosis (McFarland et al., 2013; Zanotto-Filho et al., 2017). Bacteria from the genus *Helicobacter* have long been associated with health problems such as stomach ulcers and cancers such as prostate and colon cancer (Boleij and Tjalsma, 2012). Prostate intraepithelial neoplasia and microinvasive adenocarcinoma lesions were found to be more common in mice infected with *Helicobacter hepaticus*. Lymphoid cells from these mice were able to promote the formation of neoplasia when inserted into healthy mice. These mice also displayed elevated NF-κB signaling, resulting in the increased expression of TNF-α(Akaza, 2012).

Since the brain is separated from the rest of the body by the BBB, the CNS has its own native immune cells which include glial cells, macrophages, CD8+ T cells, Tregs, CD4+ T helper (Th) cells, microglia cells, and astrocytes. These immune cells not only defend the brain from infection but are also involved in neural remodeling (Yin et al., 2017). Gut microbiota antigens activate CD4+ T cells, activating Th17 cells and immune responses (Goto et al., 2014). SCFAs can also cross the BBB and can initiate T cell differentiation in the brain among other tissue sites. SCFAs also result in increased expression of the Foxp3 transcription factor via activation of the foxp3 promoter (Kim et al., 2014). Astrocytes can also be activated by microbial metabolites by binding to aryl hydrocarbon receptors, which initiates IFN-I signaling, initiating the activation and recruitment of neurotoxic immune cells (Fearon et al., 2013).

Dysbiosis can even alter the structure of microglia, such as those observed in germ-free mice. In this case, these microglia have increased levels of receptors required for immune cell differentiation and proliferation. These include the cell surface receptors colony stimulating factor 1 receptor (CSF1R), F4/80, and CD31. It is normal to only find high levels of these receptors on the surface of immature microglia cells, with the expression decreasing as the microglia mature. Activation of GPR43 receptor on these cells by a ligand triggers an inflammatory response. This immune response is observed in mice that have received antibiotic treatment as well. Furthermore, both germ-free and antibiotic-treated mice exhibit elevated levels of microglia (Erny et al., 2015) with gene expression profiles resembling those of younger microglia (Matcovitch-Natan et al., 2016).

The immune system is primed through the activation of the type I interferon (IFN-I) cytokine signaling pathway by recognizing various PAMPs from a wide variety of pathogens including viruses, bacteria, and tumor cells.

In CNS models, IFN-1 protects against brain cancers, while also promoting dendritic cell and cytotoxic T cell maturation involved in cancer cell response (Budhwani et al., 2018; Zitvogel et al., 2015). Additionally, IFN-I induces apoptosis to regulate growth and proliferation in hematological cancers (Lee et al., 2012). The expression of IFN-1 can be influenced by the gut microbiome (Giles and Stagg, 2017) where higher levels of lactic acid bacteria stimulate TLR3 to increase INF-β secretion from dendritic cells (Metidji et al., 2015).

NEUROTRANSMITTERS IN CANCER AND THE MICROBIOME

Receptors for neurotransmitters include serpentine receptors, the G protein coupled receptors (GPCRs), and ligand-gated ion channels (LGICs). These receptors are commonly expressed on the surface of cancer cells, and the binding of ligands (neurotransmitters) to these receptors can lead to the activation of pathways that contribute to increased proliferation and migration (Hutchings et al., 2020) (Figure 9.3A). Cancer cells can promote these pathways through the production and secretion of neurotransmitters. For example, prostate cancer cells produce and secrete neurotransmitters in a similar manner to neuroendocrine cells (Jiang et al., 2019).

Serotonin or 5-hydroxytryptamine (5-HT) is a monoamine neurotransmitter that plays an active role in many biological systems including the CNS, the neuroendocrine system, the enteric nervous system (Chin et al., 2012; Yano et al., 2015), and the immune system (Kwon et al., 2019). Serotonin also plays a central role in the development and progression of multiple cancers (Figure 9.3B) (Singhal et al., 2019), including gliomas (Merzak et al., 1996), prostate cancer (Siddiqui et al., 2006), bladder cancer (Siddiqui et al., 2006), small cell lung carcinoma (Cattaneo et al., 1994), colon cancer (Tutton and Steel, 1979), breast cancer (Pai et al., 2009), and hepatocellular carcinoma (Soll et al., 2010). Serotonin signaling pathways in cancer cells lead to increased cell growth and survival and cell cycle alterations. These changes are linked to alterations in the expression of genes such as MEK-ERK1/2 and JAK2-STAT3 (Oufkir et al., 2010). Higher levels of serotonin are associated with an increase in angiogenesis (Oufkir et al., 2010; Zamani and Qu, 2012). Serotonin receptors commonly overexpressed in cancers include the 5-HT1 and 5-HT$_2$ receptors (Ataee et al., 2010; Nishikawa et al., 2010; Sonier et al., 2006) (Figure 9.3).

Despite its role in these various systems and the best-known role taking place in the brain and CNS, it is now known that up to 90% of all serotonins are synthesized in the gut (Liu et al., 2021). Dysbiosis in the gut is known to alter the synthesis, and breakdown of serotonin, leading to altered serotonin levels in both the gut and the hippocampus in mice (Yaghoubfar et al., 2020). Germ-free male mice were also found to have higher levels of serotonin in the hippocampus and higher levels of serotonin precursor in their blood (Clarke et al., 2013). Metabolites from certain bacteria have also been isolated from the feces of cancer patients with higher levels of 5-HT (Yano et al., 2015).

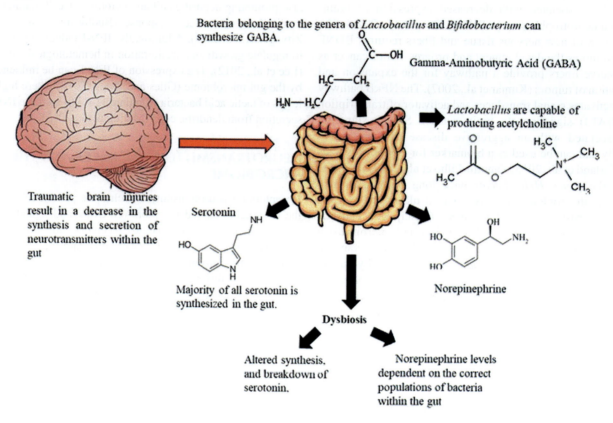
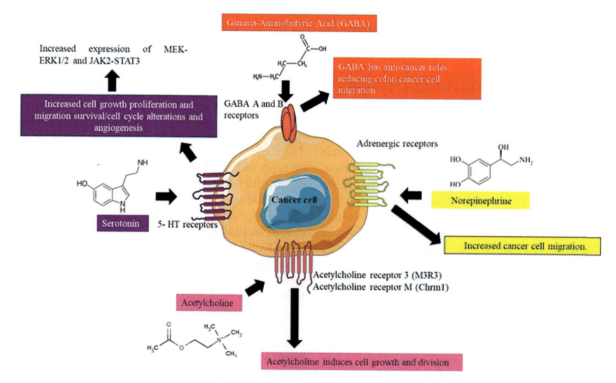

FIGURE 9.3 **The role of neurotransmitters in cancer development.** (A) Bacteria within the gut secrete a multitude of neurotransmitters including serotonin, norepinephrine, GABA, and acetylcholine. (B) These different neurotransmitters bind to receptors on the surface of cancer cells and either initiate pro-oncogenic processes or in the case of GABA are known to inhibit the formation of cancer.

It has also been demonstrated that traumatic brain injuries result in a decrease in the synthesis of secretion within the gut (Figure 9.3A). This also demonstrates the communication regarding this neurotransmitter and its related functions along the GBA (Mercado et al., 2022). As such it is not surprising that changes in the level of serotonin promote colon cancer development. However, in this case, serotonin plays an anticancer role, and colon cancer is associated with lower levels of serotonin accompanied by increased levels of DNA damage and inflammation (Sakita et al., 2019). Norepinephrine signaling promotes cancer cell migration (Joseph et al., 2002). The levels of norepinephrine and other catecholamines appear to be dependent on the correct populations of bacteria within the gut. Decreased levels of norepinephrine are seen in germ-free mice (Neufeld et al., 2011) (Figure 9.3). Another catecholamine, dopamine stimulates dopaminergic neurons as well as activating both the innate and adaptive immune systems (Ben-Shaanan et al., 2016) and is synthesized by specific gut microbes (Dinan et al., 2013). Gamma-aminobutyric acid (GABA) can be synthesized by bacteria belonging to the genera of *Lactobacillus* and *Bifidobacterium* (Barrett et al., 2012). GABA has anticancer roles, reducing colon cancer cell migration (Joseph et al., 2002) (Figure 9.3). GABA signaling is observed in both the sympathetic nervous system (SNS), and the parasympathetic nervous system (PNS). Acetylcholine induces cell growth and division (Knox et al., 2013), with multiple cancers showing increased expression levels of acetylcholine receptors such as acetylcholine receptor 3 (M3R3) in gastric cancer (Hayakawa et al., 2017) and the acetylcholine receptor M (Chrm1) muscarinic receptors on stromal cells in prostate cancer (Dobrenis et al., 2015). Bacteria of the subspecies *Lactobacillus* are capable of producing acetylcholine (Dinan et al., 2013) (Figure 9.3).

NEUROGENESIS REGULATION BY MICROBIOTA

The process of neurogenesis, which involves the creation of new nervous tissue, plays a critical role in various cancers. These cancers rely on nerve tissue for essential signals and can utilize nerves as pathways for migration and cell movement. Tumor cells release specific compounds to initiate the neurogenesis process (Entschladen et al., 2006). Once they are established, these newly formed nerve fibers release chemical messengers in the form of neurotransmitters that are capable of stimulating cancer cell growth and migration (Magnon et al., 2013). Perineural invasion (PNI) is the process where cancer cells grow around new nerves (Amit et al., 2016). Neurogenesis can be stimulated through signals that originate from the microbiome. These signaling pathways are initiated through the Toll-like receptor 2 (TLR2) signaling pathway. Using animal models, it has been observed that the supplementation of the animal model's diet with various mixtures of specific bacteria can alter the process of neurogenesis. Some bacteria populations delay or inhibit the process while others initiate it (Ait-Belgnaoui et al., 2014; Ogbonnaya et al., 2015).

Neuronal proliferation, neurogenesis, and BDNF signaling are all known to be regulated through the action of miRNAs. The transcription of these miRNAs is influenced by the microbiome. Altered levels of these miRNAs as well as the mRNAs they regulate were observed in germ-free or antibiotic treated mice (Fung et al., 2017). In another example of the role played by the GBA, gut microbe dysbiosis affected miRNA transcription in the amygdala and prefrontal cortex (Hoban et al., 2017). BDNF expression is regulated at the mRNA level through the action of miR-206-3p, a miRNA whose transcription is controlled by gut microbiota (Hoban et al., 2017; Lee et al., 2012). BDNF stimulates neuron growth both in normal brain development but also in cancer-related neurogenesis, where it is important for cancer invasion, metastasis, and cancer development and growth (reviewed in Dlamini et al., 2021).

TREATMENTS FOR CANCERS BASED ON THE MICROBIOME NEURAL INTERACTIONS

Returning the gut microbiome to a healthy balanced state involves addressing dysbiosis. Restoring a diverse and healthy gut microbiome has emerged as a potential solution for mitigating the cancer-promoting effects of an altered gut–brain axis. This can be achieved through various interventions such as dietary modifications, intake of prebiotics, utilization of postbiotics, and even fecal transplantation from individuals with a well-balanced gut (Gibson et al., 2017). While probiotics have long been marketed as general health supplements recommended after antibiotic treatment, recent research on the specific impact of different bacterial species on neurogenesis associated with cancer suggests that targeted inoculation with specific commensal microorganisms is becoming a promising approach in cancer therapy (Bashiardes et al., 2017; Routy et al., 2018). For instance, studies have examined the potential use of *Bifidobacterium longum* to inhibit the growth of colon cancer, where it was found to be effective in slowing the progression of the cancer. These studies have also indicated that supplements containing this bacterium can reduce the incidence rate of colon cancer. Moreover, these bacteria produce metabolites which prevent cell proliferation caused by azoxymethane, a genotoxic carcinogen. These metabolites are also capable of suppressing certain groups of oncoproteins (Singh et al., 1997). In mouse models with melanoma, supplementing their diet with bacteria from the genus *Bifidobacterium* was found to enhance immunotherapy treatment involving PD-L1 blockade (Sivan et al., 2015). Post-chemotherapy abdominal pain is a common side-effect of chemotherapy and occurs as a result of microbial toxicity. The resulting dysbiosis alters the effect of the gut microbiota on nerves capable of sensing pain. This pain can be treated using probiotics (Osterlund et al., 2007). Chemotherapy-induced cognitive impairment (CICI) is another complication of chemotherapy related to the GBA. The symptoms of this condition include decreased memory, attention, and concentration. It is caused by chemotherapy induced dysbiosis leading to BBB damage and neuroinflammation negatively affecting the CNS. This condition can also be treated using probiotic supplementation (Subramaniam et al., 2020).

Most treatment strategies using microbial supplementation would be used in conjunction with other treatment options. This, however, presents a problem as many treatment options used to treat cancer and secondary infections, such as chemotherapy, radiotherapy, and antibiotics, have toxic effects on the microbiome. These treatments affect those microbes already present as well as the therapeutic ones introduced. This was demonstrated in treating mice with tumors with the immunostimulatory cyclophosphamide. The effectiveness of the drug was decreased when the mice were also given antibiotics, due to a decrease in Th1 and Th17 cells following antibiotic treatment (Viaud et al., 2013).

Apart from targeting and correcting dysbiosis for therapeutic purposes, the cancer specific changes in the microbiome populations can also be used as a biomarker for diagnosis and prognosis (Wirbel et al., 2019; Nejman et al., 2020). The transcriptome or proteome of isolated gut microflora samples are one such way of determining the population composition of the gut microbiome (Poore et al., 2020). There are also limitations to the use of microbiomes as diagnostic or prognostic tools. Chief among these is the fact that signatures (transcriptomic or proteomic) may be clouded by those of the host. Another problem is the threat of contamination by the environment and other microbes not isolated from the patient. The gut brain axis is now also known to be involved in stress- and mood-related conditions (Foster et al., 2017). It has been observed that mice with a healthy gut microbiome perform well in stress and anxiety tests with fewer negative effects and outcomes. However, these positive results are not observed in every animal trial, and this points to a lack of knowledge about the interactions along the gut–brain axis (Romijn and Rucklidge, 2015).

The complex nature of the gut–brain axis means that different research approaches from those currently used are required. This is also reflected in the personal nature of the gut microbiome, with a healthy gut microbiome being specific to individuals or populations (Ngandu et al., 2015; Dardiotis et al., 2014). There is still a very limited understanding of how the gut microbiome may change over time and what influence this may have on the development of cancer. A large-scale study involving over 9000 adults of different ages, showed that the makeup of the gut microbiome changes, becoming more specific to an individual based on their lifestyle, previous infections, and life experiences (Wilmanski et al., 2021). There is also currently a limited understanding of the immunological effects of different bacteria and microbes and how these effects alter signaling along the gut–brain axis. The widespread use of animal models in the research surrounding the gut–brain axis, means that not all aspects can be tested and it is often difficult to meaningfully interpret the results in a human context (Nithianantharajah et al., 2017).

Human studies also need to be performed with more participants and over a greater length of time (Marx et al., 2020). It is also not known if any interventions can be effective

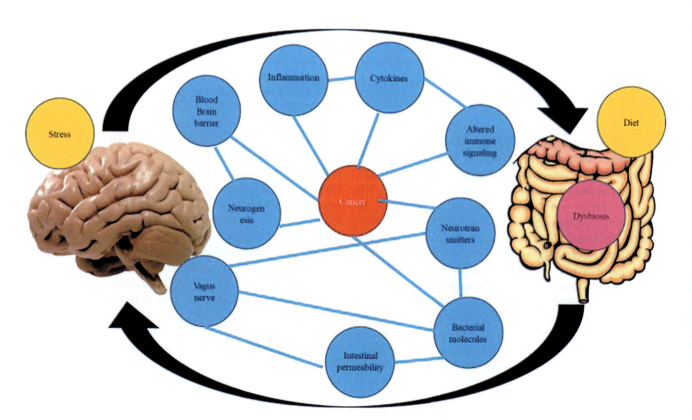

FIGURE 9.4 A summary of the factors involved in the gut–brain axis promoting cancer development. The complex interplay of the various factors involved in the gut brain axis means that any therapeutic solution will have to take the needs of the individual into account.

if an individual's diet, stress levels (both psychological and physical), and levels of physical activity are not considered. As such all of these aspects must be part of a treatment centered around the alteration of the gut microbiome (Tun et al., 2017). Another limitation is the timing of interventions, as any attempt to alter the microbiome is going to be affected by the patient's exposure to environmental factors. These can be varied and include exposure to other people and animals. This has been demonstrated in studies involving the development of the gut microbiome in infants, where even the dietary intake of the mother can affect the microbiome of a breastfeeding infant (Laforest-Lapointe et al., 2021).

CONCLUSIONS

The ability of the gut microbiome to influence the nervous system through the secretion of neurotransmitters, the immune system, and metabolites is now known to initiate cancer development and assist in its progression. Due to the nature of the nervous and immune systems these effects can be observed throughout the body and can result in the stimulation (Dardiotis et al., 2014) or inhibition of nerve function and growth. This relationship is currently being investigated for its therapeutic potential and as a basis for behavioral and cognitive functions that occur in diseases such as cancer. These strategies mainly involve altering the gut microbiota through the use of probiotics, fecal transplant or even through the use of antibiotics. All these efforts are aimed at restoring the gut microbiome to a more diverse population of microbes consisting of symbiotic and commensal bacteria while replacing or removing harmful pathogenic organisms. However, the targeting of the gut–brain axis for therapeutic reasons is limited by our current lack of knowledge and the complex interplay between various components of the gut–brain axis (Figure 9.4). An individual's microbiome depends on their life experiences and environment and a healthy microbiome will not be the same in every individual, with there being a great degree of variability amongst populations and even individuals. This means that there can be no single therapeutic solution targeting the microbiome. Rather the needs of each individual will need to be determined.

REFERENCES

AIT-BELGNAOUI, A., COLOM, A., BRANISTE, V., RAMALHO, L., MARROT, A., CARTIER, C., HOUDEAU, E., THEODOROU, V. & TOMPKINS, T. 2014. Probiotic gut effect prevents the chronic psychological stress-induced brain activity abnormality in mice. *Neurogastroenterol Motil*, 26, 510–20.

AKAZA, H. 2012. Prostate cancer chemoprevention by soy isoflavones: Role of intestinal bacteria as the "second human genome". *Cancer Sci*, 103, 969–75.

AMIT, M., NA'ARA, S. & GIL, Z. 2016. Mechanisms of cancer dissemination along nerves. *Nat Rev Cancer*, 16, 399–408.

ARUMUGAM, M., RAES, J., PELLETIER, E., LE PASLIER, D., YAMADA, T., MENDE, D. R., FERNANDES, G. R., TAP, J., BRULS, T., BATTO, J. M., BERTALAN, M., BORRUEL, N., CASELLAS, F., FERNANDEZ, L., GAUTIER, L., HANSEN, T., HATTORI, M., HAYASHI, T., KLEEREBEZEM, M., KUROKAWA, K., LECLERC, M., LEVENEZ, F., MANICHANH, C., NIELSEN, H. B., NIELSEN, T., PONS, N., POULAIN, J., QIN, J., SICHERITZ-PONTEN, T., TIMS, S., TORRENTS, D., UGARTE, E., ZOETENDAL, E. G., WANG, J., GUARNER, F., PEDERSEN, O., DE VOS, W. M., BRUNAK, S., DORÉ, J., ANTOLÍN, M., ARTIGUENAVE, F., BLOTTIERE, H. M., ALMEIDA, M., BRECHOT, C., CARA, C., CHERVAUX, C., CULTRONE, A., DELORME, C., DENARIAZ, G., DERVYN, R., FOERSTNER, K. U., FRISS, C., VAN DE GUCHTE, M., GUEDON, E., HAIMET, F., HUBER, W., VAN HYLCKAMA-VLIEG, J., JAMET, A., JUSTE, C., KACI, G., KNOL, J., LAKHDARI, O., LAYEC, S., LE ROUX, K., MAGUIN, E., MÉRIEUX, A., MELO MINARDI, R., M'RINI, C., MULLER, J., OOZEER, R., PARKHILL, J., RENAULT, P., RESCIGNO, M., SANCHEZ, N., SUNAGAWA, S., TORREJON, A., TURNER, K., VANDEMEULEBROUCK, G., VARELA, E., WINOGRADSKY, Y., ZELLER, G., WEISSENBACH, J., EHRLICH, S. D. & BORK, P. 2011. Enterotypes of the human gut microbiome. *Nature*, 473, 174–80.

ATAEE, R., AJDARY, S., REZAYAT, M., SHOKRGOZAR, M. A., SHAHRIARI, S. & ZARRINDAST, M. R. 2010. Study of 5HT3 and HT4 receptor expression in HT29 cell line and human colon adenocarcinoma tissues. *Arch Iran Med*, 13, 120–5.

ATARASHI, K., NISHIMURA, J., SHIMA, T., UMESAKI, Y., YAMAMOTO, M., ONOUE, M., YAGITA, H., ISHII, N., EVANS, R., HONDA, K. & TAKEDA, K. 2008. ATP drives lamina propria T(H)17 cell differentiation. *Nature*, 455, 808–12.

BÄCKHED, F., LEY, R. E., SONNENBURG, J. L., PETERSON, D. A. & GORDON, J. I. 2005. Host-bacterial mutualism in the human intestine. *Science*, 307, 1915–20.

BANKS, W. A. 2009. Characteristics of compounds that cross the blood-brain barrier. *BMC Neurol*, 9 (Suppl 1), S3.

BANKS, W. A. 2015. The blood-brain barrier in neuroimmunology: Tales of separation and assimilation. *Brain Behav Immun*, 44, 1–8.

BARRETT, E., ROSS, R. P., O'TOOLE, P. W., FITZGERALD, G. F. & STANTON, C. 2012. γ-Aminobutyric acid production by culturable bacteria from the human intestine. *J Appl Microbiol*, 113, 411–7.

BASHIARDES, S., TUGANBAEV, T., FEDERICI, S. & ELINAV, E. 2017. The microbiome in anti-cancer therapy. *Semin Immunol*, 32, 74–81.

BENE, K., VARGA, Z., PETROV, V. O., BOYKO, N. & RAJNAVOLGYI, E. 2017. Gut microbiota species can provoke both inflammatory and tolerogenic immune responses in human dendritic cells mediated by retinoic acid receptor alpha ligation. *Front Immunol*, 8, 427.

BEN-SHAANAN, T. L., AZULAY-DEBBY, H., DUBOVIK, T., STAROSVETSKY, E., KORIN, B., SCHILLER, M., GREEN, N. L., ADMON, Y., HAKIM, F., SHEN-ORR, S. S. & ROLLS, A. 2016. Activation of the reward system boosts innate and adaptive immunity. *Nat Med*, 22, 940–4.

BICKELS, J., KOLLENDER, Y., MERINSKY, O. & MELLER, I. 2002. Coley's toxin: Historical perspective. *Isr Med Assoc J*, 4, 471–2.

BLACHER, E., BASHIARDES, S., SHAPIRO, H., ROTHSCHILD, D., MOR, U., DORI-BACHASH, M., KLEIMEYER, C.,

MORESI, C., HARNIK, Y., ZUR, M., ZABARI, M., BRIK, R. B., KVIATCOVSKY, D., ZMORA, N., COHEN, Y., BAR, N., LEVI, I., AMAR, N., MEHLMAN, T., BRANDIS, A., BITON, I., KUPERMAN, Y., TSOORY, M., ALFAHEL, L., HARMELIN, A., SCHWARTZ, M., ISRAELSON, A., ARIKE, L., JOHANSSON, M. E. V., HANSSON, G. C., GOTKINE, M., SEGAL, E. & ELINAV, E. 2019. Potential roles of gut microbiome and metabolites in modulating ALS in mice. *Nature,* 572, 474–80.

BLECHARZ, K. G., COLLA, R., ROHDE, V. & VAJKOCZY, P. 2015. Control of the blood–brain barrier function in cancer cell metastasis. *Biol Cell,* 107, 342–71.

BOLEIJ, A. & TJALSMA, H. 2012. Gut bacteria in health and disease: A survey on the interface between intestinal microbiology and colorectal cancer. *Biol Rev Camb Philos Soc,* 87, 701–30.

BRAGANHOL, E., KUKULSKI, F., LÉVESQUE, S. A., FAUSTHER, M., LAVOIE, E. G., ZANOTTO-FILHO, A., BERGAMIN, L. S., PELLETIER, J., BAHRAMI, F., BEN YEBDRI, F., FONSECA MOREIRA, J. C., BATTASTINI, A. M. & SÉVIGNY, J. 2015. Nucleotide receptors control IL-8/CXCL8 and MCP-1/CCL2 secretions as well as proliferation in human glioma cells. *Biochim Biophys Acta,* 1852, 120–30.

BRANISTE, V., AL-ASMAKH, M., KOWAL, C., ANUAR, F., ABBASPOUR, A., TÓTH, M., KORECKA, A., BAKOCEVIC, N., NG, L. G., KUNDU, P., GULYÁS, B., HALLDIN, C., HULTENBY, K., NILSSON, H., HEBERT, H., VOLPE, B. T., DIAMOND, B. & PETTERSSON, S. 2014. The gut microbiota influences blood-brain barrier permeability in mice. *Sci Transl Med,* 6, 263ra158.

BROWNING, K. N., ZHENG, Z., GETTYS, T. W. & TRAVAGLI, R. A. 2006. Vagal afferent control of opioidergic effects in rat brainstem circuits. *J Physiol,* 575, 761–76.

BUDHWANI, M., MAZZIERI, R. & DOLCETTI, R. 2018. Plasticity of type i interferon-mediated responses in cancer therapy: From anti-tumor immunity to resistance. *Front Oncol,* 8, 322.

BUFFINGTON, S. A., DI PRISCO, G. V., AUCHTUNG, T. A., AJAMI, N. J., PETROSINO, J. F. & COSTA-MATTIOLI, M. 2016. Microbial reconstitution reverses maternal diet-induced social and synaptic deficits in offspring. *Cell,* 165, 1762–75.

BURBERRY, A., WELLS, M. F., LIMONE, F., COUTO, A., SMITH, K. S., KEANEY, J., GILLET, G., VAN GASTEL, N., WANG, J. Y., PIETILAINEN, O., QIAN, M., EGGAN, P., CANTRELL, C., MOK, J., KADIU, I., SCADDEN, D. T. & EGGAN, K. 2020. C9orf72 suppresses systemic and neural inflammation induced by gut bacteria. *Nature,* 582, 89–94.

CARABOTTI, M., SCIROCCO, A., MASELLI, M. A. & SEVERI, C. 2015. The gut-brain axis: Interactions between enteric microbiota, central and enteric nervous systems. *Ann Gastroenterol,* 28, 203–9.

CATTANEO, M. G., PALAZZI, E., BONDIOLOTTI, G. & VICENTINI, L. M. 1994. 5-HT1D receptor type is involved in stimulation of cell proliferation by serotonin in human small cell lung carcinoma. *Eur J Pharmacol,* 268, 425–30.

CHIN, A., SVEJDA, B., GUSTAFSSON, B. I., GRANLUND, A. B., SANDVIK, A. K., TIMBERLAKE, A., SUMPIO, B., PFRAGNER, R., MODLIN, I. M. & KIDD, M. 2012. The role of mechanical forces and adenosine in the regulation of intestinal enterochromaffin cell serotonin secretion. *Am J Physiol Gastrointest Liver Physiol,* 302, G397–405.

CHU, F. F., ESWORTHY, R. S., CHU, P. G., LONGMATE, J. A., HUYCKE, M. M., WILCZYNSKI, S. & DOROSHOW, J. H. 2004. Bacteria-induced intestinal cancer in mice with disrupted Gpx1 and Gpx2 genes. *Cancer Res,* 64, 962–8.

CLARKE, G., GRENHAM, S., SCULLY, P., FITZGERALD, P., MOLONEY, R. D., SHANAHAN, F., DINAN, T. G. & CRYAN, J. F. 2013. The microbiome-gut-brain axis during early life regulates the hippocampal serotonergic system in a sex-dependent manner. *Mol Psychiatry,* 18, 666–73.

COLEY, W. B. 1891. II. Contribution to the knowledge of sarcoma. *Ann Surg,* 14, 199–220.

COYTE, K. Z., SCHLUTER, J. & FOSTER, K. R. 2015. The ecology of the microbiome: Networks, competition, and stability. *Science,* 350, 663–6.

CRYAN, J. F. & DINAN, T. G. 2012. Mind-altering microorganisms: The impact of the gut microbiota on brain and behaviour. *Nat Rev Neurosci,* 13, 701–12.

CUI, J., CHEN, Y., WANG, H. Y. & WANG, R. F. 2014. Mechanisms and pathways of innate immune activation and regulation in health and cancer. *Hum Vaccin Immunother,* 10, 3270–85.

DANEMAN, R. & PRAT, A. 2015. The blood-brain barrier. *Cold Spring Harb Perspect Biol,* 7, a020412.

DARDIOTIS, E., KOSMIDIS, M. H., YANNAKOULIA, M., HADJIGEORGIOU, G. M. & SCARMEAS, N. 2014. The Hellenic Longitudinal Investigation of Aging and Diet (HELIAD): rationale, study design, and cohort description. *Neuroepidemiology,* 43, 9–14.

DE COUCK, M., CAERS, R., SPIEGEL, D. & GIDRON, Y. 2018. The role of the vagus nerve in cancer prognosis: A systematic and a comprehensive review. *J Oncol,* 2018, 1236787.

DIAZ HEIJTZ, R., WANG, S., ANUAR, F., QIAN, Y., BJÖRKHOLM, B., SAMUELSSON, A., HIBBERD, M. L., FORSSBERG, H. & PETTERSSON, S. 2011. Normal gut microbiota modulates brain development and behavior. *Proc Natl Acad Sci U S A,* 108, 3047–52.

DINAN, T. G., STANTON, C. & CRYAN, J. F. 2013. Psychobiotics: A novel class of psychotropic. *Biol Psychiatry,* 74, 720–6.

DISSING-OLESEN, L., HONG, S. & STEVENS, B. 2015. New brain lymphatic vessels drain old concepts. *EBioMedicine,* 2, 776–7.

DLAMINI, Z., MATHABE, K., PADAYACHY, L., MARIMA, R., EVANGELOU, G., SYRIGOS, K. N., BIANCHI, A., LOLAS, G. & HULL, R. 2021. Many voices in a choir: Tumor-induced neurogenesis and neuronal driven alternative splicing sound like suspects in tumor growth and dissemination. *Cancers (Basel),* 13, 2138.

DOBRENIS, K., GAUTHIER, L. R., BARROCA, V. & MAGNON, C. 2015. Granulocyte colony-stimulating factor off-target effect on nerve outgrowth promotes prostate cancer development. *Int J Cancer,* 136, 982–8.

DONOHOE, D. R., HOLLEY, D., COLLINS, L. B., MONTGOMERY, S. A., WHITMORE, A. C., HILLHOUSE, A., CURRY, K. P., RENNER, S. W., GREENWALT, A., RYAN, E. P., GODFREY, V., HEISE, M. T., THREADGILL, D. S., HAN, A., SWENBERG, J. A., THREADGILL, D. W. & BULTMAN, S. J. 2014. A gnotobiotic mouse model demonstrates that dietary fiber protects against colorectal tumorigenesis in a microbiota- and butyrate-dependent manner. *Cancer Discov,* 4, 1387–97.

DUVALLET, C., GIBBONS, S. M., GURRY, T., IRIZARRY, R. A. & ALM, E. J. 2017. Meta-analysis of gut microbiome studies identifies disease-specific and shared responses. *Nat Commun,* 8, 1784.

ELLWARDT, E., WALSH, J. T., KIPNIS, J. & ZIPP, F. 2016. Understanding the role of T cells in CNS homeostasis. *Trends Immunol,* 37, 154–65.

ENGELHARDT, B. & LIEBNER, S. 2014. Novel insights into the development and maintenance of the blood-brain barrier. *Cell Tissue Res,* 355, 687–99.

ENTSCHLADEN, F., PALM, D., LANG, K., DRELL, T. L. T. & ZAENKER, K. S. 2006. Neoneurogenesis: Tumors may initiate their own innervation by the release of neurotrophic factors in analogy to lymphangiogenesis and neoangiogenesis. *Med Hypotheses,* 67, 33–5.

ERICKSON, M. A., DOHI, K. & BANKS, W. A. 2012. Neuroinflammation: A common pathway in CNS diseases as mediated at the blood–brain barrier. *Neuroimmunomodulation,* 19, 121–30.

ERNY, D., HRABĚ DE ANGELIS, A. L., JAITIN, D., WIEGHOFER, P., STASZEWSKI, O., DAVID, E., KEREN-SHAUL, H., MAHLAKOIV, T., JAKOBSHAGEN, K., BUCH, T., SCHWIERZECK, V., UTERMÖHLEN, O., CHUN, E., GARRETT, W. S., MCCOY, K. D., DIEFENBACH, A., STAEHELI, P., STECHER, B., AMIT, I. & PRINZ, M. 2015. Host microbiota constantly control maturation and function of microglia in the CNS. *Nat Neurosci,* 18, 965–77.

FEARON, K., ARENDS, J. & BARACOS, V. 2013. Understanding the mechanisms and treatment options in cancer cachexia. *Nat Rev Clin Oncol,* 10, 90–9.

FORSYTHE, P., BIENENSTOCK, J. & KUNZE, W. A. 2014. Vagal pathways for microbiome-brain-gut axis communication. *Adv Exp Med Biol,* 817, 115–33.

FOSTER, J. A., RINAMAN, L. & CRYAN, J. F. 2017. Stress & the gut-brain axis: Regulation by the microbiome. *Neurobiol Stress,* 7, 124–36.

FUNG, T. C., OLSON, C. A. & HSIAO, E. Y. 2017. Interactions between the microbiota, immune and nervous systems in health and disease. *Nat Neurosci,* 20, 145–55.

GAREAU, M. G., WINE, E., RODRIGUES, D. M., CHO, J. H., WHARY, M. T., PHILPOTT, D. J., MACQUEEN, G. & SHERMAN, P. M. 2011. Bacterial infection causes stress-induced memory dysfunction in mice. *Gut,* 60, 307–17.

GIBSON, G. R., HUTKINS, R., SANDERS, M. E., PRESCOTT, S. L., REIMER, R. A., SALMINEN, S. J., SCOTT, K., STANTON, C., SWANSON, K. S., CANI, P. D., VERBEKE, K. & REID, G. 2017. Expert consensus document: The International Scientific Association for Probiotics and Prebiotics (ISAPP) consensus statement on the definition and scope of prebiotics. *Nat Rev Gastroenterol Hepatol,* 14, 491–502.

GIL-CRUZ, C., PEREZ-SHIBAYAMA, C., DE MARTIN, A., RONCHI, F., VAN DER BORGHT, K., NIEDERER, R., ONDER, L., LÜTGE, M., NOVKOVIC, M., NINDL, V., RAMOS, G., ARNOLDINI, M., SLACK, E. M. C., BOIVIN-JAHNS, V., JAHNS, R., WYSS, M., MOOSER, C., LAMBRECHT, B. N., MAEDER, M. T., RICKLI, H., FLATZ, L., ERIKSSON, U., GEUKING, M. B., MCCOY, K. D. & LUDEWIG, B. 2019. Microbiota-derived peptide mimics drive lethal inflammatory cardiomyopathy. *Science,* 366, 881–6.

GILES, E. M. & STAGG, A. J. 2017. Type 1 interferon in the human intestine-A co-ordinator of the immune response to the microbiota. *Inflamm Bowel Dis,* 23, 524–33.

GOTO, Y., PANEA, C., NAKATO, G., CEBULA, A., LEE, C., DIEZ, M. G., LAUFER, T. M., IGNATOWICZ, L. & IVANOV, II 2014. Segmented filamentous bacteria antigens presented by intestinal dendritic cells drive mucosal Th17 cell differentiation. *Immunity,* 40, 594–607.

GRIBBLE, F. M. & REIMANN, F. 2016. Enteroendocrine cells: Chemosensors in the intestinal epithelium. *Annu Rev Physiol,* 78, 277–99.

GRIVENNIKOV, S. I., WANG, K., MUCIDA, D., STEWART, C. A., SCHNABL, B., JAUCH, D., TANIGUCHI, K., YU, G.-Y., ÖSTERREICHER, C. H. & HUNG, K. E. J. N. 2012. Adenoma-linked barrier defects and microbial products drive IL-23/IL-17-mediated tumour growth. *Nature,* 491, 254–8.

GUR, C., IBRAHIM, Y., ISAACSON, B., YAMIN, R., ABED, J., GAMLIEL, M., ENK, J., BAR-ON, Y., STANIETSKY-KAYNAN, N., COPPENHAGEN-GLAZER, S., SHUSSMAN, N., ALMOGY, G., CUAPIO, A., HOFER, E., MEVORACH, D., TABIB, A., ORTENBERG, R., MARKEL, G., MIKLIĆ, K., JONJIC, S., BRENNAN, C. A., GARRETT, W. S., BACHRACH, G. & MANDELBOIM, O. 2015. Binding of the Fap2 protein of Fusobacterium nucleatum to human inhibitory receptor TIGIT protects tumors from immune cell attack. *Immunity,* 42, 344–55.

HAYAKAWA, Y., SAKITANI, K., KONISHI, M., ASFAHA, S., NIIKURA, R., TOMITA, H., RENZ, B. W., TAILOR, Y., MACCHINI, M., MIDDELHOFF, M., JIANG, Z., TANAKA, T., DUBEYKOVSKAYA, Z. A., KIM, W., CHEN, X., URBANSKA, A. M., NAGAR, K., WESTPHALEN, C. B., QUANTE, M., LIN, C. S., GERSHON, M. D., HARA, A., ZHAO, C. M., CHEN, D., WORTHLEY, D. L., KOIKE, K. & WANG, T. C. 2017. Nerve growth factor promotes gastric tumorigenesis through aberrant cholinergic signaling. *Cancer Cell,* 31, 21–34.

HEYM, N., HEASMAN, B. C., HUNTER, K., BLANCO, S. R., WANG, G. Y., SIEGERT, R., CLEARE, A., GIBSON, G. R., KUMARI, V. & SUMICH, A. L. 2019. The role of microbiota and inflammation in self-judgement and empathy: implications for understanding the brain-gut-microbiome axis in depression. *Psychopharmacology (Berl),* 236, 1459–70.

HOBAN, A. E., STILLING, R. M., G, M. M., MOLONEY, R. D., SHANAHAN, F., DINAN, T. G., CRYAN, J. F. & CLARKE, G. 2017. Microbial regulation of microRNA expression in the amygdala and prefrontal cortex. *Microbiome,* 5, 102.

HUTCHINGS, C., PHILLIPS, J. A. & DJAMGOZ, M. B. A. 2020. Nerve input to tumours: Pathophysiological consequences of a dynamic relationship. *Biochim Biophys Acta Rev Cancer,* 1874, 188411.

INSERRA, A., ROGERS, G. B., LICINIO, J. & WONG, M. L. 2018. The microbiota-inflammasome hypothesis of major depression. *Bioessays,* 40, e1800027.

JANG, H. M., LEE, H. J., JANG, S. E., HAN, M. J. & KIM, D. H. 2018. Evidence for interplay among antibacterial-induced gut microbiota disturbance, neuro-inflammation, and anxiety in mice. *Mucosal Immunol,* 11, 1386–97.

JIANG, S. H., ZHU, L. L., ZHANG, M., LI, R. K., YANG, Q., YAN, J. Y., ZHANG, C., YANG, J. Y., DONG, F. Y., DAI, M., HU, L. P., LI, J., LI, Q., WANG, Y. H., YANG, X. M., ZHANG, Y. L., NIE, H. Z., ZHU, L., ZHANG, X. L., TIAN, G. A., ZHANG, X. X., CAO, X. Y., TAO, L. Y., HUANG, S., JIANG, Y. S., HUA, R., QIAN LUO, K., GU, J. R., SUN, Y. W., HOU, S. &

ZHANG, Z. G. 2019. GABRP regulates chemokine signalling, macrophage recruitment and tumour progression in pancreatic cancer through tuning KCNN4-mediated Ca(2+) signalling in a GABA-independent manner. *Gut*, 68, 1994–2006.

JONES, C. B., DAVIS, C. M. & SFANOS, K. S. 2020. The potential effects of radiation on the gut-brain axis. *Radiat Res*, 193, 209–222.

JOSEPH, J., NIGGEMANN, B., ZAENKER, K. S. & ENTSCHLADEN, F. 2002. The neurotransmitter gamma-aminobutyric acid is an inhibitory regulator for the migration of SW 480 colon carcinoma cells. *Cancer Res*, 62, 6467–9.

KAMADA, N., SEO, S. U., CHEN, G. Y. & NÚÑEZ, G. 2013. Role of the gut microbiota in immunity and inflammatory disease. *Nat Rev Immunol*, 13, 321–35.

KAUFMANN, F. N., COSTA, A. P., GHISLENI, G., DIAZ, A. P., RODRIGUES, A. L. S., PELUFFO, H. & KASTER, M. P. 2017. NLRP3 inflammasome-driven pathways in depression: Clinical and preclinical findings. *Brain Behav Immun*, 64, 367–83.

KIM, C. H., PARK, J. & KIM, M. 2014. Gut microbiota-derived short-chain fatty acids, T cells, and inflammation. *Immune Netw*, 14, 277–88.

KNOX, S. M., LOMBAERT, I. M., HADDOX, C. L., ABRAMS, S. R., COTRIM, A., WILSON, A. J. & HOFFMAN, M. P. 2013. Parasympathetic stimulation improves epithelial organ regeneration. *Nat Commun*, 4, 1494.

KOSTIC, A. D., CHUN, E., ROBERTSON, L., GLICKMAN, J. N., GALLINI, C. A., MICHAUD, M., CLANCY, T. E., CHUNG, D. C., LOCHHEAD, P., HOLD, G. L., EL-OMAR, E. M., BRENNER, D., FUCHS, C. S., MEYERSON, M. & GARRETT, W. S. 2013. Fusobacterium nucleatum potentiates intestinal tumorigenesis and modulates the tumor-immune microenvironment. *Cell Host Microbe*, 14, 207–15.

KUMAR, A., GODWIN, J. W., GATES, P. B., GARZA-GARCIA, A. A. & BROCKES, J. P. 2007. Molecular basis for the nerve dependence of limb regeneration in an adult vertebrate. *Science*, 318, 772–7.

KUWAHARA, A., MATSUDA, K., KUWAHARA, Y., ASANO, S., INUI, T. & MARUNAKA, Y. 2020. Microbiota-gut-brain axis: enteroendocrine cells and the enteric nervous system form an interface between the microbiota and the central nervous system. *Biomed Res*, 41, 199–216.

KWON, Y. H., WANG, H., DENOU, E., GHIA, J. E., ROSSI, L., FONTES, M. E., BERNIER, S. P., SHAJIB, M. S., BANSKOTA, S., COLLINS, S. M., SURETTE, M. G. & KHAN, W. I. 2019. Modulation of gut microbiota composition by serotonin signaling influences intestinal immune response and susceptibility to colitis. *Cell Mol Gastroenterol Hepatol*, 7, 709–28.

LAFOREST-LAPOINTE, I., BECKER, A. B., MANDHANE, P. J., TURVEY, S. E., MORAES, T. J., SEARS, M. R., SUBBARAO, P., SYCURO, L. K., AZAD, M. B. & ARRIETA, M. C. 2021. Maternal consumption of artificially sweetened beverages during pregnancy is associated with infant gut microbiota and metabolic modifications and increased infant body mass index. *Gut Microbes*, 13, 1–15.

LEE, S. E., LI, X., KIM, J. C., LEE, J., GONZÁLEZ-NAVAJAS, J. M., HONG, S. H., PARK, I. K., RHEE, J. H. & RAZ, E. 2012. Type I interferons maintain Foxp3 expression and T-regulatory cell functions under inflammatory conditions in mice. *Gastroenterology*, 143, 145–54.

LIU, N., SUN, S., WANG, P., SUN, Y., HU, Q. & WANG, X. 2021. The mechanism of secretion and metabolism of gut-derived 5-hydroxytryptamine. *Int J Mol Sci*, 22, 7931.

LLOYD-PRICE, J., ABU-ALI, G. & HUTTENHOWER, C. 2016. The healthy human microbiome. *Genome Med*, 8, 51.

MA, Q., XING, C., LONG, W., WANG, H. Y., LIU, Q. & WANG, R. F. 2019. Impact of microbiota on central nervous system and neurological diseases: the gut-brain axis. *J Neuroinflammation*, 16, 53.

MAGNON, C., HALL, S. J., LIN, J., XUE, X., GERBER, L., FREEDLAND, S. J. & FRENETTE, P. S. 2013. Autonomic nerve development contributes to prostate cancer progression. *Science*, 341, 1236361.

MANGANI, D., WELLER, M. & ROTH, P. 2017. The network of immunosuppressive pathways in glioblastoma. *Biochem Pharmacol*, 130, 1–9.

MARX, W., SCHOLEY, A., FIRTH, J., D'CUNHA, N. M., LANE, M., HOCKEY, M., ASHTON, M. M., CRYAN, J. F., O'NEIL, A., NAUMOVSKI, N., BERK, M., DEAN, O. M. & JACKA, F. 2020. Prebiotics, probiotics, fermented foods and cognitive outcomes: A meta-analysis of randomized controlled trials. *Neurosci Biobehav Rev*, 118, 472–84.

MASANTA, W. O., HEIMESAAT, M. M., BERESWILL, S., TAREEN, A. M., LUGERT, R., GROß, U. & ZAUTNER, A. E. 2013. Modification of intestinal microbiota and its consequences for innate immune response in the pathogenesis of campylobacteriosis. *Clin Dev Immunol*, 2013, 526860.

MATCOVITCH-NATAN, O., WINTER, D. R., GILADI, A., VARGAS AGUILAR, S., SPINRAD, A., SARRAZIN, S., BEN-YEHUDA, H., DAVID, E., ZELADA GONZÁLEZ, F., PERRIN, P., KEREN-SHAUL, H., GURY, M., LARA-ASTAISO, D., THAISS, C. A., COHEN, M., BAHAR HALPERN, K., BARUCH, K., DECZKOWSKA, A., LORENZO-VIVAS, E., ITZKOVITZ, S., ELINAV, E., SIEWEKE, M. H., SCHWARTZ, M. & AMIT, I. 2016. Microglia development follows a stepwise program to regulate brain homeostasis. *Science*, 353, aad8670.

MCFARLAND, B. C., HONG, S. W., RAJBHANDARI, R., TWITTY, G. B., JR., GRAY, G. K., YU, H., BENVENISTE, E. N. & NOZELL, S. E. 2013. NF-κB-induced IL-6 ensures STAT3 activation and tumor aggressiveness in glioblastoma. *PLoS One*, 8, e78728.

MEISEL, M., HINTERLEITNER, R., PACIS, A., CHEN, L., EARLEY, Z. M., MAYASSI, T., PIERRE, J. F., ERNEST, J. D., GALIPEAU, H. J., THUILLE, N., BOUZIAT, R., BUSCARLET, M., RINGUS, D. L., WANG, Y., LI, Y., DINH, V., KIM, S. M., MCDONALD, B. D., ZURENSKI, M. A., MUSCH, M. W., FURTADO, G. C., LIRA, S. A., BAIER, G., CHANG, E. B., EREN, A. M., WEBER, C. R., BUSQUE, L., GODLEY, L. A., VERDÚ, E. F., BARREIRO, L. B. & JABRI, B. 2018. Microbial signals drive pre-leukaemic myeloproliferation in a Tet2-deficient host. *Nature*, 557, 580–4.

MERCADO, N. M., ZHANG, G., YING, Z. & GÓMEZ-PINILLA, F. 2022. Traumatic brain injury alters the gut-derived serotonergic system and associated peripheral organs. *Biochim Biophys Acta Mol Basis Dis*, 1868, 166491.

MERZAK, A., KOOCHEKPOUR, S., FILLION, M. P., FILLION, G. & PILKINGTON, G. J. 1996. Expression of serotonin receptors in human fetal astrocytes and glioma cell lines: A possible role in glioma cell proliferation and migration. *Brain Res Mol Brain Res*, 41, 1–7.

METIDJI, A., RIEDER, S. A., GLASS, D. D., CREMER, I., PUNKOSDY, G. A. & SHEVACH, E. M. 2015. IFN-α/β receptor signaling promotes regulatory T cell development and function under stress conditions. *J Immunol,* 194, 4265–76.

NEJMAN, D., LIVYATAN, I., FUKS, G., GAVERT, N., ZWANG, Y., GELLER, L. T., ROTTER-MASKOWITZ, A., WEISER, R., MALLEL, G., GIGI, E., MELTSER, A., DOUGLAS, G. M., KAMER, I., GOPALAKRISHNAN, V., DADOSH, T., LEVIN-ZAIDMAN, S., AVNET, S., ATLAN, T., COOPER, Z. A., ARORA, R., COGDILL, A. P., KHAN, M. A. W., OLOGUN, G., BUSSI, Y., WEINBERGER, A., LOTAN-POMPAN, M., GOLANI, O., PERRY, G., ROKAH, M., BAHAR-SHANY, K., ROZEMAN, E. A., BLANK, C. U., RONAI, A., SHAOUL, R., AMIT, A., DORFMAN, T., KREMER, R., COHEN, Z. R., HARNOF, S., SIEGAL, T., YEHUDA-SHNAIDMAN, E., GAL-YAM, E. N., SHAPIRA, H., BALDINI, N., LANGILLE, M. G. I., BEN-NUN, A., KAUFMAN, B., NISSAN, A., GOLAN, T., DADIANI, M., LEVANON, K., BAR, J., YUST-KATZ, S., BARSHACK, I., PEEPER, D. S., RAZ, D. J., SEGAL, E., WARGO, J. A., SANDBANK, J., SHENTAL, N. & STRAUSSMAN, R. 2020. The human tumor microbiome is composed of tumor type-specific intracellular bacteria. *Science,* 368, 973–80.

NEUFELD, K. M., KANG, N., BIENENSTOCK, J. & FOSTER, J. A. 2011. Reduced anxiety-like behavior and central neurochemical change in germ-free mice. *Neurogastroenterol Motil,* 23, 255–64, e119.

NGANDU, T., LEHTISALO, J., SOLOMON, A., LEVÄLAHTI, E., AHTILUOTO, S., ANTIKAINEN, R., BÄCKMAN, L., HÄNNINEN, T., JULA, A., LAATIKAINEN, T., LINDSTRÖM, J., MANGIALASCHE, F., PAAJANEN, T., PAJALA, S., PELTONEN, M., RAURAMAA, R., STIGSDOTTER-NEELY, A., STRANDBERG, T., TUOMILEHTO, J., SOININEN, H. & KIVIPELTO, M. 2015. A 2 year multidomain intervention of diet, exercise, cognitive training, and vascular risk monitoring versus control to prevent cognitive decline in at-risk elderly people (FINGER): A randomised controlled trial. *Lancet,* 385, 2255–63.

NISHIKAWA, T., TSUNO, N. H., SHUNO, Y., SASAKI, K., HONGO, K., OKAJI, Y., SUNAMI, E., KITAYAMA, J., TAKAHASHI, K. & NAGAWA, H. 2010. Antiangiogenic effect of a selective 5-HT4 receptor agonist. *J Surg Res,* 159, 696–704.

NITHIANANTHARAJAH, J., BALASURIYA, G. K., FRANKS, A. E. & HILL-YARDIN, E. L. 2017. Using animal models to study the role of the gut-brain axis in autism. *Curr Dev Disord Rep,* 4, 28–36.

O'KEEFE, S. J. 2016. Diet, microorganisms and their metabolites, and colon cancer. *Nat Rev Gastroenterol Hepatol,* 13, 691–706.

O'MAHONY, S. M., FELICE, V. D., NALLY, K., SAVIGNAC, H. M., CLAESSON, M. J., SCULLY, P., WOZNICKI, J., HYLAND, N. P., SHANAHAN, F., QUIGLEY, E. M., MARCHESI, J. R., O'TOOLE, P. W., DINAN, T. G. & CRYAN, J. F. 2014. Disturbance of the gut microbiota in early-life selectively affects visceral pain in adulthood without impacting cognitive or anxiety-related behaviors in male rats. *Neuroscience,* 277, 885–901.

OGBONNAYA, E. S., CLARKE, G., SHANAHAN, F., DINAN, T. G., CRYAN, J. F. & O'LEARY, O. F. 2015. Adult hippocampal neurogenesis is regulated by the microbiome. *Biol Psychiatry,* 78, e7–9.

OSTERLUND, P., RUOTSALAINEN, T., KORPELA, R., SAXELIN, M., OLLUS, A., VALTA, P., KOURI, M., ELOMAA, I. & JOENSUU, H. 2007. Lactobacillus supplementation for diarrhoea related to chemotherapy of colorectal cancer: A randomised study. *Br J Cancer,* 97, 1028–34.

OUFKIR, T., ARSENEAULT, M., SANDERSON, J. T. & VAILLANCOURT, C. 2010. The 5-HT 2A serotonin receptor enhances cell viability, affects cell cycle progression and activates MEK-ERK1/2 and JAK2-STAT3 signalling pathways in human choriocarcinoma cell lines. *Placenta,* 31, 439–47.

PAI, V. P., MARSHALL, A. M., HERNANDEZ, L. L., BUCKLEY, A. R. & HORSEMAN, N. D. 2009. Altered serotonin physiology in human breast cancers favors paradoxical growth and cell survival. *Breast Cancer Res,* 11, R81.

PALAZZO, M., BALSARI, A., ROSSINI, A., SELLERI, S., CALCATERRA, C., GARIBOLDI, S., ZANOBBIO, L., ARNABOLDI, F., SHIRAI, Y. F., SERRAO, G. & RUMIO, C. 2007. Activation of enteroendocrine cells via TLRs induces hormone, chemokine, and defensin secretion. *J Immunol,* 178, 4296–303.

PINTO-SANCHEZ, M. I., HALL, G. B., GHAJAR, K., NARDELLI, A., BOLINO, C., LAU, J. T., MARTIN, F. P., COMINETTI, O., WELSH, C., RIEDER, A., TRAYNOR, J., GREGORY, C., DE PALMA, G., PIGRAU, M., FORD, A. C., MACRI, J., BERGER, B., BERGONZELLI, G., SURETTE, M. G., COLLINS, S. M., MOAYYEDI, P. & BERCIK, P. 2017. Probiotic Bifidobacterium longum NCC3001 reduces depression scores and alters brain activity: A pilot study in patients with irritable bowel syndrome. *Gastroenterology,* 153, 448–459.e8.

POORE, G. D., KOPYLOVA, E., ZHU, Q., CARPENTER, C., FRARACCIO, S., WANDRO, S., KOSCIOLEK, T., JANSSEN, S., METCALF, J., SONG, S. J., KANBAR, J., MILLER-MONTGOMERY, S., HEATON, R., MCKAY, R., PATEL, S. P., SWAFFORD, A. D. & KNIGHT, R. 2020. Microbiome analyses of blood and tissues suggest cancer diagnostic approach. *Nature,* 579, 567–74.

PRESCOTT, S. L. & LIBERLES, S. D. 2022. Internal senses of the vagus nerve. *Neuron,* 110, 579–99.

RHEE, K. J., WU, S., WU, X., HUSO, D. L., KARIM, B., FRANCO, A. A., RABIZADEH, S., GOLUB, J. E., MATHEWS, L. E., SHIN, J., SARTOR, R. B., GOLENBOCK, D., HAMAD, A. R., GAN, C. M., HOUSSEAU, F. & SEARS, C. L. 2009. Induction of persistent colitis by a human commensal, enterotoxigenic Bacteroides fragilis, in wild-type C57BL/6 mice. *Infect Immun,* 77, 1708–18.

RIQUELME, E., ZHANG, Y., ZHANG, L., MONTIEL, M., ZOLTAN, M., DONG, W., QUESADA, P., SAHIN, I., CHANDRA, V., SAN LUCAS, A., SCHEET, P., XU, H., HANASH, S. M., FENG, L., BURKS, J. K., DO, K. A., PETERSON, C. B., NEJMAN, D., TZENG, C. D., KIM, M. P., SEARS, C. L., AJAMI, N., PETROSINO, J., WOOD, L. D., MAITRA, A., STRAUSSMAN, R., KATZ, M., WHITE, J. R., JENQ, R., WARGO, J. & MCALLISTER, F. 2019. Tumor microbiome diversity and composition influence pancreatic cancer outcomes. *Cell,* 178, 795–806.e12.

ROMIJN, A. R. & RUCKLIDGE, J. J. 2015. Systematic review of evidence to support the theory of psychobiotics. *Nutr Rev,* 73, 675–93.

ROUTY, B., GOPALAKRISHNAN, V., DAILLÈRE, R., ZITVOGEL, L., WARGO, J. A. & KROEMER, G. 2018. The gut microbiota influences anticancer immunosurveillance and general health. *Nat Rev Clin Oncol,* 15, 382–96.

SAKITA, J. Y., BADER, M., SANTOS, E. S., GARCIA, S. B., MINTO, S. B., ALENINA, N., BRUNALDI, M. O., CARVALHO, M. C., VIDOTTO, T., GASPAROTTO, B., MARTINS, R. B., SILVA, W. A., JR., BRANDÃO, M. L., LEITE, C. A., CUNHA, F. Q., KARSENTY, G., SQUIRE, J. A., UYEMURA, S. A. & KANNEN, V. 2019. Serotonin synthesis protects the mouse colonic crypt from DNA damage and colorectal tumorigenesis. *J Pathol,* 249, 102–13.

SAVIGNAC, H. M., KIELY, B., DINAN, T. G. & CRYAN, J. F. 2014. Bifidobacteria exert strain-specific effects on stress-related behavior and physiology in BALB/c mice. *Neurogastroenterol Motil,* 26, 1615–27.

SEPICH-POORE, G. D., ZITVOGEL, L., STRAUSSMAN, R., HASTY, J., WARGO, J. A. & KNIGHT, R. 2021. The microbiome and human cancer. *Science,* 371, eabc4552.

SHARON, G., GARG, N., DEBELIUS, J., KNIGHT, R., DORRESTEIN, P. C. & MAZMANIAN, S. K. 2014. Specialized metabolites from the microbiome in health and disease. *Cell Metab,* 20, 719–30.

SHERMAN, M. P., ZAGHOUANI, H. & NIKLAS, V. 2015. Gut microbiota, the immune system, and diet influence the neonatal gut-brain axis. *Pediatr Res,* 77, 127–35.

SIDDIQUI, E. J., SHABBIR, M., MIKHAILIDIS, D. P., THOMPSON, C. S. & MUMTAZ, F. H. 2006. The role of serotonin (5-hydroxytryptamine1A and 1B) receptors in prostate cancer cell proliferation. *J Urol,* 176, 1648–53.

SINGH, J., RIVENSON, A., TOMITA, M., SHIMAMURA, S., ISHIBASHI, N. & REDDY, B. S. 1997. Bifidobacterium longum, a lactic acid-producing intestinal bacterium inhibits colon cancer and modulates the intermediate biomarkers of colon carcinogenesis. *Carcinogenesis,* 18, 833–41.

SINGH, N., GURAV, A., SIVAPRAKASAM, S., BRADY, E., PADIA, R., SHI, H., THANGARAJU, M., PRASAD, P. D., MANICASSAMY, S., MUNN, D. H., LEE, J. R., OFFERMANNS, S. & GANAPATHY, V. 2014. Activation of Gpr109a, receptor for niacin and the commensal metabolite butyrate, suppresses colonic inflammation and carcinogenesis. *Immunity,* 40, 128–39.

SINGHAL, M., TURTURICE, B. A., MANZELLA, C. R., RANJAN, R., METWALLY, A. A., THEORELL, J., HUANG, Y., ALREFAI, W. A., DUDEJA, P. K., FINN, P. W., PERKINS, D. L. & GILL, R. K. 2019. Serotonin transporter deficiency is associated with dysbiosis and changes in metabolic function of the mouse intestinal microbiome. *Sci Rep,* 9, 2138.

SIVAN, A., CORRALES, L., HUBERT, N., WILLIAMS, J. B., AQUINO-MICHAELS, K., EARLEY, Z. M., BENYAMIN, F. W., LEI, Y. M., JABRI, B., ALEGRE, M. L., CHANG, E. B. & GAJEWSKI, T. F. 2015. Commensal Bifidobacterium promotes antitumor immunity and facilitates anti-PD-L1 efficacy. *Science,* 350, 1084–9.

SKONIECZNA-ŻYDECKA, K., MARLICZ, W., MISERA, A., KOULAOUZIDIS, A. & ŁONIEWSKI, I. 2018. Microbiome–The missing link in the gut-brain axis: Focus on its role in gastrointestinal and mental health. *J Clin Med,* 7, 52.

SOLL, C., JANG, J. H., RIENER, M. O., MORITZ, W., WILD, P. J., GRAF, R. & CLAVIEN, P. A. 2010. Serotonin promotes tumor growth in human hepatocellular cancer. *Hepatology,* 51, 1244–54.

SOMMER, F. & BÄCKHED, F. 2013. The gut microbiota--masters of host development and physiology. *Nat Rev Microbiol,* 11, 227–38.

SONIER, B., ARSENEAULT, M., LAVIGNE, C., OUELLETTE, R. J. & VAILLANCOURT, C. 2006. The 5-HT2A serotoninergic receptor is expressed in the MCF-7 human breast cancer cell line and reveals a mitogenic effect of serotonin. *Biochem Biophys Res Commun,* 343, 1053–9.

STARNES, C. O. 1992. Coley's toxins in perspective. *Nature,* 357, 11–2.

STILLING, R. M., VAN DE WOUW, M., CLARKE, G., STANTON, C., DINAN, T. G. & CRYAN, J. F. 2016. The neuropharmacology of butyrate: The bread and butter of the microbiota-gut-brain axis? *Neurochem Int,* 99, 110–132.

SUBRAMANIAM, C. B., BOWEN, J. M., GLADMAN, M. A., LUSTBERG, M. B., MAYO, S. J. & WARDILL, H. R. 2020. The microbiota-gut-brain axis: An emerging therapeutic target in chemotherapy-induced cognitive impairment. *Neurosci Biobehav Rev,* 116, 470–79.

SUDO, N., CHIDA, Y., AIBA, Y., SONODA, J., OYAMA, N., YU, X. N., KUBO, C. & KOGA, Y. 2004. Postnatal microbial colonization programs the hypothalamic-pituitary-adrenal system for stress response in mice. *J Physiol,* 558, 263–75.

SUN, M., WU, W., LIU, Z. & CONG, Y. 2017. Microbiota metabolite short chain fatty acids, GPCR, and inflammatory bowel diseases. *J Gastroenterol,* 52, 1–8.

TRAVAGLI, R. A. & ANSELMI, L. 2016. Vagal neurocircuitry and its influence on gastric motility. *Nat Rev Gastroenterol Hepatol,* 13, 389–401.

TUN, H. M., KONYA, T., TAKARO, T. K., BROOK, J. R., CHARI, R., FIELD, C. J., GUTTMAN, D. S., BECKER, A. B., MANDHANE, P. J., TURVEY, S. E., SUBBARAO, P., SEARS, M. R., SCOTT, J. A. & KOZYRSKYJ, A. L. 2017. Exposure to household furry pets influences the gut microbiota of infant at 3-4 months following various birth scenarios. *Microbiome,* 5, 40.

TUTTON, P. J. & STEEL, G. G. 1979. Influence of biogenic amines on the growth of xenografted human colorectal carcinomas. *Br J Cancer,* 40, 743–9.

UCHIMURA, Y., FUHRER, T., LI, H., LAWSON, M. A., ZIMMERMANN, M., YILMAZ, B., ZINDEL, J., RONCHI, F., SORRIBAS, M., HAPFELMEIER, S., GANAL-VONARBURG, S. C., GOMEZ DE AGÜERO, M., MCCOY, K. D., SAUER, U. & MACPHERSON, A. J. 2018. Antibodies set boundaries limiting microbial metabolite penetration and the resultant mammalian host response. *Immunity,* 49, 545–559.e5.

VÉTIZOU, M., PITT, J. M., DAILLÈRE, R., LEPAGE, P., WALDSCHMITT, N., FLAMENT, C., RUSAKIEWICZ, S., ROUTY, B., ROBERTI, M. P., DUONG, C. P., POIRIER-COLAME, V., ROUX, A., BECHAREF, S., FORMENTI, S., GOLDEN, E., CORDING, S., EBERL, G., SCHLITZER, A., GINHOUX, F., MANI, S., YAMAZAKI, T., JACQUELOT, N., ENOT, D. P., BÉRARD, M., NIGOU, J., OPOLON, P., EGGERMONT, A., WOERTHER, P. L., CHACHATY, E., CHAPUT, N., ROBERT, C., MATEUS, C., KROEMER, G., RAOULT, D., BONECA, I. G., CARBONNEL, F., CHAMAILLARD, M. & ZITVOGEL, L. 2015. Anticancer immunotherapy by CTLA-4 blockade relies on the gut microbiota. *Science,* 350, 1079–84.

VIAUD, S., SACCHERI, F., MIGNOT, G., YAMAZAKI, T., DAILLÈRE, R., HANNANI, D., ENOT, D. P., PFIRSCHKE, C., ENGBLOM, C., PITTET, M. J., SCHLITZER, A.,

GINHOUX, F., APETOH, L., CHACHATY, E., WOERTHER, P. L., EBERL, G., BÉRARD, M., ECOBICHON, C., CLERMONT, D., BIZET, C., GABORIAU-ROUTHIAU, V., CERF-BENSUSSAN, N., OPOLON, P., YESSAAD, N., VIVIER, E., RYFFEL, B., ELSON, C. O., DORÉ, J., KROEMER, G., LEPAGE, P., BONECA, I. G., GHIRINGHELLI, F. & ZITVOGEL, L. 2013. The intestinal microbiota modulates the anticancer immune effects of cyclophosphamide. *Science*, 342, 971–6.

WIKOFF, W. R., ANFORA, A. T., LIU, J., SCHULTZ, P. G., LESLEY, S. A., PETERS, E. C. & SIUZDAK, G. 2009. Metabolomics analysis reveals large effects of gut microflora on mammalian blood metabolites. *Proc Natl Acad Sci U S A*, 106, 3698–703.

WILMANSKI, T., DIENER, C., RAPPAPORT, N., PATWARDHAN, S., WIEDRICK, J., LAPIDUS, J., EARLS, J. C., ZIMMER, A., GLUSMAN, G., ROBINSON, M., YURKOVICH, J. T., KADO, D. M., CAULEY, J. A., ZMUDA, J., LANE, N. E., MAGIS, A. T., LOVEJOY, J. C., HOOD, L., GIBBONS, S. M., ORWOLL, E. S. & PRICE, N. D. 2021. Gut microbiome pattern reflects healthy ageing and predicts survival in humans. *Nat Metab*, 3, 274–86.

WIRBEL, J., PYL, P. T., KARTAL, E., ZYCH, K., KASHANI, A., MILANESE, A., FLECK, J. S., VOIGT, A. Y., PALLEJA, A., PONNUDURAI, R., SUNAGAWA, S., COELHO, L. P., SCHROTZ-KING, P., VOGTMANN, E., HABERMANN, N., NIMÉUS, E., THOMAS, A. M., MANGHI, P., GANDINI, S., SERRANO, D., MIZUTANI, S., SHIROMA, H., SHIBA, S., SHIBATA, T., YACHIDA, S., YAMADA, T., WALDRON, L., NACCARATI, A., SEGATA, N., SINHA, R., ULRICH, C. M., BRENNER, H., ARUMUGAM, M., BORK, P. & ZELLER, G. 2019. Meta-analysis of fecal metagenomes reveals global microbial signatures that are specific for colorectal cancer. *Nat Med*, 25, 679–89.

XAVIER, J. B., YOUNG, V. B., SKUFCA, J., GINTY, F., TESTERMAN, T., PEARSON, A. T., MACKLIN, P., MITCHELL, A., SHMULEVICH, I., XIE, L., CAPORASO, J. G., CRANDALL, K. A., SIMONE, N. L., GODOY-VITORINO, F., GRIFFIN, T. J., WHITESON, K. L., GUSTAFSON, H. H., SLADE, D. J., SCHMIDT, T. M., WALTHER-ANTONIO, M. R. S., KOREM, T., WEBB-ROBERTSON, B. M., STYCZYNSKI, M. P., JOHNSON, W. E., JOBIN, C., RIDLON, J. M., KOH, A. Y., YU, M., KELLY, L. & WARGO, J. A. 2020. The cancer microbiome: Distinguishing direct and indirect effects requires a systemic view. *Trends Cancer*, 6, 192–204.

YAGHOUBFAR, R., BEHROUZI, A., ASHRAFIAN, F., SHAHRYARI, A., MORADI, H. R., CHOOPANI, S., HADIFAR, S., VAZIRI, F., NOJOUMI, S. A., FATEH, A., KHATAMI, S. & SIADAT, S. D. 2020. Modulation of serotonin signaling/metabolism by Akkermansia muciniphila and its extracellular vesicles through the gut-brain axis in mice. *Sci Rep*, 10, 22119.

YANO, J. M., YU, K., DONALDSON, G. P., SHASTRI, G. G., ANN, P., MA, L., NAGLER, C. R., ISMAGILOV, R. F., MAZMANIAN, S. K. & HSIAO, E. Y. 2015. Indigenous bacteria from the gut microbiota regulate host serotonin biosynthesis. *Cell*, 161, 264–76.

YIN, J., VALIN, K. L., DIXON, M. L. & LEAVENWORTH, J. W. 2017. The role of microglia and macrophages in CNS homeostasis, autoimmunity, and cancer. *J Immunol Res*, 2017, 5150678.

ZAHALKA, A. H. & FRENETTE, P. S. 2020. Nerves in cancer. *Nat Rev Cancer*, 20, 143–57.

ZAMANI, A. & QU, Z. 2012. Serotonin activates angiogenic phosphorylation signaling in human endothelial cells. *FEBS Lett*, 586, 2360–5.

ZANOTTO-FILHO, A., GONÇALVES, R. M., KLAFKE, K., DE SOUZA, P. O., DILLENBURG, F. C., CARRO, L., GELAIN, D. P. & MOREIRA, J. C. 2017. Inflammatory landscape of human brain tumors reveals an NFκB dependent cytokine pathway associated with mesenchymal glioblastoma. *Cancer Lett*, 390, 176–187.

ZITVOGEL, L., GALLUZZI, L., KEPP, O., SMYTH, M. J. & KROEMER, G. 2015. Type I interferons in anticancer immunity. *Nat Rev Immunol*, 15, 405–14.

10 Gut Microbiome and Cancer-Related Inflammation

*Meshack Bida, Masibulele Nonxuba, Benny Mosoane,
Tsholofelo Kungoane, Victoria P. Belancio, and Zodwa Dlamini*

INTRODUCTION

The composition of the microorganisms within each organ system in the human body varies from individual to individual. These dynamics can be influenced by lifestyle choices, genetics, and dietary or medication intake (Francescone et al., 2014, Maynard et al., 2012, Lozupone et al., 2012). This complex ecology of the microbial community serves a critical role in human health that involves the digestion of food, production of essential high-energy metabolites, defending the host against virulent microorganisms, and maintaining immune homeostasis (Cho and Blaser, 2012, Artis, 2008). Along the gastrointestinal track (GIT), the microbiota is metabolically active and benefits the host by generating toxins that knock down virulent strains (of the same species), starving competitor organisms by metabolizing key nutrients, maintaining the integrity of the mucosal and epithelial layer, and activating the immune system (Artis, 2008, Gamage et al., 2006, Francescone et al., 2014).

Dysbiosis refers to the imbalance of the diverse microbial community. Specific pathogens may cause dysbiosis or take advantage of altered microbial ratios to cause diseases (Francescone et al., 2014). The imbalance of the ratio of certain phyla has been linked to certain GIT diseases, such that protumorigenic cytokines are upregulated, promoting carcinogenesis (Figure 10.1). Therefore, there is a need to fully understand the origins and mechanisms of dysbiosis. For instance, in cutaneous psoriasis, the ratio of Firmicutes versus Actinobacteria is increased (Yan et al., 2017) and the amount of *Fusobacteria* species in colon cancers and adenomas are enriched, often associated with chemoresistance and unfavorable prognosis (Abed et al., 2020).

Chronic infections are postulated to account for 10–20% of all cancers. Studies of molecular mechanisms underlying tumorigenesis have associated the increased risks of cancer development with persistent chronic inflammation, suggesting that their interaction is a well-orchestrated physiological process (Greten and Grivennikov, 2019). While some cancer types such as gastric cancer, hepatocellular carcinoma (HCC), and colorectal carcinoma (CRC) are preceded by hepatitis, and gastritis by *Helicobacter pylori*, respectively, the development of other cancer types is not preceded by chronic inflammation for initiation and progression (Grivennikov et al., 2010a). Instead, the growth of these tumors is said to elicit inflammation in response to anticancer treatment and associated tumor cell death (Greten and Grivennikov, 2019).

Although the concept of inflammation in promoting cancer development and progression is a well-acknowledged phenomenon, it appears that microbiota plays a modulatory role in inflammatory response even though a direct link between cancer and microbiota is not completely understood. Mouse model-based studies have previous demonstrated that uncontrolled helper-T cells (Th1) can exacerbate colitis in interleukin 10 (IL-10)-deficient mice in response to microbiota and can initiate cancer development (Kühn et al., 1993, Berg et al., 1996). Immunoregulatory cytokine, IL-10, is essential for the regulation of inflammation in the intestines of humans and mice (Gunasekera et al., 2020). The intestinal resident bacteria can generate inflated immune responses such as colitis, particularly if there is a break in key components of the immune tolerance. IL-10 knockout (KO) germ-free mice showed no colitis development and no abnormal activation of the immune system (Sellon et al., 1998). The same IL-10 KO mice readily develop invasive CRC when they are colonized by a pathogenic *NC101 Escherichia coli* strain, possibly due to increased DNA damage (Arthur et al., 2012).

Pro-inflammatory immune response can be induced by the alteration in the composition of gut microbiota by modulating mucosal toll-like receptors (TLR) responsiveness (Fang et al., 2022). Mice deficient in TLR-4 and myeloid differentiation primary response 88 (MyD88) show less susceptibility to developing colitis-associated cancers. Microbial sensing through TLR/MyD88 has been implicated in promoting CRC development (Le Noci et al., 2021, Wang et al., 2018). High levels of TLR-4 and MyD88 have been correlated with poor prognosis in human CRC (Wang et al., 2018).

The utility of antibiotics to ameliorate inflammation and limit cancer progression has consolidated the role of microbiota in cancer. When subjected to microbiota-depleting antibiotics, Nod1 KO mice that are susceptible to suffering colitis-associated tumors, showed a reduction in tumor burden (Chen et al., 2008). Antibiotic eradication of *Helicobacter pylori* in the setting of gastric mucosa-associated lymphoid tissue (MALT) lymphoma has shown improved outcomes and

Gut Microbiome and Cancer-Related Inflammation

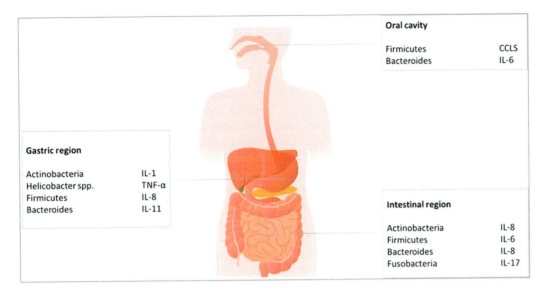

FIGURE 10.1 **The distribution of microbiota in the body and its influence on disease.** The left side shows normal bacteria in the various body organs and the strains increased in dysbiosis are in bold. The right side shows cytokines and chemokines that are upregulated with inflammation and cancer.

may cure some patients (these include *Helicobacter pylori* negative patients) (Gong et al., 2016, Chen et al., 2005).

This chapter focuses on the cross-link mechanistic channels that associate gut bacteria, chronic inflammation, and tumorigenesis and metastasis. Furthermore, the interaction between gut microbes, immune cells, and inflammatory meditators will be discussed. Lastly, the potential strategies for modulating inflammation-associated cancer risks will be explored.

INFLAMMATION AND CANCER

Based on the observation that leukocytes are frequently present in cancerous biopsy tissues, Rudolf Virchow suggested an existing relationship between inflammation and cancer in 1963 (Balkwill and Mantovani, 2001). Years later, epidemiologic studies demonstrated that chronic inflammation was accompanied by a high relative risk of developing colon, liver, and stomach cancer. About 20% of malignant cancers follow local chronic inflammation, such as gastric cancer and *Helicobacter pylori*-induced gastritis, HCC and hepatitis, CRC and IBD (Francescone et al., 2014). Host immune response and inflammation are two closely related processes which alter the tissue microenvironment by dysregulating various signaling pathways (Grivennikov et al., 2010b). In contrast to the inflammation type that precedes carcinogenesis, inflammation can be induced by a growing tumor (so-called "tumor-elicited inflammation") or results from a response to anticancer therapy and/or cell death, promoting therapeutic resistance and cancer progression (Greten and Grivennikov, 2019). For instance, when immune responsive cell infiltrated in most sporadic CRC tissues, the expression of inflammatory chemokines and cytokines were shown to have increased, although only 2% of CRCs were discovered to be preceded by inflammation associated with IBD (Hibino et al., 2021).

Accordingly, numerous tumor intrinsic factors have been suggested to inflict tumor-elicited inflammation. This includes excessive production of pro-inflammatory cytokines and chemokines, inactivation of tumor suppressors, such as *TP53*, cancer cell-autonomous effects, induction of angiogenesis, recruitment of immune cells, and the activation of *KRAS* and *MYC* oncogenes (Abed et al., 2020, Greten and Grivennikov, 2019, Wellenstein and de Visser, 2018). Moreover, bacteria and their metabolites also act as triggers of tumor-elicited inflammation.

Most solid tumors can engage immune effector cells and modulate pro-inflammatory cytokines and growth factors to regulate the progression and metastasis of the tumor. This process often exacerbates tumor spread and progression, as well as imparting anticancer therapy resistance. The colony-stimulating factor-1 (CSF-1) is an inflammatory mediator that accelerates tumor development by the recruitment of macrophages (Huang et al., 2021). Tumor expression of RAS oncogene often results in the upregulation of pro-inflammatory cytokine IL-8 in nude mouse models which results in larger tumor size, infiltration by the immune, and tumor angiogenesis (Grivennikov et al., 2010b).

INFLAMMATORY BOWEL DISEASE AND COLON CANCER RISK

IBD is a key risk factor for the development of CRC, small bowel cancer, intestinal lymphoma, and cholangiocarcinoma (Laredo et al., 2023). In IBD, proinflammatory growth factors and cytokines are upregulated; they are also highly expressed in CRC, where they are believed to influence tumor initiation, growth, and progression (Tenesa et al., 2008). In the reparative phase of inflammation, stem cells are often activated to differentiate into somatic cells and in the process may become vulnerable to mutagens which induce genetic instability, some of which may result in the initiation of tumorigenesis. These "wound healing-like" reactions stimulate pre-neoplastic proliferation in IBD associated with the loss of tissue integrity.

HEPATITIS AND CANCER RISK

The association of chronic inflammation with HCC arises from different etiologies that include hepatitis B or C infection. Accumulating evidence has shown that patients with hepatitis infection have a higher risk of developing HCC by 15–17-fold. These viruses induce hepatic inflammation and fibrosis, which culminates in cirrhosis, in which regenerative nodules are formed (El-Serag and Rudolph, 2007). According to the experimental data generated from various studies, alterations in hepatitis are critical components in promoting HCC and cholangiocarcinoma (Khalyfa et al., 2022, Fragkou et al., 2021, Massarweh and El-Serag, 2017).

The induction of chronic inflammation by hepatitis causes hepatic and biliary epithelial cell damage. Because a liver has a high regenerative capacity, this in turn, promotes cell proliferation and increases the frequency of genomic DNA mutations by damaging reactive oxygen species' DNA (Yang et al., 2019). When the high rate of cell proliferation is coupled with DNA mutation, the likelihood of malignant transformation increases. The persistence of chronic inflammation in liver cells inflicts the evasion of immune surveillance by changing the hepatic immune system. These changes include the translocation of gut-derived metabolites and pathogens to the liver, the suppression of premature hepatocellular cells by imposing oxidative stress leading to cellular damage via DNA alterations leading to HCC, the deregulation of the senescence-associated secretome, the infiltration of myeloid-derived suppressor cells, and the production of protumorigenic cytokines (Yang et al., 2019, Khalyfa et al., 2022).

CROSS-LINK BETWEEN GUT MICROBES, IMMUNE CELLS, AND INFLAMMATION IN CANCER

In normal physiology, the eubiosis of the gut microbiome is characterized by an intact healthy mucosal barrier and mucus layer, a parity of pro-inflammatory cytokines and anti-inflammatory cytokines, as well as immunoglobulin A secretions and routine immune cells surveillance (Rebersek, 2021). However, the disturbance of these parameters due to the enhanced dysbiosis between beneficial and potential gut microbials has been associated with the disruption of the intestinal mucosal or epithelial lining. This, in turn, allows an influx of gut microbials to the underlying tissue compartment, triggering the immune response to release pro-inflammatory mediators which are the risk factor for cancer development (Figure 10.2) (Francescone et al., 2014). As a result of the inflammatory response, various immune mediators and modulators communicate with each other to either directly or indirectly dictate whether inflammation will promote tumor growth or exert an antitumorigenic function (Grivennikov et al., 2010a).

In cooperation with environmental factors, microbes such as *Helicobacter pylori* can inflict chronic inflammation that affects expressions of miRNAs that are able to induce the production of numerous tumor-related mRNAs or proteins (Link et al., 2012). The events induced by chronic inflammation operate in tandem to modulate cell functions that advance gastric carcinogenesis. In pathophysiology, these microbes can produce carcinogenic metabolites to disrupt normal cellular signaling, thereby interfering with normal cell growth restrictions. Similarly, microbes can induce hormones which increase epithelial cell proliferation or directly affect the oncogenes by changing cell transformation (Zhou et al., 2022).

There are a number of studies that have identified several bacteria that influence cancer development by altering the

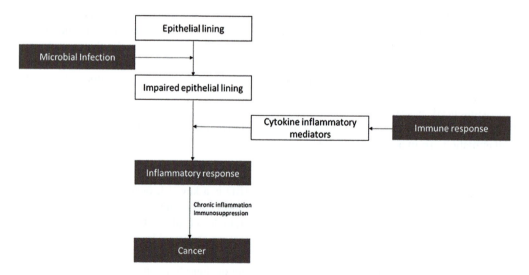

FIGURE 10.2 Schematic diagram illustrating the interplay between the microbial, immune and inflammation response, and cancer development. During microbial dysbiosis, the gut epithelial lining is often impaired, causing the invasion of microbes to the underlying epithelial lining. This in turn, triggers an immune response followed by an inflammatory response. If the inflammation persists chronically, cancer develops eventually.

TABLE 10.1
Bacteria that induce human cancers

Bacteria	Cancer	Expression	Mechanism	Function
Helicobacter pylori	Gastric cancer	High	Wnt/β-catenin pathway	Regulating cellular turnover and apoptosis
			Correa pathway	Chronic inflammatory response
Fusobacterium nucleatum	CRC	High	Invasion of CRC cells	Influencing CRC development
	OSCC	High	Invasion of OSCC cells	Pro-inflammatory cascades
Escherichia coli	CRC	Imbalance	Inducing inflammation, oxidative stress, changes in the cellular niche, interference and manipulation of the host cell cycle	Promoting cancer formation
Bacteroides fragilis	CRC	High	Inducing chronic intestinal inflammation and tissue damage	Promoting colon tumorigenesis
			Activation of Wnt/β-catenin, NFκB pathway, and Th17 adaptive immunity	Promoting colon tumorigenesis
Salmonella enterica	Gallbladder cancer	High	Activation of MAPK and AKT pathways	Cancer tumorigenesis

CRC, colorectal cancer; OSCC, oral squamous cell carcinoma; MAPK, mitogen-activated protein kinase.

host's physiology (Table 10.1). Nevertheless, bacterial characterization has not been well elucidated in human cancers owing to their low biological expression.

GUT MICROBIAL AND INFLAMMATION IN CANCER

The role of inflammation in cultivating a fertile environment for tumor development, growth, and metastasis is a well-established concept in cancer biology. As illustrated in Figure 10.3, studies have associated microbe-induced chronic inflammation with pro-tumorigenic effects (Sun et al., 2017, Gao et al., 2023, Arthur et al., 2012). Indeed, certain bacteria are suggested to induce mucosal permeability modifications to enable the translocation of bacteria and bacterial toxins, ultimately enhancing the transformation of precancerous conditions. Subsequently, local immune responses may be significantly affected, and thus affect tissue homeostasis to promote the development of cancer (Mantovani et al., 2008). Molecules of inflammatory pathways and inflammatory mediators like IL-1, tumor necrosis factor-α (TNF-α), and nitric oxide (NO) have been documented as being involved in communications between the immune cells and transforming tissue cells (Mantovani et al., 2008).

Helicobacter pylori is probably one of the most well-understood models whose infection is closely related to the development of gastric cancer. Based on the work by Marshall and Warren in 1982, *Helicobacter pylori* was described as the primary etiologic agent which causes chronic gastritis (Marshall and Warren, 1984). Years later, it was discovered that if chronic gastritis is left untreated for a lengthy period, the infection may progress through several phases, causing the bacteria to activate a cascade of histological changes from chronic superficial gastric inflammation to atrophic gastric inflammation, intestinal metaplasia, and dysplasia, before ultimately resulting in gastric cancer (Dixon et al., 1996).

Throughout the cascade of these events, gastric epithelial cells are damaged by *Helicobacter pylori* through acquiring alterations in DNA methylation and gene mutation, and exposure to chronic inflammatory microenvironment, all of which increase the risks of developing adenocarcinoma of the stomach (Kouzu et al., 2021, Wroblewski et al., 2010). *Helicobacter pylori* produces proteases, cytotoxin A, and specific phospholipases, all of which interfere with the normal function of gastric mucosal epithelial cells and compromise the integrity of intercellular tight junctions. Consequently, these actions induce inflammatory alterations by stimulating transcription and production of inflammatory cytokines (TNF-α and IL-1) within the gastric mucosa, which play a significant role in promoting the development of adenocarcinoma in the stomach (Ito et al., 2020).

Notably, *Helicobacter pylori* infection may directly spur the proliferation and invasion of gastric cancer cells via the CagA-MET pathway which in turn, may interact with host proteins to turn on downstream signaling pathways, including the NF-kB, MEK/ERK, and β-catenin pathways to induce pro-inflammatory response and cell proliferation, promoting gastric cancer initiation and progression (Kouzu et al., 2021). Also, gastric mucosa-associated lymphoid tissue lymphoma has been closely linked to persistent *Helicobacter pylori* infection (Park and Koo, 2014). Accordingly, the colonization of the stomach with *Helicobacter pylori* may trigger the upregulation of IL-8 and the activation of NF-kB to induce inflammation (Keikha and Karbalaei, 2021). These changes can lead to the production of free radicals and DNA damage in gastric cells including gastric mucosa-associated lymphoid tissues. Mutation-prone repair of this damage can lead to mutations that may promote lymphomagenesis (Keikha and Karbalaei, 2021).

Like *Helicobacter pylori*, other known bacteria have been associated with chronic inflammation and the development of

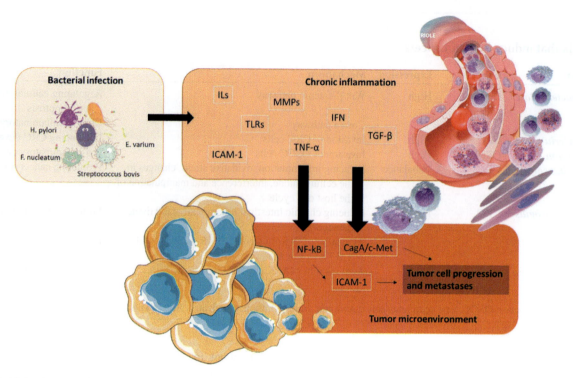

FIGURE 10.3 **An overview of the cross-link between microbial infection, chronic inflammation, and cancer.** Microbial infection within the normal tissue triggers the recruitment of inflammatory cytokines and chemokines, all of which activate several signaling pathways, such as NF-kB and CagA/c-Met, which play key roles in cultivating a fertile environment for tumor development, growth, and metastasis. CagA/c-Met: Cytotoxin-associated gene A/Mesenchymal epithelial transition factor; IFN: Interferon; ILs: Interleukins; ICAM-1: Intercellular adhesion molecule-1; MMPs: Matrix metalloproteinases; NF-κβ: nuclear factor-kappa β; TGF-β: Transforming growth factor-β; TLRs: Toll-like receptors; TNF-α: Tumor necrosis factor-α; ICAM-1: Intracellular cell adhesion molecule-1.

cancer. This includes *IFN* and CRC, *Bartonella* species and vascular tumor formation, *Salmonella typhi* and gallbladder carcinoma, and *Chlamydia pneumonia* and lung carcinoma (Vogelmann and Amieva, 2007, Shacter and Weitzman, 2002). *Fusobacterium nucleatum* is another well-known oral commensal bacterium, which has been associated with the induction of chronic inflammation that ultimately increases the risks of oral squamous cell carcinoma (SCS) (McIlvanna et al., 2021). In one study, increased levels of *Fusobacterium nucleatum* DNA were found in esophageal SCC compared to the tumor-free tissues, linking this species with poor recurrent-free survival (Yamamura et al., 2019). Before that, *Fusobacterium nucleatum* was significantly associated with CRC recurrence and resistance to chemotherapy, with the changes in the autophagy pathway considered as an underlying mechanism (Yu et al., 2017b). It was also suggested that the loss or heterogeneous expression of E-cadherin (tumor suppressor through the modulation of β-catenin pathway) in tumors with high levels of *Fusobacterium nucleatum* was associated with progressive CRC and unfavorable prognosis (Rubinstein et al., 2013).

Accumulating evidence has revealed that the alteration of bacterial species and the associated inflammatory profiles are induced in various organs, and NF-kB is considered to be a strong candidate responsible for this linkage. Moreover, the outcomes of this transcriptional factor action are pleiotropic and its deregulation has been linked to cancer (Peng et al., 2020). While its activation generally triggers acute inflammatory immune response aimed at eliminating transformed cells, the outcomes are cell-type specific and can be both pro- and anti-inflammatory (Lawrence, 2009).

Microbial and Immune Cells in Cancer

Macrophages are multipurpose immune cells that serve a protective role from infections in the host by recognizing and eliminating cancer cells. Their interplay with gut microbes is a complex and evolving area in oncology studies. It has been suggested that the immune response is influenced by the bacterial presence in a tumor microenvironment (TME) by inhibiting immune system function to promote the progression of cancer. In this regard, bacterial presence activates innate and adaptive immune cells and stimulates signaling pathways that contribute to tumorigenesis. The microbes activate Toll-like receptors (TLR) or nucleotide-binding domain and leucine-rich repeat-containing receptors (NLR) whose functions are to activate the first line of defense in response to microbial invasion and initiate a local inflammatory response. This causes the recruitment of monocytes by chemokines to the site of microbial invasion (Pushalkar et al., 2018). Subsequently, the monocytes differentiate into macrophages, which produce various bioactive mediators that promote the growth and invasive capacity of tumor cells or suppress tumor progression (Kouzu et al., 2021).

Accumulating compelling evidence indicates that the presence of bacteria, both local and distant, can impact the development of tumors. *Fusobacterium nucleatum*'s Fap2 protein, identified among tumor-promoting bacteria, was observed to interact directly with the inhibitory receptor TIGIT found in human NK cells and T cells. This interaction led to the inhibition of NK cell attacks and facilitated immune escape (Zhang et al., 2023). In preclinical models of pancreatic cancer, it was demonstrated that the presence of bacteria in tumors played a crucial role in creating an immunosuppressive tumor microenvironment (TME). This was achieved by reducing myeloid-derived suppressor cells, increasing the differentiation of M1 macrophages, promoting TH1 differentiation of CD4+ T cells, and activating CD8+ T cells, thereby promoting immune tolerance and driving pancreatic cancer initiation and progression. The removal of the microbiome reversed these effects (Pushalkar et al., 2018). The relationship between gut microbiota and immune cell composition in colorectal cancer (CRC) was explored by Kikuchi et al., who found that the gut microbiome may influence immune response suppression by decreasing M1 tumor-associated macrophages (Kikuchi et al., 2020). Additionally, Ma et al. discovered that the colonization of *Clostridium* species in the gut resulted in the synthesis of secondary bile acids, hindering NK cell activity in a C-X-C Motif Chemokine Ligand 16-dependent manner, thereby promoting hepatocellular carcinoma (HCC) progression (Ma et al., 2018).

Notably, the composition of gut microbiota plays a crucial role, as different bacterial species can exert opposing effects on tumorigenesis. In contrast to the examples of bacteria promoting tumors, some gut microbes have been shown to inhibit tumor growth. This inhibition occurs by either directly enhancing T-cells and NK cells, activating the immune cell response, or upregulating tumor antigen expression. Alternatively, these microbes can indirectly regulate the immune process and modulate the TME by stimulating the secretion of cytokines and chemokine (Zhou et al., 2023).

The enrichment of the gut with particular bacterial species like *Lactobacillus*, *Faecalibacterium*, *Akkermansia muciniphila*, and *Bifidobacterium* has been found to have a favorable effect on the response of immune check-point inhibitors (Gao et al., 2023). *Akkermansia*, in particular, was observed to enhance the immune response and preserve the integrity of the intestinal barrier (Rodrigues et al., 2022). The enrichment of *Salmonella* in the tumor microenvironment was said to stimulate the production of IL-1β by microphages and induce tumor cell apoptosis for tumor inhibition (Al-Saafeen et al., 2021). *Salmonella* can also induce the activation of microphages and NK cells through the TLR signaling pathway to enhance antitumor immunity (Al-Saafeen et al., 2021). In another study, *Lactobacillus* enhanced the production of cytokines, which in turn induced IFN-γ and the effectiveness of CD8+ T cell activation. Similarly, the expression of maturation and co-stimulation markers of dendritic cells were enhanced (Ghoneum and Felo, 2015). Because the aberrant Wnt/β-catenin signaling pathway plays a significant role in tumorigenesis, experiments have shown the inhibition of this pathway by *C. butyricum* (Li et al., 2019).

ENVIRONMENTAL IMPACT ON GUT MICROBIOTA

The digestive tract is a continuous structure starting from the mouth and ending at the anus with a diverse microbiome specific to different areas. Colonization of the mucosa by diverse microorganisms contributes to the homeostasis of the specific digestive region (Tancrede, 1992). These microorganisms exist in a symbiotic relationship that allows for the interaction and proliferation of different microbial species which maintain the physiological and defense mechanisms of the host whilst inhibiting the propagation of pathogenic organisms (Marsh and Percival, 2006). The environment in which these organisms exist plays a role in maintaining the ecosystem by providing nutrition, protection, and surfaces for attachment. These include the pH, oxygen content, and mucosal barriers within the environment that provide receptors for attachment and proliferation of certain aerobic and anaerobic microorganisms (Marsh, 2000, Tancrede, 1992). An imbalance in this homeostasis often results in the development of inflammatory diseases, which predispose to the development of carcinogenesis (Loftus et al., 2021). The role of host lifestyle such as psychosocial stress has been elucidated in dysbiosis that predisposes to carcinogenesis (Figure 10.4) (Rebersek, 2021).

The source of environmental microflora of an infant is mainly through passive transfer from caregivers through touch and kissing. This acquisition of microflora continues to occur and changes throughout life fluctuating in

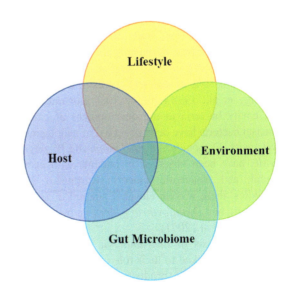

FIGURE 10.4 Four key factors involved in the imbalance of homeostasis in gut microbiome and gastrointestinal carcinogenesis are the host and the host's lifestyle, environment, and gut microbiome. Each factor has an influence on the homeostasis within the gut and must remain balances to avoid dysbiosis.

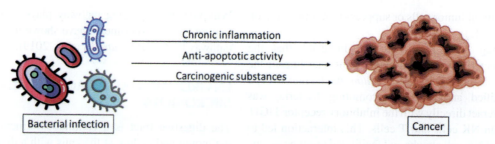

FIGURE 10.5 An overview of the influence of oral bacteria in the development of cancers, underpinning the contribution of chronic inflammation, anti-apoptotic activity, and carcinogenic substances. Bacterial infection influences tumor development, progression, and survival by stimulating chronic inflammation, sustaining anti-apoptotic activities, and secreting carcinogenic substances into the tumor microenvironment.

composition based on the age, sex, and diet of individuals (Marsh and Percival, 2006, Tuominen and Rautava, 2021). The eruption of teeth is associated with plaque accumulation and also provides an environment for microbial retention, which if uncontrolled may cause local irritation and the development of periodontal disease (Issrani et al., 2022, Keijser et al., 2008). Periodontal disease has been associated with many systemic diseases such as diabetes, obesity, cardiovascular disease, respiratory tract infections, and certain cancers (Issrani et al., 2022, Tancrede, 1992, Karpiński, 2019). These are attributed to the opportunistic pathogens that secrete endotoxin which circulates systemically or the systemic production of inflammatory mediators in response to the periodontal pathogens (Issrani et al., 2022).

Oral microflora plays a critical role in the pathogenesis of neoplasms including oral SCC, CRC and pancreatic carcinoma (Wang et al., 2021, Chen et al., 2019, Flemer et al., 2018, Tuominen and Rautava, 2021, Meurman, 2010). The most common bacteria detected in patients with oral SCC include *Streptococcus* spp., *Peptostreptococcus* spp., *Porphyromonas gingivalis*, *Prevotella* spp., and *Capnocytophaga gingivalis* (Karpiński, 2019). These organisms have been isolated in the saliva of patients with oral SCC and are predictive of cancer development in 80% of cases (Karpiński, 2019, Sun et al., 2020, Nagy et al., 1998). Figure 10.5 illustrates the effect of oral cavity bacteria in the development of cancer. Oral commensal bacteria have been observed in neoplasms outside the oral cavity. *Fusobacterium nucleatum* and *Porphyromonas gingivalis* have been observed in patients with esophageal, colorectal, and pancreatic cancers (Karpiński, 2019). In some studies, there was an elevated amount of *Bacteroides*, *Streptococcus*, and *Desulfovibrio genera* in the saliva of CRC patients (Wang et al., 2021).

The pathogenesis of microbiota in the development of carcinogenesis is linked to their role in causing local chronic inflammation with the production of cytokines by the inflammatory cells and the release of carcinogenic substances which result in a malignant phenotype (Peters et al., 2016, Wang et al., 2021, Issrani et al., 2022). Elevated levels of *F. nucleatum*, *Porphyromonas gingivalis*, *Bacteroides*, *Streptococcus*, and *Desulfovibrio genera* microorganisms in saliva and stool can be used in the diagnosis and prognosis of CRC (Flemer et al., 2018, Wang et al., 2021, Russo et al., 2018).

GUT MICROBIOME AS A SOURCE OF BIOMARKERS FOR CANCER DIAGNOSIS AND PROGNOSIS

The role of gut microbiota in cancer goes beyond treatment but also serves a diagnostic and prognostic purpose. Through CRC metagenomics investigation, bacterial biomarkers in several ethnic groups' fecal microbiomes were identified and validated (Yu et al., 2017a). Identification of fecal microbe DNA can help detect CRC early on and can serve as an essential screening tool in individuals without symptoms. In addition, the role of fecal immunohistochemistry for screening has been explored (Sun et al., 2023).

One study analyzed gut microbiota in lung cancer patients using 16S rRNA gene sequencing and found that organisms like *Veillonella*, *Enterococcus*, *Clostridiodes*, *Megasphaera*, and *Actinomyces* were increased in cancer patients compared to the cancer-free individuals (Zhao et al., 2021). These findings imply that these gut microbes and their metabolites may function as vital biomarkers and potential targets for lung cancer therapy (Zhao et al., 2021). Studies in pancreatic cancer also suggest potential signature gut microbiota. The presence of *Clostridiacea*, *Lachnospraceae*, *Veillonellaceae*, and *Odoribacter* with the absence of *Ruminococcaceae* was demonstrated in the gut of pancreatic cancer patients (Half et al., 2019). This demonstrates that the profile of gut microbiota can effectively serve as a maker of cancer, let alone early detection of cancer.

Analysis of gut microbiota in CRC patients has demonstrated a lower relative abundance of *Bacteroidetes* and *Actinobacteria* in high-risk compared to low-risk patients (Yamaoka et al., 2018), suggesting its utility as the prognostic indicator. Moreover, higher levels of *Bacteroides fragilis* and *Fusobacterium nucleatum* in the gut have been associated with poor postoperative outcomes in CRC patients (Wei et al., 2016). The ratio of *Prevotella/Bacteroides* has been associated with better efficacy of nabuliumab in hepatocellular cancer (Chung et al., 2021).

THE ROLE OF GUT MICROBIOTA IN CANCER THERAPY

The practice of combining anticancer therapy and microbes has been known for decades when inactivated *Streptococcus* is injected into cancer tissue. Many studies have demonstrated that injection or oral intake of microbial preparations can invigorate local immune response against tumors (Zbar et al., 1970, Aso and Akazan, 1992, Stebbing et al., 2012). Currently, conventional therapies in cancer patients alter the gut microbiota, which in turn affects the treatment efficacy and side effects. The use of probiotics, prebiotics, and fecal microbiota transplantation has realized some clinical efficacy.

Probiotics are instrumental to host bacterial content which when boosted in cancer patients can reactivate damaged gut microbiota in the patient. It has been demonstrated that the groundbreaking probiotic *Lactobacillus rhamnosus* GG strain (LGG), which has been researched extensively in oncology, can directly influence host cell signaling pathways such as the WNT or mTOR pathways (Stebbing et al., 2012, Taherian-Esfahani et al., 2016). By inducing Th1 immune cell polarization through DC recognition, LGG enhances the host immune system and aids in the early elimination of newly generated cancer cells by the host (Khailova et al., 2017). A combination of multiple probiotics, such as *Bifidobacterium longum* (BB536) and *Lactobacillus johnsonii* (La1), has demonstrated its ability to adhere to the colon mucosa, reduce the concentration of intestinal pathogens, and regulate the local formation of an anticancer immune environment (Gianotti et al., 2010). By reducing the proliferation of CD83-11c, CD83-HLA-DR, and CD83-123 in probiotics-receiving cohorts compared to control cohorts, this is accomplished (Cai et al., 2016).

FMT has made a recent quantum leap in cancer treatment. FMT from healthy donors corrects gut dysbiosis (Xu et al., 2022). Through the administration of oral dried capsules, gastroscopy, or colonoscopy, the manipulation of the gut microbiota can be easily and rapidly accomplished (Chin et al., 2017, van Nood et al., 2013). In melanoma patients, FMT alters gut microbiota to reprogram the TME and influence the local immune system to overcome resistance to PD-1 blockers (Davar et al., 2021).

LIMITATIONS AND FUTURE PERSPECTIVES

The gut-derived microbiota-associated carcinogenesis stems from localized chronic inflammation, the release of cytokines from the inflammatory cells, and the production of carcinogenic substances that result in a malignant transformation. There are however some questions that remain unanswered in the exploration of gut microbiome and cancer-related inflammation. Although multiple microbiome studies have revealed numerous relative proportions of bacteria in various organs between healthy individuals and cancer patients, little is known about the mechanisms underlying the maintenance and eventual alterations of these ratios in cancer patients. Cancer does not appear to follow any particular pattern. Similarly, how the host genetic makeup and environmental exposure factors fit the picture is unclear. Consequently, these obscurities draw necessity to identify relevant bacteria in humans, study their abundance and the effects of their byproducts on cancer development, and investigate their interactions with the immune system.

CONCLUSION

The pathogenesis of microbiota in the development of cancer is linked to their role in causing local chronic inflammation with the release of cytokines by the inflammatory cells as well as the production of carcinogenic substances. Moreover, inflammation can be induced by growing tumors or results from a response to anticancer therapy cell death. The role of the NF-kβ signaling pathway in chronic inflammation is realized and has also been found to be even more exaggerated in several cancers. Despite the known fact that microbes promote tumor growth and progression, microbes can modulate the tumor microenvironment to inhibit tumor growth through the activation of T cells and NK cells which increase antitumor immune response. The application of therapeutic gut microbiota to correct dysbiosis adds another avenue of cancer treatment in the field of oncology.

REFERENCES

ABED, J., MAALOUF, N., MANSON, A. L., EARL, A. M., PARHI, L., EMGÅRD, J. E. M., KLUTSTEIN, M., TAYEB, S., ALMOGY, G., ATLAN, K. A., CHAUSHU, S., ISRAELI, E., MANDELBOIM, O., GARRETT, W. S. & BACHRACH, G. 2020. Colon cancer-associated fusobacterium nucleatum may originate from the oral cavity and reach colon tumors via the circulatory system. *Front Cell Infect Microbiol*, 10, 400.

AL-SAAFEEN, B. H., FERNANDEZ-CABEZUDO, M. J. & AL-RAMADI, B. K. 2021. Integration of *Salmonella* into combination cancer therapy. *Cancers (Basel)*, 13, 3228.

ARTHUR, J. C., PEREZ-CHANONA, E., MÜHLBAUER, M., TOMKOVICH, S., URONIS, J. M., FAN, T. J., CAMPBELL, B. J., ABUJAMEL, T., DOGAN, B., ROGERS, A. B., RHODES, J. M., STINTZI, A., SIMPSON, K. W., HANSEN, J. J., KEKU, T. O., FODOR, A. A. & JOBIN, C. 2012. Intestinal inflammation targets cancer-inducing activity of the microbiota. *Science*, 338, 120–3.

ARTIS, D. 2008. Epithelial-cell recognition of commensal bacteria and maintenance of immune homeostasis in the gut. *Nat Rev Immunol*, 8, 411–20.

ASO, Y. & AKAZAN, H. 1992. Prophylactic effect of a *Lactobacillus casei* preparation on the recurrence of superficial bladder cancer. BLP Study Group. *Urol Int*, 49, 125–9.

BALKWILL, F. & MANTOVANI, A. 2001. Inflammation and cancer: back to Virchow? *Lancet*, 357, 539–45.

BERG, D. J., DAVIDSON, N., KÜHN, R., MÜLLER, W., MENON, S., HOLLAND, G., THOMPSON-SNIPES, L., LEACH, M. W. & RENNICK, D. 1996. Enterocolitis and colon cancer in interleukin-10-deficient mice are associated with aberrant cytokine production and CD4(+) TH1-like responses. *J Clin Invest*, 98, 1010–20.

CAI, S., KANDASAMY, M., RAHMAT, J. N., THAM, S. M., BAY, B. H., LEE, Y. K. & MAHENDRAN, R. 2016. Lactobacillus rhamnosus GG activation of dendritic cells and neutrophils depends on the dose and time of exposure. *J Immunol Res,* 2016, 7402760.

CHEN, G. Y., SHAW, M. H., REDONDO, G. & NÚÑEZ, G. 2008. The innate immune receptor Nod1 protects the intestine from inflammation-induced tumorigenesis. *Cancer Res,* 68, 10060–7.

CHEN, L. T., LIN, J. T., TAI, J. J., CHEN, G. H., YEH, H. Z., YANG, S. S., WANG, H. P., KUO, S. H., SHEU, B. S., JAN, C. M., WANG, W. M., WANG, T. E., WU, C. W., CHEN, C. L., SU, I. J., WHANG-PENG, J. & CHENG, A. L. 2005. Long-term results of anti-Helicobacter pylori therapy in early-stage gastric high-grade transformed MALT lymphoma. *J Natl Cancer Inst,* 97, 1345–53.

CHEN, Y., CHEN, X., YU, H., ZHOU, H. & XU, S. 2019. Oral microbiota as promising diagnostic biomarkers for gastrointestinal cancer: A systematic review. *Onco Targets Ther,* 12, 11131–44.

CHIN, S. M., SAUK, J., MAHABAMUNUGE, J., KAPLAN, J. L., HOHMANN, E. L. & KHALILI, H. 2017. Fecal microbiota transplantation for recurrent clostridium difficile infection in patients with inflammatory bowel disease: A single-center experience. *Clin Gastroenterol Hepatol,* 15, 597–99.

CHO, I. & BLASER, M. J. 2012. The human microbiome: at the interface of health and disease. *Nat Rev Genet,* 13, 260–70.

CHUNG, M. W., KIM, M. J., WON, E. J., LEE, Y. J., YUN, Y. W., CHO, S. B., JOO, Y. E., HWANG, J. E., BAE, W. K., CHUNG, I. J., SHIN, M. G. & SHIN, J. H. 2021. Gut microbiome composition can predict the response to nivolumab in advanced hepatocellular carcinoma patients. *World J Gastroenterol,* 27, 7340–49.

DAVAR, D., DZUTSEV, A. K., MCCULLOCH, J. A., RODRIGUES, R. R., CHAUVIN, J. M., MORRISON, R. M., DEBLASIO, R. N., MENNA, C., DING, Q., PAGLIANO, O., ZIDI, B., ZHANG, S., BADGER, J. H., VETIZOU, M., COLE, A. M., FERNANDES, M. R., PRESCOTT, S., COSTA, R. G. F., BALAJI, A. K., MORGUN, A., VUJKOVIC-CVIJIN, I., WANG, H., BORHANI, A. A., SCHWARTZ, M. B., DUBNER, H. M., ERNST, S. J., ROSE, A., NAJJAR, Y. G., BELKAID, Y., KIRKWOOD, J. M., TRINCHIERI, G. & ZAROUR, H. M. 2021. Fecal microbiota transplant overcomes resistance to anti-PD-1 therapy in melanoma patients. *Science,* 371, 595–602.

DIXON, M. F., GENTA, R. M., YARDLEY, J. H. & CORREA, P. 1996. Classification and grading of gastritis. The updated Sydney System. International Workshop on the Histopathology of Gastritis, Houston 1994. *Am J Surg Pathol,* 20, 1161–81.

EL-SERAG, H. B. & RUDOLPH, K. L. 2007. Hepatocellular carcinoma: epidemiology and molecular carcinogenesis. *Gastroenterology,* 132, 2557–76.

FANG, Y., YAN, C., ZHAO, Q., ZHAO, B., LIAO, Y., CHEN, Y., WANG, D. & TANG, D. 2022. The association between gut microbiota, toll-like receptors, and colorectal cancer. *Clin Med Insights Oncol,* 16, 11795549221130549.

FLEMER, B., WARREN, R. D., BARRETT, M. P., CISEK, K., DAS, A., JEFFERY, I. B., HURLEY, E., MICHEAL, O. R., SHANAHAN, F. & PAUL, W. T. 2018. The oral microbiota in colorectal cancer is distinctive and predictive. *Gut,* 67, 1454–63.

FRAGKOU, N., SIDERAS, L., PANAS, P., EMMANOUILIDES, C. & SINAKOS, E. 2021. Update on the association of hepatitis B with intrahepatic cholangiocarcinoma: Is there new evidence? *World J Gastroenterol,* 27, 4252–75.

FRANCESCONE, R., HOU, V. & GRIVENNIKOV, S. I. 2014. Microbiome, inflammation, and cancer. *Cancer J,* 20, 181–9.

GAMAGE, S. D., PATTON, A. K., STRASSER, J. E., CHALK, C. L. & WEISS, A. A. 2006. Commensal bacteria influence *Escherichia coli* O157:H7 persistence and Shiga toxin production in the mouse intestine. *Infect Immun,* 74, 1977–83.

GAO, Y., XU, P., SUN, D., JIANG, Y., LIN, X., HAN, T., YU, J., SHENG, C., CHEN, H. Y., HONG, J., CHEN, Y., XIAO, X. Y. & FANG, J. Y. 2023. Faecalibacterium prausnitzii abrogates intestinal toxicity and promotes tumor immunity to increase the efficacy of dual CTLA-4 and PD-1 checkpoint blockade. *Cancer Res,* 83, 3710–25.

GHONEUM, M. & FELO, N. 2015. Selective induction of apoptosis in human gastric cancer cells by Lactobacillus kefiri (PFT), a novel kefir product. *Oncol Rep,* 34, 1659–66.

GIANOTTI, L., MORELLI, L., GALBIATI, F., ROCCHETTI, S., COPPOLA, S., BENEDUCE, A., GILARDINI, C., ZONENSCHAIN, D., NESPOLI, A. & BRAGA, M. 2010. A randomized double-blind trial on perioperative administration of probiotics in colorectal cancer patients. *World J Gastroenterol,* 16, 167–75.

GONG, E. J., AHN, J. Y., JUNG, H. Y., PARK, H., KO, Y. B., NA, H. K., JUNG, K. W., KIM DO, H., LEE, J. H., CHOI, K. D., SONG, H. J., LEE, G. H. & KIM, J. H. 2016. Helicobacter pylori eradication therapy is effective as the initial treatment for patients with *H. pylori*-negative and disseminated gastric mucosa-associated lymphoid tissue lymphoma. *Gut Liver,* 10, 706–13.

GRETEN, F. R. & GRIVENNIKOV, S. I. 2019. Inflammation and cancer: Triggers, mechanisms, and consequences. *Immunity,* 51, 27–41.

GRIVENNIKOV, S. I., GRETEN, F. R. & KARIN, M. 2010a. Immunity, inflammation, and cancer. *Cell,* 140, 883–99.

GRIVENNIKOV, S. I., GRETEN, F. R. & KARIN, M. 2010b. Immunity, inflammation, and cancer. *Cell,* 140, 883–99.

GUNASEKERA, D. C., MA, J., VACHARATHIT, V., SHAH, P., RAMAKRISHNAN, A., UPRETY, P., SHEN, Z., SHEH, A., BRAYTON, C. F., WHARY, M. T., FOX, J. G. & BREAM, J. H. 2020. The development of colitis in Il10$^{(-/-)}$ mice is dependent on IL-22. *Mucosal Immunol,* 13, 493–506.

HALF, E., KEREN, N., RESHEF, L., DORFMAN, T., LACHTER, I., KLUGER, Y., RESHEF, N., KNOBLER, H., MAOR, Y., STEIN, A., KONIKOFF, F. M. & GOPHNA, U. 2019. Fecal microbiome signatures of pancreatic cancer patients. *Sci Rep,* 9, 16801.

HIBINO, S., KAWAZOE, T., KASAHARA, H., ITOH, S., ISHIMOTO, T., SAKATA-YANAGIMOTO, M. & TANIGUCHI, K. 2021. Inflammation-induced tumorigenesis and metastasis. *Int J Mol Sci,* 22, 5421.

HUANG, Y. K., BUSUTTIL, R. A. & BOUSSIOUTAS, A. 2021. The role of innate immune cells in tumor invasion and metastasis. *Cancers (Basel),* 13, 5885.

ISSRANI, R., REDDY, J., DABAH, T. H. E.-M., PRABHU, N., ALRUWAILI, M. K., MUNISEKHAR, M. S., ALSHAMMARI, S. M. & ALGHUMAIZ, S. F. 2022.

Exploring the mechanisms and association between oral microflora and systemic diseases. *Diagnostics*, 12, 2800.

ITO, N., TSUJIMOTO, H., UENO, H., XIE, Q. & SHINOMIYA, N. 2020. *Helicobacter pylori*-mediated immunity and signaling transduction in gastric cancer. *J Clin Med*, 9, 3699.

KARPIŃSKI, T. M. 2019. Role of oral microbiota in cancer development. *Microorganisms*, 7, 20.

KEIJSER, B., ZAURA, E., HUSE, S., VAN DER VOSSEN, J., SCHUREN, F., MONTIJN, R., TEN CATE, J. & CRIELAARD, W. 2008. Pyrosequencing analysis of the oral microflora of healthy adults. *J Dent Res*, 87, 1016–20.

KEIKHA, M. & KARBALAEI, M. 2021. Probiotics as the live microscopic fighters against *Helicobacter pylori* gastric infections. *BMC Gastroenterol*, 21, 388.

KHAILOVA, L., BAIRD, C. H., RUSH, A. A., BARNES, C. & WISCHMEYER, P. E. 2017. *Lactobacillus rhamnosus* GG treatment improves intestinal permeability and modulates inflammatory response and homeostasis of spleen and colon in experimental model of *Pseudomonas aeruginosa* pneumonia. *Clin Nutr*, 36, 1549–57.

KHALYFA, A. A., PUNATAR, S. & YARBROUGH, A. 2022. Hepatocellular carcinoma: Understanding the inflammatory implications of the microbiome. *Int J Mol Sci*, 23, 8164.

KIKUCHI, T., MIMURA, K., ASHIZAWA, M., OKAYAMA, H., ENDO, E., SAITO, K., SAKAMOTO, W., FUJITA, S., ENDO, H. & SAITO, M. 2020. Characterization of tumor-infiltrating immune cells in relation to microbiota in colorectal cancers. *Cancer Immunol Immunother*, 69, 23–32.

KOUZU, K., TSUJIMOTO, H., KISHI, Y., UENO, H. & SHINOMIYA, N. 2021. Role of microbial infection-induced inflammation in the development of gastrointestinal cancers. *Medicines (Basel)*, 8, 45.

KÜHN, R., LÖHLER, J., RENNICK, D., RAJEWSKY, K. & MÜLLER, W. 1993. Interleukin-10-deficient mice develop chronic enterocolitis. *Cell*, 75, 263–74.

LAREDO, V., GARCÍA-MATEO, S., MARTÍNEZ-DOMÍNGUEZ, S. J., LÓPEZ DE LA CRUZ, J., GARGALLO-PUYUELO, C. J. & GOMOLLÓN, F. 2023. Risk of cancer in patients with inflammatory bowel diseases and keys for patient management. *Cancers (Basel)*, 15, 871.

LAWRENCE, T. 2009. The nuclear factor NF-kappaB pathway in inflammation. *Cold Spring Harb Perspect Biol*, 1, a001651.

LE NOCI, V., BERNARDO, G., BIANCHI, F., TAGLIABUE, E., SOMMARIVA, M. & SFONDRINI, L. 2021. Toll like receptors as sensors of the tumor microbial dysbiosis: implications in cancer progression. *Front Cell Dev Biol*, 9, 732192.

LI, X., XIANG, Y., LI, F., YIN, C., LI, B. & KE, X. 2019. WNT/β-catenin signaling pathway regulating T cell-inflammation in the tumor microenvironment. *Front Immunol*, 10, 2293.

LINK, A., KUPCINSKAS, J., WEX, T. & MALFERTHEINER, P. 2012. Macro-role of microRNA in gastric cancer. *Dig Dis*, 30, 255–67.

LOFTUS, M., HASSOUNEH, S. A.-D. & YOOSEPH, S. 2021. Bacterial community structure alterations within the colorectal cancer gut microbiome. *BMC Microbiol*, 21, 1–18.

LOZUPONE, C. A., STOMBAUGH, J. I., GORDON, J. I., JANSSON, J. K. & KNIGHT, R. 2012. Diversity, stability and resilience of the human gut microbiota. *Nature*, 489, 220–30.

MA, C., HAN, M., HEINRICH, B., FU, Q., ZHANG, Q., SANDHU, M., AGDASHIAN, D., TERABE, M., BERZOFSKY, J. A., FAKO, V., RITZ, T., LONGERICH, T., THERIOT, C. M., MCCULLOCH, J. A., ROY, S., YUAN, W., THOVARAI, V., SEN, S. K., RUCHIRAWAT, M., KORANGY, F., WANG, X. W., TRINCHIERI, G. & GRETEN, T. F. 2018. Gut microbiome-mediated bile acid metabolism regulates liver cancer via NKT cells. *Science*, 360, eaan5931.

MANTOVANI, A., ALLAVENA, P., SICA, A. & BALKWILL, F. 2008. Cancer-related inflammation. *Nature*, 454, 436–44.

MARSH, P. & PERCIVAL, R. 2006. The oral microflora—friend or foe? Can we decide? *Int Dent J*, 56, 233–39.

MARSH, P. D. 2000. Role of the oral microflora in health. *Microb Ecol Health Dis*, 12, 130–37.

MARSHALL, B. J. & WARREN, J. R. 1984. Unidentified curved bacilli in the stomach of patients with gastritis and peptic ulceration. *Lancet*, 1, 1311–15.

MASSARWEH, N. N. & EL-SERAG, H. B. 2017. Epidemiology of hepatocellular carcinoma and intrahepatic cholangiocarcinoma. *Cancer Control*, 24, 1073274817729245.

MAYNARD, C. L., ELSON, C. O., HATTON, R. D. & WEAVER, C. T. 2012. Reciprocal interactions of the intestinal microbiota and immune system. *Nature*, 489, 231–41.

MCILVANNA, E., LINDEN, G. J., CRAIG, S. G., LUNDY, F. T. & JAMES, J. A. 2021. Fusobacterium nucleatum and oral cancer: A critical review. *BMC Cancer*, 21, 1212.

MEURMAN, J. H. 2010. Oral microbiota and cancer. *J Oral Microbiol*, 2, 5195.

NAGY, K. N., SONKODI, I., SZÖKE, I., NAGY, E. & NEWMAN, H. N. 1998. The microflora associated with human oral carcinomas. *Oral Oncology*, 34, 304–308.

PARK, J. B. & KOO, J. S. 2014. *Helicobacter pylori* infection in gastric mucosa-associated lymphoid tissue lymphoma. *World J Gastroenterol*, 20, 2751–9.

PENG, C., OUYANG, Y., LU, N. & LI, N. 2020. The NF-κB signaling pathway, the microbiota, and gastrointestinal tumorigenesis: recent advances. *Front Immunol*, 11, 1387.

PETERS, B. A., DOMINIANNI, C., SHAPIRO, J. A., CHURCH, T. R., WU, J., MILLER, G., YUEN, E., FREIMAN, H., LUSTBADER, I. & SALIK, J. 2016. The gut microbiota in conventional and serrated precursors of colorectal cancer. *Microbiome*, 4, 1–14.

PUSHALKAR, S., HUNDEYIN, M., DALEY, D., ZAMBIRINIS, C. P., KURZ, E., MISHRA, A., MOHAN, N., AYKUT, B., USYK, M., TORRES, L. E., WERBA, G., ZHANG, K., GUO, Y., LI, Q., AKKAD, N., LALL, S., WADOWSKI, B., GUTIERREZ, J., KOCHEN ROSSI, J. A., HERZOG, J. W., DISKIN, B., TORRES-HERNANDEZ, A., LEINWAND, J., WANG, W., TAUNK, P. S., SAVADKAR, S., JANAL, M., SAXENA, A., LI, X., COHEN, D., SARTOR, R. B., SAXENA, D. & MILLER, G. 2018. The pancreatic cancer microbiome promotes oncogenesis by induction of innate and adaptive immune suppression. *Cancer Discov*, 8, 403–16.

REBERSEK, M. 2021. Gut microbiome and its role in colorectal cancer. *BMC Cancer*, 21, 1325.

RODRIGUES, V. F., ELIAS-OLIVEIRA, J., PEREIRA Í, S., PEREIRA, J. A., BARBOSA, S. C., MACHADO, M. S. G. & CARLOS, D. 2022. Akkermansia muciniphila and gut immune system: A good friendship that attenuates inflammatory bowel disease, obesity, and diabetes. *Front Immunol*, 13, 934695.

RUBINSTEIN, M. R., WANG, X., LIU, W., HAO, Y., CAI, G. & HAN, Y. W. 2013. Fusobacterium nucleatum promotes colorectal carcinogenesis by modulating E-cadherin/β-catenin signaling via its FadA adhesin. *Cell Host Microbe*, 14, 195–206.

RUSSO, E., BACCI, G., CHIELLINI, C., FAGORZI, C., NICCOLAI, E., TADDEI, A., RICCI, F., RINGRESSI, M. N., BORRELLI, R., MELLI, F., MILOEVA, M., BECHI, P., MENGONI, A., FANI, R. & AMEDEI, A. 2018. Preliminary comparison of oral and intestinal human microbiota in patients with colorectal cancer: A pilot study. *Frontiers in Microbiology*, 8, 2699.

SELLON, R. K., TONKONOGY, S., SCHULTZ, M., DIELEMAN, L. A., GRENTHER, W., BALISH, E., RENNICK, D. M. & SARTOR, R. B. 1998. Resident enteric bacteria are necessary for development of spontaneous colitis and immune system activation in interleukin-10-deficient mice. *Infect Immun*, 66, 5224–31.

SHACTER, E. & WEITZMAN, S. A. 2002. Chronic inflammation and cancer. *Oncology (Williston Park)*, 16, 217–26, 229; discussion 230–2.

STEBBING, J., DALGLEISH, A., GIFFORD-MOORE, A., MARTIN, A., GLEESON, C., WILSON, G., BRUNET, L. R., GRANGE, J. & MUDAN, S. 2012. An intra-patient placebo-controlled phase I trial to evaluate the safety and tolerability of intradermal IMM-101 in melanoma. *Ann Oncol*, 23, 1314–19.

SUN, J., CHEN, F. & WU, G. 2023. Potential effects of gut microbiota on host cancers: focus on immunity, DNA damage, cellular pathways, and anticancer therapy. *ISME J*, 17, 1535–51.

SUN, J., TANG, Q., YU, S., XIE, M., XIE, Y., CHEN, G. & CHEN, L. 2020. Role of the oral microbiota in cancer evolution and progression. *Cancer Med*, 9, 6306–21.

SUN, M., WU, W., LIU, Z. & CONG, Y. 2017. Microbiota metabolite short chain fatty acids, GPCR, and inflammatory bowel diseases. *J Gastroenterol*, 52, 1–8.

TAHERIAN-ESFAHANI, Z., ABEDIN-DO, A., NOURI, Z., MIRFAKHRAIE, R., GHAFOURI-FARD, S. & MOTEVASELI, E. 2016. Lactobacilli differentially modulate mTOR and Wnt/ β-catenin pathways in different cancer cell lines. *Iran J Cancer Prev*, 9, e5369.

TANCREDE, C. 1992. Role of human microflora in health and disease. *Eur J Clin Microbiol Infect Dis*, 11, 1012–15.

TENESA, A., FARRINGTON, S. M., PRENDERGAST, J. G., PORTEOUS, M. E., WALKER, M., HAQ, N., BARNETSON, R. A., THEODORATOU, E., CETNARSKYJ, R., CARTWRIGHT, N., SEMPLE, C., CLARK, A. J., REID, F. J., SMITH, L. A., KAVOUSSANAKIS, K., KOESSLER, T., PHAROAH, P. D., BUCH, S., SCHAFMAYER, C., TEPEL, J., SCHREIBER, S., VÖLZKE, H., SCHMIDT, C. O., HAMPE, J., CHANG-CLAUDE, J., HOFFMEISTER, M., BRENNER, H., WILKENING, S., CANZIAN, F., CAPELLA, G., MORENO, V., DEARY, I. J., STARR, J. M., TOMLINSON, I. P., KEMP, Z., HOWARTH, K., CARVAJAL-CARMONA, L., WEBB, E., BRODERICK, P., VIJAYAKRISHNAN, J., HOULSTON, R. S., RENNERT, G., BALLINGER, D., ROZEK, L., GRUBER, S. B., MATSUDA, K., KIDOKORO, T., NAKAMURA, Y., ZANKE, B. W., GREENWOOD, C. M., RANGREJ, J., KUSTRA, R., MONTPETIT, A., HUDSON, T. J., GALLINGER, S., CAMPBELL, H. & DUNLOP, M. G. 2008. Genome-wide association scan identifies a colorectal cancer susceptibility locus on 11q23 and replicates risk loci at 8q24 and 18q21. *Nat Genet*, 40, 631–7.

TUOMINEN, H. & RAUTAVA, J. 2021. Oral microbiota and cancer development. *Pathobiology*, 88, 116–26.

VAN NOOD, E., VRIEZE, A., NIEUWDORP, M., FUENTES, S., ZOETENDAL, E. G., DE VOS, W. M., VISSER, C. E., KUIJPER, E. J., BARTELSMAN, J. F., TIJSSEN, J. G., SPEELMAN, P., DIJKGRAAF, M. G. & KELLER, J. J. 2013. Duodenal infusion of donor feces for recurrent Clostridium difficile. *N Engl J Med*, 368, 407–15.

VOGELMANN, R. & AMIEVA, M. R. 2007. The role of bacterial pathogens in cancer. *Curr Opin Microbiol*, 10, 76–81.

WANG, L., YU, K., ZHANG, X. & YU, S. 2018. Dual functional roles of the MyD88 signaling in colorectal cancer development. *Biomed Pharmacother*, 107, 177–84.

WANG, Y., ZHANG, Y., QIAN, Y., XIE, Y. H., JIANG, S. S., KANG, Z. R., CHEN, Y. X., CHEN, Z. F. & FANG, J. Y. 2021. Alterations in the oral and gut microbiome of colorectal cancer patients and association with host clinical factors. *Int J Cancer*, 149, 925–35.

WEI, Z., CAO, S., LIU, S., YAO, Z., SUN, T., LI, Y., LI, J., ZHANG, D. & ZHOU, Y. 2016. Could gut microbiota serve as prognostic biomarker associated with colorectal cancer patients' survival? A pilot study on relevant mechanism. *Oncotarget*, 7, 46158–172.

WELLENSTEIN, M. D. & DE VISSER, K. E. 2018. Cancer-cell-intrinsic mechanisms shaping the tumor immune landscape. *Immunity*, 48, 399–416.

WROBLEWSKI, L. E., PEEK, R. M., JR. & WILSON, K. T. 2010. Helicobacter pylori and gastric cancer: Factors that modulate disease risk. *Clin Microbiol Rev*, 23, 713–39.

XU, H., CAO, C., REN, Y., WENG, S., LIU, L., GUO, C., WANG, L., HAN, X., REN, J. & LIU, Z. 2022. Antitumor effects of fecal microbiota transplantation: Implications for microbiome modulation in cancer treatment. *Front Immunol*, 13, 949490.

YAMAMURA, K., IZUMI, D., KANDIMALLA, R., SONOHARA, F., BABA, Y., YOSHIDA, N., KODERA, Y., BABA, H. & GOEL, A. 2019. Intratumoral fusobacterium nucleatum levels predict therapeutic response to neoadjuvant chemotherapy in esophageal squamous cell carcinoma. *Clin Cancer Res*, 25, 6170–79.

YAMAOKA, Y., SUEHIRO, Y., HASHIMOTO, S., HOSHIDA, T., FUJIMOTO, M., WATANABE, M., IMANAGA, D., SAKAI, K., MATSUMOTO, T., NISHIOKA, M., TAKAMI, T., SUZUKI, N., HAZAMA, S., NAGANO, H., SAKAIDA, I. & YAMASAKI, T. 2018. Fusobacterium nucleatum as a prognostic marker of colorectal cancer in a Japanese population. *J Gastroenterol*, 53, 517–24.

YAN, D., ISSA, N., AFIFI, L., JEON, C., CHANG, H. W. & LIAO, W. 2017. The role of the skin and gut microbiome in psoriatic disease. *Curr Dermatol Rep*, 6, 94–103.

YANG, Y. M., KIM, S. Y. & SEKI, E. 2019. Inflammation and liver cancer: Molecular mechanisms and therapeutic targets. *Semin Liver Dis*, 39, 26–42.

YU, J., FENG, Q., WONG, S. H., ZHANG, D., LIANG, Q. Y., QIN, Y., TANG, L., ZHAO, H., STENVANG, J., LI, Y., WANG, X., XU, X., CHEN, N., WU, W. K., AL-AAMA, J., NIELSEN, H. J., KIILERICH, P., JENSEN, B. A., YAU, T. O., LAN, Z., JIA, H., LI, J., XIAO, L., LAM, T. Y., NG, S. C., CHENG, A. S., WONG, V. W., CHAN, F. K., XU, X., YANG, H., MADSEN, L., DATZ, C., TILG, H., WANG, J., BRÜNNER, N., KRISTIANSEN, K., ARUMUGAM, M., SUNG, J. J. & WANG, J. 2017a. Metagenomic analysis of faecal microbiome as a tool towards targeted non-invasive biomarkers for colorectal cancer. *Gut*, 66, 70–8.

YU, T., GUO, F., YU, Y., SUN, T., MA, D., HAN, J., QIAN, Y., KRYCZEK, I., SUN, D., NAGARSHETH, N., CHEN, Y., CHEN, H., HONG, J., ZOU, W. & FANG, J. Y. 2017b. Fusobacterium nucleatum promotes chemoresistance to colorectal cancer by modulating autophagy. *Cell,* 170, 548–563.e16.

ZBAR, B., BERNSTEIN, I., TANAKA, T. & RAPP, H. J. 1970. Tumor immunity produced by the intradermal inoculation of living tumor cells and living *Mycobacterium bovis* (strain BCG). *Science,* 170, 1217–8.

ZHANG, J., GUO, F., LI, L., ZHANG, S. & WANG, Y. 2023. Immune evasion and therapeutic opportunities based on natural killer cells. *Chin J Cancer Res,* 35, 283–98.

ZHAO, F., AN, R., WANG, L., SHAN, J. & WANG, X. 2021. Specific gut microbiome and serum metabolome changes in lung cancer patients. *Front Cell Infect Microbiol,* 11, 725284.

ZHOU, X., KANDALAI, S., HOSSAIN, F. & ZHENG, Q. 2022. Tumor microbiome metabolism: A game changer in cancer development and therapy. *Front Oncol,* 12, 933407.

ZHOU, Y., CHENG, L., LIU, L. & LI, X. 2023. NK cells are never alone: crosstalk and communication in tumour microenvironments. *Mol Cancer,* 22, 34.

11 Diet, Lifestyle, and the Gut Microbiome

Thabiso Victor Miya, Zukile Mbita, Suzana Savkovic, and Zodwa Dlamini

INTRODUCTION

Nearly 40 trillion microorganisms, including 3,000 different types of fungi, bacteria, and viruses, make up the dynamic human microbiota. It is crucial for maintaining systemic homeostasis and functional stability since it displays varying microbial richness and individual differences (Cahenzli et al., 2013, Kovatcheva-Datchary et al., 2015, Sender et al., 2016b, Adak and Khan, 2019, Martinez-Guryn et al., 2019). Over 97% of the human microbiota is found in the gastrointestinal (GI) tract, particularly in the colon (Sender et al., 2016a, Sender et al., 2016b). This microbiota, also referred to as the gut microbiota, has been well investigated and is now understood to mediate various physiological processes, including the maturation of the immune system and the creation of some nutrients (Cummings, 1983, McNeil, 1984, Adak and Khan, 2019, Gensollen et al., 2016). When the balance between the microbiota and the human host is upset, gut dysbiosis occurs. Alterations in metabolic secretory products and taxonomic composition (Figure 11.1) are examples of its symptoms. These alterations have all been related to physiological abnormalities in a variety of illnesses, including cancer (Yu and Schwabe, 2017, Tilg et al., 2018, Dejea et al., 2018, Kadosh et al., 2020, Ma et al., 2018, Meisel et al., 2018, Verstraelen, 2019, Buchta Rosean et al., 2019, Liu et al., 2020, Parida et al., 2021, Viennois et al., 2022). The role of the microbiota in maintaining health has thus been the subject of extensive research and monetary expenditure. Gut microorganisms create a variety of bioactive chemicals that can have an impact on health; some, like vitamins, are advantageous, while others are detrimental. Host immune responses, including a mucus barrier, assist in preventing potentially hazardous germs from damaging tissues along the intestine. The maintenance of a diverse and healthy population of helpful gut bacteria aids in the prevention of harmful bacteria by competing with them for food and colonization sites. Dietary modifications, especially the use of different fibers, may be one of the most effective methods to maintain a healthy gut microbial community. Probiotics, which are live beneficial bacteria, are one strategy that may help with health maintenance (Conlon and Bird, 2014). In this chapter, we discuss how dietary patterns and lifestyle can affect the function and gut microbiome composition. We also explore the potential of dietary interventions to regulate the gut microbiota and lower the risk of cancer, including Mediterranean, ketogenetic, and paleolithic diets, as well as fermented foods.

THE IMPACT OF DIET ON THE GUT MICROBIOME

Diet is one of the key variables affecting the composition of the gut microbiota (Illiano et al., 2020, Martinez et al., 2021, Weir et al., 2021). Modern diets in developed nations are typically heavier in fatty acids and fat than those of pre-agricultural people (Eaton, 2006, Westman et al., 2007). Low glycemic index foods and dietary fiber intake are also part of this diet (Dedoussis et al., 2007). This "Western diet," which is high in animal protein and saturated fatty acids (SFAs) but low in dietary fiber, is typically preferred by children from the West (US, Europe, and Canada). Unsurprisingly, the gut microbiota of children in Europe is usually rich in Enterobacteriaceae (*Escherichia* and *Shigella*), Firmicutes (*Acetitomaculum* and *Faecalibacterium*), and Gram-negative bacteria, while being depleted in Bacteroides and *Xylanibacter* bacteria, similar to that of children in rural Africa. The consumption of a Western diet also contributes to a fall in the diversity and stability of microorganisms as well as the extinction of various bacterial species (Schnorr et al., 2014), which are signs of unhealthy gut microbiota (Backhed et al., 2005). Children from an African hamlet in Burkina Faso were reported to consume a low-fat and vegetable-rich diet (De Filippo et al., 2010). The Hadza, a group of hunter-gatherers from Tanzania, were reported to have more varied and richer gut flora than urban inhabitants in Italy. The Hadza's gut microbiota contained organisms from the phylum Spirochaetes, the genera *Sphingobacteriales*, *Treponema*, *Anaerophaga*, and *Ruminobacter*, as well as the family *Veillonellaceae*. However, the same taxa were not present in the gut microbiota of the Italian participants. The microbiota of the Italian participants, on the other hand, overexpressed the phyla Firmicutes and Actinobacteria, as well as the genera *Blautia*, *Alistipes*, *Bacteroides*, and *Bifidobacterium* (Schnorr et al., 2014).

Composition of the human gut microbiota has also been discovered to be mediated by other diets. *Actinobacteria*, *Ruminococcus*, *Bacteroidetes* (*Xylanibacterium*, *Prevotella*), *Bifidobacteria*, *Lactobacilli*, *Proteobacteria*, *Blautia*, *Eubacterium rectale*, *Streptococcus*, and *Bifidobacteria* are more prevalent in diets high in digestible and non-digestible fiber as well as plant-derived carbohydrates. Additionally, it raises the Firmicutes:Bacteroides ratio and the variety of microbiota while lowering the proportions of *Enterococcus*, *Firmicutes*, *Eubacterium*, *Bacteroides*, *Clostridium* spp., *Roseburia*, and *Bacteroidaceae*. A vegetarian or vegan diet upregulates the ratio of *Bifidobacterium*, *Lactobacillus*,

Diet, Lifestyle, and the Gut Microbiome

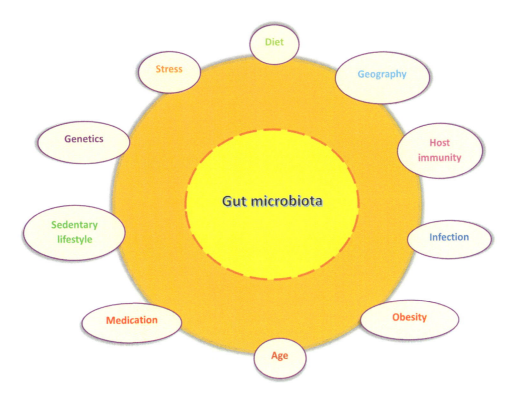

FIGURE 11.1 Several important variables that can affect the taxonomic composition of the gut microbiome and induce gut dysbiosis. These include diet, stress, genetics, age, sedentary lifestyle, and obesity.

Faecalibacterium prausnitzii, *Clostridium clostridio*, and *Bacteroides thetaiotaomicron*, while decreasing the proportions of *Bacteroides fragilis*, *Acteroides* species, *Escherichia coli*, *Clostridium perfringens*, and *Clostridium* cluster XIVa. *Firmicutes*, *Clostridium*, *Bacteroidetes*, and *Prevotella* are more prevalent, whilst *Bacillaceae* and *Proteobacteria* are less prevalent in the Mediterranean diet, which is frequently regarded as the finest diet and comprises a substantial amount of fruits, vegetables, monounsaturated fats, and grains. Lastly, a high-protein diet decreases the proportion of Firmicutes such as *Roseburia*, *Eubacterium rectale*, and *Ruminococcus bromii* and upregulates the proportion of the Bacteroides enterotypes, *Bilophila* and *Alistipes* (Pineiro and Stanton, 2007, Bonder et al., 2016, Singh et al., 2017, Sędzikowska and Szablewski, 2021).

DIETARY COMPONENTS AND THEIR EFFECTS ON THE GUT MICROBIOME

PREBIOTICS

Prebiotics are parts of indigestible foods that benefit the host by favorably mediating the growth and function of one or a few specific colonic bacteria, and thus ameliorating the health of the host (Roberfroid et al., 2010). Instead of being degraded by gastrointestinal enzymes, prebiotics are preferentially fermented by colonic bacteria. Prebiotics include a variety of substances, such as dietary polyphenols, inulin, and oligosaccharides. Inulin is a general term for β (2-1) linear fructans with varying levels of polymerization. Notably, inulin is fermented by colonic bacteria to gases and SCFAs. Different oligosaccharides, including soybean oligosaccharides (SBOSs), fructooligosaccharides (FOSs), and galactooligosaccharides (GOSs), may function as probiotics (Fatima et al., 2017). Inulin-rich vegetables like chicory and Jerusalem artichokes are thought to be prebiotic-rich diets. Beneficial bacterial populations, such as *Bifidobacteria* and *Lactobacilli*, are increased by inulin (Kleessen et al., 2007, Ramnani et al., 2010). Conversely, inulin decreases *Bacteroides* (Kleessen et al., 2007), enterococci (Kleessen et al., 1997), and facultative anaerobes (Brighenti et al., 1999) populations. Inulin has been reported to boost *Faecalibacterium prausnitzii* and *Bifidobacterium* counts in obese women while decreasing *Propionibacterium* and *Bacteroides* counts (Dewulf et al., 2013). In addition to lowering serum LDL-cholesterol and glucose levels, eating yacon syrup—which contains GOS or FOS—has been shown to reduce BMI, body weight, and waist circumference in obese adults (Genta et al., 2009). Prebiotics have been shown in numerous studies to help treat human metabolic conditions (Sędzikowska and Szablewski, 2021).

Prebiotics have also been reported to influence brain processes. The growth of beneficial bacteria like *Eubacterium rectale*, *Roseburia intestinalis*, and *Anaerostipes caccae*—which are known to manufacture butyrate—is aided by the plant polysaccharide arabinoxylan (Van den Abbeele et al., 2011). Plant polyphenols, which are present in significant proportions in vegetables, seeds, fruits, and nuts as well as in

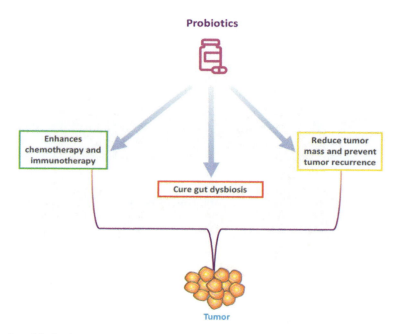

FIGURE 11.2 **The role of probiotics in cancer therapy**. Probiotics have the power to combat dysbiosis, boost the effectiveness of immunotherapy and chemotherapy, lessen tumor mass, and stop cancer recurrence.

beverages and foods including coffee, chocolate, soymilk, and red wine, have also been postulated to have prebiotic qualities. *Lactobacilli* and *Bifidobacteria* counts are increased by polyphenols, whereas *Salmonella typhimurium*, *Bacteroides*, *Staphylococcus aureus*, and *Clostridium* counts are decreased (Cuervo et al., 2014).

Probiotics

Probiotics are considered dietary supplements since they are live microbes given to the host in suitable proportions (Pineiro and Stanton, 2007). Currently, lactic acid bacteria make up the majority of bacterial probiotics sold. These include *Limosilactobacillus reuteri*, *Lactiplantibacillus plantarum*, *Lactiplantibacillus gasseri* and *Lacticaseibacillus paracasei*, *Lactiplantibacillus salivarius*, and *Bifidobacterium*, e.g., *B. lactis* (Pokrzywnicka and Gumprecht, 2016). Probiotics play a role in several processes in both humans and animals, including the immune system, metabolism, illness prevention, and anti-tumorigenic actions (Figure 11.2) (Gomes et al., 2014). Furthermore, probiotics may also affect the restoration of normal brain processes (Liu et al., 2015).

Probiotic consumption affects body weight, according to animal research. The injection of *L. plantarum* decreases adipocyte size in mice (Takemura et al., 2010), *L. paracasei* decreases fat storage (Aronsson et al., 2010), and *L. ingluviei* raises body weight (Angelakis et al., 2012). Treatment with *L. casei/paracasei*, *L. gasseri*, and *L. plantarum* showed a reduction in obesity (Chen et al., 2014a). Probiotic VSL#3 was reported to upregulate the release of GLP-1, a hormone that decreases appetite and consists of eight distinct bacterial strains from the genera *Bifidobacterium* and *Lactobacillus* (Yadav et al., 2013). Furthermore, probiotics were reported to affect mood. Administration of *B. longum* and *L. rhamnosus* in animals was reported to normalize anxiety-like behavior which is triggered by *Trichuris muris* (Bravo et al., 2011). On the other hand, treatment with *Bifidobacterium* and *Lactobacillus* has been shown to lessen anxiety symptoms in humans (Rao et al., 2009). *B. longum* and *Lactobacillus helveticus* treatment for two weeks similarly reduced depression and anxiety symptoms in healthy individuals (Messaoudi et al., 2011). They are also thought to affect the human brain, specifically those areas that manage functions linked to sensation and emotion (Tillisch et al., 2013). They have been reported to reduce BDNF levels and modify GABA levels (Bravo et al., 2011), as well as perform a variety of other activities (Sędzikowska and Szablewski, 2021). It was discovered that probiotic administration lowers LDL-cholesterol, C-reactive protein, plasma triglycerides, and total cholesterol while increasing IL-10, IGA, SCFAs, and HDL-cholesterol levels. The treatment was also associated with insulin sensitivity (Wang et al., 2012, Rajkumar et al., 2014, Foligné et al., 2016). Probiotics boost the abundance of helpful gut bacteria, e.g., *Lactobacilli* and *Bifidobacteria*, while drastically decreasing the counts of enteropathogens, e.g., *H. pylori* and *E. coli* (Liu et al., 2010, Yang and Sheu, 2012).

Antibiotics

The human gut microbiota composition is significantly impacted by antibiotics, with some taxa taking months to recover after treatment (Dethlefsen and Relman, 2011). A five-day antibiotic course could lead the human intestinal microbiota to take up to four weeks to return to a regular state, and some taxa may take up to six months to return to their pre-treatment proportions. The main outcomes of antibiotic treatment are a reduction in the variety and/or abundance of Bacteroides and a reduction in the equilibrium of the population (Dethlefsen et al., 2008). The infant gut microbiota of mothers who received gentamycin and ampicillin within 48 hours of giving birth had greater *Proteobacteria* counts and lower Actinobacteria and the genus *Lactobacillus* counts than infants of mothers who did not receive the medications. The recovery process was still not complete after eight weeks, and the *Proteobacteria* level remained high (Fouhy et al., 2012). Several additional antibiotics have also been discovered to affect the gut microbiome of the infant. For instance, administration of cephalexin decreases *Bifidobacterium* levels while increasing *Enterobacteriaceae* and *Enterococcus* levels (Tanaka et al., 2009), and vancomycin therapy given intravenously for six weeks was seen to change *Lactobacillus* levels (Thuny et al., 2010). The overgrowth of *Clostridium difficile* induced by antibiotic therapy in infants can result in antibiotic-associated diarrhea (McFarland, 2008). Animal studies have supported several of these observations (Yu et al., 2014). Notably, it has been shown that administering antibiotics to animals causes them to have more *Candida albicans* in their GI tracts (Noverr et al., 2005). The microbiota in the human gut is impacted by the drug metformin, which is routinely recommended to people with type 2 diabetes. *Escherichia* counts and serum metformin levels had a positive and negative correlation, respectively (Forslund et al., 2015, Mardinoglu et al., 2016). Moreover, it has been asserted that metformin may benefit patients by elevating butyrate and propionate production levels (Mardinoglu et al., 2016).

DIETARY FAT

A healthy adult human diet must include dietary fat, however, due to its high-calorie content, it should be ingested in moderation. Saturated, unsaturated, and trans fats are the three main forms of fat. Unsaturated fats are sometimes referred to as "good fats" since they have been linked with a reduced risk of heart disease and obesity. Contrarily, saturated and trans fats have the opposite relationship and are utilized in numerous processed foods that are part of the Western diet to ameliorate shelf life, taste, and texture (Waldman et al., 2018). The impact of a high-fat diet (HFD) on the human gut microbiota is less well understood, even though fat has received more research than any other dietary element regarding the development of cancer (Newsome et al., 2023). A randomized, controlled feeding trial on healthy young Chinese adults (18–35 years old; <28 kg/m² BMI) demonstrated that eating extra fat has a deleterious impact on the makeup of the gut microbiota, host biology, and microbial metabolites (Wan et al., 2019, Wan et al., 2020). In this six-month experiment, individuals were given either an HFD (40% fat) or an isocaloric low-fat diet (LFD; 20% fat). The diets differed in their fat-to-carbohydrate ratio, principally because soybean oil was used in place of carbohydrates while having the same amount of protein in each. Neither meal intervention significantly modified the fecal microbiota structure (beta-diversity) from the baseline after six months. However, the LFD improved the Shannon Index for microbiota alpha-diversity and boosted the growth of the genera Faecalibacterium and Blautia, which are known to comprise bacteria that digest complex carbohydrates to synthesize the SCFA butyrate. In contrast, the HFD reduced the relative abundance of *Faecalibacterium* and increased the relative abundance of bacteria like *Lactobacillus*, *Bifidobacterium*, *Clostridium*, *Bacteroides*, and *Alistipes*, the majority of which synthesize bile salt hydrolases (BSH), enzymes that catalyze the hydrolysis of conjugated primary bile acids (BAs). In addition to other metabolites, diets with different fat contents significantly affected BAs and SCFAs, which were linked with changes in certain bacterial taxa. Butyrate levels in particular rose during the LFD while falling during the HFD in terms of fecal SCFA levels. The HFD intervention was found to result in higher levels of secondary BAs like taurodeoxycholic acid (TDCA) and deoxycholic acid (DCA). Based on the composition of the microbiota determined using 16S rRNA gene sequencing, it was predicted that the microbiota connected to HFD would have more proinflammatory genes, such as those involved in the synthesis of lipopolysaccharide (LPS) and the metabolism of arachidonic acid. The increased plasma levels of inflammatory markers like thromboxane B2, C-reactive protein, prostaglandin E2, and leukotriene B4 in individuals following the HFD consistently demonstrated a mild systemic inflammatory response. Notably, unsaturated fatty acids from soybean oil were added to the HFD utilized in the Chinese dietary intervention experiment. This is different from the typical Western diet, which has a lot of saturated fats that are largely derived from animal sources. However, meals high in animal-based fat were linked in studies involving healthy Africans and Americans to similar alterations in microbial activities linked to BA and SCFA metabolism as well as the development of a mild host inflammatory response. (David et al., 2014, O'Keefe et al., 2015). It is crucial to remember that there were diets with low and high fat contents in these two tests (David et al., 2014, O'Keefe et al., 2015), and they also differed significantly in other nutrients like fiber, carbohydrates, minerals, and vitamins, which may induce some of the reported effects on the host and the microbiota. For instance, a reduced intake of complex carbohydrates, which serve as the substrates for bacterial fermentation, is likely a factor in the reduction of SCFAs associated with HFD. All things considered, it seems that increased dietary fat consumption routinely regulated the activities of the gut microbiota, such as reducing SCFA synthesis increasing BA metabolism, and triggering inflammatory reactions in humans (Newsome et al., 2023).

DIETARY FIBERS

The impact of fiber intake on the gut microbiota will vary depending on the type of fiber consumed because dietary fiber has a broad meaning (Holscher, 2017). Dietary fibers (DFs) are carbohydrates that are not absorbed or digested in the human small intestine and have ten or more monomeric units (MUs)

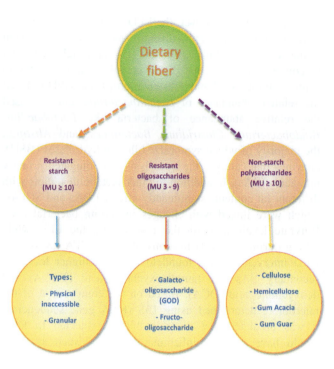

FIGURE 11.3 A schematic diagram showing three types of fibers classified by the number of monomeric units (MUs). These are resistant starch with MU ≥ 10, resistant oligosaccharides with MU 3-9, and lastly non-starch polysaccharides with MU ≥ 10.

but also the beneficial effects of consumption (McRorie and Fahey, 2013). Insoluble fibers like cellulose, are frequently poorly fermented by gut microbes. However, their consumption in the diet accelerates gut transit time, which decreases the amount of time that colonic bacteria have to ferment undigested food (Titgemeyer et al., 1991). Although psyllium is a nonfermentable fiber as well, it has special therapeutic advantages due to its high solubility and viscosity, including better glycemic management and lower blood cholesterol levels (McRorie and Fahey, 2013, McRorie Jr, 2015). Examples of highly fermentable fibers with high levels of viscosity and solubility are pectins and β-glucan (McRorie and Fahey, 2013). Whole grains like barley (β-glucan) and oats, and fruits like apples (pectin) naturally contain these fibers in the diet (Schieber et al., 2001, Elleuch et al., 2011). It is also believed that psyllium, pectin, and β-glucans' physiological benefits which include slower glucose absorption and bile acid binding have an impact on the gut flora. Resistant maltodextrins, inulin, polydextrose, soluble corn fiber, and resistant starch are non-viscous, soluble fibers that are easily digested by GI bacteria (Martínez et al., 2010, Holscher et al., 2015a, Holscher et al., 2015b).

Cholesterol

The average dietary consumption of cholesterol in Western countries has alarmingly increased over the past 20 years and only recently has a daily intake cap been created. Saturated fat and cholesterol are typically ingested together, and foods like processed carbohydrates, high-fat dairy products, and animal meat are particularly rich in cholesterol (Carson et al., 2020). There has not yet been any research on how dietary cholesterol affects the microbiome specifically in humans (Newsome et al., 2023). Nevertheless, recent research revealed that some members of the human gut microbiota can mediate homeostasis of the host cholesterol by metabolically converting cholesterol into coprostanol (Kenny et al., 2020), and cholesterol sulfate (Le et al., 2022, Yao et al., 2022).

Salt

The processed and preserved foods that constitute a significant portion of the Western diet frequently include high salt levels, but the effects of this extra salt consumption on human gut microbiota remain unknown (Newsome et al., 2023). Increased salt consumption from 6 to ~13.8 g NaCl/day for 14 days in a study involving 12 healthy participants removed certain *Lactobacillus* species from the gut (Wilck et al., 2017). Although this experiment was brief and constrained by the small number of participants, salt inhibition of *Lactobacillus* was replicated in various mice investigations. It is yet unknown why excessive dietary salt affects *Lactobacillus* in particular. Reduced *Lactobacillus* (tryptophan metabolizers) was thought to be the cause of the systemic and intestinal inflammatory reactions brought on by a high-salt diet (HSD), which led to a shortage of Th17-inducing indole metabolites (Wilck et al., 2017, Miranda et al., 2018).

(Figure 11.3). This is according to the Codex Alimentarius Commission. DFs fall into the following groups: (1) polymers of consumed carbohydrates that occur spontaneously in food; (2) edible carbohydrate polymers created by physical, enzymatic, or chemical methods from food basic materials and that have been shown through generally accepted scientific research to have beneficial physiological effects; and (3) synthesized edible carbohydrate polymers that have been shown through generally accepted scientific research to have beneficial physiological effects (Committee, 2010). Dietary fibers are classified using a variety of categories since they are heterogeneous. These categories include origin, chemical makeup, and physical characteristics, with further subcategorization based on the level of polymerization (e.g., length of the chain). Notably, each one of these characteristics may affect microbial fermentation. Plant-based fibers can be divided into types that come from cereals and other grains, fruits, legumes, nuts, fruits, and vegetables, as well as other sources (Holscher, 2017). Notably, the fibers found in various plant species will, however, differ in their physicochemical characteristics and chemical compositions (Schieber et al., 2001, Elleuch et al., 2011, McRorie and Fahey, 2013). Bananas, for instance, have resistant starch and fructans of the inulin type, whereas apples have pectin. Therefore, diets high in plant-based foods offer a variety of dietary fibers, supporting a microbiota with a more varied composition (Bourquin et al., 1993, Bourquin et al., 1996).

The viscosity, solubility, and fermentability of fibers are physicochemical features that affect fermentation only,

LIFESTYLE FACTORS AND THE GUT MICROBIOME

STRESS AND SLEEP

Chronic and acute stress have opposing effects on health, ranging from immunosuppression to immune system activation, respectively. Through the brain-gut microbiota axis, stress consequently affects not just the brain but also other systems like the GI tract and the immune system (Cryan and Dinan, 2012). Virus-free mouse models provided the first proof that gut bacteria affect neurological development by showing an accelerated stress response. This study improved our knowledge of the crucial roles that gut microbes play in brain circuits that are involved in motor control, anxiety, and social behavior (Heijtz et al., 2011, Desbonnet et al., 2014). In addition to creating neurotransmitters and SCFAs, gut bacteria additionally promote the synthesis of cytokines from immune cells, subsequently affecting brain activity via the vagus nerve. Similarly, the brain and the hypothalamus-pituitary-adrenal axis both govern the gut microbiota composition (Cryan and Dinan, 2012). Therefore, a stressful stimulus outside the body can affect how the brain and gut microbiota work. Stressful factors can be both physiological and psychological. Extreme physical exercise, such as that involved in military training, can induce physiological stress. This sort of training involves intense exercise as well as dealing with extreme weather (cold or hot), psychological stress, and lack of sleep because of the strict discipline expected by the military. The effects on the GI tract can be severe and include dysbiosis, inflammation, and intestinal barrier permeability damage (Karl et al., 2017). On the other hand, it is well-recognized that lack of sleep induces stress on the body. It induces a disruption in circadian rhythm, which affects the action of various hormones (Garaulet et al., 2013) and gut microbes (Liang and FitzGerald, 2017), as well as an increase in several proinflammatory cytokines, like IL-1 and IL-6 (Li et al., 2017b). Greater proportions of *Erysipelotrichaceae* and *Coriobacteriaceae* have been shown by the scant scientific evidence in healthy individuals, even after a 48-hour sleep restriction (only 4 hours of sleep per day) (Benedict et al., 2016).

Increased performance in cognitive activities and higher concentrations of bacteria from the *Lentisphaerae* phyla and Verrucomicrobia have both been linked to enhanced sleep quality. The specific mechanisms underlying how sleep affects the gut microbiota are as yet unknown. However, identification of microbial metabolites interacting with the brain-gut microbiota axis may shed light on this matter (Redondo-Useros et al., 2020). For instance, different bacterial species can synthesize important neurotransmitters that play a role in the process of sleep (Yunes et al., 2016, Valles-Colomer et al., 2019), for instance, serotonin and γ-aminobutyric acid (GABA) (Gottesmann, 2002, Ursin, 2002).

In terms of psychological stress, mental illnesses like depression share a high frequency of intestinal problems like irritable bowel syndrome (IBS) (Skonieczna-Żydecka et al., 2018), and the efficacy of certain probiotic strains in alleviating anxiety and stress symptoms (dubbed psychobiotics) has confirmed the strong link between the brain and the gut microbiota in illness conditions. (Taylor et al., 2020a). Depression and anxiety are signs of personality and mood problems, which have also been associated with worsening GI symptoms and modifications in the gut flora of healthy people. One study, for example, discovered a sex-dependent link between nutrition, gut microbiome, and mental problems. *Lactobacillus* was shown to be inversely associated with male depression levels, whilst *Bifidobacterium* was found to be inversely related to female anxiety levels (Taylor et al., 2020a). Notably, due to their abilities to improve mood and their beneficial effects on the brain-gut microbiota axis, the species of *Bifidobacterium* spp. and *Lactobacillus* spp. are regarded as psychobiotic species (Sarkar et al., 2016). According to the Kim et al. study, which discovered an association between *Gammaproteobacteria* and *Peptostreptococcaceae* and neuroticism, which is a personality trait linked to an elevated risk of anxiety disorders, *Peptostreptococcaceae* levels also increased along with anxiety symptoms. Furthermore, Proteobacteria levels and low conscientiousness were positively associated (Kim et al., 2018). However, because these studies are cross-sectional, it is challenging to establish a causal connection. Negative emotions have impacts on health that go beyond the GI tract. This is according to a study by Sutin and colleagues who discovered a link between chronic inflammation, neuroticism, low conscientiousness, and the activation of the hypothalamic-pituitary-adrenocortical (HPA) axis (Sutin et al., 2010). Furthermore, given the accumulating data pointing to a sex-specific pattern in the brain and gut microbiota interactions, it is necessary to create adequate interventional studies utilizing appropriate mental health surveys, psychological therapy, and metagenomic techniques (Audet, 2019) and the fact that emotional conditions are sharply rising (Baxter et al., 2013). This is to identify the precise mechanisms at play and to enhance the lives of men and women who appear to be in good health but have severe emotional anguish (Redondo-Useros et al., 2020).

EXERCISE

An increased risk of various affluent diseases, such as obesity, diabetes, asthma, and cardiovascular disease (CVD), is linked to a sedentary lifestyle, which is a key contributor to morbidity in developed Western cultures (Biswas et al., 2015, Same et al., 2016, Wilmot et al., 2012, Chen et al., 2014b). There is recent data that suggests the gut microbiota has a significant impact on these disorders (Koeth et al., 2013, Tang et al., 2013, Tang and Hazen, 2017, Woting et al., 2014, Utzschneider et al., 2016, Turnbaugh et al., 2006, Williams et al., 2016, Wang et al., 2011, Zhernakova et al., 2016). Conversely, exercise has been found to improve human health, which is likely due in major part to the regulation of the gut microbiota composition (Redondo-Useros et al., 2020). The microbiota composition of rugby players is healthier in comparison to inactive people. Rugby players particularly have higher levels of Akkermansia and α-diversity. Protein consumption and values of α-diversity were associated, demonstrating that both diet and exercise have a significant effect on the gut microbiota makeup (Clarke et al., 2014). Similarly, compared to sedentary women, active women showed greater numbers of several beneficial bacteria (*Roseburia hominis*, *F. prausnitzii A*, and *Muciniphila*) (Bressa et al., 2017). However, dietary patterns can have a greater effect on intestinal microbiota compared to exercise. Nevertheless, there has not been much research on how exercise affects it alone. As a result, Cronin and colleagues investigated how the microbiota of inactive people changed after an 8-week intervention that included moderate exercise and protein dietary supplements. The primary finding implied that moderate exercise has no impact on untrained individuals because neither the variety of bacteria nor the concentrations of the bacterial taxa under study changed (Cronin et al., 2018). These findings contradict what was previously reported in subjects who were physically active, indicating that the degree of exercise has a different impact on the gut microbiota. As a result of years of optimal nutrition and an increased level of physical fitness over time, elite athletes do indeed appear to have a gut microbiota that supports metabolism (Cronin et al., 2017). One way that moderate exercise may alter gut microbes is by decreasing the degree of intestinal permeability (IP), maintaining mucosal thickness, reducing the pace of bacterial translocation, as well as increasing the synthesis of antimicrobial proteins like defensins (Luo et al., 2014). However, other researchers have suggested the existence of a muscle-microbiota axis because muscles include TLR-4 and TLR-5 receptors, which can be triggered by circulating LPS from gut bacteria and cause the muscle to create inflammatory cytokines. Additionally, as evidenced by the greater levels of butyrate, which helps to regulate lipids, cholesterol, and glucose in the muscle, moderate physical activity can alter bacterial functioning. Additionally, moderate exercise can increase levels of specific lymphocyte populations and gut IgA, decrease intestinal transit time, and do all of these things at the same time, all of which may affect the gut microbiota composition (Luo et al., 2014).

TOBACCO CONSUMPTION

Although tobacco consumption does not seem to have an impact on the gut microbiota, there is evidence that smokers with Crohn's disease demonstrated reduced bacterial diversity and lower levels of *Enterorhabdus*, *Gordonibacter*, and *Collinsella* in contrast to non-smokers, which casts doubt on the possibility that smoking and microbiota are connected (Opstelten et al., 2016). In addition, quitting smoking for eight weeks can change the gut microbiota of healthy people who smoke. Furthermore, it raises bacterial diversity and the proportions of Firmicutes and Actinobacteria while lowering those of Proteobacteria and Bacteroidetes. The small sample size and the presence of additional possible factors that were not controlled may have limited the strength of these results, even though dietary intake was under control and was not linked with changes in the microbiome. Although the processes linking tobacco smoking to modifications in the gut microbiota are poorly understood, potential linked routes include changes in mucosal immunity and IP (Biedermann et al., 2013). The upsurge in the use of tobacco from early life, combined with the commonly known negative effects of tobacco on the course of intestinal disorders (Berkowitz et al., 2018), makes this an essential subject of research about the microbiome (Redondo-Useros et al., 2020).

ALCOHOL CONSUMPTION

Alcohol has known negative effects on health (Redondo-Useros et al., 2020). Alcohol misuse is linked to several inflammatory illnesses, including mental, intestinal, and liver disorders (Erol and Karpyak, 2015, Sæther et al., 2019). The increase in gut dysbiosis is one of the hypothesized mechanisms correlating alcohol consumption to the formation of inflammatory diseases. The gut microbiota of alcoholics differs from healthy controls by having higher amounts of Proteobacteria and lower levels of Bacteroidetes (Mutlu et al., 2012). Increased proinflammatory cytokines and plasma endotoxin (LPS) representing intestinal barrier disruption, are other characteristics of alcoholic patients (Mutlu et al., 2012, Tsuruya et al., 2016). Leclercq and colleagues demonstrated that IP facilitates interactions between the lamina propia's immune cells and the lumen gut microbiota. In return, this enabled the emergence of either proinflammatory or anti-inflammatory responses (Leclercq et al., 2014). In comparison to alcoholics with reduced IP and healthy controls, alcoholic individuals with high permeability demonstrated significant reductions in the overall bacterial levels and the *Ruminococcaceae* family as well as increased concentrations of *Blautia* and *Lachnospiraceae*. Alcoholics who were still drinking and those who had been sober for more than a month were both included in the dysbiotic group, indicating that dysbiosis is sustained throughout time. Additionally, *Ruminococcaceae* species, *Bifidobacterium*, and *Lactobacillus* increased following alcohol abstinence. This indicated their potential roles in IP recovery. The authors proposed that gut proteolytic fermentation metabolites, including indolic compounds, branched-chain FAs, and potentially hazardous metabolites including sulfur-containing and phenolic compounds, may be the result of inflammation and failure of the gut barrier (Leclercq et al., 2014).

DIETARY INTERVENTIONS FOR MODULATING THE GUT MICROBIOME AND REDUCING CANCER RISK

MEDITERRANEAN DIET

The Mediterranean diet (MD) is a dietary pattern followed by many populations residing in the Mediterranean Basin (Klement and Pazienza, 2019). The MD enhances general health status and lowers the risk of non-communicable diseases (NCDs), in addition to being acknowledged by UNESCO as a cultural treasure of humanity (Martinez-Lacoba et al., 2018). The MD characteristics comprise the following components: (i) high intake of nuts, seeds, legumes, fruits, vegetables, and cereals

TABLE 11.1
Nutritional features of a typical Mediterranean diet

Ingredients	Consumption frequency
Seeds, nuts, honey, dry fruits	Regular basis (typically as snacks)
Poultry (chicken, eggs)	Low to moderate
Processed and red meats	Very low
Wine	Low to moderate (occasionally, especially with evening meals)
Various fresh salads, vegetables, and fruits	Daily basis (seasonal varieties)
Various minimally processed or unprocessed legumes, cereals, and whole grains	Regular staple
Minimally processed or unprocessed yogurt and cheese	Low to moderate
Seafood (seaweeds, oysters, fish)	Low to moderate
Fish oil; extra-virgin olive oil	The main source of fat rich in mono- and poly-SFAs; low in saturated fat

(mainly whole grains); (ii) reduced intake of meat, sweets, and saturated fats; (iii) large consumption of unsaturated fat, especially from olive oil; (iv) moderate wine consumption; and (v) medium-low consumption of dairy items, mostly cheese and yogurt (Table 11.1) (Del Chierico et al., 2014, Ostan et al., 2015). Since a low consumption of SFAs and a high consumption of poly- and monounsaturated fatty acids have been linked to reduced inflammatory signaling (Wisniewski et al., 2019), and a high consumption of microbiota-accessible carbohydrates with the synthesis of SCDAs, features (i)–(iii) are thus regarded as key features for the prevention of NCDs via microbiota effects, since low consumption of SFAs and high consumption of poly- and monounsaturated fatty acids were linked to a lower inflammatory signaling (Wisniewski et al., 2019), and high consumption of microbiota-accessible carbohydrates was linked to the synthesis of SCFAs.

Higher fecal levels of SCFA were consistently discovered in individuals who adhered more closely to the MD. This was in particular with the intake of legumes, fruits, and vegetables, and independent from the overall dietary character (omnivore, vegetarian, or vegan) (Garcia-Mantrana et al., 2018; Trajkovska Petkoska and Trajkovska-Broach, 2021). The microbial features in individuals following the MD are therefore believed to prevent carcinogenesis. This is in addition to other mechanisms like high micronutrient and polyphenol consumption (Ostan et al., 2015). Interestingly, just after two weeks of consuming a low-fiber (12 g/day) and a high-fat (52% energy) Western diet, the prevalence of the *Fusobacterium nucleatum*—common in human colorectal carcinomas and linked with their development—was reported to increase (O'Keefe et al., 2015).

The MD pattern does, however, seem to have cancer-preventing properties outside of the gut. Data from the EPIC research study demonstrated that the MD is linked to a 33% lower risk of gastric cancer (Bamia et al., 2013). According to findings from the MOLI-SANI trial, circulating inflammatory markers like leukocytes, platelet counts, C-reactive protein (CRP), and granulocyte/lymphocyte ratio were shown to be lower (Bonaccio et al., 2017). The granulocyte/lymphocyte ratio particularly serves as an independent predictor of tumorigenesis, progression, and metastasis. Additionally, it was linked to a worse prognosis in cancer (Reuter et al., 2010). Shivley and colleagues recently demonstrated that eating the MD for 31 months induced a change in the microbiome of female monkeys' mammary glands, particularly with a ten-fold increase in *Lactobacillus* levels in comparison to monkeys fed a Western diet. This change was also followed by an increase in breast bile acid metabolites and a reduction in reactive oxygen species (ROS) metabolites (Shively et al., 2018). This study shows that altering the local microbiota by dietary choices can reduce the chance of carcinogenesis in organs other than the gut. In summary, the MD pattern is linked to favorable microbiome-related characteristics inside and outside the gut, and therefore it might serve as a preventative strategy against NCDs, such as cancer (Klement and Pazienza, 2019).

KETOGENIC DIET

Ketogenic diets (KDs) are a specific kind of low-carbohydrate diet in which the amount of carbohydrates is reduced to such a degree (about 50 g/day) that the resulting low insulin concentrations and modestly high cortisol levels trigger the liver to produce ketone bodies (Klement and Pazienza, 2019). KDs may support metabolic health and protection against cancer and other NCDs via a variety of methods, including: (i) reduction of insulin levels; (ii) increasing the oxidation of the substrate in the mitochondria, which leads to a slight persistent increase in the generation of ROS in the mitochondria and a hormetic anti-oxidative adaptation; and (iii) specific anti-inflammatory and anti-oxidative properties of the HDACi ketone body β-hydroxybutyrate (Miller et al., 2018). Nevertheless, there is no evidence that KD can support a healthy microbiota and gut metabolome. It may be plausible that high consumption of non-starchy vegetables, monounsaturated fatty acids, and n-3 PUFAs would be advantageous for improving gut health in cancer prevention (Klement and Pazienza, 2019). A composition like this might be typical, for example, of the Spanish Mediterranean KD (Pérez-Guisado et al., 2008). Furthermore, because butyrate and β-hydroxybutyrate are structurally and functionally similar, increased systemic quantities of the latter may reduce the relevance of microbial butyrate synthesis (Klement and Pazienza, 2019).

KDs have been demonstrated to reduce cancer cell glycolysis and proliferation in most preclinical tumor models. Additionally, certain discoveries have also shown the transfer of such anti-tumor properties to patients (Klement, 2017, Weber et al., 2018). However, the microbiota's potential function in mediating the anti-tumor effects of KDs has yet to be studied. Notably, no research has been conducted yet into the possibility that the microbiota might be involved in modulating the anti-tumor effects of KDs (Klement and Pazienza, 2019). Given the findings of recent research showing a significant function for the gut microbiota in reducing the symptoms of three major neurological disorders, namely; infantile refractory epilepsy (Xie et al., 2017), autism (Newell et al., 2016), and multiple sclerosis (Swidsinski et al., 2017), such a role seems plausible. KD dramatically raised the Firmicutes/Bacteroidetes ratio, which is normally low in autism spectrum disorder. It also regulated the excess of the mucin-degrading bacterium *A. muciniphila* in the BTBRT$^{+tf/j}$ mouse model of autism spectrum condition (Newell et al., 2016). KD initially reduced overall gut bacterial concentrations in multiple sclerosis patients during the first few weeks. However, when kept up for six months, it was able to bring the microbial fermentative mass back to levels comparable to those in healthy controls (Swidsinski et al., 2017). Lastly, KD considerably altered the gut microbiota composition toward that of healthy controls in infants with refractory epilepsy. This led to a majority of cases of decreased seizure frequency: *Bacteroides* and *Prevotella* levels escalated, but *Cronobacter* levels declined by almost 50% (Xie et al., 2017). All three studies show that KD can reverse the dysbiosis linked to a variety of neurological diseases. It remains to be seen if cancer patients can likewise experience such beneficial outcomes (Klement and Pazienza, 2019).

Paleolithic Diet

Evolutionary medicine offers a framework for the conventional explanation for the rise in NCDs, which holds that a poor adaptation to the modern lifestyle results in disease. Within this framework, diet is crucial, and the phrase "Paleolithic diet" or "Paleo diet" (PD) was used to describe a contemporary diet that resembles the Old Stone Age diet of our predecessors, which historically covers the majority of human life (Lemke et al., 2016). PD of the modern era usually comprises the following features: (i) high fruits, vegetables, spices, and herbs consumption; (ii) moderate-to-high intake of fish, eggs, lean meats, and organs; (iii) minimal consumption of seeds and nuts; (iv) absence of all grains, processed foods, dairy items, legumes, and plant oils (except coconut and olive oil), as well as nightshades in some PD variations. The latter attribute (iv) differentiates the PD from the majority of other dietary patterns and may contribute to the PD's superiority over other "healthy" diets, including the MD, in small randomized studies (Spreadbury, 2012, Manheimer et al., 2015). Notably, legumes and grains have been linked to intestinal barrier disruption and the promotion of auto-immune and inflammatory and auto-immune NCDs such as obesity and cancer (Carrera-Bastos et al., 2011, Spreadbury, 2012, De Punder and Pruimboom, 2013). Indeed, there are various regimens for treating auto-immune disorders that are based on PD and also focus on the exclusion of specific food groups that are common in the Western diet (Lee et al., 2017, Konijeti et al., 2017). A PD also ensures that microbiota-accessible carbohydrates are consumed at a high rate, which is expected to improve the diversity of the gut microbiome (Wahls, 2018). Indeed, the microbiome of the Hadza hunter-gatherers from Tanzania, who still eat foods that would have been available to early humans in Africa during the Paleolithic era, has been proven to be far more diversified than that of metropolitan Italians. In particular, Firmicutes (72 ± 1.9%) and Bacteroidetes (17 ± 1.1%) dominated at the phylum level, followed by Proteobacteria (6 ± 1.2%) and Spirochaetes (3 ± 0.9%), which were substantially enriched in contrast to Italians (Schnorr et al., 2014). Nevertheless, the evolutionary viewpoint would also imply that the Hadza microbiota is tailored to their way of life as equatorial hunter-gatherers. On the other hand, populations farther from the equator, such as those in Europe, would have a different "optimal" ancestral microbiome. This is because the diets of non-equatorial hunter-gatherers are lower in fiber and carbohydrates (Ruscio, 2017). A recent study looked at healthy Italians who had been on a contemporary PD for more than a year. Firmicutes (65.1 ± 2.1%) and Bacteroidetes (24.6 ± 2.2%) were the two most prevalent phyla in the gut microbiome, followed by Proteobacteria (4.4 ± 1.6%), Actinobacteria (3.4 ± 0.8%), and Verrucomicrobia (1.2 ± 0.5%). Lachnospiraceae, Ruminococcaceae, Prevotellaceae, and Bacteroidaceae were the most prevalent bacteria at the family level, whereas *Faecalibacterium*, *Bacteroides*, and *Pervotella* dominated at the genus level (Barone et al., 2019). The microbiome diversity from the PD was significantly higher and equivalent to that of Hadza hunter-gatherers when compared to Italians who followed the MD. This study is significant as it demonstrates how switching back to a contemporary PD devoid of grains, refined sugar, dairy, and other processed foods might help reverse microbiome diversity loss in Western nations. Future clinical research looking at PDs as a possible anti-inflammatory adjuvant to cancer therapy would be interesting given their link with increased microbiome diversity and their suspected anti-inflammatory characteristics (Klement and Pazienza, 2019). The effectiveness of a ketogenic variant of a PD against tumorigenesis was recently illustrated by many case reports published by a Hungarian group (Tóth and Clemens, 2016, Tóth and Clemens, 2017, Tóth et al., 2018), highlighting the potential of this strategy (Klement and Pazienza, 2019).

LOW-CARBOHYDRATE DIET

Another dietary option associated with weight loss and ameliorated health markers is limiting carbohydrates (Sackner-Bernstein et al., 2015). From an evolutionary perspective, a low-carbohydrate diet (<40% of energy) would have been usual and would have prevented hyperglycemia and hyperinsulinemia, both of which raise the risk of cancer (Fine, 2013). The percentage of several bacterial phyla was unaffected by a low-carbohydrate, high-protein diet for weight loss in overweight individuals, however, *E. rectale* and *Collinsella aerofaciens* relatives were dramatically reduced (Walker et al., 2011). Conversely, diets with high levels of complex carbohydrates upregulated levels of beneficial Bifidobacteria like the subspecies *Bifidobacterium breve*, *Bifidobacterium longum*, and *Bifidobacterium thetaiotaomicron*. It also decreased the expansion of opportunistic species, such as *Enterobacteriaceae* and *Mycobacterium avium* subspecies *paratuberculosis* (Pokusaeva et al., 2011).

On the other hand, a condition known as "carbotoxicity" is known to result from consuming an excessive amount of refined sugar, which has harmful consequences on human health (Kroemer et al., 2018), enhancing bile production to promote the growth of harmful bacteria like *Clostridium perfringens* and *Clostridium decile* (Berg et al., 2012). Furthermore, evidence points to the possibility that sugar molecules control the microbiota. This results in the establishment of a Westernized microbiome characterized by a significant loss of diversity in the gut microbiome (Payne et al., 2012, Segata, 2015). It is commonly known that tumor cells primarily obtain their energy from glycolysis and glucose and that dietary sugar can increase the risk of tumorigenesis (Healy et al., 2016). A novel method to reduce cardiotoxicity is to substitute resistant starch for digestible carbohydrates. In a pancreatic cancer mouse model, resistant starch reduced tumor growth and altered the composition of the microbiota. It did this by stimulating the growth of proinflammation-fighting bacteria while suppressing the growth of anti-inflammatory ones. In particular, proinflammatory microorganisms like *Bacteroides acidifaciens*, *Clostridium cocleatum*, *Escherichia coli*, and *Ruminococcus gnavus* significantly decreased in pancreatic cancer-bearing mice fed a high-fiber diet, while butyrate-producing bacteria like *Lachnospiraceae* increased. These results suggest that, assuming a causal mechanism connecting microbiota to carcinogenesis, customized dietary patterns with a beneficial effect on the gut microbial communities can function in combination with traditional anti-cancer medications (Panebianco et al., 2017).

FERMENTED FOODS

Foods produced through beneficial microbial growth and enzymatic food component transformations are referred to as fermented meals and beverages by the International Scientific Association for Probiotics and Prebiotics (ISAPP) (Marco et al., 2021). Some examples of foods that have gone through fermentation and encompass living organisms include sour cream, kimchi, most cheeses, yogurt, sauerkraut, natto, kombucha, miso, some beers, kefir, and unheated (raw) fermented sausages (like salami). Fermented foods frequently have a high concentration of living microorganisms when served raw and have a long history of being suitable for consumption (Marco et al., 2021). Substantial amounts of live lactic acid bacteria (LAB) can be consumed through fermented foods such as cheeses and yogurt, which are necessary for the development of fermented meals. A thorough genome-wide analysis of 9445 human fecal sample metagenomes revealed that the frequency of LAB species was frequently low and linked with lifestyle, age, and location (Pasolli et al., 2020). Similar LAB strains have been found in food and gut microbiomes, suggesting that fermented foods might be the main source of the LAB located in the microbiome. Even though fermented foods include living bacteria that reach the gut microbiota alive (Dal Bello et al., 2003), it is critical to emphasize that they are unlikely to survive and have a significant impact on the microbial population as a whole because they are not adapted to the gut (Walter et al., 2018). As a result, it is believed that the metabolites synthesized by these species, which are abundant in fermented foods, are the active components that provide any beneficial effects (Taylor et al., 2020b).

Although the microorganisms found in fermented foods are unlikely to have a significant effect on the formation of the gut microbiome, there is growing evidence suggesting that they can alter the host together with its immune system. In a 17-week randomized prospective study (n = 18) in which participants increased their baseline average consumption of fermented foods from 0.4 ± 0.6 to 6.3 ± 2.9 servings/day, it was discovered that a diet high in fermented foods steadily increased the diversity of the gut microbiome. It also downregulated inflammatory markers in the blood (Wastyk et al., 2021). Yogurt intake was linked with a higher relative abundance of organisms used as yogurt starters (*Bifidobacterium animalis* subsp. *lactis* and *Streptococcus thermophilus*) in individuals who had ameliorated metabolic health as measured by lower visceral fat. (Le Roy et al., 2022). Milk fermentation byproducts like branched chain hydroxy acids (BCHA) are abundant in yogurt (Daniel et al., 2022). According to recent studies in mice, giving the equivalent of two servings of yogurt daily prevented hepatic steatosis and insulin resistance in cases of diet-induced obesity. Changes in the composition of the gut microbiome and the maintenance of BCHA levels—which are typically decreased in diet-induced obesity—both had an impact on this. (Daniel et al., 2022). Despite the conflicting and limited evidence to the contrary, fermented foods are a culturally acceptable and safe route for live microbes to briefly reside and travel through the human alimentary canal, thus impacting the immune system. Due to their low pH and distinct preparation mechanisms, which expose consumers to microbe species that are not usually in the food chain, fermented foods may have health benefits (Hitch et al., 2022).

FASTING

Fasting is a pattern of dieting that involves abstinence from any solid food for a set amount of time. It has been followed for millennia, mostly as a religious observance, and unintentionally for millions of years during the evolution of humans, influencing human metabolic flexibility in the process (Freese et al., 2017). Scientists support fasting diets because of the related health benefits, which go beyond weight loss (Mattson et al., 2014). Several studies have shown that fasting, temporary calorie restriction, or protein-restricted meals had positive effects on mice models of specific forms of cancer (Brandhorst et al., 2013, Fontana et al., 2013, Panebianco et al., 2017) as well as reducing side effects of chemotherapy on patients (Safdie et al., 2009, Brandhorst et al., 2013). The gut microbiota is certainly one of the key mechanisms through which fasting produces metabolic benefits. For instance, every-other-day fasting (EODF) therapy altered the gut microbiota composition compared to control mice given access to food at will, increasing the amounts of Firmicutes while reducing the majority of other phyla and, subsequently, increasing SCFA synthesis (Li et al., 2017a).

Fasting boosts mitochondrial uncoupling in colon cancer models. It also induces an anti-Warburg effect, which raises oxygen intake but lowers ATP generation (Bianchi et al., 2015). Fasting ameliorates tumor-bearing survival and it is safe, feasible, and well tolerated. This is shown by the fact that most mice had smaller tumors compared to controls when combined with standard treatments (temozolomide, gemcitabine) (Safdie et al., 2012, Panebianco et al., 2017). Withholding food lowers the quantity of possibly harmful Proteobacteria while raising the levels of *Akkermansia muciniphila* (Zheng et al., 2018). Patients with metastatic melanoma who also have high *A. muciniphila* prevalence respond well to anti-PD1 therapy. These findings highlight the significance of the microbiota in immunotherapy (Matson et al., 2018).

Nevertheless, fasting can exacerbate cachexia syndrome, a disease that affects around 50% of cancer patients. In one study, colon cancer-bearing mice predisposed to cachexia were given *Lactobacillus reuteri* in drinking water. This was to test the hypothesis that changing the gut microbiota could decrease cachexia. It was previously reported that administering prebiotics and probiotics ameliorates therapeutic responses and reduces toxic side effects (Yoo and Kim, 2016). In comparison with animals not receiving *L. reuteri* supplementation, the body weight and mass of the gastrocnemius muscles were both raised. Moreover, neutrophil levels, a sign of systemic inflammation, were also decreased in these mice (Varian et al., 2016).

CHALLENGES AND LIMITATIONS OF DIETARY INTERVENTIONS FOR MODULATING THE GUT MICROBIOME AND REDUCING CANCER RISK

Although several pre-clinical mouse models have shown how nutrition influences the generation of microbe metabolites and how these may affect the host immune system and cancer, translating this knowledge to people is difficult. Genetic variation, geographical distance, gut composition of the microbiome, and dietary compliance variations are obstacles that induce heterogeneous responses in human interventional trials. These factors are frequently absent in genetically and environmentally engineered mice. More crucially, studies on high-salt diets utilizing concentrations far higher than those found in a Western diet show that many dietary regimens delivered to mice are not physiologically applicable to humans. The most substantial evidence for a connection between food and the development of cancer comes from interventional trials that involved modifying single, strictly regulated components while also keeping an eye on changes in the microbiota and downstream metabolites (Newsome et al., 2023). Despite sharing some traits with a Western diet, such as being high in fat, a healthy diet like the MD affects the microbiota and produces bioactivities that may help reduce the occurrence of cancer (Schwingshackl and Hoffmann, 2016, Mentella et al., 2019, Nagpal et al., 2019). Fecal analyses are commonly used in studies on the effects of diet, although they have the intrinsic limitation of not taking into consideration regional variations in the GI tract's microbial-derived nutrition metabolism, such as those in the ileum, ascending/descending colon, cecum, etc. In the past, tumor research has primarily focused on the proximal vs. distal colon, which is still a narrow range. In contrast, human dietary studies rarely use healthy tissue biopsies. The geography of the digestive tract may be partially captured by tissue biopsy. The impact of dietary modifications on the microbial and nutritional profiles along the digestive tract must be investigated in future research. Additionally, dietary regimens in the case of carcinogenesis and progression can vary. This depends on whether the microbiota is present or absent in extraintestinal sites of carcinogenesis, therefore this should also be investigated (Newsome et al., 2023).

CONCLUSION AND FUTURE PERSPECTIVES

This chapter aimed to give a thorough overview of how dietary patterns, and to a lesser extent, lifestyle can have crucial and far-reaching effects on human health. It also showed how these effects are significantly modulated by the gut microorganisms that live in the GI tract. Despite recent considerable advances in the comprehension of the complexity of gut microbial communities, additional research is required to determine the precise roles played by microorganisms in maintaining (or adversely affecting) the integrity of tissues both outside and within the gut. To achieve the required changes in microbial communities, products, and health consequences, it is also necessary to determine which dietary components serve as substrates for the microorganisms. The process of determining what makes up a healthy population of gut microorganisms will be particularly difficult. There may be links between specific microbial population profiles and certain diseases and disorders. It is frequently difficult to determine what causes these profiles, whether diet, genetic predisposition, environmental/lifestyle factors, or modified microbial populations are to blame for the illness. Although dietary modifications can have a substantial influence, sometimes they will not be enough to transform the microbial populations in a way that promotes improved health. It might be necessary to utilize probiotics and other techniques. Early detection and prevention of the appearance of hazardous microbial profiles and their effects may be possible. The starting point is understanding the ontogenesis of the gut microbial population profiles and how this influences the immune system development. In this regard, it will be crucial to identify the variables that control how our human microbial communities evolve in infancy (Conlon and Bird, 2014).

Dietary habits discussed in this chapter show promise for preventing cancer and enhancing general health. By mediating an eubiotic microbiota, these effects are at least partially regulated. Evidence exists that supports the fact that such dietary microbiome manipulation may have beneficial synergistic effects during cancer treatment. Though equivalent at the phylum level, the microbiota of mice used in much of the research in this area so far is unique at lower taxonomic levels. Therefore, clinical research is warranted to support the function of microbiome regulation in cancer treatment that these animal data suggest. However, the "fast food culture" in industrialized nations is characterized by the Western diet, high sugar levels, processed foods, and low in fiber. Additionally, it has a strong association with dysbiosis, microbial diversity loss, and an elevated risk of cancer, cardiovascular disease, metabolic syndrome, and obesity. There is substantial evidence that promote a new food culture centered on restricting dietary excess and favoring locally grown fresh and natural foods would be beneficial for each individual's microbiota. Even though eubiosis may be highly dependent on a person's environment, it can be challenging to ascertain general microbial composition (Klement and Pazienza, 2019).

REFERENCES

ADAK, A. & KHAN, M. R. 2019. An insight into gut microbiota and its functionalities. *Cellular and Molecular Life Sciences,* 76, 473–493.

ANGELAKIS, E., BASTELICA, D., AMARA, A. B., EL FILALI, A., DUTOUR, A., MEGE, J.-L., ALESSI, M.-C. & RAOULT, D. 2012. An evaluation of the effects of Lactobacillus ingluviei on body weight, the intestinal microbiome, and metabolism in mice. *Microbial Pathogenesis,* 52, 61–68.

ARONSSON, L., HUANG, Y., PARINI, P., KORACH-ANDRÉ, M., HÅKANSSON, J., GUSTAFSSON, J.-Å., PETTERSSON, S., ARULAMPALAM, V. & RAFTER, J. 2010. Decreased fat storage by Lactobacillus paracasei is associated with increased levels of angiopoietin-like 4 protein (ANGPTL4). *PloS One,* 5, e13087.

AUDET, M.-C. 2019. Stress-induced disturbances along the gut microbiota-immune-brain axis and implications for mental health: Does sex matter? *Frontiers in Neuroendocrinology,* 54, 100772.

BACKHED, F., LEY, R. E., SONNENBURG, J. L., PETERSON, D. A. & GORDON, J. I. 2005. Host-bacterial mutualism in the human intestine. *Science,* 307, 1915–1920.

BAMIA, C., LAGIOU, P., BUCKLAND, G., GRIONI, S., AGNOLI, C., TAYLOR, A. J., DAHM, C. C., OVERVAD, K., OLSEN, A. & TJØNNELAND, A. 2013. Mediterranean diet and colorectal cancer risk: Results from a European cohort. *European Journal of Epidemiology,* 28, 317–328.

BARONE, M., TURRONI, S., RAMPELLI, S., SOVERINI, M., D'AMICO, F., BIAGI, E., BRIGIDI, P., TROIANI, E. & CANDELA, M. 2019. Gut microbiome response to a modern Paleolithic diet in a Western lifestyle context. *PLoS One,* 14, e0220619.

BAXTER, A. J., SCOTT, K. M., VOS, T. & WHITEFORD, H. A. 2013. Global prevalence of anxiety disorders: A systematic review and meta-regression. *Psychological Medicine,* 43, 897–910.

BENEDICT, C., VOGEL, H., JONAS, W., WOTING, A., BLAUT, M., SCHÜRMANN, A. & CEDERNAES, J. 2016. Gut microbiota and glucometabolic alterations in response to recurrent partial sleep deprivation in normal-weight young individuals. *Molecular Metabolism,* 5, 1175–1186.

BERG, A. M., KELLY, C. P. & FARRAYE, F. A. 2012. Clostridium difficile infection in the inflammatory bowel disease patient. *Inflammatory Bowel Diseases,* 19, 194–204.

BERKOWITZ, L., SCHULTZ, B. M., SALAZAR, G. A., PARDO-ROA, C., SEBASTIÁN, V. P., ÁLVAREZ-LOBOS, M. M. & BUENO, S. M. 2018. Impact of cigarette smoking on the gastrointestinal tract inflammation: Opposing effects in Crohn's disease and ulcerative colitis. *Frontiers in Immunology,* 9, 74.

BIANCHI, G., MARTELLA, R., RAVERA, S., MARINI, C., CAPITANIO, S., ORENGO, A., EMIONITE, L., LAVARELLO, C., AMARO, A. & PETRETTO, A. 2015. Fasting induces anti-Warburg effect that increases respiration but reduces ATP-synthesis to promote apoptosis in colon cancer models. *Oncotarget,* 6, 11806.

BIEDERMANN, L., ZEITZ, J., MWINYI, J., SUTTER-MINDER, E., REHMAN, A., OTT, S. J., STEURER-STEY, C., FREI, A., FREI, P. & SCHARL, M. 2013. Smoking cessation induces profound changes in the composition of the intestinal microbiota in humans. *PloS One,* 8, e59260.

BISWAS, A., OH, P. I., FAULKNER, G. E., BAJAJ, R. R., SILVER, M. A., MITCHELL, M. S. & ALTER, D. A. 2015. Sedentary time and its association with risk for disease incidence, mortality, and hospitalization in adults: A systematic review and meta-analysis. *Annals of Internal Medicine,* 162, 123–132.

BONACCIO, M., POUNIS, G., CERLETTI, C., DONATI, M. B., IACOVIELLO, L., DE GAETANO, G. & INVESTIGATORS, M. S. S. 2017. Mediterranean diet, dietary polyphenols and low grade inflammation: Results from the MOLI-SANI study. *British Journal of Clinical Pharmacology,* 83, 107–113.

BONDER, M. J., TIGCHELAAR, E. F., CAI, X., TRYNKA, G., CENIT, M. C., HRDLICKOVA, B., ZHONG, H., VATANEN, T., GEVERS, D. & WIJMENGA, C. 2016. The influence of a short-term gluten-free diet on the human gut microbiome. *Genome Medicine,* 8, 1–11.

BOURQUIN, L. D., TITGEMEYER, E. C. & FAHEY JR, G. C. 1993. Vegetable fiber fermentation by human fecal bacteria: Cell wall polysaccharide disappearance and short-chain fatty acid production during in vitro fermentation and water-holding capacity of unfermented residues. *The Journal of Nutrition,* 123, 860–869.

BOURQUIN, L. D., TITGEMEYER, E. C. & FAHEY JR, G. C. 1996. Fermentation of various dietary fiber sources by human fecal bacteria. *Nutrition Research*, 16, 1119–1131.

BRANDHORST, S., WEI, M., HWANG, S., MORGAN, T. E. & LONGO, V. D. 2013. Short-term calorie and protein restriction provide partial protection from chemotoxicity but do not delay glioma progression. *Experimental Gerontology*, 48, 1120–1128.

BRAVO, J. A., FORSYTHE, P., CHEW, M. V., ESCARAVAGE, E., SAVIGNAC, H. M., DINAN, T. G., BIENENSTOCK, J. & CRYAN, J. F. 2011. Ingestion of Lactobacillus strain regulates emotional behavior and central GABA receptor expression in a mouse via the vagus nerve. *Proceedings of the National Academy of Sciences*, 108, 16050–16055.

BRESSA, C., BAILÉN-ANDRINO, M., PÉREZ-SANTIAGO, J., GONZÁLEZ-SOLTERO, R., PÉREZ, M., MONTALVO-LOMINCHAR, M. G., MATÉ-MUÑOZ, J. L., DOMÍNGUEZ, R., MORENO, D. & LARROSA, M. 2017. Differences in gut microbiota profile between women with active lifestyle and sedentary women. *PloS One*, 12, e0171352.

BRIGHENTI, F., CASIRAGHI, M., CANZI, E. & FERRARI, A. 1999. Effect of consumption of a ready-to-eat breakfast cereal containing inulin on the intestinal milieu and blood lipids in healthy male volunteers. *European Journal of Clinical Nutrition*, 53, 726–733.

BUCHTA ROSEAN, C., BOSTIC, R. R., FEREY, J. C., FENG, T.-Y., AZAR, F. N., TUNG, K. S., DOZMOROV, M. G., SMIRNOVA, E., BOS, P. D. & RUTKOWSKI, M. R. 2019. Preexisting commensal dysbiosis is a host-intrinsic regulator of tissue inflammation and tumor cell dissemination in hormone receptor–positive breast cancer. *Cancer Research*, 79, 3662–3675.

CAHENZLI, J., KÖLLER, Y., WYSS, M., GEUKING, M. B. & MCCOY, K. D. 2013. Intestinal microbial diversity during early-life colonization shapes long-term IgE levels. *Cell Host & Microbe*, 14, 559–570.

CARRERA-BASTOS, P., FONTES-VILLALBA, M., O'KEEFE, J. H., LINDEBERG, S. & CORDAIN, L. 2011. The western diet and lifestyle and diseases of civilization. *Research Reports in Clinical Cardiology*, 15–35.

CARSON, J. A. S., LICHTENSTEIN, A. H., ANDERSON, C. A., APPEL, L. J., KRIS-ETHERTON, P. M., MEYER, K. A., PETERSEN, K., POLONSKY, T. & VAN HORN, L. 2020. Dietary cholesterol and cardiovascular risk: A science advisory from the American Heart Association. *Circulation*, 141, e39–e53.

CHEN, D., YANG, Z., CHEN, X., HUANG, Y., YIN, B., GUO, F., ZHAO, H., ZHAO, T., QU, H. & HUANG, J. 2014a. The effect of Lactobacillus rhamnosus hsryfm 1301 on the intestinal microbiota of a hyperlipidemic rat model. *BMC Complementary and Alternative Medicine*, 14, 1–9.

CHEN, Y.-C., TU, Y.-K., HUANG, K.-C., CHEN, P.-C., CHU, D.-C. & LEE, Y. L. 2014b. Pathway from central obesity to childhood asthma. Physical fitness and sedentary time are leading factors. *American Journal of Respiratory and Critical Care Medicine*, 189, 1194–1203.

CLARKE, S. F., MURPHY, E. F., O'SULLIVAN, O., LUCEY, A. J., HUMPHREYS, M., HOGAN, A., HAYES, P., O'REILLY, M., JEFFERY, I. B. & WOOD-MARTIN, R. 2014. Exercise and associated dietary extremes impact on gut microbial diversity. *Gut*, 63, 1913–1920.

COMMITTEE, C. A. 2010. *Guidelines on Nutrition Labelling CAC/GL 2-1985 as Last Amended 2010*. Joint FAO/WHO Food Standards Programme, Secretariat of the Codex Alimentarius Commission. Rome, Italy: FAO.

CONLON, M. A. & BIRD, A. R. 2014. The impact of diet and lifestyle on gut microbiota and human health. *Nutrients*, 7, 17–44.

CRONIN, O., BARTON, W., SKUSE, P., PENNEY, N. C., GARCIA-PEREZ, I., MURPHY, E. F., WOODS, T., NUGENT, H., FANNING, A. & MELGAR, S. 2018. A prospective metagenomic and metabolomic analysis of the impact of exercise and/or whey protein supplementation on the gut microbiome of sedentary adults. *MSystems*, 3, e00044–18.

CRONIN, O., O'SULLIVAN, O., BARTON, W., COTTER, P. D., MOLLOY, M. G. & SHANAHAN, F. 2017. *Gut Microbiota: Implications for Sports and Exercise Medicine*. BMJ Publishing Group Ltd and British Association of Sport and Exercise Medicine.

CRYAN, J. F. & DINAN, T. G. 2012. Mind-altering microorganisms: The impact of the gut microbiota on brain and behaviour. *Nature Reviews Neuroscience*, 13, 701–712.

CUERVO, A., VALDÉS, L., SALAZAR, N., DE LOS REYES-GAVILAN, C. G., RUAS-MADIEDO, P., GUEIMONDE, M. & GONZALEZ, S. 2014. Pilot study of diet and microbiota: Interactive associations of fibers and polyphenols with human intestinal bacteria. *Journal of Agricultural and Food Chemistry*, 62, 5330–5336.

CUMMINGS, J. 1983. Fermentation in the human large intestine: Evidence and implications for health. *The Lancet*, 321, 1206–1209.

DAL BELLO, F., WALTER, J., HAMMES, W. & HERTEL, C. 2003. Increased complexity of the species composition of lactic acid bacteria in human feces revealed by alternative incubation condition. *Microbial Ecology*, 455–463.

DANIEL, N., NACHBAR, R. T., TRAN, T. T. T., OUELLETTE, A., VARIN, T. V., COTILLARD, A., QUINQUIS, L., GAGNÉ, A., ST-PIERRE, P. & TROTTIER, J. 2022. Gut microbiota and fermentation-derived branched chain hydroxy acids mediate health benefits of yogurt consumption in obese mice. *Nature Communications*, 13, 1343.

DAVID, L. A., MAURICE, C. F., CARMODY, R. N., GOOTENBERG, D. B., BUTTON, J. E., WOLFE, B. E., LING, A. V., DEVLIN, A. S., VARMA, Y. & FISCHBACH, M. A. 2014. Diet rapidly and reproducibly alters the human gut microbiome. *Nature*, 505, 559–563.

DE FILIPPO, C., CAVALIERI, D., DI PAOLA, M., RAMAZZOTTI, M., POULLET, J. B., MASSART, S., COLLINI, S., PIERACCINI, G. & LIONETTI, P. 2010. Impact of diet in shaping gut microbiota revealed by a comparative study in children from Europe and rural Africa. *Proceedings of the National Academy of Sciences*, 107, 14691–14696.

DE PUNDER, K. & PRUIMBOOM, L. 2013. The dietary intake of wheat and other cereal grains and their role in inflammation. *Nutrients*, 5, 771–787.

DEDOUSSIS, G. V., KALIORA, A. C. & PANAGIOTAKOS, D. B. 2007. Genes, diet and type 2 diabetes mellitus: A review. *The Review of Diabetic Studies*, 4, 13.

DEJEA, C. M., FATHI, P., CRAIG, J. M., BOLEIJ, A., TADDESE, R., GEIS, A. L., WU, X., DESTEFANO SHIELDS, C. E., HECHENBLEIKNER, E. M. & HUSO, D. L. 2018. Patients with familial adenomatous polyposis harbor colonic biofilms containing tumorigenic bacteria. *Science*, 359, 592–597.

DEL CHIERICO, F., VERNOCCHI, P., DALLAPICCOLA, B. & PUTIGNANI, L. 2014. Mediterranean diet and health: Food effects on gut microbiota and disease control. *International Journal of Molecular Sciences*, 15, 11678–11699.

DESBONNET, L., CLARKE, G., SHANAHAN, F., DINAN, T. G. & CRYAN, J. 2014. Microbiota is essential for social development in the mouse. *Molecular Psychiatry*, 19, 146–148.

DETHLEFSEN, L. & RELMAN, D. A. 2011. Incomplete recovery and individualized responses of the human distal gut microbiota to repeated antibiotic perturbation. *Proceedings of the National Academy of Sciences*, 108, 4554–4561.

DETHLEFSEN, L., HUSE, S., SOGIN, M. L. & RELMAN, D. A. 2008. The pervasive effects of an antibiotic on the human gut microbiota, as revealed by deep 16S rRNA sequencing. *PLoS Biology*, 6, e280.

DEWULF, E. M., CANI, P. D., CLAUS, S. P., FUENTES, S., PUYLAERT, P. G., NEYRINCK, A. M., BINDELS, L. B., DE VOS, W. M., GIBSON, G. R. & THISSEN, J.-P. 2013. Insight into the prebiotic concept: Lessons from an exploratory, double blind intervention study with inulin-type fructans in obese women. *Gut*, 62, 1112–1121.

EATON, S. B. 2006. The ancestral human diet: What was it and should it be a paradigm for contemporary nutrition? *Proceedings of the Nutrition Society*, 65, 1–6.

ELLEUCH, M., BEDIGIAN, D., ROISEUX, O., BESBES, S., BLECKER, C. & ATTIA, H. 2011. Dietary fibre and fibre-rich by-products of food processing: Characterisation, technological functionality and commercial applications: A review. *Food Chemistry*, 124, 411–421.

EROL, A. & KARPYAK, V. M. 2015. Sex and gender-related differences in alcohol use and its consequences: Contemporary knowledge and future research considerations. *Drug and Alcohol Dependence*, 156, 1–13.

FATIMA, N., AKHTAR, T. & SHEIKH, N. 2017. Prebiotics: A novel approach to treat hepatocellular carcinoma. *Canadian Journal of Gastroenterology and Hepatology*, 2017, 6238106.

FINE, E. J. 2013. An evolutionary and mechanistic perspective on dietary carbohydrate restriction in cancer prevention. *Journal of Evolution and Health: A Joint Publication of the Ancestral Health Society and the Society for Evolutionary Medicine and Health*, 1.

FOLIGNÉ, B., PARAYRE, S., CHEDDANI, R., FAMELART, M.-H., MADEC, M.-N., PLÉ, C., BRETON, J., DEWULF, J., JAN, G. & DEUTSCH, S.-M. 2016. Immunomodulation properties of multi-species fermented milks. *Food Microbiology*, 53, 60–69.

FONTANA, L., ADELAIYE, R. M., RASTELLI, A. L., MILES, K. M., CIAMPORCERO, E., LONGO, V. D., NGUYEN, H., VESSELLA, R. & PILI, R. 2013. Dietary protein restriction inhibits tumor growth in human xenograft models of prostate and breast cancer. *Oncotarget*, 4, 2451.

FORSLUND, K., HILDEBRAND, F., NIELSEN, T., FALONY, G., LE CHATELIER, E., SUNAGAWA, S., PRIFTI, E., VIEIRA-SILVA, S., GUDMUNDSDOTTIR, V. & KROGH PEDERSEN, H. 2015. Disentangling type 2 diabetes and metformin treatment signatures in the human gut microbiota. *Nature*, 528, 262–266.

FOUHY, F., GUINANE, C. M., HUSSEY, S., WALL, R., RYAN, C. A., DEMPSEY, E. M., MURPHY, B., ROSS, R. P., FITZGERALD, G. F. & STANTON, C. 2012. High-throughput sequencing reveals the incomplete, short-term recovery of infant gut microbiota following parenteral antibiotic treatment with ampicillin and gentamicin. *Antimicrobial Agents and Chemotherapy*, 56, 5811–5820.

FREESE, J., KLEMENT, R. J., RUIZ-NÚÑEZ, B., SCHWARZ, S. & LÖTZERICH, H. 2017. The sedentary (r) evolution: Have we lost our metabolic flexibility? *F1000Research*, 6, 1787.

GARAULET, M., GÓMEZ-ABELLÁN, P., ALBURQUERQUE-BÉJAR, J. J., LEE, Y.-C., ORDOVÁS, J. M. & SCHEER, F. A. 2013. Timing of food intake predicts weight loss effectiveness. *International Journal of Obesity*, 37, 604–611.

GARCIA-MANTRANA, I., SELMA-ROYO, M., ALCANTARA, C. & COLLADO, M. C. 2018. Shifts on gut microbiota associated to mediterranean diet adherence and specific dietary intakes on general adult population. *Frontiers in microbiology*, 9, 890.

GENSOLLEN, T., IYER, S. S., KASPER, D. L. & BLUMBERG, R. S. 2016. How colonization by microbiota in early life shapes the immune system. *Science*, 352, 539–544.

GENTA, S., CABRERA, W., HABIB, N., PONS, J., CARILLO, I. M., GRAU, A. & SÁNCHEZ, S. 2009. Yacon syrup: Beneficial effects on obesity and insulin resistance in humans. *Clinical Nutrition*, 28, 182–187.

GOMES, A. C., BUENO, A. A., DE SOUZA, R. G. M. & MOTA, J. F. 2014. Gut microbiota, probiotics and diabetes. *Nutrition Journal*, 13, 1–13.

GOTTESMANN, C. 2002. GABA mechanisms and sleep. *Neuroscience*, 111, 231–239.

HEALY, M. E., LAHIRI, S., HARGETT, S. R., CHOW, J. D., BYRNE, F. L., BREEN, D. S., KENWOOD, B. M., TADDEO, E. P., LACKNER, C. & CALDWELL, S. H. 2016. Dietary sugar intake increases liver tumor incidence in female mice. *Scientific Reports*, 6, 22292.

HEIJTZ, R. D., WANG, S., ANUAR, F., QIAN, Y., BJÖRKHOLM, B., SAMUELSSON, A., HIBBERD, M. L., FORSSBERG, H. & PETTERSSON, S. 2011. Normal gut microbiota modulates brain development and behavior. *Proceedings of the National Academy of Sciences*, 108, 3047–3052.

HITCH, T. C., HALL, L. J., WALSH, S. K., LEVENTHAL, G. E., SLACK, E., DE WOUTERS, T., WALTER, J. & CLAVEL, T. 2022. Microbiome-based interventions to modulate gut ecology and the immune system. *Mucosal Immunology*, 15, 1095–1113.

HOLSCHER, H. D. 2017. Dietary fiber and prebiotics and the gastrointestinal microbiota. *Gut Microbes*, 8, 172–184.

HOLSCHER, H. D., BAUER, L. L., GOURINENI, V., PELKMAN, C. L., FAHEY JR, G. C. & SWANSON, K. S. 2015a. Agave inulin supplementation affects the fecal microbiota of healthy adults participating in a randomized, double-blind, placebo-controlled, crossover trial. *The Journal of Nutrition*, 145, 2025–2032.

HOLSCHER, H. D., CAPORASO, J. G., HOODA, S., BRULC, J. M., FAHEY JR, G. C. & SWANSON, K. S. 2015b. Fiber supplementation influences phylogenetic structure and functional capacity of the human intestinal microbiome: Follow-up of a randomized controlled trial. *The American Journal of Clinical Nutrition*, 101, 55–64.

ILLIANO, P., BRAMBILLA, R. & PAROLINI, C. 2020. The mutual interplay of gut microbiota, diet and human disease. *The FEBS Journal*, 287, 833–855.

KADOSH, E., SNIR-ALKALAY, I., VENKATACHALAM, A., MAY, S., LASRY, A., ELYADA, E., ZINGER, A., SHAHAM,

M., VAALANI, G. & MERNBERGER, M. 2020. The gut microbiome switches mutant p53 from tumour-suppressive to oncogenic. *Nature,* 586, 133–138.

KARL, J. P., MARGOLIS, L. M., MADSLIEN, E. H., MURPHY, N. E., CASTELLANI, J. W., GUNDERSEN, Y., HOKE, A. V., LEVANGIE, M. W., KUMAR, R. & CHAKRABORTY, N. 2017. Changes in intestinal microbiota composition and metabolism coincide with increased intestinal permeability in young adults under prolonged physiological stress. *American Journal of Physiology-Gastrointestinal and Liver Physiology,* 312, G559-G571.

KENNY, D. J., PLICHTA, D. R., SHUNGIN, D., KOPPEL, N., HALL, A. B., FU, B., VASAN, R. S., SHAW, S. Y., VLAMAKIS, H. & BALSKUS, E. P. 2020. Cholesterol metabolism by uncultured human gut bacteria influences host cholesterol level. *Cell Host & Microbe,* 28, 245–257.e6.

KIM, H.-N., YUN, Y., RYU, S., CHANG, Y., KWON, M.-J., CHO, J., SHIN, H. & KIM, H.-L. 2018. Correlation between gut microbiota and personality in adults: A cross-sectional study. *Brain, Behavior, and Immunity,* 69, 374–385.

KLEESSEN, B., SCHWARZ, S., BOEHM, A., FUHRMANN, H., RICHTER, A., HENLE, T. & KRUEGER, M. 2007. Jerusalem artichoke and chicory inulin in bakery products affect faecal microbiota of healthy volunteers. *British Journal of Nutrition,* 98, 540–549.

KLEESSEN, B., SYKURA, B., ZUNFT, H.-J. & BLAUT, M. 1997. Effects of inulin and lactose on fecal microflora, microbial activity, and bowel habit in elderly constipated persons. *The American Journal of Clinical Nutrition,* 65, 1397–1402.

KLEMENT, R. J. & PAZIENZA, V. 2019. Impact of different types of diet on gut microbiota profiles and cancer prevention and treatment. *Medicina,* 55, 84.

KLEMENT, R. J. 2017. Beneficial effects of ketogenic diets for cancer patients: A realist review with focus on evidence and confirmation. *Medical Oncology,* 34, 1–15.

KOETH, R. A., WANG, Z., LEVISON, B. S., BUFFA, J. A., ORG, E., SHEEHY, B. T., BRITT, E. B., FU, X., WU, Y. & LI, L. 2013. Intestinal microbiota metabolism of L-carnitine, a nutrient in red meat, promotes atherosclerosis. *Nature Medicine,* 19, 576–585.

KONIJETI, G. G., KIM, N., LEWIS, J. D., GROVEN, S., CHANDRASEKARAN, A., GRANDHE, S., DIAMANT, C., SINGH, E., OLIVEIRA, G. & WANG, X. 2017. Efficacy of the autoimmune protocol diet for inflammatory bowel disease. *Inflammatory Bowel Diseases,* 23, 2054–2060.

KOVATCHEVA-DATCHARY, P., NILSSON, A., AKRAMI, R., LEE, Y. S., DE VADDER, F., ARORA, T., HALLEN, A., MARTENS, E., BJÖRCK, I. & BÄCKHED, F. 2015. Dietary fiber-induced improvement in glucose metabolism is associated with increased abundance of Prevotella. *Cell Metabolism,* 22, 971–982.

KROEMER, G., LÓPEZ-OTÍN, C., MADEO, F. & DE CABO, R. 2018. Carbotoxicity—noxious effects of carbohydrates. *Cell,* 175, 605–614.

LE ROY, C. I., KURILSHIKOV, A., LEEMING, E. R., VISCONTI, A., BOWYER, R. C., MENNI, C., FALCHI, M., KOUTNIKOVA, H., VEIGA, P. & ZHERNAKOVA, A. 2022. Yoghurt consumption is associated with changes in the composition of the human gut microbiome and metabolome. *BMC Microbiology,* 22, 1–12.

LE, H. H., LEE, M.-T., BESLER, K. R., COMRIE, J. M. & JOHNSON, E. L. 2022. Characterization of interactions of dietary cholesterol with the murine and human gut microbiome. *Nature Microbiology,* 7, 1390–1403.

LECLERCQ, S., MATAMOROS, S., CANI, P. D., NEYRINCK, A. M., JAMAR, F., STÄRKEL, P., WINDEY, K., TREMAROLI, V., BÄCKHED, F. & VERBEKE, K. 2014. Intestinal permeability, gut-bacterial dysbiosis, and behavioral markers of alcohol-dependence severity. *Proceedings of the National Academy of Sciences,* 111, E4485–E4493.

LEE, J. E., BISHT, B., HALL, M. J., RUBENSTEIN, L. M., LOUISON, R., KLEIN, D. T. & WAHLS, T. L. 2017. A multimodal, nonpharmacologic intervention improves mood and cognitive function in people with multiple sclerosis. *Journal of the American College of Nutrition,* 36, 150–168.

LEMKE, D., KLEMENT, R., PAUL, S. & SPITZ, J. 2016. Die Paläoernährung und ihr Stellenwert für die Prävention und Behandlung chronischer Krankheiten. *Aktuelle Ernährungsmedizin,* 41, 437–449.

LI, G., XIE, C., LU, S., NICHOLS, R. G., TIAN, Y., LI, L., PATEL, D., MA, Y., BROCKER, C. N. & YAN, T. 2017a. Intermittent fasting promotes white adipose browning and decreases obesity by shaping the gut microbiota. *Cell Metabolism,* 26, 672–685. e4.

LI, H.-L., LU, L., WANG, X.-S., QIN, L.-Y., WANG, P., QIU, S.-P., WU, H., HUANG, F., ZHANG, B.-B. & SHI, H.-L. 2017b. Alteration of gut microbiota and inflammatory cytokine/chemokine profiles in 5-fluorouracil induced intestinal mucositis. *Frontiers in Cellular and Infection Microbiology,* 7, 455.

LIANG, X. & FITZGERALD, G. A. 2017. Timing the microbes: The circadian rhythm of the gut microbiome. *Journal of Biological Rhythms,* 32, 505–515.

LIU, J.-E., ZHANG, Y., ZHANG, J., DONG, P.-L., CHEN, M. & DUAN, Z.-P. 2010. Probiotic yogurt effects on intestinal flora of patients with chronic liver disease. *Nursing Research,* 59, 426–432.

LIU, N.-N., MA, Q., GE, Y., YI, C.-X., WEI, L.-Q., TAN, J.-C., CHU, Q., LI, J.-Q., ZHANG, P. & WANG, H. 2020. Microbiome dysbiosis in lung cancer: From composition to therapy. *NPJ Precision Oncology,* 4, 33.

LIU, X., CAO, S. & ZHANG, X. 2015. Modulation of gut microbiota–brain axis by probiotics, prebiotics, and diet. *Journal of Agricultural and Food Chemistry,* 63, 7885–7895.

LUO, B., XIANG, D., NIEMAN, D. C. & CHEN, P. 2014. The effects of moderate exercise on chronic stress-induced intestinal barrier dysfunction and antimicrobial defense. *Brain, Behavior, and Immunity,* 39, 99–106.

MA, C., HAN, M., HEINRICH, B., FU, Q., ZHANG, Q., SANDHU, M., AGDASHIAN, D., TERABE, M., BERZOFSKY, J. A. & FAKO, V. 2018. Gut microbiome–mediated bile acid metabolism regulates liver cancer via NKT cells. *Science,* 360, eaan5931.

MANHEIMER, E. W., VAN ZUUREN, E. J., FEDOROWICZ, Z. & PIJL, H. 2015. Paleolithic nutrition for metabolic syndrome: Systematic review and meta-analysis. *The American Journal of Clinical Nutrition,* 102, 922–932.

MARCO, M. L., SANDERS, M. E., GÄNZLE, M., ARRIETA, M. C., COTTER, P. D., DE VUYST, L., HILL, C., HOLZAPFEL, W., LEBEER, S. & MERENSTEIN, D. 2021. The International Scientific Association for Probiotics and Prebiotics (ISAPP) consensus statement on fermented foods. *Nature Reviews Gastroenterology & Hepatology,* 18, 196–208.

MARDINOGLU, A., BOREN, J. & SMITH, U. 2016. Confounding effects of metformin on the human gut microbiome in type 2 diabetes. *Cell Metabolism*, 23, 10–12.

MARTÍNEZ, I., KIM, J., DUFFY, P. R., SCHLEGEL, V. L. & WALTER, J. 2010. Resistant starches types 2 and 4 have differential effects on the composition of the fecal microbiota in human subjects. *PloS One*, 5, e15046.

MARTINEZ, J. E., KAHANA, D. D., GHUMAN, S., WILSON, H. P., WILSON, J., KIM, S. C., LAGISHETTY, V., JACOBS, J. P., SINHA-HIKIM, A. P. & FRIEDMAN, T. C. 2021. Unhealthy lifestyle and gut dysbiosis: A better understanding of the effects of poor diet and nicotine on the intestinal microbiome. *Frontiers in Endocrinology*, 12, 667066.

MARTINEZ-GURYN, K., LEONE, V. & CHANG, E. B. 2019. Regional diversity of the gastrointestinal microbiome. *Cell Host & Microbe*, 26, 314–324.

MARTINEZ-LACOBA, R., PARDO-GARCIA, I., AMO-SAUS, E. & ESCRIBANO-SOTOS, F. 2018. Mediterranean diet and health outcomes: A systematic meta-review. *European Journal of Public Health*, 28, 955–961.

MATSON, V., FESSLER, J., BAO, R., CHONGSUWAT, T., ZHA, Y., ALEGRE, M.-L., LUKE, J. J. & GAJEWSKI, T. F. 2018. The commensal microbiome is associated with anti–PD-1 efficacy in metastatic melanoma patients. *Science*, 359, 104–108.

MATTSON, M. P., ALLISON, D. B., FONTANA, L., HARVIE, M., LONGO, V. D., MALAISSE, W. J., MOSLEY, M., NOTTERPEK, L., RAVUSSIN, E. & SCHEER, F. A. 2014. Meal frequency and timing in health and disease. *Proceedings of the National Academy of Sciences*, 111, 16647–16653.

MCFARLAND, L. V. 2008. Antibiotic-associated diarrhea: epidemiology, trends and treatment. *Future Microbiology*, 3, 563–578.

MCNEIL, N. 1984. The contribution of the large intestine to energy supplies in man. *The American Journal of Clinical Nutrition*, 39, 338–342.

MCRORIE JR, J. 2015. Psyllium is not fermented in the human gut. *Neurogastroenterology and Motility: The Official Journal of the European Gastrointestinal Motility Society*, 27, 1681–1682.

MCRORIE, J. W. & FAHEY, G. C. 2013. A review of gastrointestinal physiology and the mechanisms underlying the health benefits of dietary fiber: Matching an effective fiber with specific patient needs. *Clinical Nursing Studies*, 1, 82–92.

MEISEL, M., HINTERLEITNER, R., PACIS, A., CHEN, L., EARLEY, Z. M., MAYASSI, T., PIERRE, J. F., ERNEST, J. D., GALIPEAU, H. J. & THUILLE, N. 2018. Microbial signals drive pre-leukaemic myeloproliferation in a Tet2-deficient host. *Nature*, 557, 580–584.

MENTELLA, M. C., SCALDAFERRI, F., RICCI, C., GASBARRINI, A. & MIGGIANO, G. A. D. 2019. Cancer and mediterranean diet: A review. *Nutrients*, 11, 2059.

MESSAOUDI, M., LALONDE, R., VIOLLE, N., JAVELOT, H., DESOR, D., NEJDI, A., BISSON, J.-F., ROUGEOT, C., PICHELIN, M. & CAZAUBIEL, M. 2011. Assessment of psychotropic-like properties of a probiotic formulation (Lactobacillus helveticus R0052 and Bifidobacterium longum R0175) in rats and human subjects. *British Journal of Nutrition*, 105, 755–764.

MILLER, V. J., VILLAMENA, F. A. & VOLEK, J. S. 2018. Nutritional ketosis and mitohormesis: Potential implications for mitochondrial function and human health. *Journal of Nutrition and Metabolism*, 2018, 5157645.

MIRANDA, P. M., DE PALMA, G., SERKIS, V., LU, J., LOUIS-AUGUSTE, M. P., MCCARVILLE, J. L., VERDU, E. F., COLLINS, S. M. & BERCIK, P. 2018. High salt diet exacerbates colitis in mice by decreasing Lactobacillus levels and butyrate production. *Microbiome*, 6, 1–17.

MUTLU, E. A., GILLEVET, P. M., RANGWALA, H., SIKAROODI, M., NAQVI, A., ENGEN, P. A., KWASNY, M., LAU, C. K. & KESHAVARZIAN, A. 2012. Colonic microbiome is altered in alcoholism. *American Journal of Physiology-Gastrointestinal and Liver Physiology*, 302, G966–G978.

NAGPAL, R., SHIVELY, C. A., REGISTER, T. C., CRAFT, S. & YADAV, H. 2019. Gut microbiome-Mediterranean diet interactions in improving host health. *F1000Research*, 8, 699.

NEWELL, C., BOMHOF, M. R., REIMER, R. A., HITTEL, D. S., RHO, J. M. & SHEARER, J. 2016. Ketogenic diet modifies the gut microbiota in a murine model of autism spectrum disorder. *Molecular Autism*, 7, 1–6.

NEWSOME, R., YANG, Y. & JOBIN, C. Western diet influences on microbiome and carcinogenesis. Seminars in Immunology, 2023, Elsevier, 101756.

NOVERR, M. C., FALKOWSKI, N. R., MCDONALD, R. A., MCKENZIE, A. N. & HUFFNAGLE, G. B. 2005. Development of allergic airway disease in mice following antibiotic therapy and fungal microbiota increase: Role of host genetics, antigen, and interleukin-13. *Infection and Immunity*, 73, 30–38.

O'KEEFE, S. J., LI, J. V., LAHTI, L., OU, J., CARBONERO, F., MOHAMMED, K., POSMA, J. M., KINROSS, J., WAHL, E. & RUDER, E. 2015. Fat, fibre and cancer risk in African Americans and rural Africans. *Nature Communications*, 6, 1–14.

OPSTELTEN, J. L., PLASSAIS, J., VAN MIL, S. W., ACHOURI, E., PICHAUD, M., SIERSEMA, P. D., OLDENBURG, B. & CERVINO, A. C. 2016. Gut microbial diversity is reduced in smokers with Crohn's disease. *Inflammatory Bowel Diseases*, 22, 2070–2077.

OSTAN, R., LANZARINI, C., PINI, E., SCURTI, M., VIANELLO, D., BERTARELLI, C., FABBRI, C., IZZI, M., PALMAS, G. & BIONDI, F. 2015. Inflammaging and cancer: A challenge for the Mediterranean diet. *Nutrients*, 7, 2589–2621.

PANEBIANCO, C., ADAMBERG, K., ADAMBERG, S., SARACINO, C., JAAGURA, M., KOLK, K., DI CHIO, A. G., GRAZIANO, P., VILU, R. & PAZIENZA, V. 2017. Engineered resistant-starch (ERS) diet shapes colon microbiota profile in parallel with the retardation of tumor growth in in vitro and in vivo pancreatic cancer models. *Nutrients*, 9, 331.

PARIDA, S., WU, S., SIDDHARTH, S., WANG, G., MUNIRAJ, N., NAGALINGAM, A., HUM, C., MISTRIOTIS, P., HAO, H. & TALBOT JR, C. C. 2021. A procarcinogenic colon microbe promotes breast tumorigenesis and metastatic progression and concomitantly activates notch and β-catenin axes. *Cancer Discovery*, 11, 1138–1157.

PASOLLI, E., DE FILIPPIS, F., MAURIELLO, I. E., CUMBO, F., WALSH, A. M., LEECH, J., COTTER, P. D., SEGATA, N. & ERCOLINI, D. 2020. Large-scale genome-wide analysis links lactic acid bacteria from food with the gut microbiome. *Nature Communications*, 11, 2610.

PAYNE, A., CHASSARD, C. & LACROIX, C. 2012. Gut microbial adaptation to dietary consumption of fructose, artificial sweeteners and sugar alcohols: Implications for host–microbe interactions contributing to obesity. *Obesity Reviews*, 13, 799–809.

PÉREZ-GUISADO, J., MUÑOZ-SERRANO, A. & ALONSO-MORAGA, Á. 2008. Spanish Ketogenic Mediterranean Diet: A healthy cardiovascular diet for weight loss. *Nutrition Journal*, 7, 1–7.

PINEIRO, M. & STANTON, C. 2007. Probiotic bacteria: legislative framework—requirements to evidence basis. *The Journal of Nutrition*, 137, 850S–853S.

POKRZYWNICKA, P. & GUMPRECHT, J. 2016. Intestinal microbiota and its relationship with diabetes and obesity. *Clinical Diabetology*, 5, 164–172.

POKUSAEVA, K., FITZGERALD, G. F. & VAN SINDEREN, D. 2011. Carbohydrate metabolism in Bifidobacteria. *Genes & Nutrition*, 6, 285–306.

RAJKUMAR, H., MAHMOOD, N., KUMAR, M., VARIKUTI, S. R., CHALLA, H. R. & MYAKALA, S. P. 2014. Effect of probiotic (VSL# 3) and omega-3 on lipid profile, insulin sensitivity, inflammatory markers, and gut colonization in overweight adults: A randomized, controlled trial. *Mediators of Inflammation*, 2014, 348959.

RAMNANI, P., GAUDIER, E., BINGHAM, M., VAN BRUGGEN, P., TUOHY, K. M. & GIBSON, G. R. 2010. Prebiotic effect of fruit and vegetable shots containing Jerusalem artichoke inulin: A human intervention study. *British Journal of Nutrition*, 104, 233–240.

RAO, A. V., BESTED, A. C., BEAULNE, T. M., KATZMAN, M. A., IORIO, C., BERARDI, J. M. & LOGAN, A. C. 2009. A randomized, double-blind, placebo-controlled pilot study of a probiotic in emotional symptoms of chronic fatigue syndrome. *Gut Pathogens*, 1, 1–6.

REDONDO-USEROS, N., NOVA, E., GONZÁLEZ-ZANCADA, N., DÍAZ, L. E., GÓMEZ-MARTÍNEZ, S. & MARCOS, A. 2020. Microbiota and lifestyle: A special focus on diet. *Nutrients*, 12, 1776.

REUTER, S., GUPTA, S. C., CHATURVEDI, M. M. & AGGARWAL, B. B. 2010. Oxidative stress, inflammation, and cancer: How are they linked? *Free Radical Biology and Medicine*, 49, 1603–1616.

ROBERFROID, M., GIBSON, G. R., HOYLES, L., MCCARTNEY, A. L., RASTALL, R., ROWLAND, I., WOLVERS, D., WATZL, B., SZAJEWSKA, H. & STAHL, B. 2010. Prebiotic effects: Metabolic and health benefits. *British Journal of Nutrition*, 104, S1–S63.

RUSCIO, M. 2017. Do you really want a hunter-gatherer microbiota? Perils and pitfalls for your gut. *Journal of Evolution and Health: A Joint Publication of the Ancestral Health Society and the Society for Evolutionary Medicine and Health*, 2.

SACKNER-BERNSTEIN, J., KANTER, D. & KAUL, S. 2015. Dietary intervention for overweight and obese adults: Comparison of low-carbohydrate and low-fat diets. A meta-analysis. *PloS One*, 10, e0139817.

SÆTHER, S. M. M., KNAPSTAD, M., ASKELAND, K. G. & SKOGEN, J. C. 2019. Alcohol consumption, life satisfaction and mental health among Norwegian college and university students. *Addictive Behaviors Reports*, 10, 100216.

SAFDIE, F. M., DORFF, T., QUINN, D., FONTANA, L., WEI, M., LEE, C., COHEN, P. & LONGO, V. D. 2009. Fasting and cancer treatment in humans: A case series report. *Aging (Albany NY)*, 1, 988.

SAFDIE, F., BRANDHORST, S., WEI, M., WANG, W., LEE, C., HWANG, S., CONTI, P. S., CHEN, T. C. & LONGO, V. D. 2012. Fasting enhances the response of glioma to chemo-and radiotherapy. PloS One, 7, e44603.

SAME, R. V., FELDMAN, D. I., SHAH, N., MARTIN, S. S., AL RIFAI, M., BLAHA, M. J., GRAHAM, G. & AHMED, H. M. 2016. Relationship between sedentary behavior and cardiovascular risk. *Current Cardiology Reports*, 18, 1–7.

SARKAR, A., LEHTO, S. M., HARTY, S., DINAN, T. G., CRYAN, J. F. & BURNET, P. W. 2016. Psychobiotics and the manipulation of bacteria–gut–brain signals. *Trends in Neurosciences*, 39, 763–781.

SCHIEBER, A., STINTZING, F. C. & CARLE, R. 2001. By-products of plant food processing as a source of functional compounds—recent developments. *Trends in Food Science & Technology*, 12, 401–413.

SCHNORR, S. L., CANDELA, M., RAMPELLI, S., CENTANNI, M., CONSOLANDI, C., BASAGLIA, G., TURRONI, S., BIAGI, E., PEANO, C. & SEVERGNINI, M. 2014. Gut microbiome of the Hadza hunter-gatherers. *Nature Communications*, 5, 3654.

SCHWINGSHACKL, L. & HOFFMANN, G. 2016. Does a Mediterranean-type diet reduce cancer risk? *Current Nutrition Reports*, 5, 9–17.

SĘDZIKOWSKA, A. & SZABLEWSKI, L. 2021. Human gut microbiota in health and selected cancers. *International Journal of Molecular Sciences*, 22, 13440.

SEGATA, N. 2015. Gut microbiome: Westernization and the disappearance of intestinal diversity. *Current Biology*, 25, R611–R613.

SENDER, R., FUCHS, S. & MILO, R. 2016a. Are we really vastly outnumbered? Revisiting the ratio of bacterial to host cells in humans. *Cell*, 164, 337–340.

SENDER, R., FUCHS, S. & MILO, R. 2016b. Revised estimates for the number of human and bacteria cells in the body. *PLoS Biology*, 14, e1002533.

SHIVELY, C. A., REGISTER, T. C., APPT, S. E., CLARKSON, T. B., UBERSEDER, B., CLEAR, K. Y., WILSON, A. S., CHIBA, A., TOOZE, J. A. & COOK, K. L. 2018. Consumption of Mediterranean versus Western diet leads to distinct mammary gland microbiome populations. *Cell Reports*, 25, 47–56. e3.

SINGH, R. K., CHANG, H.-W., YAN, D., LEE, K. M., UCMAK, D., WONG, K., ABROUK, M., FARAHNIK, B., NAKAMURA, M. & ZHU, T. H. 2017. Influence of diet on the gut microbiome and implications for human health. *Journal of Translational Medicine*, 15, 1–17.

SKONIECZNA-ŻYDECKA, K., MARLICZ, W., MISERA, A., KOULAOUZIDIS, A. & ŁONIEWSKI, I. 2018. Microbiome—the missing link in the gut-brain axis: Focus on its role in gastrointestinal and mental health. *Journal of Clinical Medicine*, 7, 521.

SPREADBURY, I. 2012. Comparison with ancestral diets suggests dense acellular carbohydrates promote an inflammatory microbiota, and may be the primary dietary cause of leptin resistance and obesity. *Diabetes, Metabolic Syndrome and Obesity: Targets and Therapy*, 5, 175–189.

SUTIN, A. R., TERRACCIANO, A., DEIANA, B., NAITZA, S., FERRUCCI, L., UDA, M., SCHLESSINGER, D. & COSTA, P. 2010. High neuroticism and low conscientiousness are associated with interleukin-6. *Psychological Medicine*, 40, 1485–1493.

SWIDSINSKI, A., DÖRFFEL, Y., LOENING-BAUCKE, V., GILLE, C., GÖKTAS, Ö., REIßHAUER, A., NEUHAUS,

J., WEYLANDT, K.-H., GUSCHIN, A. & BOCK, M. 2017. Reduced mass and diversity of the colonic microbiome in patients with multiple sclerosis and their improvement with ketogenic diet. *Frontiers in Microbiology*, 8, 1141.

TAKEMURA, N., OKUBO, T. & SONOYAMA, K. 2010. Lactobacillus plantarum strain No. 14 reduces adipocyte size in mice fed high-fat diet. *Experimental Biology and Medicine*, 235, 849–856.

TANAKA, S., KOBAYASHI, T., SONGJINDA, P., TATEYAMA, A., TSUBOUCHI, M., KIYOHARA, C., SHIRAKAWA, T., SONOMOTO, K. & NAKAYAMA, J. 2009. Influence of antibiotic exposure in the early postnatal period on the development of intestinal microbiota. *FEMS Immunology & Medical Microbiology*, 56, 80–87.

TANG, W. W. & HAZEN, S. L. 2017. Microbiome, trimethylamine N-oxide, and cardiometabolic disease. *Translational Research*, 179, 108–115.

TANG, W. W., WANG, Z., LEVISON, B. S., KOETH, R. A., BRITT, E. B., FU, X., WU, Y. & HAZEN, S. L. 2013. Intestinal microbial metabolism of phosphatidylcholine and cardiovascular risk. *New England Journal of Medicine*, 368, 1575–1584.

TAYLOR, A. M., THOMPSON, S. V., EDWARDS, C. G., MUSAAD, S. M., KHAN, N. A. & HOLSCHER, H. D. 2020a. Associations among diet, the gastrointestinal microbiota, and negative emotional states in adults. *Nutritional Neuroscience*, 23, 983–992.

TAYLOR, B. C., LEJZEROWICZ, F., POIREL, M., SHAFFER, J. P., JIANG, L., AKSENOV, A., LITWIN, N., HUMPHREY, G., MARTINO, C. & MILLER-MONTGOMERY, S. 2020b. Consumption of fermented foods is associated with systematic differences in the gut microbiome and metabolome. *Msystems*, 5, e00901– e00919.

THUNY, F., RICHET, H., CASALTA, J.-P., ANGELAKIS, E., HABIB, G. & RAOULT, D. 2010. Vancomycin treatment of infective endocarditis is linked with recently acquired obesity. *PLoS Oone*, 5, e9074.

TILG, H., ADOLPH, T. E., GERNER, R. R. & MOSCHEN, A. R. 2018. The intestinal microbiota in colorectal cancer. *Cancer Cell*, 33, 954–964.

TILLISCH, K., LABUS, J., KILPATRICK, L., JIANG, Z., STAINS, J., EBRAT, B., GUYONNET, D., LEGRAIN–RASPAUD, S., TROTIN, B. & NALIBOFF, B. 2013. Consumption of fermented milk product with probiotic modulates brain activity. *Gastroenterology*, 144, 1394–1401.e4.

TITGEMEYER, E. C., BOURQUIN, L. D., FAHEY JR, G. C. & GARLEB, K. A. 1991. Fermentability of various fiber sources by human fecal bacteria in vitro. *The American Journal of Clinical Nutrition*, 53, 1418–1424.

TÓTH, C. & CLEMENS, Z. 2016. Halted progression of soft palate cancer in a patient treated with the paleolithic ketogenic diet alone: A 20-months follow-up. *American Journal of Medical Case Reports*, 4, 288–92.

TÓTH, C. & CLEMENS, Z. 2017. Treatment of rectal cancer with the paleolithic ketogenic diet: A 24-months follow-up. *American Journal of Medical Case Reports*, 5, 205–16.

TÓTH, C., SCHIMMER, Z. C. M. & CLEMENS, Z. 2018. Complete cessation of recurrent cervical intraepithelial neoplasia (CIN) by the paleolithic ketogenic diet: A case report. *Journal of Cancer Research Treatment*, 6, 1–5.

TRAJKOVSKA PETKOSKA, A. & TRAJKOVSKA-BROACH, A. 2021. Mediterranean diet—A healthy dietary pattern and lifestyle for strong immunity. *Analysis of Infectious Disease Problems (Covid-19) and Their Global Impact*, 279–305.

TSURUYA, A., KUWAHARA, A., SAITO, Y., YAMAGUCHI, H., TSUBO, T., SUGA, S., INAI, M., AOKI, Y., TAKAHASHI, S. & TSUTSUMI, E. 2016. Ecophysiological consequences of alcoholism on human gut microbiota: Implications for ethanol-related pathogenesis of colon cancer. *Scientific Reports*, 6, 27923.

TURNBAUGH, P. J., LEY, R. E., MAHOWALD, M. A., MAGRINI, V., MARDIS, E. R. & GORDON, J. I. 2006. An obesity-associated gut microbiome with increased capacity for energy harvest. *Nature*, 444, 1027–1031.

URSIN, R. 2002. Serotonin and sleep. *Sleep Medicine Reviews*, 6, 55–67.

UTZSCHNEIDER, K. M., KRATZ, M., DAMMAN, C. J. & HULLARG, M. 2016. Mechanisms linking the gut microbiome and glucose metabolism. *The Journal of Clinical Endocrinology & Metabolism*, 101, 1445–1454.

VALLES-COLOMER, M., FALONY, G., DARZI, Y., TIGCHELAAR, E. F., WANG, J., TITO, R. Y., SCHIWECK, C., KURILSHIKOV, A., JOOSSENS, M. & WIJMENGA, C. 2019. The neuroactive potential of the human gut microbiota in quality of life and depression. *Nature Microbiology*, 4, 623–632.

VAN DEN ABBEELE, P., GÉRARD, P., RABOT, S., BRUNEAU, A., EL AIDY, S., DERRIEN, M., KLEEREBEZEM, M., ZOETENDAL, E. G., SMIDT, H. & VERSTRAETE, W. 2011. Arabinoxylans and inulin differentially modulate the mucosal and luminal gut microbiota and mucin-degradation in humanized rats. *Environmental Microbiology*, 13, 2667–2680.

VARIAN, B. J., GOURESHETTI, S., POUTAHIDIS, T., LAKRITZ, J. R., LEVKOVICH, T., KWOK, C., TELIOUSIS, K., IBRAHIM, Y. M., MIRABAL, S. & ERDMAN, S. E. 2016. Beneficial bacteria inhibit cachexia. *Oncotarget*, 7, 11803.

VERSTRAELEN, H. 2019. Of microbes and women: BRCA1, vaginal microbiota, and ovarian cancer. *The Lancet Oncology*, 20, 1049–1051.

VIENNOIS, E., GEWIRTZ, A. T. & CHASSAING, B. 2022. Connecting the dots: Dietary fat, microbiota dysbiosis, altered metabolome, and colon cancer. *Gastroenterology*, 162, 38–39.

WAHLS, T. L. 2018. Feeding your microbiome well. *Journal of Evolution and Health: A Joint Publication of the Ancestral Health Society and the Society for Evolutionary Medicine and Health*, 2.

WALDMAN, H. S., KRINGS, B. M., SMITH, J. W. & MCALLISTER, M. J. 2018. A shift toward a high-fat diet in the current metabolic paradigm: A new perspective. *Nutrition*, 46, 33–35.

WALKER, A. W., INCE, J., DUNCAN, S. H., WEBSTER, L. M., HOLTROP, G., ZE, X., BROWN, D., STARES, M. D., SCOTT, P. & BERGERAT, A. 2011. Dominant and diet-responsive groups of bacteria within the human colonic microbiota. *The ISME Journal*, 5, 220–230.

WALTER, J., MALDONADO-GÓMEZ, M. X. & MARTÍNEZ, I. 2018. To engraft or not to engraft: An ecological framework for gut microbiome modulation with live microbes. *Current Opinion in Biotechnology*, 49, 129–139.

WAN, Y., WANG, F., YUAN, J., LI, J., JIANG, D., ZHANG, J., LI, H., WANG, R., TANG, J. & HUANG, T. 2019. Effects of dietary fat on gut microbiota and faecal metabolites, and their relationship with cardiometabolic risk factors: A 6-month randomised controlled-feeding trial. *Gut*, 68, 1417–1429.

WAN, Y., YUAN, J., LI, J., LI, H., ZHANG, J., TANG, J., NI, Y., HUANG, T., WANG, F. & ZHAO, F. 2020. Unconjugated and secondary bile acid profiles in response to higher-fat, lower-carbohydrate diet and associated with related gut microbiota: A 6-month randomized controlled-feeding trial. *Clinical Nutrition,* 39, 395–404.

WANG, S., ZHU, H., LU, C., KANG, Z., LUO, Y., FENG, L. & LU, X. 2012. Fermented milk supplemented with probiotics and prebiotics can effectively alter the intestinal microbiota and immunity of host animals. *Journal of Dairy Science,* 95, 4813–4822.

WANG, Z., KLIPFELL, E., BENNETT, B. J., KOETH, R., LEVISON, B. S., DUGAR, B., FELDSTEIN, A. E., BRITT, E. B., FU, X. & CHUNG, Y.-M. 2011. Gut flora metabolism of phosphatidylcholine promotes cardiovascular disease. *Nature,* 472, 57–63.

WASTYK, H. C., FRAGIADAKIS, G. K., PERELMAN, D., DAHAN, D., MERRILL, B. D., FEIQIAO, B. Y., TOPF, M., GONZALEZ, C. G., VAN TREUREN, W. & HAN, S. 2021. Gut-microbiota-targeted diets modulate human immune status. *Cell,* 184, 4137–4153. e14.

WEBER, D. D., AMINAZDEH-GOHARI, S. & KOFLER, B. 2018. Ketogenic diet in cancer therapy. *Aging (Albany NY),* 10, 164.

WEIR, T. L., TRIKHA, S. R. J. & THOMPSON, H. J. Diet and cancer risk reduction: The role of diet-microbiota interactions and microbial metabolites. *Seminars in Cancer Biology,* 2021. Elsevier, 53–60.

WESTMAN, E. C., FEINMAN, R. D., MAVROPOULOS, J. C., VERNON, M. C., VOLEK, J. S., WORTMAN, J. A., YANCY, W. S. & PHINNEY, S. D. 2007. Low-carbohydrate nutrition and metabolism. *The American Journal of Clinical Nutrition,* 86, 276–284.

WILCK, N., MATUS, M. G., KEARNEY, S. M., OLESEN, S. W., FORSLUND, K., BARTOLOMAEUS, H., HAASE, S., MÄHLER, A., BALOGH, A. & MARKÓ, L. 2017. Salt-responsive gut commensal modulates TH17 axis and disease. *Nature,* 551, 585–589.

WILLIAMS, N. C., JOHNSON, M. A., SHAW, D. E., SPENDLOVE, I., VULEVIC, J., SHARPE, G. R. & HUNTER, K. A. 2016. A prebiotic galactooligosaccharide mixture reduces severity of hyperpnoea-induced bronchoconstriction and markers of airway inflammation. *British Journal of Nutrition,* 116, 798–804.

WILMOT, E. G., EDWARDSON, C. L., ACHANA, F. A., DAVIES, M. J., GORELY, T., GRAY, L. J., KHUNTI, K., YATES, T. & BIDDLE, S. J. 2012. Sedentary time in adults and the association with diabetes, cardiovascular disease and death: Systematic review and meta-analysis. *Diabetologia,* 55, 2895–2905.

WISNIEWSKI, P. J., DOWDEN, R. A. & CAMPBELL, S. C. 2019. Role of dietary lipids in modulating inflammation through the gut microbiota. *Nutrients,* 11, 117.

WOTING, A., PFEIFFER, N., LOH, G., KLAUS, S. & BLAUT, M. 2014. Clostridium ramosum promotes high-fat diet-induced obesity in gnotobiotic mouse models. *MBio,* 5, e01530–14.

XIE, G., ZHOU, Q., QIU, C.-Z., DAI, W.-K., WANG, H.-P., LI, Y.-H., LIAO, J.-X., LU, X.-G., LIN, S.-F. & YE, J.-H. 2017. Ketogenic diet poses a significant effect on imbalanced gut microbiota in infants with refractory epilepsy. *World Journal of Gastroenterology,* 23, 6164.

YADAV, H., LEE, J.-H., LLOYD, J., WALTER, P. & RANE, S. G. 2013. Beneficial metabolic effects of a probiotic via butyrate-induced GLP-1 hormone secretion. *Journal of Biological Chemistry,* 288, 25088–25097.

YANG, Y. J. & SHEU, B. S. 2012. Probiotics-containing yogurts suppress Helicobacter pylori load and modify immune response and intestinal microbiota in the *Helicobacter pylori*-infected children. *Helicobacter,* 17, 297–304.

YAO, L., D'AGOSTINO, G. D., PARK, J., HANG, S., ADHIKARI, A. A., ZHANG, Y., LI, W., AVILA-PACHECO, J., BAE, S. & CLISH, C. B. 2022. A biosynthetic pathway for the selective sulfonation of steroidal metabolites by human gut bacteria. *Nature Microbiology,* 7, 1404–1418.

YOO, J. Y. & KIM, S. S. 2016. Probiotics and prebiotics: Present status and future perspectives on metabolic disorders. *Nutrients,* 8, 173.

YU, L. C.-H., SHIH, Y.-A., WU, L.-L., LIN, Y.-D., KUO, W.-T., PENG, W.-H., LU, K.-S., WEI, S.-C., TURNER, J. R. & NI, Y.-H. 2014. Enteric dysbiosis promotes antibiotic-resistant bacterial infection: Systemic dissemination of resistant and commensal bacteria through epithelial transcytosis. *American Journal of Physiology-Gastrointestinal and Liver Physiology,* 307, G824–G835.

YU, L.-X. & SCHWABE, R. F. 2017. The gut microbiome and liver cancer: Mechanisms and clinical translation. *Nature reviews Gastroenterology & Hepatology,* 14, 527–539.

YUNES, R., POLUEKTOVA, E., DYACHKOVA, M., KLIMINA, K., KOVTUN, A., AVERINA, O., ORLOVA, V. & DANILENKO, V. 2016. GABA production and structure of gadB/gadC genes in Lactobacillus and Bifidobacterium strains from human microbiota. *Anaerobe,* 42, 197–204.

ZHENG, X., ZHOU, K., ZHANG, Y., HAN, X., ZHAO, A., LIU, J., QU, C., GE, K., HUANG, F. & HERNANDEZ, B. 2018. Food withdrawal alters the gut microbiota and metabolome in mice. *The FASEB Journal,* 32, 4878.

ZHERNAKOVA, A., KURILSHIKOV, A., BONDER, M. J., TIGCHELAAR, E. F., SCHIRMER, M., VATANEN, T., MUJAGIC, Z., VILA, A. V., FALONY, G. & VIEIRA-SILVA, S. 2016. Population-based metagenomics analysis reveals markers for gut microbiome composition and diversity. *Science,* 352, 565–569.

12 Microbiome Dynamics in Pediatric Solid Tumors: Challenges and Opportunities

Michelle McCabe, Dineo Disenyane, Lindie Lamola, Botle Precious Damane, Demetra Demetriou, Thabiso Victor Miya, Talent Chipiti, Lloyd Mabonga, Ellen Mapunda, and Zodwa Dlamini

INTRODUCTION

The human microbiome consists of approximately 39 trillion microorganisms, comprising nearly 3,000 species of bacteria, archaea, viruses, and fungi (Sender, Fuchs and Milo, 2016; Zhao et al., 2023). The human microbiota is found on the skin, upper respiratory tract, gastrointestinal tract, and genital tracts (Huttenhower et al., 2012; Lloyd-Price, Abu-Ali and Huttenhower, 2016; Gebrayel et al., 2022). The majority (~95%) of normal human microbiota is found in the intestine (gut) and mainly consists of the phyla Bacteroidetes, Firmicutes, and Actinobacteria, which are essential in maintaining gut homeostasis (Tap et al., 2009; Jandhyala et al., 2015; Dupont et al., 2020; Stojanov, Berlec and Štrukelj, 2020). Gut microbiota has been found to play a significant role in an array of normal biological functions involved in the digestive, metabolic, immune, and nervous systems (Jandhyala et al., 2015; Kho and Lal, 2018). This includes a protective function against pathogenic organisms, diseases, vaccines, and drug metabolic responses (Wiertsema et al., 2021). Genetic predispositions to certain diseases have also shown to have an effect on microbiome shaping in a few animal model studies, increasing distinct microbiota involved in certain mechanisms such as hyper- or hypo-methylation (Allen and Sears, 2019; Cahana and Iraqi, 2020). Epigenetic mutations have shown to lead to the loss of the second functional alleles in genetic diseases such as Lynch Syndrome (*MSH*2 gene) and leukemia (*PAX5* gene) (Allen and Sears, 2019; Vicente-Dueñas et al., 2020). Bacteria, such as *Escherichia coli* (*E. coli*) that harbors a pathogenic island, polyketide synthase (pks), which expresses enzymes that synthesize an alkylating compound—colibactin (genotoxin)—along with enterotoxigenic *Bacteroides fragilis*, have shown to induce double-stranded DNA breaks and enhance DNA damage and tumor development in colorectal cancer (CRC) mouse models (Dougherty and Jobin, 2023; Lichtenstern and Lamichhane-Khadka, 2023). A few studies have shown a protective effect of an increase in commensal butyrate-producing microbes (e.g. Firmicutes), against the genomic or epigenomic altering microbes in disease models such as leukemia and CRC mouse models (Cohen et al., 2019; Singh et al., 2023). Increased longitudinal studies are needed to establish if targeted microbiome alterations in children predisposed to genetic disorders can serve as a potential prevention strategy.

Gut microbiome research in children has been limited, mainly due to small population cohorts. Thus far research has shed considerable light on the microbiome's important role in the maturity of the immune and nervous systems, and the overall growth in child to adult development (Hollister et al., 2015; Derrien, Alvarez and de Vos, 2019). Studies have also illustrated the microbiota taxonomy in healthy children is unique when compared to healthy adult microbiota, and displays functionally distinct roles, suggesting the gut microbiome develops slowly overtime toward adulthood (Nash, Frank and Friedman, 2017; Derrien, Alvarez and de Vos, 2019; Niu et al., 2020; Radjabzadeh et al., 2020). In many illnesses, a shift in organism composition, metabolites, vesicles, etc. has been illustrated in the gut, and associated with many chronic conditions such as allergies, asthma, diabetes, inflammatory bowel disease, and even cancer (Yassour et al., 2016; Quaglio et al., 2022; Saeed et al., 2022). The gut microbiome has also been established as a key regulator in the development and progression of cancer, and certain bacteria in the gut are linked to oncology therapeutic efficacies and side effects (Bhatt, Redinbo and Bultman, 2017; Masetti et al., 2021).

This chapter focuses on healthy microbiome symbiosis as well as dysbiosis in children, with the main emphasis on the differences in pediatric versus adult microbiota composition, modulation of the immune system, susceptibility of the microbiome to pediatric cancer, treatment responses, and microbiome-based interventions to assist in improving treatment efficacy and outcomes in pediatric cancer.

THE UNIQUE GUT MICROBIOME DEVELOPMENT IN CHILDREN

From the time of birth, some researchers propose even during the perinatal stages, the gut microbiota develops and conditions important physiological systems (i.e., metabolic, nerve, immune, etc.), essential for healthy life maintenance throughout the human being's life span. Not many microbiome studies have been conducted in children between the ages of 3 and pre-adolescent years (mainly due to ethical implications and challenges in obtaining stool samples), and research conducted in children below the age of 3 years demonstrates the human microbiome is already shaped early in life (by 3 years of age), and influenced by factors dependent on gestational periods, type of delivery—vaginal/cesarean (Figure 12.1), breast- or formula-fed, antibiotic treatments, etc. (Wen and Duffy, 2017; Davis et al., 2020; Barnett et al., 2023).

More recently, evidence from globally represented population cohorts of older children: 3–12 years of age, suggests the well-established microbiome evolves slowly with the host over a longer period (~10 years) and this developmental and shaping process is critical for healthy gut microbiota homeostasis and particularly for later stages in life (Hollister et al., 2015; Derrien, Alvarez and de Vos, 2019; Dogra et al., 2021). Significant variations (e.g., diet, treatment, stress, antibiotics, etc.) during this process and stage of microbiome development could have a negative effect on the host in subsequent years. This malleability of the microbiota in response to the diet could also assist in interventions to promote health or prevent disease later in life (Derrien, Alvarez and de Vos, 2019).

VARYING GUT MICROBIOTA COMPOSITION IN CHILDREN AND ADULTS

For future microbiota interventions to reduce disease risk and maintain health, an in-depth understanding of the gut microbiota population and host pathway interactions are required in both the early and later stages of life. Microbiota diversity in the gut has been linked to peak metabolic and immune function and has been shown to prevent disease development in adults (Hills et al., 2019). Amplified or improved molecular ability however has not been directly proportional to an increased variation of microbial species, indicating much more research into the functional abilities of different microbial species is needed (Rinninella et al., 2019). Microbiome diversity has been shown to increase with age until it plateaus into a well-established diversified microbiota in the adult stage of life (Derrien, Alvarez and de Vos, 2019) (Figure 12.2).

In the first year of a child's life, microbiota consists mainly of *Akkermansia muciniphila, Bacteroides, Veillonella,*

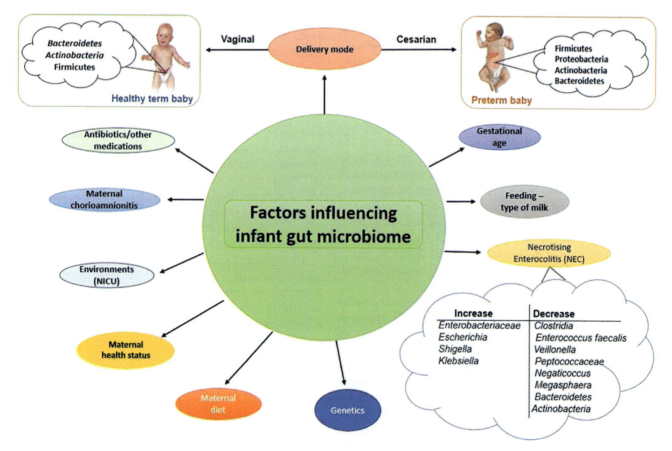

FIGURE 12.1 **Factors influencing the gut microbiome in infants in early life.** The gut microbial composition rapidly changes during childhood due to maternal microbiome composition, delivery method, infant feeding mode, antibiotic use, and other environmental factors. Necrotizing enterocolitis in infancy has been linked to disruptions in the gut flora. Understanding the influence of maternal-to-infant transmission of dysbiotic microorganisms and subsequently regulating newborn early colonization or rectifying early-life gut dysbiosis may thus be a promising technique for overcoming chronic health issues.

Clostridium coccoides, and *Clostridium botulinum* species (Yatsunenko et al., 2012; Rinninella et al., 2019). In the mature adult gut microbiome, the structure is dominated by Firmicutes (*Lachnospiraceae* and *Ruminococcaceae*), Bacteroidetes (*Bacteroidaceae, Prevotellaceae,* and *Rikenellaceae*), and Actinobacteria (*Bifidobacteriaceae* and *Coriobacteriaceae*) (Table 12.1). Literature shows at approximately 3 years of age a child's gut microbiota composition and diversity are almost identical to an adult's (Hills et al., 2019). Microbiota profiles are unique to individuals, and ages and populations from various countries around the world have displayed distinctive gut microbiota signatures due to specific dietary and cultural habits, the environment, lifestyle, physiology, and unique genetic factors (Turnbaugh et al., 2009; Yu et al., 2023). A study by Fallani et al. (2011) illustrated infants in the North of Europe were linked with increased levels of *Bifidobacteria*, whereas higher quantities of Bacteroides and Lactobacilli were seen in children from the south of Europe. Diets rich in natural fiber and carbohydrates were also associated with raised Firmicutes and *Prevotella*, however, increased consumption of animal products showed escalated levels of Bacteroidetes (Fallani et al., 2011; Koren et al., 2013). *Prevotella* was seen predominantly in the African population individuals compared to those of European ancestry, and Bacteroidetes were most commonly found in the gut microbiome of American and Western world populations (De Filippo et al., 2010). Older people from the seventh decade of life showed decreased gut microbiota composition, which could be attributed to less variation in diets in older aged people. Reduced variation in microbiota related to decreased digestive, metabolism, and immune function, with a specific decrease in the *Bifidobacterium* population (involved in immunomodulation and metabolic activity), and an increase in communities such as *Clostridium* and Proteobacteria were observed (Guigoz, Doré and Schiffrin, 2008; Rinninella et al., 2019).

GUT MICROBIOME IMPACT ON THE IMMUNE SYSTEM IN CHILDREN

The interaction between early life microbiota and the development of the immune system is quite complex. The introduction to microorganisms (either pathogenic or normal microbiota) early in an infant's life shapes the intrinsic immune system response to identify one's own (personal/normal) flora from foreign and pathogenic microorganisms (Fragkou et al., 2021). Neonates who are delivered via the birth canal (exposed to maternal vaginal microbiota) and breastfed during infancy (minimum of 6 months) has shown to have up to 20% reduction in risk to developing certain types of diseases such as the hematological malignancies (i.e., acute lymphoblastic leukemia (ALL)), compared to cesarean mode of delivery and formula-fed infants (Dunn et al., 2017).

Breast milk has been shown to modulate optimal immune function in infants, through specific nutrients, antibodies, anti-inflammatory molecules, oligosaccharides, and lactoferrin (Quitadamo, Comegna and Cristalli, 2021). Postpartum colostrum secreted by mothers in the first few days is concentrated with critical innate and adaptive immune function compounds, such as secretory IgA, leukocytes and lactoferrin, oligosaccharides, sodium, chloride, and magnesium. Later stage milk production has been found to contain increased levels of calcium, lactose, protein, and potassium, indicating a higher level of immune protection in the first stages of life compared to more nutritional goals in subsequent milk secretion. Maternal-milk microbiome has been shown to profile the gut microbiome in the newborn, while the milk oligosaccharides allow the microbiota to flourish within the gut, modulate intestinal epithelial cell response, and enable development of the immune system. Milk oligosaccharides are the main components for the saccharolytic intestinal microbiome to grow, and crucial for the development of the *Bifidobacteria* to dominate the gut of healthy breastfed infants (Sánchez et al., 2021). Formula-fed infants however demonstrate decreased *Bifidobacterium* species, and a greater alpha-diversity in gastrointestinal bacteria, such as *Veillonella* and *Clostridioides, Escherichia coli,* and *Clostridium difficile* (Wang et al., 2020; Ruiz-Ojeda et al., 2023).

In addition, distinctively *Propionibacterium, Streptococcus,* and *Finegoldia* genera and bacteria of the Clostridiales order had higher relative abundance in the breastfed group, compared to the formula-fed group with higher levels of the Enterobacteriaceae family, the Enterococcus, and Bacilli class (Wang et al., 2020). Research has shown a type of feedback link which exists between maternal-skin, maternal-milk, and baby's saliva during feeding, interchanging microbiota, pathogens, immunological molecules, compounds and nutrients according to growth and immunological requirements of the infant (Al-Shehri et al., 2015). A small cohort of ten formula-fed and ten MOM-fed preterm infants, found a similar alpha-diversity but a significantly different beta-diversity of the gut microbiota between the two groups (Wang et al., 2020). Alpha-diversity is a measurement of the depth of taxa (n=) or its consistency (the relative abundance) of an average sample within a certain environment, whereas beta-diversity measures the variability in the taxa community among samples within an environment (Derrien, Alvarez and de Vos, 2019; Walters and Martiny, 2020).

The overuse of antibiotics has led to the selection of resistant opportunistic pathogens which have accumulated to an alarming level in the human body, loss of basic physiological equilibria, strongly influencing the immune system, and is believed to be the promoter of long-term diseases (Francino, 2016; Langdon, Crook and Dantas, 2016). Figure 12.3 shows a summary of key clinical research comparing the gut microbiota of pre-school and school-age children to that of adults.

TABLE 12.1
Microbiota variations within individuals

		Microbial abundance					
		Actinobacteria	Firmicutes	Bacteroides	Fusobacteria	Proteobacteria	References
Gut tract anatomical part	Small intestines		*Lactobacillus*			*Enterobacteriaceae*	(Chu et al., 2017; Hills et al., 2019)
	Collon		*Lachnospiraceae ruminococcaceae*	*Bacteroidaceae Prevotellaceae Rikenellaceae*			(Chu et al., 2017; Hills et al., 2019)
Gestational	Preterm birth (<37 weeks of gestation)	*Bifidobacterium* spp. (decreased) *Atopobium* spp. (decreased)	Firmicutes (decreased) (non-secretor mothers) *Lactobacillus* (increased) *Rumonicoccus Lachinospiraceae Peptostreptococcaceae Clostridiaceae*	*Bacteroides* (increased) (non-secretor mothers)		*Enterobacteriaceae* (increased) *Enterococcus* spp. (increased)	(Gibson et al., 2016)
	Full term birth	*Bifidobacterium* spp. (increased)	*Rumonicoccus Lachinospiraceae Peptostreptococcaceae Clostridiaceae*	*Bacteroidetes* (increased)		*Enterobacteriaceae*	(Gibson et al., 2016)
Delivery method	Vaginal delivery	*Bifidobacterium Bifidobacterium* spp. (increased) *Longum* (increased) *Catenulutum* (increased)	*Lactobacillus* (increased) *Staphylococcus* (increased) *Streptococcus* (increased)	*Prevotella Bacteroides fragilis* (increased)	*Sneathia* (increased)	*Escherichia* (increased)	(Dominguez-Bello et al., 2010; Dunn et al., 2017)
	C-section	*Corynebacterium* (increased) *Propionibacterium* (increased)	*Staphylococcus* (increased)	*Bacteroides* (decreased)		*Escherichia* (decreased) *Shigella* (decreased)	(Dominguez-Bello et al., 2010; Chu et al., 2016; Dunn et al., 2017)
Feeding	Breast milk	*Bifidobacterium* spp. (increased)	*Lactobacillus* (increased) *Staphylococcus* (increased)			*Enterococcus* (increased)	(Harmsen et al., 2000; Morelli 2008; Biesbroek et al., 2014; Sánchez et al., 2021)
	Artificial milk	*Bifidobacterium* spp. (increased)	*Clostridium* (increased) *Clostridium difficile* (increased) *Lactobacillus* (increased)	*Bacteroides* (increased)		*Escherichia* (increased)	(Wang et al., 2020; Ruiz-Ojeda et al., 2023)

Microbiome Dynamics in Pediatric Solid Tumors

Age				
Introduction of solid foods	*Bifidobacterium* spp. (increased)	*Firmicutes* (increased) *Lactobacilli* (increased) *Clostridium coccoides* (increased)	*Bacteroides* (increased) *Bacteroidetes* (increased)		(Hills et al., 2019)
Childhood (First year of life)	*Bifidobacterium* spp.	*Veillonella* *C. coccoides* *C. botulinum*	*Bacteroides*		(Yatsunenko et al., 2012; Rinninella et al., 2019)
2-3 years old to adult	*Bifidobacterium* spp. *Coriobacteriaceae*	*Lachnospiraceae* *Ruminococcaceae*	*Bacteroidaceae* *Prevotellaceae* *Rikenellaceae*	*Fusobacteria*	*Proteobacteria*	(Hills et al., 2019)
Over 70	*Bifidobacteriaceae* (decreased)	*Clostridium* (decreased)			*Proteobacteria* (increased)	(Guigoz, Doré and Schiffrin, 2008; Rinninella et al., 2019)

Note: Adapted from Rinninella et al., 2019.

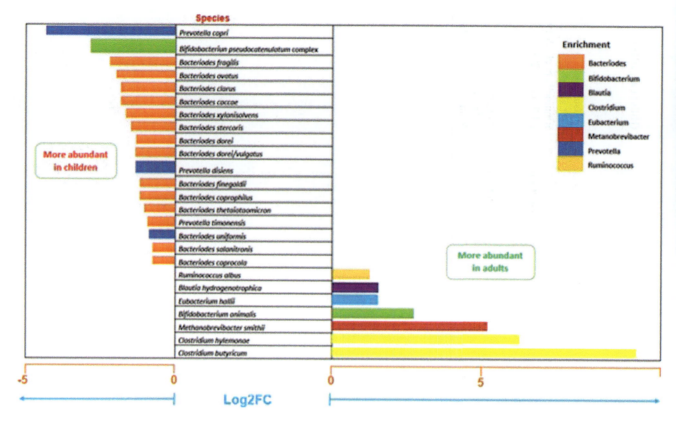

FIGURE 12.2 **Varying gut microbiota composition in children and adults.** Microbiome diversity has been shown to increase with age until it plateaus into a well-established diversified microbiota in the adult stage of life.

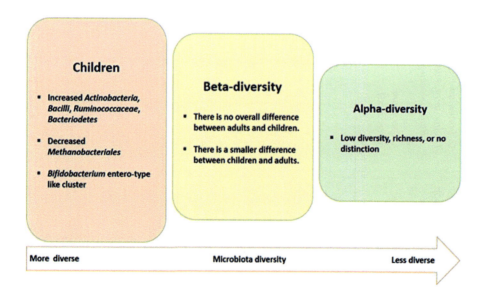

FIGURE 12.3 **A summary of key clinical research comparing the gut microbiota of pre-school and school-age children to that of adults.** Gut microbiota formation and maturation is a highly dynamic process that can be influenced by varied prenatal circumstances. Bacterial alpha-diversity and functional complexity grow with age, although interindividual differences (beta-diversity) diminish. The colonization pattern is determined by age. Intra-group gut microbiota commonality is higher in children than in adults, implying that children's microbiota is more diverse than that of adults.

Significance of nutrition in shaping the gut microbiome in pre- and postnatal stages

Multiple lifestyle factors are associated with gut microbiome diversity, including physical activity, diet (increased intake of fruit and vegetables), and decreased consumption of fast foods and sugar-loaded drinks (Manor et al., 2020). Interestingly, studies have also indicated maternal nutrition during pregnancy also has an impact on the growth and development of the fetus *in utero*,

Microbiome Dynamics in Pediatric Solid Tumors

suggesting a negative maternal microbiome effect can stunt fetal growth, cause immune dysfunction and metabolism defects, etc. (Moossavi et al., 2019; Robertson et al., 2019; Tian et al., 2023). Biogeographical maternal microbiota data has shown microbiota profiling in pregnant women is unique compared to women not pregnant, and the microbial composition changes throughout pregnancy (Robertson et al., 2019). This suggests the prenatal microbiota may play an important role in the *in utero* environment that influences both the duration of pregnancy and the trajectory of fetal growth and development (Gorczyca et al., 2022). Maternal microbiota during pregnancy is shaped by environmental factors such as diet, antibiotic intake, stress, etc. (Edwards, Cunningham and Dunlop, 2017).

More recent research of bacteria in the meconium has shed light on an already present microbiome *in utero*, colonized by bacteria found in the placenta, amniotic fluid, and the umbilical cord (Walker et al., 2017; Olaniyi et al., 2020; Turunen et al., 2021). Another interesting observation in animal studies of pregnant mice and monkeys fed with a high-fat Western diet, illustrated alteration in both the maternal and neonate gut microbiome, with a lower overall bacterial abundance (alpha diversity), and increased Firmicutes compared to Bacteroidetes bacteria (Ma et al., 2014; Contu et al., 2019; Elsakr et al., 2019). In addition, a change in immune system development was also noted in neonates exposed to western diets compared to balanced diet control groups (Ma et al., 2014). In the primate study, lower *Campylobacter* levels were seen and associated with increased gastrointestinal disorders such as irritable bowel syndrome. Figure 12.4 shows the significance of nutrition in shaping the gut microbiome in pre- and postnatal stages.

Interestingly, despite changing the neonate's diet to a low-fat diet after weaning, the altered gut microbiome shaped during the high-fat diet exposure prenatally persisted even in the postnatal stages. Unfortunately, not many gestational dietary studies have been conducted in humans, however in one study where diets differed considerably from the average (high-fat versus balanced), the meconium microbiome in the uterus differed considerably, with a significant reduction in *Bacteroides* in neonates exposed to prenatal high-fat intake diet (Chu et al., 2016). In both gestational dietary studies in humans and primates, negative effects were seen in infants independent of maternal obesity status, demonstrating diet has a fundamental influence on shaping the fetal gut microbiome (Ma et al., 2014).

GUT MICROBIOME IMPACT ON CANCER SUSCEPTIBILITY AND DEVELOPMENT IN CHILDREN

Most of the microbes found in the gut have an impact on the host and disease states. Through the interactions of the gut

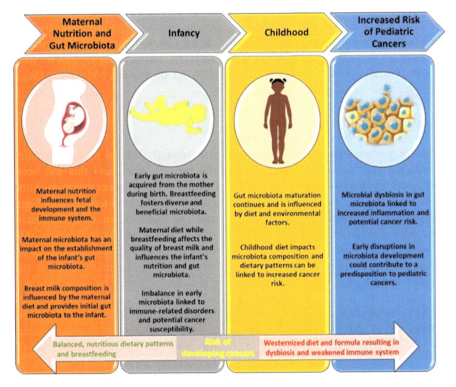

FIGURE 12.4 **The significance of nutrition in shaping the gut microbiome in pre-and postnatal stages.** Nutrition and the gut microbiome have a complex, primarily symbiotic interaction with the human host, which is responsible for a variety of health effects. This link begins early in life, possibly as early as pregnancy, when maternal diet and intestinal flora seed the fetus' microbiota and boost immune cell growth in utero. Dysbiosis caused by early life traumas such as malnutrition forms the foundation for persistent GI illnesses. This bidirectional contact opens new possibilities for dietary treatments of disorders that were previously thought to be unrelated to GI health.

microbiota with cells of the gut wall, the microbiome can act as an antigen and directly and indirectly induce immune processes and modify gene expression. A balance between the gut and microbiota is needed to maintain homeostasis. When there is a dissemblance, the function of the microbiota on the host changes. This change is termed dysbiosis. Dysbiosis can be involved in physiological processes that can lead to changes in metabolism and immune responses. In addition, it can influence processes that are involved in inflammation and lead to neoplastic and non-neoplastic diseases (Sági et al., 2022).

CARCINOGENESIS AND PEDIATRIC SPECIFICITIES

Several mechanisms have been proposed that implicate the gut microbiome with carcinogenesis, thus resulting in dysbiosis (Vimal, Himal and Kannan, 2020). Firstly, the microbiome can regulate and change cell proliferation and apoptosis by harming host DNA and subsequently intervening in signaling pathways that lead to carcinogenesis (Bhatt, Redinbo and Bultman, 2017). Secondly, chronic inflammation can also lead to malignancies, and the microbiome can completely evade the immune system which can transition into carcinogenic states (Bhatt, Redinbo and Bultman, 2017; Lazar et al., 2018). Research has shown these types of mechanisms are facilitated by *Fusobacterium nucleatum*, and the interactions lead to the inhibition of NK cell cytotoxicity and lymphocyte cell activity (Zhao et al., 2022). A third alternative mechanism identified is the negative effect of harmful metabolite production by microbiota on the immune system (Belkaid and Hand, 2014). A study by Amitay et al. showed that children who were not breastfed were at an increased risk of developing hematolymphoid neoplasms (Amitay and Keinan-Boker, 2015). In contrast, the gut microbiome of children who are breastfed comprised predominantly of *Lactobacillus, Staphylococcus*, and *Bifidobacterium*, when compared to those who are not breastfed mainly consisted of *Roseburia, Clostridium*, and *Anaerostipes* in their microbiota. Thus dysbiosis can lead to the development of various disease states ranging from inflammatory and immunological disorders to cancer. Other microbial populations associated with cancer include *Bacteroides, Escherichia*, Acinetobacter, and *Fusobacterium* (Kostic et al., 2012). In addition, microbiota populations dominant in *Bacteroides, Parabacteroides, Alistipes*, and *Akkermansia* have been linked to high tumor burden, in contrast to *Clostridiales* Cluster XIVa associated with lower risk for tumor development (Baxter et al., 2014).

THE INTERACTION OF THE GUT MICROBIOME AND SYSTEMIC TREATMENTS IN CHILDREN

It is widely known that cancer therapy, inclusive of chemotherapy, radiotherapy, and immunotherapy, can interact with and affect the gut microbiome negatively and thus lead to dysbiosis (Kunika, Frey and Rangrez, 2023). This interaction is dependent on the composition of the gut microbiome. Dysbiosis can also affect the metabolism of chemotherapeutic agents (Wei, Wen and Xian, 2021). Firstly, literature suggests that the gut microbiome plays a significant role in in the potency and efficacy of cancer drugs, such as irinotecan (Roy and Trinchieri, 2017; Rebersek, 2021). Secondly, gut microbiome is important in antitumor therapy, with the response and metabolism of certain immune checkpoints inhibitors dependent on certain microbiota (Aghamajidi and Vareki, 2022). Thus, the composition of gut microbiome can either increase or decrease toxic side effects and improve or worsen the efficacy of some oncologic therapies (Kunika, Frey and Rangrez, 2023). Numerous studies show that oncological treatment pharmacodynamics can change the structure of the gut microbiome, and lead to potential toxicity. In one study of patients who were treated with chemotherapy for ALL, the gut microbiome profile varied in patients when compared to controls (Sági et al., 2022). Patients with ALL had an increase of certain bacteria, specifically Bacteroidetes phylum, before chemotherapy was started in comparison to after chemotherapy (Sági et al., 2022). According to literature the gut microbiome is reduced post chemotherapy when compared to pre-chemotherapy (Huang et al., 2012; Wei, Wen and Xian, 2021). Some bacteria, e.g., *Bacteroides*, were greatly reduced while others increased, e.g., Clostridiaceae and Streptococcaceae (Sági et al., 2022). Cancer therapy shows acute and chronic complications which are physical and psychological (Stein, Syrjala and Andrykowski, 2008). Physical complications of oncological therapies include mucosal barrier injury and mucositis which can lead to sepsis, organ failure, and possible death. Other studies have also shown that in patients who received chemotherapy, 22.4% had posttraumatic stress disorder, depression, and anxiety (Sági et al., 2022).

CHRONIC TOXIC EFFECT OF CHEMOTHERAPY ON THE MICROBIOME

The overall survival of cancer patient has improved over the last 50 years, and this has been attributed mostly to improvement of cancer therapies. Another important factor to consider is the long-term effect of surviving cancer patients and the high rate of chronic toxicity after chemotherapy (Stein, Syrjala and Andrykowski, 2008). Even though cancer therapy alters the microbiome during treatment, the long-term effect on the microbiome is still under investigation. Study findings thus far show long-term effects in surviving ALL patients include obesity and metabolic disorders (Barnea et al., 2015). One study showed that treatment-related dysbiosis predisposed patients to obesity due to the reduction in *Faecalibacterium* (Breton, Galmiche and Déchelotte, 2022). Other studies demonstrate decreased attention span, concentration, process, and reaction time (Tooley, 2020; Oldacres et al., 2023). Researchers have proposed different possibilities to alter the gut microbiome profile positively in order to potentially prevent future acute and chronic side effects. An example of such interventions is the introduction of prebiotics to boost proliferation of good bacteria (probiotics) thus restoring a balanced gut microbiome. In one study cohort, 60 patients with acute leukemia were given probiotics (containing *Lactobacillus rhamnaosus*), and evidently less therapeutic side effects were observed in comparison to the control group (Zhou, Zhou and Zhang, 2022).

CHEMOTHERAPEUTIC EFFECTS ON THE GUT MICROBIOME AND OUTCOMES FOR PEDIATRIC ONCOLOGY PATIENTS

Changes in the gut microbiota have been shown to affect the metabolism, toxicity, and efficacy of drugs (Huang et al., 2022). This highlights the importance of a symbiotic relationship between the microbiota and its host. Chemotherapy is used as one of the first-line treatments for cancers. Chemotherapeutic agents indiscriminately affect certain healthy cells, leading to several side effects, such as intestinal mucositis, myelosuppression, alopecia, and bone loss (Sagi et al., 2022). According to some reports adverse drug reactions have been observed in about 40% of patients receiving standard doses of chemotherapy and 100% of patients receiving high-dose chemotherapy, these side effects include, but are not limited to, vomiting, abdominal pain, diarrhea, and mucositis (Ervin et al., 2020). Mucositis can affect both the oral cavity and intestine and represents one of the most common side effects of chemotherapy. The development of mucositis involves the chemotherapeutic drug, the immune system, and gut microbes resulting in a loss of mucosal integrity (Wei et al., 2021). Intestinal mucositis has been shown to have a negative effect on the quality of life of the patient as well as a negative impact on treatment outcome (Wei et al., 2021). The relationship between gut microbiota dysbiosis and chemotherapy-induced intestinal mucositis has drawn much attention for research recently (Ervin et al., 2020).

Long-Term Outcomes for Pediatric Oncology Patients

In pediatric oncology, understanding and managing the long-term effects of chemotherapy on the gut microbiome is crucial for improving treatment outcomes and the overall well-being of patients. Research should focus on the personalized approaches to address these issues based on each child's unique circumstances. Not many studies have investigated long-term effects of chemotherapy on the microbiome. A study by Chua et al. (2020) investigated the changes in the microbiome in children with ALL. The study was well constructed as they reported on data collected prior to the commencement of the therapy, during, and nine months after chemotherapy administration (Chua et al., 2020). According to this pilot study, which was made up of seven cases and controls, before chemotherapy was introduced, there was noticeable variability among the cases (individuals with ALL) in terms of the types of species which were in abundance, when compared to the controls (Chua et al., 2020). According to the report, Bacteroidetes phylum and *Bacteroides* genus were the most abundant and a notable decrease was recorded during the administration of chemotherapy. However, according to the study, following the administration and halting of the chemotherapy, the microbiota between the cases and controls were similar. Of note, which was reported in the study, is that before the commencement of the chemotherapy, some of the cases had a composition of the microbiota that was slightly different from the rest of the case group, and they state that this may be attributable to antibiotics which the cases may have been administered prior the ALL diagnosis (Chua et al., 2020).

However, even though antibiotics are well-known causes of alterations in the microbiome, studies have suggested that they are not the only contributors, factors such as the changes in the immune system, severity of disease (in this instance ALL), ethnicity, infections, and intensity of the treatment have also been implicated and studies investigating these co-factors should be conducted (Chua et al., 2020). In the meantime, the impact on the microbiota may lead to long-term dysbiosis, and further research over longer periods is required to determine whether the observed dysbiosis is permanent or may be restored over time. The early years of life are a crucial period for microbiome development. Disruptions in the microbiome during childhood could have long-term health consequences, potentially impacting immune function and metabolic health.

CONSEQUENCES OF TREATMENT AND GUT MICROBIOME DYSBIOSIS

Dysbiosis can result from compositional changes at the phylum level, for instance, Bacteroidetes species may be reduced compared to Firmicutes species, or from a change in abundance of one or more species. Dysbiosis may also result from the changes in virulence properties by specific bacterial species within a microbiome, and the activities of these virulent phenotypes subsequently change host pathology (Manos, 2022). Several studies have investigated the changes of intestinal microbiota following chemotherapy treatment. Some reports have shown that the abundances of specific species (i.e., Firmicutes and Actinobacteria) had significantly decreased while other species such as Proteobacteria increased following the chemotherapy introduction (Ervin, Ramanan and Bhatt, 2020). While other reports showed that chemotherapy influenced occurrence of intestinal domination, which is the occupation of at least 30% of the microbiota by a single predominating bacterial taxon. In some instances, the domination events were caused by opportunistic pathogenic bacteria, such as *Staphylococcus, Enterobacter,* and *Escherichia* (Ervin, Ramanan and Bhatt, 2020).

Drug Metabolism and the Gut Microbiome

The microbiome is involved in the metabolism of drugs and nutrients. Alterations in the microbiome can affect how the body processes drugs (Leardini et al., 2022). The gut microbiome encodes enzymes capable of metabolizing

TABLE 12.2
The effects of gut microbiota on the efficacy and toxicity of anticancer drugs

Anticancer drugs	Gut microbiome	Potential mechanisms	Effects	References
Effects of microbiota on the efficacy of anticancer drugs				
Oxaliplatin	Ileal microbiota (e.g., B. fragilis)	Immunomodulation	Enhanced efficacy	Iida et al. 2013
5-Fluorouracil	F. nucleatum	Immunomodulation	Drug resistance	Yu et al. 2017
Capecitabine	Bacterial uridine phosphorylase	Enzymatic degradation	Decreased efficacy	Javdan et al. 2020
Gemcitabine	Bacterial cytidine deaminase	Enzymatic degradation	Drug resistance	Guenther et al. 2020
Immune Checkpoint	A. muciniphila, Burkholderiales, B. adolescentis, B. fragilis, B. longum, B. thetaiotaomicron, E. faecium, E. hirae, Faecalibacterium, F. nucleatum, Lachnospiraceae, Prevotella, Ruminococcaceae	Immunomodulation	Enhanced efficacy	Huang et al. 2022
Effects of microbiota on toxicity of anticancer drugs				
Oxaliplatin	Commensal microbiota	Mechanism still Unclear	Neurotoxicity	Iida et al. 2013
5-Fluorouracil	F. nucleatum P. oris	Bacterial dysbiosis	Oral mucositis	Yu et al. 2017; Scott et al. 2017
Irinotecan	Bacterial β-glucuronidase	Enzymatic degradation	Gastrointestinal toxicity	Huang et al. 2022
EGFR inhibitor	Skin microbiota	Bacterial dysbiosis	Skin toxicity	Huang et al. 2022
Immune checkpoint inhibitor	Bacterial polyamine transport system	Immunomodulation	Immune related adverse effects	Huang et al. 2022

many drugs. According to the literature, more than 60 drugs/compounds are known to undergo direct and indirect gut microbial modifications (Ervin, Ramanan and Bhatt, 2020). As such, the microbiome can alter the activity of drugs, these changes seem to have an impact on the efficacy as well as toxicity of the drug, which in turn could cause adverse drug reactions (Table 12.2) (Huang et al., 2022) As explored in a review by Huang et al. (2022), research in pharmacomicrobiomics is an emerging field aiming to investigate the role of microbiome compositional and functional variations on drug efficacy, toxicity, and pharmacokinetics (Huang et al., 2022). The authors suggest that the research can make use of the human microbiome to predict treatment response, improve the efficacy of the drugs, and reduce adverse drug reactions. More research is warranted in this field.

MICROBIOME-BASED INTERVENTIONS, TAILORED TO THE PEDIATRIC POPULATION IMPROVE TREATMENT EFFICACY AND REDUCE TREATMENT-RELATED COMPLICATIONS

In recent decades, understanding the role of the intestinal microbial community playing an important role in health and disease has increased. The intestinal microbial community in a state of delicate balance is now widely recognized to maintain health. The importance of precision medicine/personalized therapy can be extended to the individualized tailored administration of probiotics and prebiotics to influence the effect or response of future cancer therapeutics (Kashyap et al., 2017). Probiotics are active microorganisms that colonize the human intestines and change the composition of the microbiota of the host (Wang, Zhang and Zhang, 2021). The use of probiotics to regulate intestinal microbiota to improve host immunity has been investigated greatly in recent times. Evidence shows that probiotics play significant roles in gut microbiota composition, which can improve the host's immune system and responses (Wang, Zhang and Zhang, 2021).

Research on the role of probiotics and their ability to prevent chemotherapy-induced gut toxicity, chemotherapy-induced diarrhea, etc. would be beneficial. Prebiotics are another element to consider in treatment interventions. Prebiotics are defined as nondigestible dietary fibers that are fermented by gut bacteria. Prebiotics have a beneficial effect on the gut microbiome by selectively driving the growth and activity of commensal microbes, such as *Lactobacillus* and *Bifidobacterium* (Davani-Davari et al., 2019; Bedu-Ferrari et al., 2022). The research on the beneficial effects of prebiotics is restricted to how they exhibit anticancer effects, and currently, there is limited understanding of how prebiotics influence chemotherapy-induced toxicity or chemosensitivity (Batista et al., 2020). More studies are required to explore the benefits of pre- and probiotics, especially in childhood cancer cases. Fecal microbiota transplantation (FMT) is an alternative and the most direct way to alter gut microbiota composition. Studies have shown the potential of FMT in alleviating cancer-associated dysbiosis and chemotherapy-associated complications (Chen et al., 2019). Additionally, FMT could enhance the efficacy of cancer immunotherapy, thus remarkably affecting clinical outcomes and therefore a

LIMITATIONS

The number of studies on the gut microbiome is increasing, yet little is known about the relationship between gut microbiota and pediatric tumors, especially pediatric solid tumors. The very small number of patients (cohorts) and the challenges associated with sample collection make it challenging to investigate (Sági et al., 2022). Additionally, to prevent infections, children with solid tumors frequently receive chemotherapy, radiation therapy, and intensive antibiotic prophylaxis (Kurt et al., 2008). Studies on cancer treatment toxicities have linked gut microbiota, primarily in adult patients; however, there are few studies on pediatric cancer patients (Roy and Trinchieri, 2017; Bhuta et al., 2019; Wen, Jin and Chen, 2019). The development of more individualized and effective therapy in pediatric oncology will require the completion of more trials with larger cohorts. The standard course of treatment for pediatric cancer patients is complex and aggressive anticancer therapy, which frequently results in myelosuppression and involves radiation, chemotherapy, and surgery. Both directly and indirectly, these treatment modalities impact the gut microbiome and have a significant impact on the entire body, including the gastrointestinal system, liver, and bone marrow. Considerable research of illness development, treatment efficacy, staging, or side effect manifestations attests to the significance of the gut microbiota. Further research is needed in determining an individual's microbiome profile for improved and more effective cancer surveillance, diagnostics, prognosis, and tailored treatment prediction (Sági et al., 2022).

Chemotherapies are toxic substances that typically affect every cell in the body, including cancerous cells; they are not limited to particular types of cancer. The majority of chemotherapy patients deal with long-term physical and psychological side effects and therapy-related problems. Patients are at risk for obesity and metabolic syndrome, which can result in serious side effects like heart disease (Nottage et al., 2014; Zhang et al., 2014; Saultier et al., 2016). An important therapeutic approach for several cancers is allogeneic hematopoietic stem cell transplantation or allo-HSCT. Graft-versus-host disease, however, is one of its most serious side effects. Multiple organs, including the gastrointestinal tract, might be impacted by GVHD (Ferrara, 1993). Chemotherapy and radiation before allo-HSCT can compromise the gut epithelium's barrier integrity. This compromised intestinal barrier allows bacteria and their byproducts to move around and trigger the innate immune system, which in turn triggers alloreactive donor T-cells and the development of GVHD (Shono and Van Den Brink, 2018). Furthermore, a decrease in bacterial diversity may result in a higher death rate in GVHD (Taur et al., 2014).

Sustainability is the primary obstacle facing therapies centered on the microbiota. Long-term dedication is necessary to obtain the therapeutic effects of changes to the microbiome brought about by probiotic and prebiotic supplements, a balanced diet, exercise, and FMT (Vrieze et al., 2012; Clarke et al., 2014; Sheflin et al., 2016; Kootte et al., 2017; Krumbeck et al., 2018; Tandon et al., 2019; Kassaian et al., 2020). Children will not always find it easy to adhere to a balanced diet or exercise. Children diagnosed with or surviving cancer should receive comprehensive care that includes targeted interventions to treat microbial dysbiosis.

CONCLUSION AND FUTURE PERSPECTIVES

The relationship between pediatric tumors, especially pediatric solid tumors, and the gut microbiome is still unclear despite the increasing number of publications on this topic. The relatively small number of patient cohorts and the challenges associated with sample collection make the study challenging. Pediatric solid tumors account for 60% of all pediatric tumors (Dome et al., 2019). Patients with pediatric cancer typically get sophisticated and intensive anticancer therapy, which frequently results in myelosuppression and includes radiation, chemotherapy, and surgery (Mohiuddin, Zaky and Cortes, 2023). The gut microbiota is impacted both directly and indirectly by these treatments, which have a significant impact on the entire body, including the gastrointestinal tract, liver, and bone marrow (Weersma, Zhernakova and Fu, 2020). Multiple research projects about the development of diseases, the effectiveness of therapy, staging, or side effect manifestations support the significance of the gut microbiome (Shreiner, Kao and Young, 2015). Further research is needed, but eventually, it might be possible to determine a person's microbiome profile before beginning anticancer therapy to forecast efficacy or select a suitable and personalized course of treatment (Behrouzi, Nafari and Siadat, 2019). Additionally, microbiomes may be utilized as a biomarker (Zwezerijnen-Jiwa et al., 2023). The question of whether dysbiosis promotes or results from neoplasms is yet unsolved (Thomas and Jobin, 2015). The pediatric oncology population has been the subject of few microbiome investigations, and further research involving larger cohorts is required to facilitate the development of more personalized and efficacious therapy in pediatric cancer (Sági et al., 2022).

REFERENCES

Aghamajidi, A. and Vareki, S. M. (2022) 'The effect of the gut microbiota on systemic and anti-tumor immunity and response to systemic therapy against cancer', *Cancers*, 14(15), pp. 1–20. doi: 10.3390/cancers14153563.

Allen, J. and Sears, C. L. (2019) 'Impact of the gut microbiome on the genome and epigenome of colon epithelial cells: Contributions to colorectal cancer development', *Genome Medicine*. BioMed Central Ltd. doi: 10.1186/s13073-019-0621-2.

Al-Shehri, S. S. et al. (2015) 'Breastmilk-saliva interactions boost innate immunity by regulating the oral microbiome in early infancy', *PLoS One*, 10(9), pp. 1–19. doi: 10.1371/journal.pone.0135047.

Amitay, E. L. and Keinan-Boker, L. (2015) 'Breastfeeding and childhood leukemia incidence: a meta-analysis and systematic review', *JAMA Pediatrics*, 169(6), pp. 1–9. doi: 10.1001/jamapediatrics.2015.1025.

Barnea, D. et al. (2015) 'Obesity and metabolic disease after childhood cancer', *Oncology (Williston Park)*, 29(11), pp. 849–855.

Barnett, D. J. M. et al. (2023) 'Human milk oligosaccharides, antimicrobial drugs, and the gut microbiota of term neonates: observations from the KOALA birth cohort study', *Gut Microbes*, 15(1). doi: 10.1080/19490976.2022.2164152.

Batista, V. L. et al. (2020) 'Probiotics, prebiotics, synbiotics, and paraprobiotics as a therapeutic alternative for intestinal mucositis', *Frontiers in Microbiology*, 11(September). doi: 10.3389/fmicb.2020.544490.

Baxter, N. T. et al. (2014) 'Structure of the gut microbiome following colonization with human feces determines colonic tumor burden', *Microbiome*, 2(1), pp. 1–11. doi: 10.1186/2049-2618-2-20.

Bedu-Ferrari, C. et al. (2022) 'Prebiotics and the human gut microbiota: from breakdown mechanisms to the impact on metabolic health', *Nutrients*, 14(10), pp. 1–23. doi: 10.3390/nu14102096.

Behrouzi, A., Nafari, A. H. and Siadat, S. D. (2019) 'The significance of microbiome in personalized medicine', *Clinical and Translational Medicine*, 8(1). doi: 10.1186/s40169-019-0232-y.

Belkaid, Y. and Hand, T. W. (2014) 'Role of the microbiota in immunity and inflammation', *Cell*, 157(1), pp. 121–141. doi: 10.1016/j.cell.2014.03.011.

Bhatt, A. P., Redinbo, M. R. and Bultman, S. J. (2017) 'The role of the microbiome in cancer development and therapy', *CA: A Cancer Journal for Clinicians*, 67(4), pp. 326–344. doi: 10.3322/caac.21398.

Bhuta, R. et al. (2019) 'The gut microbiome and pediatric cancer: current research and gaps in knowledge', *Journal of the National Cancer Institute – Monographs*, 2019(54), pp. 169–173. doi: 10.1093/jncimonographs/lgz026.

Biesbroek, G. et al. (2014) 'Early respiratory microbiota composition determines bacterial succession patterns and respiratory health in children', *American Journal of Respiratory and Critical Care Medicine*, 190(11), pp. 1283–1292. doi: 10.1164/rccm.201407-1240OC.

Breton, J., Galmiche, M. and Déchelotte, P. (2022) 'Dysbiotic gut bacteria in obesity: an overview of the metabolic mechanisms and therapeutic perspectives of next-generation probiotics', *Microorganisms*, 10(2). doi: 10.3390/microorganisms10020452.

Cahana, I. and Iraqi, F. A. (2020) 'Impact of host genetics on gut microbiome: take-home lessons from human and mouse studies', *Animal Models and Experimental Medicine*, 3(3), pp. 229–236. doi: 10.1002/ame2.12134.

Chen, D. et al. (2019) 'Fecal microbiota transplantation in cancer management: current status and perspectives', *International Journal of Cancer*, 145(8), pp. 2021–2031. doi: 10.1002/ijc.32003.

Chu, D. M. et al. (2016) 'The early infant gut microbiome varies in association with a maternal high-fat diet', *Genome Medicine*, 8(1), pp. 1–12. doi: 10.1186/s13073-016-0330-z.

Chu, D. M., Ma, J., Prince, A. L., Anthony, K. M., Seferovic, M. D. and Aagaard, K. M. (2017) 'Maturation of the infant microbiome community structure and function across multiple body sites and in relation to mode of delivery', *Nature Medicine*, 23(3), pp. 314–326.

Chua, L. L. et al. (2020) 'Temporal changes in gut microbiota profile in children with acute lymphoblastic leukemia prior to commencement-, during-, and post-cessation of chemotherapy', *BMC Cancer*, 20(1), pp. 1–11. doi: 10.1186/s12885-020-6654-5.

Clarke, G. et al. (2014) 'Minireview: gut microbiota: the neglected endocrine organ', *Molecular Endocrinology*, 28(8), pp. 1221–1238. doi: 10.1210/me.2014-1108.

Cohen, L. J. et al. (2019) 'Genetic factors and the intestinal microbiome guide development of microbe-based therapies for inflammatory bowel diseases', *Gastroenterology*, 156(8), pp. 2174–2189. doi: 10.1053/j.gastro.2019.03.017.

Contu, L. et al. (2019) 'Pre- and post-natal high fat feeding differentially affects the structure and integrity of the neurovascular unit of 16-month old male and female mice', *Frontiers in Neuroscience*, 13(October), pp. 1–17. doi: 10.3389/fnins.2019.01045.

Davani-Davari, D. et al. (2019) 'Prebiotics: definition, types, sources, mechanisms, and clinical applications', *Foods*, 8(3), pp. 1–27. doi: 10.3390/foods8030092.

Davis, E. C. et al. (2020) 'Microbiome composition in pediatric populations from birth to adolescence: impact of diet and prebiotic and probiotic interventions', *Digestive Diseases and Sciences*, 65(3), pp. 706–722. doi: 10.1007/s10620-020-06092-x.

Derrien, M., Alvarez, A. S. and de Vos, W. M. (2019) 'The gut microbiota in the first decade of life', *Trends in Microbiology*, 27(12), pp. 997–1010. doi: 10.1016/j.tim.2019.08.001.

Dogra, S. K. et al. (2021) 'Nurturing the early life gut microbiome and immune maturation for long term health', *Microorganisms*, 9(10). doi: 10.3390/microorganisms9102110.

Dome, J. S. et al. (2019) 'Pediatric solid tumors'. In *Abeloff's Clinical Oncology*. 6th ed. Elsevier Inc. doi: 10.1016/B978-0-323-47674-4.00092-X.

Dominguez-Bello, M. G., Costello, E. K., Contreras, M., Magris, M., Hidalgo, G., Fierer, N. and Knight, R. (2010) 'Delivery mode shapes the acquisition and structure of the initial microbiota across multiple body habitats in newborns', *Proceeding of the National Academcy Science of the United States of America*, 107(26), 11971–11975.

Dougherty, M. W. and Jobin, C. (2023) 'Intestinal bacteria and colorectal cancer: etiology and treatment', *Gut Microbes*. doi: 10.1080/19490976.2023.2185028.

Dunn, A. B. et al. (2017) 'The maternal infant microbiome: considerations for labor and birth', *MCN*, 42(6), pp. 1–7.

Dupont, H. L. et al. (2020) 'The intestinal microbiome in human health and disease', *Transactions of the American Clinical and Climatological Association*, 131(5), pp. 178–197. Available at: http://www.ncbi.nlm.nih.gov/pubmed/32675857%0A http://www.pubmedcentral.nih.gov/artic lerender.fcgi?artid= PMC7358474.

Edwards, S. M. et al. (2017) 'The maternal gut microbiome during pregnancy', *MCN The American Journal of Maternal/Child Nursing*, 42(6), pp. 310–316. doi: 10.1097/NMC.0000000000000372.

Edwards, S. M., Cunningham, S. A. and Dunlop, A. L. (2017) *Edwards-2017-R-Maternal- Microbiome-Pregnancy*, pp. 1–7.

Elsakr, J. M. et al. (2019) 'Maternal Western-style diet affects offspring islet composition and function in a non-human primate model of maternal over-nutrition', *Molecular Metabolism*, 25(April), pp. 73–82. doi: 10.1016/j.molmet.2019.03.010.

Ervin, S. M., Ramanan, S. V. and Bhatt, A. P. (2020) 'Relationship between the gut microbiome and systemic chemotherapy', *Digestive Diseases and Sciences*, 65(3), pp. 874–884. doi: 10.1007/s10620-020-06119-3.

Fallani, M. et al. (2011) 'Determinants of the human infant intestinal microbiota after the introduction of first complementary foods in infant samples from five European centres', *Microbiology*, 157(5), pp. 1385–1392. doi: 10.1099/mic.0.042143-0.

Ferrara, J. L. M. (1993) 'Cytokine dysregulation as a mechanism of graft versus host disease', *Current Opinion in Immunology*, 5(5), pp. 794–799. doi: 10.1016/0952- 7915(93)90139-J.

De Filippo, C. et al. (2010) 'Impact of diet in shaping gut microbiota revealed by a comparative study in children from Europe and rural Africa', *Proceedings of the National Academy of Sciences of the United States of America*, 107(33), pp. 14691–14696. doi: 10.1073/pnas.1005963107.

Fragkou, P. C. et al. (2021) 'Impact of early life nutrition on children's immune system and noncommunicable diseases through its effects on the bacterial microbiome, virome and mycobiome', *Frontiers in Immunology*, 12(March), pp. 1–8. doi: 10.3389/fimmu.2021.644269.

Francino, M. P. (2016) 'Antibiotics and the human gut microbiome: dysbioses and accumulation of resistances', *Frontiers in Microbiology*, 6(JAN), pp. 1–11. doi: 10.3389/fmicb.2015.01543.

Gebrayel, P. et al. (2022) 'Microbiota medicine: towards clinical revolution', *Journal of Translational Medicine*, 20(1), pp. 1–20. doi: 10.1186/s12967-022-03296-9.

Gorczyca, K. et al. (2022) 'Changes in the gut microbiome and pathologies in pregnancy', *International Journal of Environmental Research and Public Health*, 19(16). doi: 10.3390/ijerph19169961.

Gibson, M. K., Wang, B., Ahmadi, S., Burnham, C. A., Tarr, P. I., Warner, B. B. and Dantas, G. (2016) 'Developmental dynamics of the preterm infant gut microbiota and antibiotic resistome', *Nature Microbiology*, 1, p. 16024.

Guenther, M., Haas, M., Heinemann, V., Kruger, S., Westphalen, C. B., von Bergwelt- Baildon, M., Mayerle, J., Werner, J., Kirchner, T., Boeck, S. and Ormanns, S. (2020) 'Bacterial lipopolysaccharide as negative predictor of gemcitabine efficacy in advanced pancreatic cancer – translational results from the AIO-PK0104 Phase 3 study', *British Journal of Cancer*, 123(9), pp. 1370–1376.

Guigoz, Y., Doré, J. and Schiffrin, E. J. (2008) 'The inflammatory status of old age can be nurtured from the intestinal environment', *Current Opinion in Clinical Nutrition and Metabolic Care*, 11(1), pp. 13–20. doi: 10.1097/MCO.0b013e3282f2bfdf.

Harmsen, H. J. M., Wildeboer-Veloo, A. C. M., Raangs, G. C., Wagendorp, A. A., Klijn, N., Bindels, J. G. and Welling, G. W. (2000). 'Analysis of intestinal flora development in breast-fed and formula-fed infants by using molecular identification and detection methods', *Journal of Pediatric Gastroenterology and Nutrition*, 30(1), pp. 61–67.

Hills, R. D. et al. (2019) 'Gut microbiome: profound implications for diet and disease', *Nutrients*, 11(7), pp. 1–40. doi: 10.3390/nu11071613.

Hollister, E. B. et al. (2015) 'Structure and function of the healthy pre-adolescent pediatric gut microbiome', *Microbiome*, pp. 1–13. doi: 10.1186/s40168-015-0101-x.

Huang, J., Liu, W., Kang, W., He, Y., Yang, R., Mou, X. and Zhao, W. (2022), 'Effects of microbiota on anticancer drugs: current knowledge and potential applications', *EBioMedicine*, 83, p. 104197.

Huang, Y. et al. (2012) 'Effect of high-dose methotrexate chemotherapy on intestinal Bifidobacteria, Lactobacillus and Escherichia coli in children with acute lymphoblastic leukemia', *Experimental Biology and Medicine*, 237(3), pp. 305–311. doi: 10.1258/ebm.2011.011297.

Huttenhower, C. et al. (2012) 'Structure, function and diversity of the healthy human microbiome', *Nature*, 486(7402), pp. 207–214. doi: 10.1038/nature11234.

Iida, N., Dzutsev, A., Stewart, C. A., Smith, L., Bouladoux, N., Weingarten, R. A., Molina, D. A., Salcedo, R., Back, T., Cramer, S., Dai, R. M., Kiu, H., Cardone, M., Naik, S., Patri, A. K., Wang, E., Marincola, F. M., Frank, K. M., Belkaid, Y., Trinchieri, G. and Goldszmid, R. S. (2013) 'Commensal bacteria control cancer response to therapy by modulating the tumor microenvironment', *Science*, 342(6161), pp. 967–70.

Jandhyala, S. M. et al. (2015) 'Role of the normal gut microbiota', *World Journal of Gastroenterology*, 21(29), pp. 8836–8847. doi: 10.3748/wjg.v21.i29.8787.

Javdan, B., Lopez, J. G., Chankhamjon, P., Lee, Y. J., Hull, R., Wu, Q., Wang, X., Chatterjee, S. and Donia, M. S. (2020). 'Personalized mapping of drug metabolism by the human gut microbiome', *Cell*, 181(7), pp. 1661–1679.e22.

Kashyap, P. C. et al. (2017) 'Microbiome at the frontier of personalized medicine', *Mayo Clinic Proceedings*, 92(12), pp. 1855–1864. doi: 10.1016/j.mayocp.2017.10.004.

Kassaian, N. et al. (2020) 'The effects of 6 mo of supplementation with probiotics and synbiotics on gut microbiota in the adults with prediabetes: a double blind randomized clinical trial', *Nutrition*, 79–80, p. 110854. doi: 10.1016/j.nut.2020.110854.

Kho, Z. Y. and Lal, S. K. (2018) 'The human gut microbiome – a potential controller of wellness and disease', *Frontiers in Microbiology*, 9(AUG), pp. 1–23. doi: 10.3389/fmicb.2018.01835.

Kootte, R. S. et al. (2017) 'Improvement of insulin sensitivity after lean donor feces in metabolic syndrome is driven by baseline intestinal microbiota composition', *Cell Metabolism*, 26(4), pp. 611–619.e6. doi: 10.1016/j.cmet.2017.09.008.

Koren, O. et al. (2013) 'A guide to enterotypes across the human body: meta-analysis of microbial community structures in human microbiome datasets', *PLoS Computational Biology*, 9(1). doi: 10.1371/journal.pcbi.1002863.

Kostic, A. D. et al. (2012) 'Genomic analysis identifies association of Fusobacterium with colorectal carcinoma', *Genome Research*, 22, pp. 292–298. doi: 10.1101/gr.126573.111.292.

Krumbeck, J. A. et al. (2018) 'Probiotic Bifidobacterium strains and galactooligosaccharides improve intestinal barrier function in obese adults but show no synergism when used together as synbiotics', *Microbiome*, 6(121). doi: https://doi.org/10.1186/s40168-018- 0494-4.

Kunika, Frey, N. and Rangrez, A. Y. (2023) 'Exploring the involvement of gut microbiota in cancer therapy-induced cardiotoxicity', *International Journal of Molecular Sciences*, 24(8). doi: 10.3390/ijms24087261.

Kurt, B. et al. (2008) 'Prophylactic antibiotics reduce morbidity due to septicemia during intensive treatment for pediatric acute myeloid leukemia', *Cancer*, 113(2), pp. 376–382. doi: 10.1002/cncr.23563.

Langdon, A., Crook, N. and Dantas, G. (2016) 'The effects of antibiotics on the microbiome throughout development and alternative approaches for therapeutic modulation', *Genome Medicine*, 8(1). doi: 10.1186/s13073-016-0294-z.

Lazar, V. et al. (2018) 'Aspects of gut microbiota and immune system interactions in infectious diseases, immunopathology, and cancer', *Frontiers in Immunology*, 9(AUG), pp. 1–18. doi: 10.3389/fimmu.2018.01830.

Leardini, D. et al. (2022) 'Pharmacomicrobiomics in pediatric oncology: the complex interplay between commonly used drugs and gut microbiome', *International Journal of Molecular Sciences*, 23(23). doi: 10.3390/ijms232315387.

Lichtenstern, C. R. and Lamichhane-Khadka, R. (2023) 'A tale of two bacteria – Bacteroides fragilis, Escherichia coli, and colorectal cancer', *Frontiers in Bacteriology*, 2. doi: 10.3389/fbrio.2023.1229077.

Lloyd-Price, J., Abu-Ali, G. and Huttenhower, C. (2016) 'The healthy human microbiome', *Genome Medicine*, 8(1), pp. 1–11. doi: 10.1186/s13073-016-0307-y.

Ma, J. et al. (2014) 'High-fat maternal diet during pregnancy persistently alters the offspring microbiome in a primate model', *Nature Communications*, 5(May). doi: 10.1038/ncomms4889.

Manor, O. et al. (2020) 'Health and disease markers correlate with gut microbiome composition across thousands of people', *Nature Communications*, 11(1), pp. 1–12. doi: 10.1038/s41467-020-18871-1.

Manos, J. (2022) 'The human microbiome in disease and pathology', *Apmis*, 130(12), pp. 690–705. doi: 10.1111/apm.13225.

Masetti, R. et al. (2021) 'Gut microbiome in pediatric acute leukemia: from predisposition to cure', *Blood Advances*, 5(22), pp. 4619–4629. doi: 10.1182/bloodadvances.2021005129.

Mohiuddin, S., Zaky, W. and Cortes, J. (2023) 'Overview of pediatric cancers', In *Perioperative Care of the Cancer Patient*, Elsevier, pp. 491–497. doi: https://doi.org/10.1016/B978-0-323-69584-8.00045-1.

Moossavi, S. et al. (2019) 'Composition and variation of the human milk microbiota are influenced by maternal and early-life factors', *Cell Host and Microbe*, 25(2), pp. 324–335.e4. doi: 10.1016/j.chom.2019.01.011.

Morelli, L. (2008) 'Postnatal development of intestinal microflora as influenced by infant nutrition', *Journal of Nutrition*, 138(9), pp. 1791S–1795S.

Nash, M. J., Frank, D. N. and Friedman, J. E. (2017) 'Early microbes modify immune system development and metabolic homeostasis-the "Restaurant" hypothesis revisited', *Frontiers in Endocrinology*, 8(DEC), pp. 1–7. doi: 10.3389/fendo.2017.00349.

Niu, J. et al. (2020) 'Evolution of the gut microbiome in early childhood: a cross-sectional study of Chinese children', *Frontiers in Microbiology*, 11(April), pp. 1–16. doi: 10.3389/fmicb.2020.00439.

Nottage, K. A. et al. (2014) 'Metabolic syndrome and cardiovascular risk among long-term survivors of acute lymphoblastic leukaemia – from the St. Jude lifetime cohort', *British Journal of Haematology*, 165(3), pp. 364–374. doi: 10.1111/bjh.12754.

Olaniyi, K. S. et al. (2020) 'Placental microbial colonization and its association with pre-eclampsia', *Frontiers in Cellular and Infection Microbiology*, 10(August), pp. 1–11. doi: 10.3389/fcimb.2020.00413.

Oldacres, L. et al. (2023) 'Interventions promoting cognitive function in patients experiencing cancer related cognitive impairment: a systematic review', *Psycho-Oncology*, 32(2), pp. 214–228. doi: 10.1002/pon.6073.

Quaglio, A. E. V. et al. (2022) 'Gut microbiota, inflammatory bowel disease and colorectal cancer', *World Journal of Gastroenterology*, 28(30), pp. 4053–4060. doi: 10.3748/wjg.v28.i30.4053.

Quitadamo, P. A., Comegna, L. and Cristalli, P. (2021) 'Anti-infective, anti-inflammatory, and immunomodulatory properties of breast milk factors for the protection of infants in the pandemic from COVID-19', *Frontiers in Public Health*, 8(March), pp. 1–29. doi: 10.3389/fpubh.2020.589736.

Radjabzadeh, D. et al. (2020) 'Diversity, compositional and functional differences between gut microbiota of children and adults', *Scientific Reports*, 10(1), pp. 1–13. doi: 10.1038/s41598-020-57734-z.

Rebersek, M. (2021) 'Gut microbiome and its role in colorectal cancer', *BMC Cancer*, 21(1), pp. 1–13. doi: 10.1186/s12885-021-09054-2.

Rinninella, E. et al. (2019) 'What is the healthy gut microbiota composition? A changing ecosystem across age, environment, diet, and diseases', *Microorganisms*, 7(1). doi: 10.3390/microorganisms7010014.

Robertson, R. C. et al. (2019) 'The human microbiome and child growth – first 1000 days and beyond', *Trends in Microbiology*, 27(2), pp. 131–147. doi: 10.1016/j.tim.2018.09.008.

Ronan, V., Yeasin, R. and Claud, E. C. (2021) 'Childhood development and the microbiome—the intestinal microbiota in maintenance of health and development of disease during childhood development', *Gastroenterology*, 160(2), pp. 495–506. doi: 10.1053/j.gastro.2020.08.065.

Roy, S. and Trinchieri, G. (2017) 'Microbiota: a key orchestrator of cancer therapy', *Nature Reviews Cancer*, 17(5), pp. 271–285. doi: 10.1038/nrc.2017.13.

Ruiz-Ojeda, F. J. et al. (2023) 'Effects of a novel infant formula on the fecal microbiota in the first six months of life: the INNOVA 2020 study', *International Journal of Molecular Sciences*, 24(3). doi: 10.3390/ijms24033034.

Saeed, N. K. et al. (2022) 'Gut microbiota in various childhood disorders: implication and indications', *World Journal of Gastroenterology*, 28(18), pp. 1875–1901. doi: 10.3748/wjg.v28.i18.1875.

Sági, V. et al. (2022) 'The influence of the gut microbiome in paediatric cancer origin and treatment', *Antibiotics*, 11(11). doi: 10.3390/antibiotics11111521.

Sánchez, C. et al. (2021) 'Human milk oligosaccharides (HMOs) and infant microbiota: a scoping review', *Foods*, 10(6), pp. 1–18. doi: 10.3390/foods10061429.

Saultier, P. et al. (2016) 'Metabolic syndrome in long-term survivors of childhood acute leukemia treated without hematopoietic stem cell transplantation: an L.E.A. study', *Haematologica*, 101(12), pp. 1603–1610. doi: 10.3324/haematol.2016.148908.

Scott, T. A., Quintaneiro, L. M., Norvaisas, P., Lui, P. P., Wilson, M. P., Leung, K. Y., Herrera-Dominguez, L., Sudiwala, S., Pessia, A., Clayton, P. T., Bryson, K., Velagapudi, V., Mills, P. B., Typas, A., Greene, N. D. E. and Cabreiro, F. (2017) 'Host-microbe co-metabolism dictates cancer drug efficacy in C. elegans', *Cell*, 169(3), 442-456.e18.

Sender, R., Fuchs, S. and Milo, R. (2016) 'Revised estimates for the number of human and bacteria cells in the body', *PLoS Biology*, 14(8), pp. 1–21. doi: 10.1371/journal.pbio.1002533.

Sheflin, A. et al. (2016) 'Dietary supplementation with rice bran or navy bean alters gut bacterial metabolism in colorectal cancer survivors. Molecular Nutrition & Food Research, 2017, 61, 1500905', *Molecular Nutrition & Food Research*, 61, p. 1500905. doi: https://doi.org/10.1002/mnfr.201500905.

Shono, Y. and Van Den Brink, M. R. M. (2018) 'Gut microbiota injury in allogeneic haematopoietic stem cell transplantation', *Nature Reviews Cancer*, 18(5), pp. 283–295. doi: 10.1038/nrc.2018.10.

Shreiner, A. B., Kao, J. Y. and Young, V. B. (2015) 'The gut microbiome in health and in disease', *Current Opinion in Gastroenterology*, 31(1), pp. 69–75. doi: 10.1097/MOG.0000000000000139.

Singh, V. et al. (2023) 'Butyrate producers, "The Sentinel of Gut": Their intestinal significance with and beyond butyrate, and prospective use as microbial therapeutics', *Frontiers in Microbiology*. doi: 10.3389/fmicb.2022.1103836.

Stein, K. D., Syrjala, K. L. and Andrykowski, M. A. (2008) 'Physical and psychological long-term and late effects of cancer', *Cancer*, 112(11 SUPPL.), pp. 2577–2592. doi: 10.1002/cncr.23448.

Stojanov, S., Berlec, A. and Štrukelj, B. (2020) 'The influence of probiotics on the firmicutes/bacteroidetes ratio in the treatment of obesity and inflammatory bowel disease', *Microorganisms*, 8(11), pp. 1–16. doi: 10.3390/microorganisms8111715.

Tandon, D. et al. (2019) 'A prospective randomized, double-blind, placebo-controlled, dose- response relationship study to investigate efficacy of fructo-oligosaccharides (FOS) on human gut microflora', *Scientific Reports*, 9(1), pp. 1–15. doi: 10.1038/s41598- 019-41837-3.

Tap, J. et al. (2009) 'Towards the human intestinal microbiota phylogenetic core', *Environmental Microbiology*, 11(10), pp. 2574–2584. doi: 10.1111/j.1462- 2920.2009.01982.x.

Taur, Y. et al. (2014) 'The effects of intestinal tract bacterial diversity on mortality following allogeneic hematopoietic stem cell transplantation', *Blood*, 124(7), pp. 1174–1182. doi: 10.1182/blood-2014-02-554725.

Thomas, R. M. and Jobin, C. (2015) 'The microbiome and cancer: is the "Oncobiome" mirage real?', *Trends in Cancer*, 1(1), pp. 24–35. doi: 10.1016/j.trecan.2015.07.005.

Tian, M. et al. (2023) 'Maternal microbe-specific modulation of the offspring microbiome and development during pregnancy and lactation', *Gut Microbes*, 15(1), pp. 1–24. doi: 10.1080/19490976.2023.2206505.

Tooley, K. L. (2020) 'Effects of the human gut microbiota on cognitive performance, brain structure and function: a narrative review', *Nutrients*, 12(10), pp. 1–17. doi: 10.3390/nu12103009.

Turnbaugh, P. J. et al. (2009) 'The effect of diet on the human gut microbiome: a metagenomic analysis in humanized gnotobiotic mice', *Science Translational Medicine*, 1(6). doi: 10.1126/scitranslmed.3000322.

Turunen, J. et al. (2021) 'Presence of distinctive microbiome in the first-pass meconium of newborn infants', *Scientific Reports*, 11(1), pp. 1–12. doi: 10.1038/s41598-021-98951-4.

Vimal, J., Himal, I. and Kannan, S. (2020) 'Role of microbial dysbiosis in carcinogenesis & cancer therapies', *Indian Journal of Medical Research*, 152, pp. 553–561. doi: DOI: 10.4103/ijmr.IJMR_1026_18.

Vrieze, A. et al. (2012) 'Transfer of intestinal microbiota from lean donors increases insulin sensitivity in individuals with metabolic syndrome', *Gastroenterology*, 143(4), pp. 913–916.e7. doi: 10.1053/j.gastro.2012.06.031.

Walker, R. W. et al. (2017) 'The prenatal gut microbiome: are we colonized with bacteria in utero?', *Pediatric Obesity*, 12, pp. 3–17. doi: 10.1111/ijpo.12217.

Walters, K. E. and Martiny, J. B. H. (2020) 'Alpha-, beta-, and gamma-diversity of bacteria varies across habitats', *PLoS One*, 15(9 September), pp. 1–17. doi: 10.1371/journal.pone.0233872.

Wang, X., Zhang, P. and Zhang, X. (2021) 'Probiotics regulate gut microbiota: an effective method to improve immunity', *Molecules*, 26(19), pp. 1–15. doi: 10.3390/molecules26196076.

Wang, Z. et al. (2020) 'Comparing gut microbiome in mothers' own breast milk- and formula-fed moderate-late preterm infants', *Frontiers in Microbiology*, 11(May), pp. 1–13. doi: 10.3389/fmicb.2020.00891.

Weersma, R. K., Zhernakova, A. and Fu, J. (2020) 'Interaction between drugs and the gut microbiome', *Gut*, 69(8), pp. 1510–1519. doi: 10.1136/gutjnl-2019-320204.

Wei, L., Wen, X. Sen and Xian, C. J. (2021) 'Chemotherapy-induced intestinal microbiota dysbiosis impairs mucosal homeostasis by modulating toll-like receptor signaling pathways', *International Journal of Molecular Sciences*, 22(17). doi: 10.3390/ijms22179474.

Wen, L. and Duffy, A. (2017) 'Factors influencing the gut microbiota, inflammation, and type 2 diabetes', *Journal of Nutrition*, 147(7), pp. 1468S–1475S. doi: 10.3945/jn.116.240754.

Wen, Y., Jin, R. and Chen, H. (2019) 'Interactions between gut microbiota and acute childhood leukemia', *Frontiers in Microbiology*, 10(JUN), pp. 1–7. doi: 10.3389/fmicb.2019.01300.

Wiertsema, S. P. et al. (2021) 'The interplay between the gut microbiome and the immune system in the context of infectious diseases throughout life and the role of nutrition in optimizing treatment strategies', *Nutrients*, 13(3), pp. 1–14. doi: 10.3390/nu13030886.

Yassour, M. et al. (2016) 'Natural history of the infant gut microbiome and impact of antibiotic treatment on bacterial strain diversity and stability', *Science Translational Medicine*, 8(343). doi: 10.1126/scitranslmed.aad0917.

Yatsunenko, T. et al. (2012) 'Human gut microbiome viewed across age and geography', *Nature*, 486(7402), pp. 222–227. doi: 10.1038/nature11053.

Yu, Z. et al. (2023) 'Greater alteration of gut microbiota occurs in childhood obesity than in adulthood obesity', *Frontiers in Pediatrics*, 11(January), pp. 1–5. doi: 10.3389/fped.2023.1087401.

Yu, T., Guo, F., Yu, Y., Sun, T., Ma, D., Han, J., Qian, Y., Kryczek, I., Sun, D., Nagarsheth, N., Chen, Y., Chen, H., Hong, J., Zou, W. and Fang, J. Y. (2017) '*Fusobacterium nucleatum* promotes chemoresistance to colorectal cancer by modulating autophagy', *Cell*, 170(3), 548–563.e16.

Zhang, F. F. et al. (2014) 'Obesity in pediatric ALL survivors: a meta-analysis', *Pediatrics*, 133(3), pp. 704–715e. doi: 10.1542/peds.2013-3332.

Zhang, J. et al. (2022) 'Cancer immunotherapy: fecal microbiota transplantation brings light', *Current Treatment Options in Oncology*, 23(12), pp. 1777–1792. doi: 10.1007/s11864-022-01027-2.

Zhao, L. Y. et al. (2023) 'Role of the gut microbiota in anticancer therapy: from molecular mechanisms to clinical applications', *Signal Transduction and Targeted Therapy*, 8(1). doi: 10.1038/s41392-023-01406-7.

Zhao, T. et al. (2022) 'Fusobacterium nucleatum: a new player in regulation of cancer development and therapeutic response',

Cancer Drug Resistance, 5(4), pp. 436–450. doi: 10.20517/cdr.2021.144.

Zhou, Y., Zhou, C. and Zhang, A. (2022) 'Gut microbiota in acute leukemia: current evidence and future directions', *Frontiers in Microbiology*, 13(December), pp. 1–14. doi: 10.3389/fmicb.2022.1045497.

Zwezerijnen-Jiwa, F. H. et al. (2023) 'A systematic review of microbiome-derived biomarkers for early colorectal cancer detection', *Neoplasia*, 36(October 2022). doi: 10.1016/j.neo.2022.100868.

13 Gut Microbiome and Systemic Side Effects of Cancer Therapies

Richard Khanyile, Lloyd Mabonga, and Zodwa Dlamini

INTRODUCTION

The development of cancer treatment options, such as radiotherapy, chemotherapy, surgery, and immunotherapy, has been the subject of enormous interest in recent decades. As a result, the mortality and morbidity rates associated with several types of cancer have been considerably lowered (Kunika et al. 2023; Santucci et al. 2022). The advantages of these cancer treatments are indisputably plain and beyond doubt. However, the advantages of traditional anticancer treatments have always been accompanied by significant systemic side effects. Thus high-quality, in-depth biological insights into the underpinning biological processes and causative agents have indicated potential relationships between cancer therapy and gut dysbiosis. Traditional anticancer therapy toxicity is linked to the gut microbiome, and related toxicity may be mitigated by adjusting the gut microbiota's constituents. For customized attenuation of these adverse events, it is especially crucial to comprehend the connection between various microorganisms and the side effects of conventional anticancer therapy (Kunika et al. 2023).

The human digestive system is home to trillions of various kinds of microorganisms, which are commonly referred to as the gut microbiome. Humans and bacteria have coevolved, and microbial populations have a significant function in human health, according to Groussin et al. (2020). Recent technological advances have resulted in a tremendous improvement in our comprehension of the gut microbiome. It has been established that the microbiome influences both health and disease progression, including cancer. Multiple investigations have suggested that the gut microbiota may be a possible target in cancer therapy modulation, potentially increasing the efficacy of cancer therapies. Changes in the composition of the microbiome have been associated with long-term cancer therapy side effects such as acute gastrointestinal toxicity and dysbiosis (as shown in Figure 13.1). As a result, the gut microbiota develops along with the host and sits at the crossroads of numerous anticancer and oncogenic metabolic processes, immunological functions, and inflammatory mechanisms in cancer (Nicholson et al. 2012).

Numerous research investigations have found a link between gut microbiota, genotoxins, and proinflammatory responses in carcinogenesis (Rajagopala et al. 2017). Along the same trajectory, it has been demonstrated that the gut microbiota can modify how the body responds to cancer therapies via a variety of mechanisms such as immunological interactions, xenometabolism, and community structure changes (Perez-Chanona and Trinchieri, 2016). These and other studies corroborate the gut microbiome-cancer axis, and a deeper comprehension of these intricate connections could eventually contribute to new and improved cancer therapies (Sepich-Poore et al. 2021; Alexander et al. 2017). In cancer patients, the link between the microbiome and cancer therapy is poorly known. In this chapter, we discuss the connection between treatment-related microbial changes and systemic side effects of cancer therapies. A deeper understanding of the link between the gut microbiome and radiotherapy, chemotherapy, surgery, and immunotherapy may help lower the risk of fatal side effects.

GUT MICROBIOTA AND IMMUNOTHERAPY

The gut microbiota, which produces a myriad of small molecules and metabolites, plays an essential role in multiple human physiological processes, including metabolism, inflammation, immunity, and neurology (Chrysostomu et al. 2023). Immunotherapy has revolutionized cancer treatment. Immunotherapy is based on blocking receptors that dampen T-cell activation. The common receptors are programmed cell death receptors (PD-L1/PD-1 receptors) and cytotoxic T lymphocyte associated antigen-4 (CTLA-4/CD28) receptors. The drugs that inhibit these receptors are called check-point inhibitors. Immunotherapy causes multiple immune-related side effects like colitis (Chrysostomu et al. 2023).

Immunotherapy-induced colitis often presents with nonspecific symptoms such as abdominal pain and diarrhea or sometimes with severe symptoms such as blood in stool or ileus (Sehgal and Khanna 2021). Colitis-resistant patients had greater numbers of Bacteroidetes, which may have limited inflammation by supporting a differentiating pathway to a Treg phenotype, while patients with increased number of *Faecalibacterium* and other Firmicutes had increased rate of colitis (Sehgal and Khanna 2021). This is a clear indication that gut microbiota can fuel systemic inflammatory cells and factors. The interplay between immunotherapy and gut microbiota worsens or attenuates the immune-related side effects of immunotherapy. More studies are needed to unravel the interplay between gut microbiota and immunotherapy (Sehgal and Khanna 2021).

DOI: 10.1201/9781032706450-13

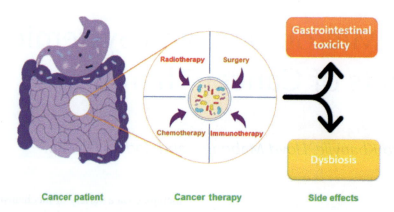

FIGURE 13.1 **Gut microbiome and systemic side effects of cancer therapies.** Changes in the composition of the microbiome have been associated with long-term cancer therapy side effects such as acute gastrointestinal toxicity and dysbiosis. As a result, the gut microbiota develops along with the host and sits at the crossroads of numerous anticancer and oncogenic metabolic processes, immunological functions, and inflammatory mechanisms in cancer (Nicholson et al. 2012). Along the same trajectory, it has been demonstrated that the gut microbiota can modify how the body responds to cancer therapies via a variety of mechanisms such as immunological interactions, xenometabolism, and community structure changes (Perez-Chanona and Trinchieri, 2016). A deeper understanding of the link between the gut microbiome and radiotherapy, chemotherapy, surgery, and immunotherapy may help lower the risk of fatal side effects.

GUT MICROBIOTA AND CHEMOTHERAPY

The human gut microbiota is a complex ecosystem containing bacteria, viruses, fungi, and yeasts (Fernandes et al. 2022). The interaction between the gut microbiota and chemotherapy determines the efficacy and the toxicity of chemotherapy (Li et al. 2016). Chemotherapy is the synthetic chemical drugs that kill or inhibit tumor cell growth. Chemotherapy affects the rapidly dividing cells, as tumor cells are known to divide rapidly. Normal mucosal cells also divide rapidly leading to them being affected by chemotherapy. Chemotherapies are classified according to mechanisms of actions through which they interact with the gut microbiota as highlighted below.

Topoisomerase I inhibitor, e.g., irinotecan, is a class of chemotherapy that inhibits topoisomerase I enzyme, which is important in the modulation of DNA topology to maintain chromosome superstructure and integrity (Vos et al. 2011). It has been shown that after receiving irinotecan the intestinal microenvironment is changed. This leads to increased harmful bacteria and reduced chemotherapy efficacy and increased toxicity. This disharmony is called microbial-host-irinotecan axis imbalance (Hofseth et al. 2020). Irinotecan induces proinflammatory cytokines like interleukin-6 (IL-6), tumor necrosis factor alpha, and IL-8 (Lin et al. 2012). It has been also observed that irinotecan treatment at the dose of 125 mg/kg over 3 days leads to a significant change in gut microbiota with an increase of *Enterobacter* and *Clostridium* species (Lin et al. 2012), while Wang et al. observed similar changes in mice (Wang et al. 2012).

The reasons for the observed changes are multifactorial. One of the reasons is that the increase in proinflammatory factors leads to a reduced number of adhesion sites and nutrition, leading to decreased gut microbiota (Stringer, 2013). The other reason is that the intestinal microbes produce the enzyme *β-glucuronidase* which can cleave the glucuronide molecule from less toxic metabolite of irinotecan leading to reactivated and toxic irinotecan (Takasuna et al. 1996). Gut microbiota produces metabolites like short-chain fatty acids which protect the gut and lead to what is called irinotecan detoxification, while also producing *β-glucuronidase* which is associated with irinotecan toxicity (Gallotti et al. 2021).

Alkylating agents, like cyclophosphamide, are used in most cancers. Cyclophosphamide is immunogenic by inducing TH1 and TH17 while inhibiting tumor growth (Ghiringhelli and Apetoh 2014). Cyclophosphamide destroys intestinal mucosa leading to the translocation of Gram-positive bacteria to lymphoid organs. These Gram-positive bacteria induce TH1 and TH17 immune cells which leads to improved antitumor effects of cyclophosphamide (Viaud et al. 2013). Cyclophosphamide also produces reactive oxygen species which reduce antioxidants, superoxide dismutase (SOD), and peroyhydrogenase (CAT) (Puertollano et al. 2011). Oxidative stress and inflammatory response lead to changes in the intestinal microenvironment and gut microbiota (Xu et al. 2023).

Antimetabolite agents, like 5-fluoro-uracil (5-FU), are the most commonly used in clinical oncology practice. 5-FU induces inflammation through neutrophil infiltration and secretion of inflammatory factors (Justino et al. 2015) leading to gut ecological imbalance. Probiotics can reduce 5-FU-induced intestinal mucositis by stabilizing the gut microbiota (Justino et al. 2015). It has been shown that the fecal flora in the stomach, jejunum, and colon change after 5-FU treatment (Liu, 2023). After 48–72 hours of 5-FU treatment, *Escherichia coli* and *Clostridium* are increased in the colon. This might lead to both local and systemic sepsis. Chen et al. (2020), through fecal microbiota transportation, demonstrated that the gut microbiota plays an important role in the regulation of muscle metabolism and promoting muscle energy production in 5-FU-induced malnutrition rats. This indicates that gut microbiota homeostasis can mitigate against 5-FU-induced muscle wasting (Chen et al. 2020).

Platinum-based agents, like cisplatin and oxaliplatin, are used in many cancer treatment combinations or as single agents. The known side effects are nausea and vomiting, mucositis, myelosuppression, mechanical hyperalgesia, renal failure, and many more. The role of the gut microbiota in worsening or reducing some of these side effects has been investigated. Hsiao et al. (2021) assessed the role of *Lactobacillus reuteri* and *Clostridium butyricum* (LCs) in renal failure. LCs in the gut microbiota lead to decreased inflammation. LCs supplementation has led to decreased microphages and neutrophils infiltration of the intestinal mucosa and less inflammation in the kidneys. LCs prevent goblet cell damage and gut-derived endogenous endotoxin production in rats treated with cisplatin. LCs also improve intestinal permeability in rats treated with cisplatin (Hsiao et al. 2021). Oxaliplatin changes the intestinal microbiota and promotes the development of chemotherapy-induced mechanical hyperalgesia. Gut microbiota plays a role in oxaliplatin-induced mechanical hyperalgesia. More studies are needed to assess the role of microbiota in mechanical hyperalgesia caused by other chemotherapies (Liu et al. 2023).

Antimicrotubules agents, like taxanes (paclitaxel and docetaxel), are anticancer drugs that are used in many cancer treatments. Paclitaxel is a natural anticancer drug that is widely used in the treatment of breast cancer, ovarian cancer, lung cancer, and many other cancers (Liu et al. 2023). The interplay between paclitaxel and microbiota, in the manifestation of some of the side effects of paclitaxel, has been investigated. In mice treated with paclitaxel, this chemotherapy affected the microbes and the lining of the gut. These changes caused inflammation in the surrounding tissues, which in turn produced signals that promote inflammation in the brain (Loman et al. 2019). Inflammation in the brain leads to fatigue, weight loss, and cognitive impairment. This is the first study to focus on microbial-gut-brain axis (Loman et al. 2019). Inflammation and microglial activation modulate higher order brain function, including cognitive performance (Loman et al. 2019).

In short, chemotherapy affects the gut microbiota leading to modulation of both local and systemic side effects of chemotherapy. The evidence from animal models requires specific focused attention in a proper clinical setting. A balanced gut microbiota is important in the management of chemotherapy side effects.

GUT MICROBIOTA AND RADIOTHERAPY

Although there has been a lot of interest in the recent discovery that the gut microbiota plays a role in radiotherapy, little is understood about how the microbiota controls the body's reaction to radiation. It has been generally found that there is a bidirectional function to the interaction between radiation and the gut microbiota. The bidirectional effects affect how well anticancer treatments work by upsetting the microbiome environment and generating dysbiosis. The gut microbiome's diversity and abundance are significantly altered by radiation (Kim et al. 2015).

A clinical investigation by Nam et al. (2013) found that after pelvic radiation, the makeup of the gut microbiome changed overall, with a 10% reduction in Firmicutes and a 3% rise in Fusobacterium phyla. Bacteroidales (Bacteroidaceae, Rikenellaceae, Bacteroides) were found to be comparatively more common in patients with non-CR (complete response) than in those with CR, according to a study that examined 45 fecal samples from patients with rectal cancer prior to concurrent chemoradiation. Improvement in the CR rate was associated with *Duodenibacillus massiliensis* (Jang et al. 2020).

Increases in *Bacteroides* and Enterobacteriaceae and decreases in *Bifidobacterium*, *Faecalibacterium prausnitzii*, and *Clostridium* cluster XIVa are the most notable alterations in the gut microbiota linked to radiation therapy (Touchefeu et al. 2014). Normal and pathological immune responses to radiation therapy can also be influenced by gut bacteria. According to one study, a variety of processes known as "TIMER"—translocation, immunomodulation, metabolism, enzymatic degradation, and reduced diversity—allow gut bacteria to influence the consequences of cancer therapy (Alexander et al. 2017).

Higher alpha-diversity in the tumor microbiome of patients who had long-term survival revealed an intra-tumoral microbiome signature (*Pseudoxanthomonas-Streptomyces-Saccharopolyspora-Bacillus clausii*) that was highly suggestive of long-term succession in both the identification and verification cohorts, according to a study by Riquelme and colleagues (2019). Fecal microbiota transplantation (FMT) studies including human donors from short-term, long-term, or control groups altered both tumor growth and tumor immune infiltration. This allowed for the differential modulation of the tumor microbiome. Thus it becomes sense to speculate that the gut microbiota also affects how radiation stimulates the immune system (Riquelme et al. 2019).

Radiotherapy has the potential to alter the microbiome of a tumor, leading to an imbalance between pro- and anti-inflammatory cells and the cytokines that accompany them. The gut microbiota can be kept in balance by oral probiotics, prebiotics, medication therapies, and FMT, which can then alter the tumor microenvironment (Liu et al. 2021). Additional gut microbiome-related mechanisms that control the radiation response are highlighted in Figure 13.2 and include the regulation of autophagy, FIAF production, circadian rhythms, autophagy control, inflammation, butyrate and short-chain fatty acid (SCFA) synthesis, and fibroblasts linked to cancer, among other things (Liu et al. 2021).

Using mouse models of B16-OVA melanoma and TC-1 lung/cervical cancer, one group investigated whether the gut microbiota might regulate the antitumor immune reactions after radiation to non-gut organs. They discovered that the antibiotic vancomycin, which acts on gut bacteria, strengthened the radiation-induced antitumor immune response and impeded tumor growth. According to Uribe-Herranz et al. (2020), this

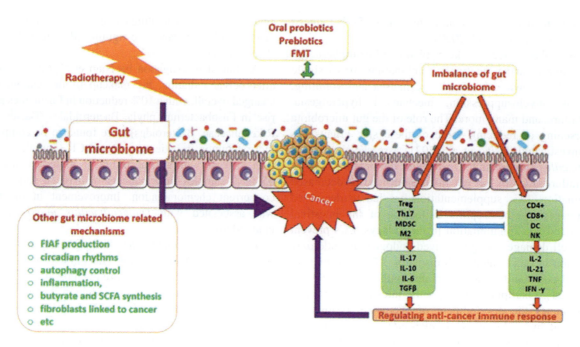

FIGURE 13.2 **The implications of the gut microbiome in regulating radiotherapy response.** Radiotherapy has the potential to alter the microbiome of a tumor, leading to an imbalance between pro- and anti-inflammatory cells and the cytokines that accompany them. The gut microbiota can be kept in balance by oral probiotics, prebiotics, medication therapies, and FMT, which can then alter the tumor microenvironment (Liu et al. 2021). Additional gut microbiome-related mechanisms that control the radiation response include the regulation of autophagy, FIAF production, circadian rhythms, autophagy control, inflammation, butyrate and SCFA synthesis, and fibroblasts linked to cancer, among other things. TGF, tumor growth factor; MDSC, myeloid-derived suppressor cells; NK, natural killer cells; RT, radiation; TNF, tumor necrosis factor; IFN, interferon; FMT, fecal microbial transplant; FIAF, fasting-induced adipose factor; SCFA, short-chain fatty acids.

synergy required interferon-γ and the cross-presentation of tumor-specific antigens to cytolytic CD8 + T cells. This team found that radiotherapy's anticancer activity was increased when vancomycin-sensitive bacteria were eliminated. In a mouse model treated with antibiotics, Cui et al. (2017) reported a relationship between intestine bacterial composition and radiosensitivity. The mice treated with antibiotics had a considerably greater survival rate following irradiation, and their intestinal bacterial composition differed markedly from that of the control group.

Suggestive evidence of a relationship between radiation sensitivity and the makeup of the gut microbiome exists, based on data from clinical research and mice models. It has been demonstrated that the timing of radiation therapy influences both local control and toxicity in patients with lung cancer (Chan et al. 2017). *Fusobacterium nucleatum* has been demonstrated to play a role in chemoresistance to colorectal cancer by inducing autophagy, which is regulated by the gut microbiome. In this context, a hypothesis has been put out linking radioresistance to autophagy regulation. Nevertheless, Yu et al. (2017) report that no research has been published so far regarding the possible impacts of gut microbiota composition on radiosensitivity through autophagy modulation.

Tumor radiation resistance or sensitivity may potentially be influenced by inflammation. Cancer-associated fibroblasts, a constituent of the tumor microenvironment, play a role in immune modulation, including inflammation, as well as tumor initiation, progression, metastasis, and angiogenesis. Radiation stimulates TGF-β1 expression, which in turn activates cancer-associated fibroblasts. Additionally, CD4+ T helper cells and CD8+ cytotoxic T cells are important modulators of the inflammatory process. When combined, the immune system's complicated inflammatory responses to an irradiation tumor and the surrounding stroma are neither entirely immunosuppressive nor completely immunostimulatory (Liu et al. 2021).

Angiopoietin-like 4 (ANGPTL4), or fasting-induced adipose factor (FIAF), is a secreted protein that is generated from epithelial cells and is regulated by the microbiota. This study on the microbial regulation of intestinal radiosensitivity linked FIAF to radioresistance. Liu et al. (2021) suggested FIAF might be helpful as a radioprotector for the gut. In colorectal cancer cell lines, it was discovered that *Escherichia coli*, *Clostridium perfringens*, *Enterococcus faecalis*, and *Bacteroides thetaiotaomicron* controlled the production of FIAF. Peroxisome proliferator-activated receptors control the transcription of ANGPTL4 in response to bacteria that generate short-chain fatty acids. *Bifidobacterium*, *Lactobacillus*, and *Streptococcus* spp. are probiotic bacteria that have been demonstrated to promote ANGPTL4 expression. As a result, the authors hypothesized that giving these probiotics may alter FIAF production and hence potentially impact the progression of colorectal cancer (Liu et al. 2021).

Gastrointestinal mucositis is a profoundly serious side effect of radiation that can result in major losses in standard of life as well as treatment postponements or dose decreases which can affect the results of treatment (Touchefeu et al. 2014). Radiation-induced diarrhea is prevalent, involving over 80% of cancer patients receiving pelvic radiation (Demers et al. 2014). However, some patients develop severe diarrhea after radiotherapy, implying that personalized treatment strategies are vital to enhance the results of therapy. The use of biomarkers to identify patients who tolerate treatment from those at increased risk for developing acute toxicities is indispensable (Liu et al. 2021).

Patients with radiation-induced diarrhea have more alterations in the gut microbiome ecosystem than those without the condition, and so the gut microbiome appears to be critical for radiation-induced diarrhea protection (Wang et al. 2015). Patients with diarrhea had higher levels of *Bacteroides*, *Dialister*, *Veillonella*, and unclassified bacterial species, but their levels of *Clostridium* XI and XVIII, *Faecalibacterium*, *Oscillibacter*, *Parabacteroides*, and *Prevotella* were lower (Wang et al. 2015). According to Neemann and Freifeld (2017), patients undergoing radiotherapy had a significant frequency of *Clostridium difficile* infection, which is associated with a high fatality rate. According to research, the overall makeup of the gut microbiota can be utilized as a predictive marker for the development of radiotherapy-induced diarrhea and exhaustion (Al-Qadami et al. 2019).

Pathobiology of gastrointestinal mucositis research has discovered that the gut microbiota plays a role in the pathophysiology of radiotherapy-induced gastrointestinal mucositis. Radiation causes tissue damage, which is followed by an increase in inflammation and the generation of proinflammatory cytokines. Because of interactions with microbial compounds that traverse the broken epithelium, this causes ulceration and increased inflammation. The healing stage encompasses extracellular matrix signaling, epithelial cell proliferation, and mucosal integrity restoration (Liu et al. 2021).

The gut microbiome influences the pathogenesis of radiation-induced gastrointestinal mucositis by modulating oxidative stress and inflammatory processes, intestinal permeability, mucus layer composition, epithelial repair and resistance to harmful stimuli, and the expression and release of immune effector molecules in the intestine (Touchefeu et al. 2014). Radiation-induced gastrointestinal mucositis can be influenced by the gut microbiota via two processes, namely translocation and dysbiosis (illustrated in Figure 13.3). Radiation damages the intestinal walls and mucus layer, leading to the translocation of bacteria and the elicitation of a response of inflammatory nature. Dysbiosis can affect both local and systemic immune responses, whether triggered by radiation or other reasons. TLR activation of NF-κB signaling, which is required for the safeguarding of the gut from radiation-induced apoptosis, is another putative mechanism by which TLR has radiation-protective effects (Liu et al. 2021).

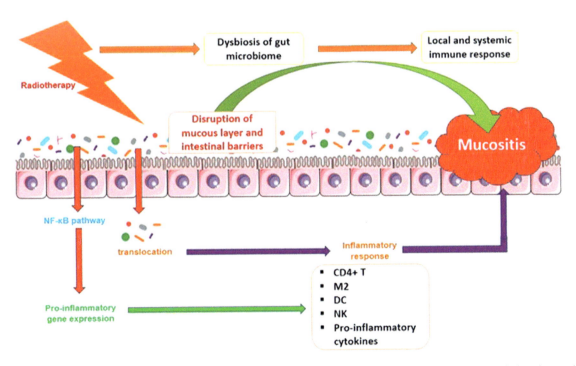

FIGURE 13.3 **The gut microbiome's putative pathways in radiation-induced intestinal mucositis.** Radiation-induced gastrointestinal mucositis can be influenced by the gut microbiota primarily through two mechanisms: translocation and dysbiosis. Radiation damages the intestinal walls and mucus layer, leading to bacterial translocation and the elicitation of an inflammatory response. Dysbiosis can affect both local and systemic immune responses, whether triggered by radiation or other reasons. TLR activation of NF-κB signaling, which is required for the safeguarding of the gut from radiation-induced apoptosis, is another putative mechanism by which TLR has radiation-protective effects. RT, radiotherapy; TLR, toll-like receptor; NF-κB, nuclear factor-kappa B; DC, dendritic cells; NK, natural killer cells.

Alterations in the microbiota are major causal factors in radiation enteropathy's harmful effects. Several investigations have revealed that radiation alters the microbial composition of the stomach (Mitra et al. 2020). Numerous clinical investigations of the microbiome before and after irradiation for gynecologic or lower gastrointestinal tract cancer revealed that radiation causes significant alterations in the microbiome profile, including a reduction in variance in the gastrointestinal and colonic microbiota. Patients with gastrointestinal or gynecologic cancer who had diarrhea after irradiation showed less variation than those who did not (Mitra et al. 2020). Table 13.1 summarizes the key findings of the gut microbiome and radiotherapy toxicity.

To maintain intestinal homeostasis, gut microbiota interactions with TLRs are generated on epithelial and immune cells. The depletion of the gut microbiota in mice by broad-spectrum antibiotics has been linked to an elevated susceptibility to methotrexate-induced gastrointestinal damage, which is inhibited by TLR2 ligand delivery. TLR4 deletion mice have been demonstrated to diminish irinotecan-associated pain and gastrointestinal toxicity. Membrane lipopolysaccharide in Gram-negative bacteria, has been shown to help safeguard intestinal crypts by inducing cyclooxygenase-2 and the synthesis of prostaglandins (Wardill et al. 2016).

Lipopolysaccharide activation of TLR4-expressing cells results in the discharge of tumor necrosis factor (TNF)-α, which engages with the TNF receptor on the exterior of subepithelial fibroblasts, resulting in the generation of prostaglandins and a decrease in radiation-induced apoptosis of epithelial stem cells (Wardill et al. 2016). The activation of TLR by means of nuclear factor-kappa B (NF-κB) signaling is another putative mechanism by which TLR has radiation-protective effects. NF-κB signaling is required for the safeguarding of the gut against radiation-induced apoptosis. Activation of NF-κB also promotes lipopolysaccharide's radioprotective properties, implying that TLRs may regulate the intestinal reaction to radiation-induced epithelium degradation via the NF-κB pathway (Liu et al. 2021).

Radiotherapy causes improper regulation of the gut microbiota, which has a detrimental effect on the variety and quantity of gut bacterial diversity, potentially resulting in the enrichment of detrimental microbiota (*Fusobacterium* and *Proteobacterium*) and an overall reduction in helpful microbiota (*Bifidobacterium* and *Faecalibacterium*) (Kunika et al. 2023; Fernandes et al. 2022a; Li et al. 2021a, b). In pelvic chemotherapy and radiotherapy (CRT), the gut microbiome composition altered significantly, with an upsurge in Proteobacteria and a decline in Clostridiales, however, following CRT the gut microbiome composition altered, with a boost in *Bacteroides* species (Li et al. 2021). Radiotherapy may contribute to intestinal radiation-induced damage by modifying bacteria that generate SCFAs. The influence of SCFAs on the incidence of different illnesses remains unknown (Li et al. 2021).

CANCER SURGERY

Postoperative complications from cancer surgery, particularly surgical excision of gastrointestinal cancer

TABLE 13.1

The gut microbiome and radiotherapy toxicity

Radiotherapy	Key findings	References
Pelvic 45–50 Gy/25 fractions/5 weeks	Patients exhibiting diarrhea showed a progressive modification in microbial diversity	Manichanh et al. 2008
Pelvic 50.4 Gy/25 fractions/5 weeks	Most patients suffered diarrhea symptom with dramatic change of gut microbial community after radiotherapy	Nam et al. 2013
Pelvic 50.4 Gy/ 25 fractions/5 weeks	Microbial diversity, richness, and the Firmicutes/Bacteroidetes ratio were significantly altered prior to radiotherapy in patients who later developed diarrhea.	Wang et al. 2015
Definitive radiation therapy, including external beam RT and brachytherapy	Patients with high toxicity demonstrated different compositional changes during CRT in addition to compositional differences in Clostridia species.	Wang et al. 2015
4 fractions of 550 cGy with 24 h intervals	Adherent microbiota from RP differed from those in uninvolved segments and was associated with tissue damage.	Wang et al. 2015
A whole-body dose of 0, 5 or 12 Gy X rays using an X-RAD 320 X-ray irradiator	Statistically significant changes in the microbial-derived products such as pipecolic acid, glutaconic acid, urobilinogen, and homogentisic acid.	Wang et al. 2015
14 Gy total body at 0.96 cGy/min	Lipopolysaccharide is radioprotective in the mouse intestine through a prostaglandin-dependent pathway.	
12 Gy total body gamma irradiation	TNFR1 and COX-2 expression to subepithelial fibroblasts plays an intermediate role in LPS-induced radioprotection in the intestine.	Riehl et al. 2004
8 Gy gamma irradiation	Selective preactivation of NF-kappa B through IKK in intestinal epithelial cells could provide a therapeutic modality that allows higher doses of radiation to be tolerated during cancer RT.	Egan et al. 2004

with alimentary reconstruction, are widespread, with infections at the surgical site and anastomotic leakage being the most common. Despite advances in preoperative planning, surgical methods, and postoperative care, anastomotic leaks and infections following surgery still occur with catastrophic consequences, including acute peritonitis and even death (Fernandes et al. 2022b). Patients often receive preoperative bowel preparation to clear their colon of feces and antibiotics to avert infection and minimize the likelihood of these two problems following surgery. These methods clearly minimize the likelihood of postoperative problems by decreasing the amount of the important bacteria in the patient's gut. Metabolism after gastrectomy is linked to changes in microbial function, such as organic compound production and nutrition transport (Erawijantari et al. 2020). Related research has found that the composition of the intestinal microbiota can predict short-term prognosis after gastrointestinal cancer surgery (El Bairi et al. 2020). Low microbial diversity and mucin-degrading *Lachnospiraceae* and *Bacteroidaceae* members, for example, are linked to postoperative anastomotic leaks (van Praagh et al. 2019).

Surgical site infections are brought about by a variety of causes, including the emergence of drug-resistant and virulent microbes because of globalization, antibiotic exposure, and the use of lengthy and invasive therapies (Alverdy et al. 2017). Is there a commensal bacterium that promotes anastomosis recovery and inhibits surgical site infections? There is evidence that some probiotics can prevent pathogenic bacteria linked to postoperative infections. Some *Bifidobacterium* and *Lactobacillus* strains, for example, may prevent the proliferation of clinically isolated methicillin-resistant *Staphylococcus aureus*, a multidrug resistant microorganism that is an essential nosocomial pathogen and is associated with postoperative infections, by means of cell competitive exclusion as well as inhibitor production. In the future, developing microbial therapeutics to improve postoperative prognosis by addressing these associated microbes may not be implausible (Zhao et al. 2023).

LIMITATIONS AND OUTLOOK

In general, numerous gut microbiota have a regulatory function in tumor therapy, including increasing patients' sensitivity to immunotherapy, minimizing chemotherapeutic drug adverse effects, and lessening radiation damage. The consequences of other mucosal barrier bacteria on the body, on the other hand, are still unknown. Previous research has identified gut microbial processes that influence carcinogenesis, inflammation, immunology, and therapeutic response at the local level. However, it is still unknown how bacteria colonizing remote epithelial barriers govern not solely carcinogenesis and immunology, but also numerous organ's physiological activities. The majority of studies on how microbiome impact cancer therapy have been conducted in mice, and translating these findings from academia to the clinic remains a hurdle (Ma et al. 2019).

The shift in the monogenus is not sufficient to clarify the mechanisms underlying the associated alterations in the body. The gut microbiota has an impact on the entire body. Although mice implanted with human microbiota exhibit pathological and immunological responses reminiscent of humans, they are not identical. The impact of the microbiome on treatment efficacy, as well as the interaction between the patient's microbiome and cancer therapy efficacy, should be investigated further in the future, particularly in conjunction with immune checkpoint blockade (Ma et al. 2019). Mechanistic investigations will most likely discover pathways for cancer therapy and enable direct manipulation of cancer medication efficacy without affecting the microbiota. Further research on the relationship between the immune response and the microbiome should be done on other cancer types in the future to reveal the underlying mechanisms of the immune system's response, which may be controlled without changing the microbiome. Influenced by the impacts of the gut microbiome manipulating inflammatory variables or the immune system's reaction by modulating inflammatory variables may be a better strategy to improve cancer therapy efficacy. Some metabolites, such as inosine, can influence cancer treatment success, and this effect is independent of the microbiome (Yu et al. 2021).

In mouse models, the byproduct of inosine generated by the microbiome was found to regulate the effectiveness of cancer therapy without altering the microbiome (Mager et al. 2020), and it may be employed as an adjuvant drug for many types of cancer therapy in the future. The use of certain metabolites generated by the gut microbiome could substitute for the microbiome's role. The safety and effectiveness should be investigated progressively through various cancer types and clinical trials. Further investigation should be conducted on the intricate structure of the effects generated by inosine or various other metabolites, which may be dependent on studies on the interplay between the immune response and microbiome-derived metabolites (Yu et al. 2021).

Discovering a way to control the transfer of microbial community and microbiota-derived metabolic products may be another avenue for future studies to investigate the connection that exists between the microbiota of the gut and locally resident microbial community or intratumor microbiota, potentially representing yet another significant mechanism of the influence caused by the gut microbiome on cancer therapies. The relationship between the immune response and metabolism should be studied in neurobiological investigations regarding the influence of the locally resident microbiome on the tumor microenvironment. Until now, conducting research on the manipulation of locally resident microbiota may have been a straightforward strategy to improve cancer therapy efficacy (Yu et al. 2021).

CONCLUSION

Cancer patients experience a wide range of short- and long-term systemic side effects linked to gastrointestinal toxicity.

Preclinical and clinical research has demonstrated that the subject could serve as a crucial mediator of how the body responds to cancer therapy. Clinical trials on a considerable number of cancer survivors are of vital importance to open new avenues for microbiota-mediated therapeutics to stop or reduce the long-term negative effects of cancer therapy. In the future, treatments may make use of approaches that allow for more exact regulation of microbiota composition, such as the relative proportion of a certain bacterial genus in the microbiome. Personalized biomarkers are desperately required to detect dysbiotic situations connected to unfavorable or poor cancer therapy outcomes and to pinpoint microbial targets that can be changed (Kunika et al. 2023; Santucci et al. 2022).

Improving cancer survivors' physical well-being necessitates an in-depth knowledge of the effects of altered gut microbiota on immunological and metabolic pathways. We can only improve the controlled functioning of the intestinal microbiota and improve cancer therapy potential by comprehending completely which gut microbes and their metabolic processes or product(s) may be manipulated (Zhao et al. 2023). Overall, the goal of the chapter was to shed light on the potential complicated interplay between the gut microbiome and the systemic side effects linked to cancer therapy, as well as to propose prospective avenues for future investigations in this important field. Direct proof corroborating suggested postulations and speculations, however, is yet lacking. More study is required to investigate further the relationship between the gut microbiota and cancer therapies, which could lead to novel therapeutic prospects and the development of predictive biomarkers.

REFERENCES

Alexander, J. L., Wilson, I. D., Teare, J., Marchesi, J. R., Nicholson, J. K. & Kinross, J. M. (2017). Gut microbiota modulation of chemotherapy efficacy and toxicity. *Nat Rev Gastroenterol Hepatol*, 14(6), 356–65.

Al-Qadami, G., Van Sebille, Y., Le, H. & Bowen, J. (2019). Gut microbiota: implications for radiotherapy response and radiotherapy-induced mucositis. *Expert Rev Gastroenterol Hepatol*, 13(5), 485–96.

Alverdy, J. C., Hyoju, S. K., Weigerinck, M. & Gilbert, J. A. (2017). The gut microbiome and the mechanism of surgical infection. *Br J Surg*, 104, e14–23.

Chan, S., Rowbottom, L., McDonald, R., Bjarnason, G. A., Tsao, M., Danjoux, C., Barnes, E., Popovic, M., Lam, H., DeAngelis, C. & Chow, E. (2017). Does the time of radiotherapy affect treatment outcomes? A review of the literature. *Clin Oncol (R Coll Radiol)*, 29(4), 231–8.

Chen, H., Xu, C., Zhang, F., Liu, Y., Guo, Y. & Yao, Q. (2020). The gut microbiota attenuates muscle wasting by regulating energy metabolism in chemotherapy-induced malnutrition rats. *Ca Chem Pharm*, 85(6), 1049–62. doi:10.1007/s00280-020-04060-w

Chrysostomou, D., Roberts, L. A., Marchesi, J. R. & Kinross, J. M. (2023). Gut microbiota modulation of efficacy and toxicity of cancer chemotherapy and immunotherapy. *Gastroenterology*, 164(2), 198–213. doi:10.1053/j.gastro.2022.10.018

Cui, M., Xiao, H., Li, Y., Zhou, L., Zhao, S., Luo, D., Zheng, Q., Dong, J., Zhao, Y., Zhang, X., Zhang, J., Lu, L., Wang, H. & Fan, S. (2017). Faecal microbiota transplantation protects against radiation-induced toxicity. *EMBO Mol Med*, 9(4), 448–61.

Demers, M., Dagnault, A. & Desjardins, J. (2014). A randomized double-blind controlled trial: impact of probiotics on diarrhea in patients treated with pelvic radiation. *Clin Nutr*, 33(5), 761–7.

Egan, L. J., Eckmann, L., Greten, F. R., Chae, S., Li, Z. W., Myhre, G. M., Robine, S., Karin, M. & Kagnoff, M. F. (2004). IκB-kinaseβ-dependent NF-κB activation provides radioprotection to the intestinal epithelium. *Proc Natl Acad Sci USA*, 101(8), 2452–7.

El Bairi, K., Jabi, R., Trapani, D., Boutallaka, H., Ouled Amar Bencheikh, B., Bouziane, M., Amrani, M., Afqir, S. & Maleb, A. (2020). Can the microbiota predict response to systemic cancer therapy, surgical outcomes, and survival? The answer is in the gut. *Expert Rev Clin Pharmacol*, 13, 403–421.

Erawijantari, P. P., Mizutani, S., Shiroma, H., Shiba, S., Nakajima, T., Sakamoto, T., Saito, Y., Fukuda, S., Yachida, S. & Yamada, T. (2020). Influence of gastrectomy for gastric cancer treatment on faecal microbiome and metabolome profiles. *Gut*, 69, 1404–1415.

Fernandes, A., Oliveira, A., Guedes, C., Fernandes, R., Soares, R. & Barata, P. (2022a). Effect of radium-223 on the gut microbiota of prostate cancer patients: a Pilot case series study. *Curr Issues Mol Biol*, 44, 4950–4959.

Fernandes, M. R., Aggarwal, P., Costa, R. G. F., Cole, A. M. & Trinchieri, G. (2022b) Targeting the gut microbiota for cancer therapy. *Nat Rev Cancer*, 22(12), 703–22. doi:10.1038/s41568-022-00513-x

Gallotti, B., Galvao, I., Leles, G., Quintanilha, M., Souza, R., Miranda, V., Rocha, V. M., Trindade, L. M., Jesus, L. C. L., Mendes, V., Andre, L. C., d'Auriol-Souza, M. M., Azevedo, V., Cardoso, V. N., Martins, F. S. & Vieira, A. T. (2021). Effects of dietary fibre intake in chemotherapy-induced mucositis in murine model. *Br J Nutrition*, 126(6), 853–64.

Ghiringhelli, F., Apetoh, L. (2014). The interplay between the immune system and chemotherapy: emerging methods for optimizing therapy. *Expert Rev Clin Immunology*, 10(1), 19–30.

Groussin, M., Mazel, F. & Alm, E. J. (2020). Co-evolution and co-speciation of host-gut bacteria systems. *Cell Host Microbe*, 28, 12–22.

Hofseth, L. J., Hebert, J. R., Chanda, A., Chen, H., Love, B. L., Pena, M. M., Murphy, E. A., Sajish, M., Sheth, A., Buckhaults, P. J., Berger, F. J. (2020) Early-onset colorectal cancer: initial clues and current views. *Nat Rev Gastroenterol Hepatol*, 17(6), 352–64.

Hsiao, Y-P., Chen, H-L., Tsai, J-N., Lin, M-Y., Liao, J-W., Wei, M-S., Ko, J-L., Ou, C-C. (2021). Administration of Lactobacillus reuteri combined with Clostridium butyricum attenuates cisplatin-induced renal damage by gut microbiota reconstitution, increasing butyric acid production, and suppressing renal inflammation. *Nutrients*, 13(8), 2792.

Jang, B. S., Chang, J. H., Chie, E. K., Kim, K., Park, J. W., Kim, M. J., Song, E. J., Nam, Y. D., Kang, S. W., Jeong, S. Y. & Kim, H. J. (2020). Gut microbiome composition is associated with a pathologic response after preoperative chemoradiation in patients with rectal cancer. *Int J Radiat Oncol Biol Phys*, 107(4), 736–46.

Justino, P. F., Melo, L. F., Nogueira, A. F., Morais, C. M., Mendes, W. O., Franco, A. X., Souza, E. P., Ribeiro, R. A., Souza, M. H. L. P., Marcos, P. & Soares, G. (2015). Regulatory role of Lactobacillus acidophilus on inflammation and gastric dysmotility in intestinal mucositis induced by 5-fluorouracil in mice. *Cancer Chemother Pharmacol*, 75, 559–67.

Kim, Y. S., Kim, J. & Park, S. J. (2015). High-throughput 16S rRNA gene sequencing reveals alterations of mouse intestinal microbiota after radiotherapy. *Anaerobe*, 33, 1–7.

Kunika, Frey N. & Rangrez, A. Y. (2023). Exploring the involvement of gut microbiota in cancer therapy-induced cardiotoxicity. *Int J Mol Sci*, 24(8), 7261.

Li, H., He, J. & Jia, W. (2016). The influence of gut microbiota on drug metabolism and toxicity. *Expert Opinion Drug Metabol Toxicol*, 12(1), 31–40. doi:10.1517/17425255.2016.1121234

Li, Y., Zhang, Y., Wei, K., He, J., Ding, N., Hua, J., Zhou, T., Niu, F., Zhou, G., Shi, T., Zhang, L. & Liu Y. (2021a). Review: effect of gut microbiota and its metabolite SCFAs on radiation-induced intestinal injury. *Front Cell Infect Microbiol*, 11, 577236.

Lin, X. B., Dieleman, L. A., Ketabi, A., Bibova, I., Sawyer, M. B., Xue, H., Field, C. J., Baracos, B. E. & Gänzle, M. E. (2012). Irinotecan (CPT-11) chemotherapy alters intestinal microbiota in tumour bearing rats. *PLoS One*, 7(7), e39764.

Liu, J., Liu, C. & Yue, J. (2021). Radiotherapy and the gut microbiome: facts and fiction. *Radiat Oncol*, 16, 9.

Liu, L., Wu, Q., Chen, Y., Ren, H., Zhang, Q., Yang, H., Zhang, W., Ding, T., Wang, S., Zhang, Y., Liu, Y. & Sun, J. (2023). Gut microbiota in chronic pain: novel insights into mechanisms and promising therapeutic strategies. *Int Immunopharmacol*, 115, 109685.

Loman, B., Jordan, K., Haynes, B., Bailey, M. & Pyter, L. (2019). Chemotherapy-induced neuroinflammation is associated with disrupted colonic and bacterial homeostasis in female mice. *Sci Rep*, 9(1), 16490.

Ma, W., Mao, Q., Xia, W., Dong, G., Yu, C. & Jiang, F. (2019). Gut microbiota shapes the efficiency of cancer therapy. *Front Microbiol*, 10, 1050.

Mager, L. F., Burkhard, R., Pett, N., Cooke, N. C. A., Brown, K., Ramay, H., Paik, S., Stagg, J., Groves, R. A., Gallo M., Lewis I. A., Geuking, M. B. & McCoy, K. D. (2020). Microbiome-derived inosine modulates response to checkpoint inhibitor immunotherapy. *Science*, 369(6510), 1481.

Manichanh, C., Varela, E., Martinez, C., Antolin, M., Llopis, M., Doré, J., Giralt, J., Guarner, F. & Malagelada, J. R. (2008). The gut microbiota predispose to the pathophysiology of acute postradiotherapy diarrhea. *Am J Gastroenterol*, 103(7), 1754–61.

Mitra, A., Grossman Biegert, G. W., Delgado, A. Y., Karpinets, T. V., Solley, T. N., Mezzari, M. P., Yoshida-Court, K., Petrosino, J. F., Mikkelson, M. D., Lin, L., Eifel, P., Zhang, J., Ramondetta, L. M., Jhingran, A., Sims, T. T., Schmeler, K., Okhuysen, P., Colbert, L. E. & Klopp, A. H. (2020). Microbial diversity and composition is associated with patient-reported toxicity during chemoradiation therapy for cervical cancer. *Int J Radiat Oncol Biol Phys*, 107(1), 163–71.

Nam, Y. D., Kim, H. J., Seo, J. G., Kang, S. W. & Bae, J. W. (2013). Impact of pelvic radiotherapy on gut microbiota of gynecological cancer patients revealed by massive pyrosequencing. *PLoS One*, 8(12), e82659.

Neemann, K. & Freifeld, A. (2017). Clostridium difficile-associated diarrhea in the oncology patient. *J Oncol Pract*, 13(1), 25–30.

Nicholson, J. K., Holmes, E., Kinross, J., Burcelin, R., Gibson, G., Jia, W. & Pettersson, S. (2012). Host-gut microbiota metabolic interactions. *Science*, 336, 1262–67.

Perez-Chanona, E. & Trinchieri, G. (2016). The role of microbiota in cancer therapy. *Curr. Opin Immunol*, 39, 75–81.

Puertollano, M. A., Puertollano, E., Alvarez de Cienfuegos, G. & de Pablo M. A. (2011). Dietary antioxidants: immunity and host defense. *Current Topics Med Chem*, 11(14), 1752–66.

Rajagopala, S. V., Vashee, S., Oldfield, L. M., Suzuki, Y., Venter, J. C., Telenti, A. & Nelson, K. E. (2017). The human microbiome and cancer the human microbiome and cancer. *Cancer Prev. Res*, 10, 226–34.

Riehl, T. E., Newberry, R. D., Lorenz, R. G. & Stenson, W. F. (2004). TNFR1 mediates the radioprotective effects of lipopolysaccharide in the mouse intestine. *Am J Physiol Gastrointest Liver Physiol*, 286(1), G166–73.

Riquelme, E., Zhang, Y., Zhang, L., Montiel, M., Zoltan, M., Dong, W., Quesada, P., Sahin, I., Chandra, V., San Lucas, A., Scheet, P., Xu, H., Hanash, S. M., Feng, L., Burks, J. K., Do, K. A., Peterson, C. B., Nejman, D., Tzeng, C. D., Kim, M. P., Sears, C. L., Ajami, N., Petrosino, J., Wood, L. D., Maitra, A., Straussman, R., Katz, M., White, J. R., Jenq, R., Wargo, J. & McAllister, F. (2019). Tumor microbiome diversity and composition influence pancreatic cancer outcomes. *Cell*, 178(4), 795–806.e12.

Santucci, C., Patel, L., Malvezzi, M., Wojtyla, C., La Vecchia, C., Negri, E. & Bertuccio, P. (2022). Persisting cancer mortality gap between western and eastern Europe. *Eur J Cancer*, 165, 1–12.

Sehgal, K. & Khanna, S. (2021). Gut microbiome and checkpoint inhibitor colitis. *Intestinal Res*, 19(4), 360–4.

Sepich-Poore, G. D., Zitvogel, L., Straussman, R., Hasty, J., Wargo, J. A. & Knight, R. (2021). The microbiome and human cancer. *Science*, 371, eabc4552.

Stringer, A. M. (2013). Interaction between host cells and microbes in chemotherapy-induced mucositis. *Nutrients*. 5(5), 1488–99.

Takasuna, K., Hagiwara, T., Hirohashi, M., Kato, M., Nomura, M., Nagai, E., Yokoi, T. & Kamataki, T. (1996). Involvement of β-glucuronidase in intestinal microflora in the intestinal toxicity of the antitumor camptothecin derivative irinotecan hydrochloride (CPT-11) in rats. *Cancer Research*, 56(16), 3752–7.

Touchefeu, Y., Montassier, E., Nieman, K., Gastinne, T., Potel, G., Bruley des Varannes, S., Le Vacon, F. & de La Cochetière, M. F. (2014). Systematic review: the role of the gut microbiota in chemotherapy- or radiation-induced gastrointestinal mucositis: current evidence and potential clinical applications. *Aliment Pharmacol Ther*, 40(5), 409–21.

Uribe-Herranz, M., Rafail, S., Beghi, S., Gil-de-Gómez, L., Verginadis, I., Bittinger, K., Pustylnikov, S., Pierini, S., Perales-Linares, R., Blair, I. A., Mesaros, C. A., Snyder, N. W., Bushman, F., Koumenis, C. & Facciabene, A. (2020). Gut microbiota modulate dendritic cell antigen presentation and radiotherapy-induced antitumor immune response. *J Clin Invest*, 130(1), 466–79.

van Praagh, J. B., de Goffau, M. C., Bakker, I. S., van Goor, H., Harmsen, H. J. M., Olinga, P. & Havenga, K. (2019). Mucus microbiome of anastomotic tissue during surgery has predictive value for colorectal anastomotic leakage. *Ann. Surg*, 269, 911–16.

Viaud, S., Saccheri, F., Mignot, G., Yamazaki, T., Daillère, R., Hannani, D., Enot, D. P., Pfirschke, C., Engblom, C., Pittet, M. J., Schlitzer, A., Ginhoux, F., Apetoh, L., Chachaty, E., Woerther, P.-L., Eberl, Gerard., Ecobichon, C., Clermont, D., Bizet, C., Gaboriau-Routhiau, V., Cerf-Bensussan, N., Opolon, P., Yessaad, N., Vivier, E., Ryffel, B., Elson, C. O., Dore, J., Kroemer, G., Lepage, P., Boneca, I. G., Ghiringhelli, F. & Zitvogel, L. (2013). The intestinal microbiota modulates the anticancer immune effects of cyclophosphamide. *Science*, 342(6161), 971–6.

Vos, S. M., Tretter, E. M., Schmidt, B. H. & Berger, J. M. (2011). All tangled up: how cells direct, manage and exploit topoisomerase function. *Nat Rev Mol Cell Biol*, 12(12), 827–41. doi:10.1038/nrm3228

Wang, A., Ling, Z., Yang, Z., Kiela, P. R., Wang, T., Wang, C., Cao, L., Geng, F., Shen, M., Ran, X., Su, Y., Cheng, T. & Wang, J. (2015). Gut microbial dysbiosis may predict diarrhea and fatigue in patients undergoing pelvic cancer radiotherapy: a pilot study. *PLoS One*, 10(5), e0126312.

Wang, T., Cai, G., Qiu, Y., Fei, N., Zhang, M., Pang, X., Jia, W., Cai, S. & Zhao, L. (2012). Structural segregation of gut microbiota between colorectal cancer patients and healthy volunteers. *ISME J*, 6(2), 320–9.

Wardill, H. R., Gibson, R. J., Van Sebille, Y. Z. A., Secombe, K. R., Coller, J. K., White, I. A., Manavis, J., Hutchinson, M. R., Staikopoulos, V., Logan, R. M. & Bowen, J. M. (2016). Irinotecan-induced gastrointestinal dysfunction and pain are mediated by common TLR4-dependent mechanisms. *Mol Cancer Ther*, 15(6), 1376–86.

Xu, J., Xu, J., Shi, T., Zhang, Y., Chen, F., Yang, C., Guo, X., Liu, G., Shao, D., Leong, K. W. & Nie, G. (2023). Probiotic-inspired nanomedicine restores intestinal homeostasis in colitis by regulating redox balance, immune responses, and the gut microbiome. *Advan Mater*, 35(3), 2207890.

Yu, M., Jia, H., Zhou, C., Yang, Y., Zhao, Y., Yang, M. & Zou, Z. (2017). Variations in gut microbiota and fecal metabolic phenotype associated with depression by 16S rRNA gene sequencing and LC/MS-based metabolomics. *J Pharm Biomed Anal*, 138, 231–39.

Yu, Z. K., Xie, R. L., You, R., Liu, Y., Chen, X., Chen, M. & Huang, P. (2021). The role of the bacterial microbiome in the treatment of cancer. *BMC Cancer*, 21, 934.

Zhao, X., Wang, J. R., Dadu, R., Busaidy, N. L., Xu, L., Learned, K. O., Chasen, N. N., Vu, T., Maniakas, A., Eguia, A. A., Diersing, J., Gross, N. D., Goepfert, R., Lai, S. Y., Hofmann, M. C., Ferrarotto, R., Lu, C., Gunn, G. B., Spiotto, M. T., Subbiah, V., Williams, M. D., Cabanillas, M. E. & Zafereo, M. E. (2023). Surgery after BRAF-directed therapy is associated with improved survival in BRAFV600E mutant anaplastic thyroid cancer: a single-center retrospective cohort study. *Thyroid*, 33(4), 484–91.

14 Gut Microbiome and Precision Medicine in Cancer

Langanani Mbodi, Aristotelis Chatziioannou, and Zodwa Dlamini

INTRODUCTION

Metabolomics, defined as "the comprehensive analysis of metabolites in a biological specimen," is an emerging technology that perhaps holds a long-awaited promise to ignite the full practice of precision medicine. Metabolites have long been used as a diagnostic aid for complex metabolic diseases such as those including inborn errors of metabolism (Clish, 2015; Dettmer et al., 2007). The metabolites are regulated through genetic factors and hence these can be used as potential disease treatment targets (Chu et al., 2021).

Precision oncology, also termed personalized medicine in cancer medicine, can be defined as "an innovative approach to tailoring disease prevention and treatment that considers differences in individuals' genes, environment, and lifestyle factors." It provides for targeted therapy based on the molecular and clinical profiles of each individual cancer type (Pfohl et al., 2021). The traditional therapeutic strategy of a "one-size-fits-all" assumed in most medical treatments programs, which is based on historic evidence of treating the "average patient," is only successful in some but not all patients. It therefore makes sense that in order to improve patients' outcome, there is a need to eradicate or modify this wasteful modality that is in most instances associated with poor outcome.

Artificial intelligence (AI), defined as "a branch of computer science which deals with the simulation of intelligent behavior in computers" (Hamet & Tremblay, 2017), relies on the computers following some specific and directed algorithms established by humans and/or learned by computer methods in order to support decisions or aid in the execution of certain tasks. Machine learning (ML) is a subfield of AI that represents processes by which a computer can, over time, improve its own performance by continuously incorporating and adding on newly generated data into an existing iterative model. It has three commonly applied algorithms: (1) supervised learning; (2) unsupervised learning; and (3) reinforcement learning (Hamet & Tremblay, 2017).

The human microbiome provides a much-needed variety of physiological functions in the human body in areas where they colonize. They provide molecular signaling as well as a variety of metabolic functions. They also provide a protective function against invasion by pathogens. Researchers have for decades documented how the state of microbiomes in a body system affects health, determines health, regulates disease, and can protect against cancers (Puschhof & Elinev, 2023). There is increasing understanding and evidence on how microbiomes affect health. This plethora of new information demands that microbiomes data should form the basis of precision medicine (Figure 14.1). The introduction of next-generation sequencing (NGS) strategies has enabled the study of microbiomes networks and their genomes, parallel to that of human genetics, to unlock the genetic codes and discover treatment opportunities. Scientists and clinicians now routinely use human genomic information for cancer patients' diagnosis and care. (Panthee et al., 2022). Can microbiomes in general and gut microbiome be incorporated into routine diagnosis and care? How far away are we and what are the obstacles to overcome?

The gut microbiome (GM) is considered a key contributor in maintaining homeostasis and other physiological functions of the host. The study of gut microbiomes dates back to the 1800s when the German pediatrician Theodor Escherich reported on his study of the "human gut flora" and the findings of the organisms that became known as *Escherichia coli* and *Bifidobacterium animalis* in the gut of newborns. These were then known as the good bacteria that colonize the gut at birth. Further research on GM developed since that period (D'Amico et al., 2022).

The gut microbiome is a complex system with bacteria, archaebacteria (microorganisms considered to be an ancient form of life that evolved separately from bacteria and algae), fungi, and viruses in a likely 1:1 ratio with human cells. It is estimated that microbiomes have 150–500 times more genes than the host (D'Amico et al., 2022; Candela et al., 2012).

OMICS IN THE GUT MICROBIOME

Advances in environmental microbial genomics have led to a better understanding of the interaction between microbiomes and the host. The use of metagenomic and metataxonomic sequencing data together with other omics has increased although still poses challenges.

The "omics" technologies for microbiome analysis have grown in scope and evolved over the years and more data have been produced for better understanding of the gut microbiome in cancer and in the promotion of precision medicine (Whon et al., 2021). Gut microbiomes have emerged as biomarkers for disease phenotypical classification, disease prognostication, and evaluation of response to treatment. This is observed in

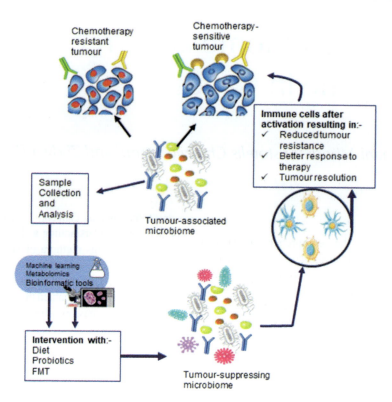

FIGURE 14.1 Elaborates how gut microbiomes contribute to cancer onset, the response to anticancer therapy, and how such processes can be engineered to develop a personalized microbiome-based treatment plan. An imbalance in microbiomes or metabolites of the microbiomes may contribute to carcinogenesis. An analysis of stools using a sequence-based approach, metabolomics, and bioinformatics is used to collect, synthesize, and analyze microbiomes and cancer as well as to design cancer treatments, such as through activation of the host immune system (e.g., prebiotics, probiotics, and FMT).

relation to changes and fluctuations in microbes' colonies in various diseases including cancer (Behrouzi et al., 2019). Examples of microbiomes used as diagnostic tests include the use of *F. nucleatum* as a diagnostic marker via FadA adhesin in colorectal cancer and the association of *Clostridium difficile* (*C. difficile*) infection with reduced microbial diversity and prediction of disease. The use of fecal microbiota transplantation (FMT) in the treatment of *C. difficile* showed 90% effectiveness in clinical state of disease although this was not tested on cancer or cancer risk patients (Paolli et al., 2016).

The principal component analysis or hierarchical clustering in conjunction with mass spectrometry can be used to mine data on microbes in any organ system. The data repositories are then used to enhance the identification of the spectrum of the microbiomes over time. An example of the use of these techniques is in the identification of metabolic biomarkers for cancers in organ systems, such as colorectal, pancreatic, lung, breast, gastric, ovarian, and prostate cancers (Puchades-Carrasco and Pineda-Lucena, 2017). Figure 14.2 shows the basic steps followed during metabolomics studies.

THE ROLE OF THE MICROBIOME IN TUMOR ONSET

During the human life span, microbiomes can respond, protect, and adapt to changes in endogenous and exogenous changes such as diet, lifestyle, and environmental changes. This is because they can move between states whilst preserving diversity, stability, and the interactions between each other and also the host. However, there are conditions that cause dysbiosis and result in the progression of disease (Fassarella et al. 2021; D'Amico et al., 2022) (Figure 14.3).

Carcinogenesis is the process of gradual accumulation and random genetic and epigenetic mutations that may take up to a decade depending on the rate of mutation. Several factors that may result in microbiome deterioration and dysfunction have been found to be associated with colorectal cancers, as an example (Bhatt et al., 2017). The presence of microbiomes in certain gut cancers such as colorectal cancers, even though not causative, are essential. There is a known signaling process between local bacteria quorum-sensing peptides (QSPs) and cancer cells irrespective of how the host-microbiome reaction is to the cancer pathology. An example is the synthesis of the *Bacillus*-derived QSPs that are produced during physiological stress over the microbiome. These can induce invasive cancer cells through a process known as epithelial mesenchymal-like that is involved in metastasis. The involvement of the QSPs is in the metastasis of the cancer as well as the angiogenesis which forms the basis of metastasis and perhaps tumor resistance to chemotherapy (Behrouzi et al., 2019; Wynendaele et al., 2015). Cellular exposure to chronic inflammation and inflammatory changes such as reactive oxygen and nitrogen

Gut Microbiome and Precision Medicine in Cancer

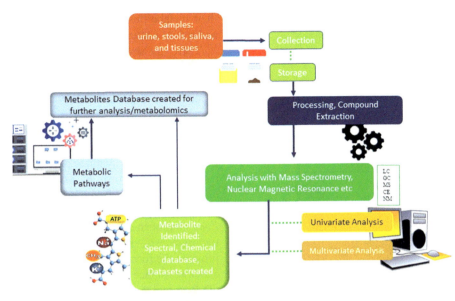

FIGURE 14.2 Flow diagram of basic steps to follow when conducting metabolomics studies. LC, liquid chromatography; MS, mass spectrometry; CE, capillary electrophoresis; GC, gas chromatography; NMR, nuclear magnetic resonance.

species and inflammatory factors such as cytokines and chemokines play a role in tumor growth and metastasis. The high prevalence of microbes such as *Fusobacterium nucleatum* (*F. nucleatum*) and NFκB signaling within the tumor environment during this chronic inflammation are the drivers of the malignant conversion. The NFκB is also capable of regulating the survival-triggering genes within cancer cells, and inflammatory-inducing genes within the host microenvironment (Behrouzi et al., 2019). An adhesion molecule in *F. nucleatum*, FadA binds to the TIGIT (limiter of innate and adaptive immunity) inhibitory receptors in natural killer cells (NKC) and inhibits cytotoxic activity, which helps invade the immune system in cancer cells. When bacteria are exposed to the CD4 T cells, they gain the ability to produce cytokines that induce tumor progression (Gur et al., 2015). Another gut bacteria, enterotoxigenic *Bacteroides fragilis* is known to lead to inflammation and induce colitis, as well as induce tumors in multiple intestinal neoplasia. This is through the STAT3 signaling which results in the production of IL-17 and IL-22 (Jiang et al., 2013; Behrouzi et al., 2019).

Obesity also results in dysbiosis, which, in combination with changes in the intestinal epithelium, results in increased permeability to microbials. This activates the immune cells and the release of pro-inflammatory cytokines, such as TNF and IL-6, and results in tumorigenesis (Louis et al., 2014; Behrouzi et al., 2019).

THE GUT MICROBIOME AND COLORECTAL CANCER

There is a documented link between microbiomes and malignancies. Most of the studies were conducted on the association between the microbiome and the gastrointestinal malignancies (liver, hepatobiliary, etc.) in general and colorectal cancer specifically. Colorectal cancer poses a

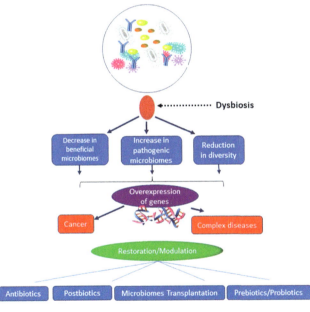

FIGURE 14.3 Some of the processes behind various types of tumors and the distinct features of microbiome of health and cancer. Multiple factors result in dysbiosis which manifests as a reduction in number and diversity of the microbiota. This results in the loss of microbiomes that are beneficial in the gut/colon environment and the host in general. Depending on the nature and extent of overexpression, this may result in the development of either a complex and chronic disease state or cancer formation. With adequate modulation, it is argued that the gut microbiota environment and functioning can be restored.

public health problem due to its significant morbidity and high mortality with epidemiological evidence of it being the second commonest cause of death in young people (Baba et al., 2017; Wei et al., 2019). The abundance of *F. nucleatum* is associated

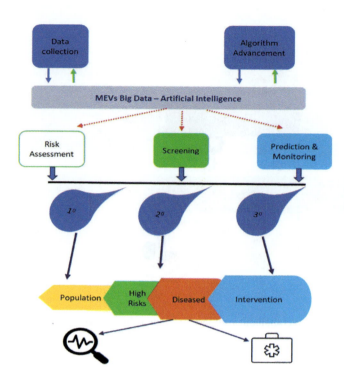

FIGURE 14.4 The application of microbial maximal extractable values (MEVs) for precision medicine, including that of risk assessment, screening, prediction, and monitoring, based on analysis through an artificial intelligence (AI) algorithm on human MEV big data and clinical data. The outcome being preventive therapy and therapeutics based on the response prediction and monitoring. (1^0, primary prevention strategy; 2^0, secondary prevention strategy; 3^0, tertiary prevention strategy.)

with intramucosal carcinomas in advanced stages. This is a multi-stepped pathogenesis that includes genetic alterations, and changes in genetic instability associated with metabolic and metagenomic shifts resulting in polypoid adenomas, carcinomas, and advanced stages of the disease. These microbial and metabolomic changes may occur early in the pathogenesis pathway and they may also be associated with the increase of *Atopobium parvulum* and *Acintomyces ondontolyticus*. The formation of antibodies against MEVs that are useful in the diagnosis of the disease, and the processes involved in the homeostasis of the gut by microbiota are complex (Yang et al., 2022; Lee et al., 2021). Figure 14.4 and Figure 14.5 elaborate some of the pathways and organisms/microbiomes involved as well as risk factors. Figure 14.5 also summarizes some of the mechanisms of therapeutic microbiota in the restoration of gut microbiome homeostasis and the effect on colorectal cancer carcinogenesis through both the immune-mediated and non-immune-mediated mechanisms.

The short-chain fatty acids (SCFAs) (acetate, propionate, and butyrate) are used by colonocytes for energy, whereas the colorectal cells undergo aerobic glycolysis instead. Hence, SCFAs play a major role in cellular homeostasis.

Mucosal dysfunctions induce epithelial-to-mesenchymal transition, increase permeability, result in loss of tight-junction proteins, and result in translocation of bacteria and their metabolites with the resultant increase in inflammation and risk of carcinogenesis (Martin & Jiang, 2009).

There are several species of bacteria that are implicated as causative in colorectal cancer. They facilitate the intestinal microbial ecosystem implicated in tumor proliferation, induction of a pro-inflammatory state, and evasion of anti-tumor activity. These species include, but are not limited to, *F. nucleatum*, *Streptococcus gallolyticus* (previous name *Streptococcus bovis* type 1), enterotoxic strains of *Bacterioides fragilis*, polyketide synthase positive (PKS^{+ve}) strains of *E. coli* (produces colibactin), *E. faecalis*, and *Peptostreptococcus anaerobius* (Chung et al., 2018; Long et al., 2019; Dai et al., 2018). A toxic polyketide-peptide, colibactin, produced by *E. coli* has been shown to induce DNA strand breaks, promote tumorigenesis, increase rates of cellular mutations, and promote the formation of tumors. *F. nucleatum* also promotes chemoresistance in CRC cells through Toll-like receptor 4 (TLR4), which renders the tumor resistant to cell death and finally treatment failure (Lee et al., 2021).

MICROBIAL EXTRACELLULAR VESICLES AS BIOMARKERS

Microbial extracellular vesicles (MEVs) used as biomarkers in liquid biopsy, also known as fluid biopsy or fluid phase biopsy, entails the sampling and analysis of nonsolid biological tissue. MEVs biomarkers are used in AI-based analysis of clinical and MEV data for the development of close to accurate prediction of pathology. Microbiomes are able to initiate cell-to-cell communication through the release of MEVs that circulate throughout the host's body and are excreted though the gut in feces. Taxonomy information of MEVs is harbored on the 16S rDNA which differs between different regions (V1-V3, V3-V4, etc.) (Yang et al., 2022).

THE GUT MICROBIOME AND IMMUNE CHECKPOINT INHIBITION

The treatment landscape for cancer has changed drastically since the discovery of immune checkpoints, with an immune checkpoint inhibitor (ICI), such as programmed death-ligand 1 (PD-L1), programmed cell death protein-1 (PD-1), and cytotoxic T-lymphocyte-associated protein-4 (CTLA4). In some centers, immune checkpoints have become a standard of care (Lee et al., 2021).

Because the efficacy of ICIs varies in patients, tumor histological type and organ affected, genetic engineering in the form of tumor-related biomarkers needs to be developed to ensure personalized treatment targeting the host genetic immune factors as well as tumor response (tumor-related biomarkers) (Ascierto et al., 2019; Ribas & Wolchok, 2018).

Gut microbiomes play a role in modulating the efficacy of anti-CTLA4 and anti-PD-1-based treatments in reducing tumor growth. Enriching the gut microbiome with *B. fragilis*, *Burkholderia cepacian*, and *Bifidobacterium* spp. significantly enhances these antibodies in cancer treatment through boosting T cell response, improving dendritic cell function,

Gut Microbiome and Precision Medicine in Cancer

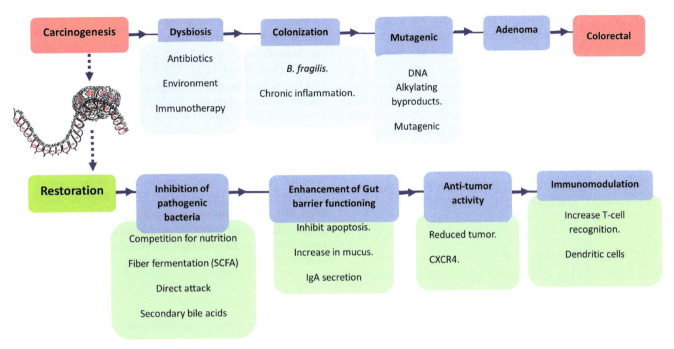

FIGURE 14.5 Summary of the mechanisms of microbiota on the gut, homeostasis, and the impact on colorectal cancer through different mechanisms. Microbiota may also restore the gut's mechanism for prevention of cancer, i.e., through enhancing gut barrier functioning, immunomodulation, promotion of inhibition of pathogenic bacterial colonization, and histopathological complexes.

and enhancing CD8+ T cell accumulation within the tumor-inhibiting growth (Sivan et al., 2015; Vetizou et al., 2015; Lee et al., 2021). ICIs such as anti-CTLA4 are associated with adverse effects such as high grade toxicity. The use of oral gavage with *B. fragilis* and *B. cepacia* reduces the toxicity and makes ICIs more tolerable. Therefore, GM is not only used as treatment for cancer but also to reduce delays and dropout that may be associated with adverse effects (Frankel et al., 2017; Larkin & Wolchok, 2015; Chapun et al., 2017).

In patients with colorectal cancer, it was found that there was a depletion of the bacterial species *B. animalis*, *Lachnospiraceae* spp., and *S. thermophiles*, which are thought to exert a protective function to the colon against cancer. A metabolite inosine, produced by *Bifidobacterium pseudolongum*, enhances the effect of ICIs (Chapun et al., 2017).

MICROBIOME AND MACHINE LEARNING

The application of Machine Learning to metagenomics has led to the identification of microbial species and biomarkers for cancer diagnosis. The combination of microbiomes data, patient genetic information, and available omics data such as transcriptomics, proteomics, and metabolomics, gives a picture of the complexity of the cancer disease and an opportunity for a personalized therapeutic approach (Mathieu et al., 2022). When machine learning is trained to predict microbiome-drug interaction for therapeutic solutions, such as identification of certain microbiomes as biomarkers of pre-cancer and cancer, it makes it more relevant to be used in this expanding research area of microbiomes. ML is also able to identify microbiomes associated with cancer progression and response to therapy. Machine learning through large data sets can identify the new probiotics which have therapeutic compounds to be evaluated for their therapeutic potential. There are drug databases such as the Drugbug database which have been used to evaluate the bacteria that metabolize a certain group of drugs and to evaluate the metabolites. The databases then afford the machine to learn and exploit chemical compounds that are based on microbial metabolism. Machine learning can classify patients into low- and high-risk groups based on patients' characteristics and microbiome profile. They can also guide the design of microbiome-targeted therapy (Namkung, 2020).

Machine learning in clinical oncology practice has been applied successfully through algorithms in relation to protein structures and function, oncology drug discovery, and cancer detection (D'Amico et al., 2022).

THE ROLE OF MICROBIOME IN PRECISION MEDICINE (DIAGNOSIS AND PERSONALIZED TREATMENT)

The diagnosis of anti-tumor pathogenic Th17 cells and Th1 immune cells response to anti-cancer resistance through identification of bacterial translocation is key not only for the diagnosis of resistance but also for modification and improvement of treatment response through restoration of the translocation effect of drugs such as cyclophosphamide. *Enterococcus hirae* and *Baresiella intestinihominis* bacteria gavage treatment successfully restores drug response (Fong et al., 2020).

Gut microbiome, through substantially enhancing PD1-based immunotherapy and inhibition of tumor growth, assists in enhancing immunotherapy drugs for cancer treatment and mediating immune activation in response to anticancer drugs. Probiotics such as *Bifidobacterium* spp. and *Akkermansia muciniphilia* have helped scientists understand how immune response is mediated by microbiomes and the administration of probiotics in patients with colorectal cancer (Sivan et al., 2015; Fong et al., 2020).

MANIPULATING THE GUT MICROBIOTA AS A POTENTIAL THERAPEUTIC STRATEGY

Fecal Microbiota Transplantation

Fecal microbiota is a therapeutic process of manipulating or replacing the gut microbiome to restore the microbiome flora health. Patients with diseases caused by *C. difficile* infection can be transplanted with a microbiome harvested from healthy individuals in order to resolve symptoms or prevent further diseases (Oh et al., 2023; Scott et al., 2015).

Patients who are on antibiotics are at risk of *C. difficile* infections. However, the risk is more than six-fold in patients on chemotherapy and radiation and in patients with colorectal cancer (Van Nood et al., 2013; Cammarota et al., 2015). FMT may also be done through a process known as washed microbiota transplantation (WMT), where microfiltration and centrifugation are done (Oh et al., 2023; Scott et al., 2015).

Bacteria that are genetically modified or engineered for specific biological functions, such as immune regulation, toxin metabolism, and anti-pathogen colonization, do so by targeting specific genes and improving the microbiome composition (Sood et al., 2019; Lythgoe et al., 2022; Oh et al., 2023; Scott et al., 2015). The immune checkpoint inhibitors are influenced by gut microbiome composition and hence FMT modifies ICPI responsiveness and relevance in precision oncology (Lythgoe et al., 2022; Oh et al., 2023; Scott et al., 2015) (Figure 14.6).

Probiotic Supplementation

Probiotics are capable of restoring host microbial communities and offer the competitive exclusion of pathogens whilst improving the barrier functioning of the gut. They also

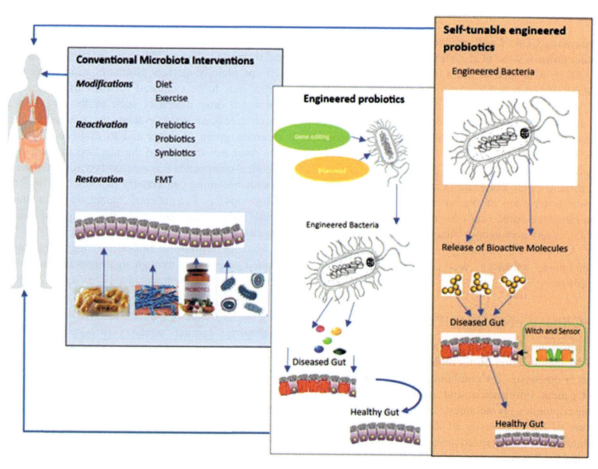

FIGURE 14.6 **The role of gut microbiota-targeted interventions through microbiome genetic engineering, probiotics and the effect on bioactive molecules and the health and disease stage of the host organism.** Genetic engineering offers solutions to both the treatment of dysbiosis and the restoration of gut microbiota to prevent cancer. Engineered bacteria are self-sustainable and through a biochemical sensor activate the release of bioactive molecules. This process offers long-term protection and enhancement of response to chemotherapy.

generate metabolites that influence metabolism. Probiotics are designed as either homogenous or heterogenous with *Bifidobacterium*, *Lactobacillus*, and *Saccharomyces* spp. as well as several species under investigation (*Faecalibacterium prausnitzii*, *Akkermansia muciniphila*, and *Clostridia* spp.) (Wieërs et al., 2020). Probiotics significantly contribute to a reduction in inflammatory markers and hence inflammation-prone cancers including colorectal cancers (Kassaian et al., 2020; Oh et al., 2023; Scott et al., 2015).

Diet and Prebiotics

A diet rich in animal proteins and saturated fats is associated with reduced diversity and complexity of microbiomes. Plant-derived diets with complex carbohydrates (prebiotics) are associated with high diversity and are protective (Oh et al., 2023).

Engineered bacteria can sense and respond to microenvironmental signals associated with more precise and effective treatment of diseases. Precision medicine uses strategies such as diet modifications, exercise, use of prebiotics, probiotics, synbiotics, postbiotics, and fecal microbiota transplantation to modify the function of the gut microbiomes (Omer et al., 2022).

CHALLENGES OF THE USE OF THE MICROBIOME IN PRECISION MEDICINE

Because disease associated with the microbiome may be a product of a single gene disorder or a result of function from one strain of microorganism, it may be easy to treat with a supplementation of a metabolite of a single gene. However, diseases may be a result of mirroring by phenotypes of the specific microbiome but involving many of its genes as opposed to being caused by multiple organisms (Buffington et al., 2016). When these are supplemented, they may require multiple bacterial species. Although diseases and cancers may be associated with certain microbiomes, microbiome metabolites, and/or microbiome deficiencies or mutations, association does not imply causality and therefore certain interventions such as FMT and probiotics may not always be effective to restore the environment and prevent or treat the malignancy (Petrosino, 2018).

CONCLUSION

Exploration of the gut microbiome will afford scientists and oncologists to design specific treatment modalities for patients' cancers without applying the principles of one size fits all. The use of immune therapy requires the application of proteomics, microbiomics, and precision medicine in the treatment, enhancing the response and prevention of colorectal cancer.

Immuno-oncology as a specialized field promises to be the next big thing. The role of microbiomes in inflammatory conditions that may result in cancer and the impact that restoration of the dysbiosis or addition of probiotics and microbiome implantation play in protection against colorectal cancer will continue to be explored in different subsets of research (human and animal). To effectively apply precision medicine principles, we need to understand the effects of gut microbiota efficacy and the toxicity of the chemotherapeutic drugs. The use of machine learning on genetic engineering will drive the principle of a "rational donor selection" in fecal microbiome transplant and lead to improved efficacy.

REFERENCES

Ascierto PA, Long GV, Robert C, Brady B, Dutriaux C, Di Giacomo AM, et al. (2019). Survival outcomes in patients with previously untreated BRAF wild-type advanced melanoma treated with nivolumab therapy: three-year follow-up of a randomized Phase 3 trial. *JAMA Oncol.* 5: 187–194.

Baba Y, Iwatsuki M, Yoshida N, Watanabe M, & Baba H. (2017). Review of the gut microbiome and esophageal cancer: pathogenesis and potential clinical implications. *Ann Gastroenterol Surg.* 1: 99–104.

Behrouzi A, Nafari AH, & Siadat SD. (2019). The significance of microbiome in personalized medicine. *Clin Trans Med.* 8: 16. https://doi.org/10.1186/s40169-019-0232-y

Bhatt AP, Redinbo MR, & Bultman SJ. (2017). The role of the microbiome in cancer development and therapy. *CA Cancer J Clin.* 67(4): 326–344. doi: 10.3322/caac.21398 PMID: 28481406y.

Buffington SA, Di Prisco GV, Auchtung TA, Ajami NJ, Petrosino JF, & Costa-Mattioli M. (2016). Microbial reconstitution reverses maternal diet-induced social and synaptic deficits in offspring. *Cell.* 165: 1762–1775. doi: 10.1016/j.cell.2016.06.001

Cammarota G, Masucci L, Ianiro G, Bibbò S, Dinoi G, Costamagna G, et al. (2015). Randomised clinical trial: faecal microbiota transplantation by colonoscopy vs. vancomycin for the treatment of recurrent *Clostridium difficile* infection. *Aliment Pharmacol Ther.* 41: 835–843. https://doi.org/10.1111/apt.13144

Candela M, Biagi E, Maccaferri S, Turroni S, & Brigidi P. (2012). Intestinal microbiota is a plastic factor responding to environmental changes. *Trends Microbiol.* 20(8): 385–391. http://dx.doi.org/10.1016/j.tim.2012.05.003

Chaput N, Lepage P, Coutzac C, Soularue E, Le Roux K, Monot C, et al. (2017). Baseline gut microbiota predicts clinical response and colitis in metastatic melanoma patients treated with ipilimumab. *Ann Oncol.* 28: 1368–1379.

Chu X, Jaeger M, Beumer J, Bakker OB, Aguirre-Gamboa R, & Oosting M. (2021). Integration of metabolomics, genomics, and immune phenotypes reveals the causal roles of metabolites in disease. *Genome Biol.* 22: 1–22.

Chung L, Thiele Orberg E, Geis AL, Chan JL, Fu K, DeStefano Shields CE, et al. (2018). *Bacteroides fragilis* toxin coordinates a pro-carcinogenic inflammatory cascade via targeting of colonic epithelial cells. *Cell Host Microbe.* 23: 203–214.e5.

Clish C. (2015). Metabolomics: an emerging but powerful tool for precision medicine. *Cold Spring Harb Mol Case Stud.* 1: a000588. https://bit.ly/3gOX3is.

D'Amico F, Barone M, Tavella T, Rampelli S, Brigidi P, & Turroni S. (2022). Host microbiomes in tumor precision medicine: How far are we? *Current Med Chem.* 29(18): 3202–3230. https://doi.org/10.2174/0929867329666220105121754

Dai Z, Coker OO, Nakatsu G, Wu WKK, Zhao L, Chen Z, et al. (2018). Multi-cohort analysis of colorectal cancer metagenome identified altered bacteria across populations and universal bacterial markers. *Microbiome*. 6: 70.

Dettmer K, Aronov PA & Hammock BD. (2007). Mass spectrometry-based metabolomics. *Mass Spectrometry Rev.* 26: 51–78.

Fassarella M, Blaak EE, Penders J, Nauta A, Smidt H, & Zoetendal EG. (2021). Gut microbiome stability and resilience: elucidating the response to perturbations in order to modulate gut health. *Gut.* 70(3): 595–605. http://dx.doi.org/10.1136/gutjnl-2020-321747.

Fong W, Li Q, & Yu J. (2020). Gut microbiota modulation: a novel strategy for prevention and treatment of colorectal cancer. *Oncogene.* 39: 4925–4943. https://doi.org/10.1038/s41388-020-1341-1

Frankel AE, Coughlin LA, Kim J, Froehlich TW, Xie Y, Frenkel EP, et al. (2017). Metagenomic shotgun sequencing and unbiased metabolomic profiling identify specific human gut microbiota and metabolites associated with immune checkpoint therapy efficacy in melanoma patients. *Neoplasia.* 19: 848–855.

Gur C, Ibrahim Y, Isaacson B, Yamin R, Abed J, Gamliel M, et al. (2015). Binding of the Fap2 protein of Fusobacterium nucleatum to human inhibitory receptor TIGIT protects tumors from immune cell attack. *Immunity.* 42(2): 344–355. https://doi.org/10.1016/j.immuni.2015.01.010

Hamet P & Tremblay J. (2017). Artificial intelligence in medicine. *Metabolism.* 69: S36–S40.

Jiang R, Wang H, Deng L, Hou J, Shi R, Yao M, et al. (2013). IL-22 is related to development of human colon cancer by activation of STAT3. *BMC Cancer.* 13: 59. https://doi.org/10.1186/1471-2407-13-59

Kassaian N, Feizi A, Rostami S, Aminorroaya A, Yaran M, & Amini M. (2020). The effects of 6 mo of supplementation with probiotics and synbiotics on gut microbiota in the adults with prediabetes: a double blind randomized clinical trial. *Nutrition.* 79–80: 110854. doi: 10.1016/j.nut.2020.110854

Larkin J, Hodi FS, & Wolchok JD. (2015). Combined nivolumab and ipilimumab or monotherapy in untreated melanoma. *N Engl J Med.* 373: 1270–1271.

Lee KA, Luong MK, Shaw H, Nathan P, Bataille V & Spector TD. (2021). The gut microbiome: what the oncologist ought to know. *Br J Cancer.* 125: 1197–1209. https://doi.org/10.1038/s41416-021-01467-x

Long X, Wong CC, Tong L, Chu ESH, Ho Szeto C, Go MYY, et al. (2019). *Peptostreptococcus anaerobius* promotes colorectal carcinogenesis and modulates tumour immunity. *Nat Microbiol.* 4: 2319–2330.

Louis P, Hold GL, & Flint HJ. (2014). The gut microbiota, bacterial metabolites and colorectal cancer. *Nat Rev.* 12: 661–672.

Lythgoe MP, Ghani R, Mullish BH, Marchesi JR, & Krell J. (2022). The potential of fecal microbiota transplantation in oncology. *Trends Microbiol.* 30(1): 10–12. https://doi.org/10.1016/j.tim.2021.10.003

Martin TA, & Jiang WG. (2009). Loss of tight junction barrier function and its role in cancer metastasis. *Biochim Biophys Acta.* 1788: 872–891.

Mathieu A, Leclercq M, Sanabria M, Perin O, & Droit A. (2022). Machine learning and deep learning applications in metagenomic taxonomy and functional annotation. *Frontiers Microbiol.* 13: 811495. https://doi.org/10.3389/fmicb.2022.811495

Namkung J. (2020). Machine learning methods for microbiome studies. *J Microbiol.* 58(3): 206–216. https://doi.org/10.1007/s12275-020-0066-8

Oh L, Ab Rahman S, Dubinsky K, Azanan MS, & Ariffin H. (2023). Manipulating the gut microbiome as a therapeutic strategy to mitigate late effects in childhood cancer survivors. *Technol Cancer Res Treatment.* 22: 15330338221149799. https://doi.org/10.1177/15330338221149799)

Omer R, Mohsin MZ, Mohsin A, Mushtaq BS, Huang X, Guo M, et al. (2022). Engineered bacteria-based living materials for biotherapeutic applications. *Frontiers in Bioengineering and Biotechnology*, 10: 870675. https://doi.org/10.3389/fbioe.2022.870675

Panthee B, Gyawali S, Panthee P, & Techato, K. (2022). Environmental and human microbiome for health. *Life (Basel, Switzerland).* 12(3): 456. https://doi.org/10.3390/life12030456

Pasolli E, Truong DT, Malik F, Waldron L, & Segata N. (2016). Machine learning meta-analysis of large metagenomic datasets: tools and biological insights. *PLoS Comput Biol.* 12: e1004977.

Petrosino JF. (2018). The microbiome in precision medicine: the way forward. *Genome Med.* 10(1): 12. https://doi.org/10.1186/s13073-018-0525-6

Pfohl U, Pflaume A, Regenbrecht M, Finkler S, Graf Adelmann Q, Reinhard C, et al. (2021). Precision oncology beyond genomics: the future is here-it is just not evenly distributed. *Cells.* 10: 928.

Puchades-Carrasco L, & Pineda-Lucena A. (2017). Metabolomics applications in precision medicine: an oncological perspective. *Current Topics in Medicinal Chemistry*, 17(24): 2740–2751. https://doi.org/10.2174/1568026617666170707120034

Puschhof J, & Elinav E. (2023) Human microbiome research: growing pains and future promises. *PLOS Biol.* 21(3): e3002053. https://doi.org/10.1371/journal.pbio.3002053

Ribas A, & Wolchok JD. (2018). Cancer immunotherapy using checkpoint blockade. *Science.* 359: 1350–1355.

Scott KP, Antoine JM, Midtvedt T, & van Hemert S. (2015). Manipulating the gut microbiota to maintain health and treat disease. *Microbial Ecol Health Dis.* 26: 25877. https://doi.org/10.3402/mehd.v26.25877

Sivan A, Corrales L, Hubert N, Williams JB, Aquino-Michaels K, Earley ZM, et al. (2015). Commensal Bifidobacterium promotes antitumor immunity and facilitates anti–PD-L1 efficacy. *Science.* 350: 1084–1089.

Sood A, Mahajan R, Singh A, Midha V, Mehta V, Narang V, et al. (2019). Role of faecal microbiota transplantation for maintenance of remission in patients with ulcerative colitis: a pilot study. *J Crohn's Colitis.* 13:1311–7. doi: 10.1093/ecco-jcc/jjz060.

van Nood E, Vrieze A, Nieuwdorp M, Fuentes S, Zoetendal EG, de Vos WM, et al. (2013). Duodenal infusion of donor feces for recurrent Clostridium difficile. *N Engl J Med.* 368(5): 407–415. doi.org/10.1056/NEJMoa1205037

Vétizou M, Pitt JM, Daillère R, Lepage P, Waldschmitt N, Flament C, et al. (2015). Anticancer immunotherapy by CTLA-4 blockade relies on the gut microbiota. *Science.* 350: 1079–1084.

Whon TW, Shin NR, Kim JY, & Roh SW. (2021). Omics in gut microbiome analysis. *J Microbiol.* 59(3): 292–297. https://doi.org/10.1007/s12275-021-1004-0

Wei M-Y, Shi S, Liang C, Meng Q-C, Hua J, Zhang Y-Y, et al. (2019). The microbiota and microbiome in pancreatic cancer: more influential than expected. *Mol Cancer.* 18: 97.

Wieërs G, Belkhir L, Enaud R, Leclercq S, Philippart de Foy JM, Dequenne I, et al. (2020). How probiotics affect the microbiota. *Front Cellular Infect Microbiol.* 9: 454. https://doi.org/10.3389/fcimb.2019.00454

Wynendaele E, Verbeke F, D'Hondt M, Hendrix A, Van De Wiele C, Burvenich C, et al. (2015). Crosstalk between the microbiome and cancer cells by quorum sensing peptides. *Peptides.* 64: 40–48. https://doi.org/10.1016/j.peptides.2014.12.009

Yang J, Shin TS, Kim JS, Jee Y-K, & Kim Y-K. (2022). A new horizon of precision medicine: combination of the microbiome and extracellular vesicles. *Exp Mol Med.* 54: 466–482. https://doi.org/10.1038/s12276-022-00748-6

15 Therapeutic Potential of the Gut Virome in Cancer

Zilungile Mkhize-Kwitshana, Pragalathan Naidoo, Rene Khan, Andreas M. Kaufmann, and Zodwa Dlamini

INTRODUCTION

Advances in technology, including metagenomic sequencing, bioinformatic analyses, and molecular biology techniques have accelerated the understanding of the landscape of the human gut microbiome, particularly the bacterial kingdom. It was only in 2003 that Breitbart and colleagues took advantage of these enablers to extend the insights of gut microbiome beyond the bacteria to include the viral community and it has been confirmed that a variety of gut viral species including viruses that infect human cells, bacterial and plant cells constitute the human gut virome (Breitbart et al., 2003; Liang and Bushman, 2021). The gastrointestinal (GI) tract harbors the highest number of viruses across the human body and is estimated to have approximately 10^9–10^{10} viral particles per gram of feces (Cao et al., 2022). A record 189,680 viral DNA genome data, approximating 54,118 species of viruses, has been published from analysis of 11,810 publicly available human stool metagenomes (Nayfach et al., 2021), demonstrating the vast diversity of the gut virome.

The gut virome is mainly colonized by bacteriophages (97.7%) followed by eukaryotic viruses (2.1%) and archaeal viruses (0.1%) (Popgeorgiev et al., 2013). The different families of viruses colonizing the human gut virome are: (i) dsDNA viral families (*Adenoviridae*, *Herpesviridae*, *Iridoviridae*, *Marseilleviridae*, *Myoviridae*, *Podoviridae*, *Polyomaviridae*, *Poxviridae*, and *Siphoviridae*); (ii) ssDNA viral families (*Anelloviridae*, *Circoviridae*, *Inoviridae*, and *Microviridae*); (iii) (+) ssRNA viral families (*Astroviridae*, *Caliciviridae*, *Coronaviridae*, *Picornaviridae*, and *Virgaviridae*); and (iv) dsRNA viral families (*Picobirnaviridae* and *Reoviridae*) (Popgeorgiev et al., 2013) (Figure 15.1). The different viral genera and species from the above-mentioned viral families and their morphology are summarized in Table 15.1.

The gut virome has been shown to play an important role in the regulation of human health and disease, similar to the known influence of bacterial microbiota. The modulatory mechanisms are orchestrated mainly through the interactions between virus/phage-bacteria and between virus/phage-host immune system (Liang and Bushman, 2021). Depending on the life cycle and environmental conditions, phages can lyse (lytic cycle) their bacterial hosts and can facilitate horizontal virome gene transfer which results in phenotypic changes in the coexisting bacterial hosts. This implies that the phages will determine the bacterial composition and function (Broecker and Moelling, 2021). Bacteriophages also interact and shape the innate and humoral immune system of the host both locally in the gut and systemically, thereby playing a role in maintaining immune homeostasis. The intricate details of the roles played by the gut virome in immune homeostasis in disease and health are reviewed elsewhere (Cao et al., 2022) and do not form part of this section.

Regarding cancer, accumulative evidence suggests that some members of the gut virome contribute to oncogenesis, particularly gastrointestinal tumors, through various mechanisms. Examples include *Epstein-Barr* virus-induced mutagenesis resulting in oncogenic transformation in intestinal cells (Umakanthan and Bukelo, 2021) and *Inovirus*-induced bacterial biofilms resulting in colon carcinogenesis (Johnson et al., 2015a). Likewise, some of the virome families have the potential to promote antitumor responses, providing an opportunity for manipulation of the virome to modulate antitumor immune responses for cancer immunotherapy.

Given the relative inefficiencies associated with current cancer treatments, scientists are actively engaged with designing and testing new treatment methods that are specific to cancer cells and deliver potent tumor toxicity with minimal side effects (Cao et al., 2020). The use of immunotherapy in recent decades has provided an alternative treatment that uses the patient's own immune system to target cancer cells, but the 10–30% effectiveness requires urgent improvement (Zhao et al., 2021, Cao et al., 2020). The potential for virotherapy was first proposed in 1910, but with the recent clinical trials and FDA-approved drug, research into this relatively unchartered field has gained momentum. Virotherapy has a two-fold application, viz. viral immunotherapy and oncolytic virotherapy. Viral immunotherapy uses genetically modified viruses to stimulate the immune system, while oncolytic virotherapy uses oncolytic viruses to directly target and kill cancer cells (Rahman and McFadden, 2021) (Figure 15.2). These newer therapies have been shown to be effective for malignant tumors, offering hope to cancer patients.

Therapeutic Potential of the Gut Virome in Cancer

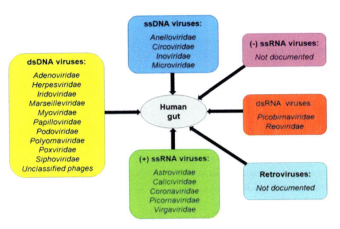

FIGURE 15.1 Summary of dsDNA, ssDNA, dsRNA, (+) ssRNA, (-) ssRNA and Retrovirus viral families found in the human gut. There are numerous types of viruses found in the gut virome.

This chapter explores the therapeutic potential of the gut virome in cancer treatment. It discusses the role of phage therapy, oncolytic viruses, and the manipulation of the virome to modulate antitumor immune responses. The chapter also highlights ongoing research efforts and the challenges associated with harnessing the therapeutic potential of the gut virome in personalized cancer therapies.

PHAGE THERAPY

Overview

Bacteriophages (or phages) are viruses that infect and replicate in bacterial cells. Phages replicate and multiply exponentially in the host bacterium by lytic (lytic phages lyse the bacterial cell to release progeny viruses) or lysogenic (lysogenic or temperate phages incorporate their nucleic acid within the host bacterial cell and replicate together with the host, resulting in the host bacteria acquiring new characteristic properties and features) mode (Sharma et al., 2017).

Over 97.7% of the gut virome contains phages (Zhang and Wang, 2023). The most dominant family of phages in the human gut are dsDNA phages (*Ackermannviridae*, *Corticoviridae*, *Myoviridae*, *Plasmaviridae*, *Podoviridae*, *Siphoviridae*, and *Tectiviridae*) and ssDNA phages (*Inoviridae* and *Microviridae*) (Dion et al., 2020). A study by Shkoporov et al. (2019) found the order *Caudovirales* (*Podoviridae* (5.0%), *Myoviridae* (8.3%), *Siphoviridae* (12.7%) and *crAss-like phages* (21.2%)), family *Microviridae* (31.0%), *Inoviridae* (0.1%) and others to be the most dominant inhabitants in the phageome (Shkoporov et al., 2019). Zhao et al. (2019) investigated the abundance of phages from different sections of the intestine. When compared to the terminal ileum, the proximal colon had a higher abundance of *Siphoviridae*, *Myoviridae* and *Microviridae*, while the distal colon and rectum had a higher abundance of both *Microviridae* and *Siphoviridae* and *Microviridae* only, respectively (Zhao et al., 2019).

Phages can regulate the composition of the intestinal microbiota through: (i) *Predation:* Phages can target a specific bacterium of interest for "predation" due to their ability to identify and recognize specific receptors located on the bacterial surface. (ii) *Lysogenic conversion:* Temperate phages can transfer genetic information with special functions to the host bacterium to enhance the host survival rate (Xu et al., 2022). (iii) *Seesaw effect (ebb and flow phenomenon):* When exposed to antibacterial drugs, bacterial strains can evolve and become drug resistant under genetic selection and in the process become phage sensitive. Likewise, bacterial exposure to phage conditions can lead to a loss in antimicrobial resistance after genetic selection. (iv) *Epithelial defense:* Phages have the ability to phagocytize and lyse harmful bacteria in addition to decreasing their colonization on the surface of the intestinal mucus layer (Xu et al., 2022).

Intestinal phages can also regulate immune responses and maintain immune homeostasis. Pathogen-associated molecular patterns, or PAMPs, are produced during phage-induced lysis. PAMPs can translocate into the mucosal barrier of the intestine and in the process activate immune responses (Sinha and Maurice, 2019, Xu et al., 2022). Phage-mediated immune responses, which are generated when phages interact with the mucosal barrier, can promote innate immunity and acquired immunity to protect commensal bacteria located in the upper layer of mucus and to promote killing of invasive pathogens located in the deepest mucus, respectively (Barr et al., 2013, Xu et al., 2022). Phages can stimulate the proliferation of CD4+ and CD8+ T lymphocytes in Peyer's patch by activating intestinal immunity via the Toll-like receptor 9-dependent interferon signaling pathway (Gogokhia et al., 2019). Phages can also promote phagocytosis of bacteria by stimulating and activating macrophages (Van Belleghem et al., 2019), express proteins that display immunoglobulin-type domains and C-type lectin folds which interferes with O-glycosylated MUC2 mucin expression in the colon (Gogokhia et al., 2019), and display immunoglobulin-type folds which are also found in T cell receptors and antibodies (Van Belleghem et al., 2019). Adhesion proteins produced by *Escherichia coli* phages can bind to lipopolysaccharide, which in turn regulates the lipopolysaccharide-mediated inflammatory response (Górski et al., 2012). *Escherichia coli* phages can also have an immunosuppressive effect and prevent the expansion of intestinal immune cells (Górski et al., 2012).

Phage therapy, which involves the use of bacteriophages to treat bacterial infections, is not typically used as a direct treatment for cancer. However, there is some research exploring the potential role of phage therapy in cancer-related areas, mainly through the modulation of the gut microbiota and the immune system. Phage therapy may indirectly impact cancer by: (i) *Regulating the composition of the gut microbiota in cancer patients:* The gut microbiota plays a crucial role in human health, and alterations in the gut microbiome have been associated with various diseases, including cancer. Phages are a part of the gut microbiota, and phage therapy

TABLE 15.1

Summary of the major viral genera/species colonizing the human gut

Viral family	Viral genera/species	Morphology	References
		dsDNA viral group	
Adenoviridae	- Enteric adenovirus 40, 41	- Viral particle size: 70–100 nm. - Virion: naked. - Number of capsomers: 252 (240 hexons and 12 pentons). - Capsid symmetry: icosahedral. - Molecular weight of nucleic acid in virion: $20-30 \times 10^6$	(Nicklin et al., 2005)
Herpesviridae	- Epstein-Barr virus - Human cytomegalovirus	- Viral particle size: 90–130 nm. - Virion: enveloped. - Number of capsomers: 162 (240 hexons and 12 pentons). - Capsid symmetry: icosahedral. - Molecular weight of nucleic acid in virion: $90-130 \times 10^6$	(Francki et al., 1991)
Myoviridae	- Bacillus phage G - phiBCD7 - phiP-SSM4	- Viral particle size: 80–455 nm × 16–20 nm - Virion: naked. - Number of capsomers: 72 capsomers (60 hexamers and 12 pentamers; T = 7). - Capsid symmetry: icosahedral. - Molecular weight of nucleic acid in virion: $44-70 \times 10^6$	(Francki et al., 1991)
Papillomaviridae	- Human papillomavirus 6, 18, 66	- Viral particle size: 80–455 nm × 16–20 nm - Virion: naked. - Number of capsomers: 72 capsomers (60 hexamers and 12 pentamers; T = 7). - Capsid symmetry: icosahedral. - Molecular weight of nucleic acid in virion: $44-70 \times 10^6$	(Abouelkhair and Kennedy, 2022)
Podoviridae	- Enterobacteria phage P22 - Phage T3	- Viral particle size: Isometric head (60 nm in diameter) and short tail (17 nm x 8 nm) with 6 short fibers. - Virion: naked. - Number of capsomers: 72 (T = 7). - Capsid symmetry: icosahedral. - Molecular weight of nucleic acid in virion: 25×10^6	(Francki et al., 1991)
Polyomaviridae	- Human polyomavirus 1 (BK virus) - Human polyomavirus 9, 12 - Human polyomavirus 2 (JC virus or John Cunningham virus) - Simian virus 40 (SV40 virus)	- Viral particle size: 40–50 nm. - Virion: naked. - Number of capsomers: 72. - Capsid symmetry: icosahedral. - Molecular weight of nucleic acid in virion: 5×10^6	(Abouelkhair and Kennedy, 2022)
Poxviridae	- Newcastle disease virus	- Viral particle size: 230 nm × 400 nm. - Virion: complex coats. - Numbers of capsomers: 72. - Capsid symmetry: complex. - Molecular weight of nucleic acid in virion: $130-200 \times 10^6$	(Francki et al., 1991)
Siphoviridae	- Clostridium phage phiCP39-O - Listeria phage A118 - Mycobacterium phage Athena - Phage PA6 - Phage SM - phiCP39-O - phiE125 Lactococcus phage BIL285	- Viral particle size: Isometric head (60 nm in diameter), and flexible tail (150 nm × 8 nm) with short terminal/subterminal tail fibers. - Virion: naked. - Numbers of capsomers: 72 (T = 7). - Capsid symmetry: icosahedral. - Molecular weight of nucleic acid in virion: 33×10^6	(Francki et al., 1991)
Iridoviridae	Lymphocystis disease virus	- Viral particle size: 125–300 nm in diameter. - Virion: naked particles and enveloped virions. - Numbers of capsomers: 12 pentasymmetrons and 20 trisymmetrons (T = 147). - Capsid symmetry: icosahedral. - Molecular weight of nucleic acid in virion: $100-250 \times 10^6$	(Francki et al., 1991)
		ssDNA viral group	
Anelloviridae	- Torque teno virus (TTV virus)	- Viral particle size: 18–30 nm in diameter. - Virion: naked. - Number of capsomers: 12 pentameric capsomers. - Capsid symmetry: icosahedral. - Molecular weight of nucleic acid in virion: $2-3.9 \times 10^6$	(Simmonds and Sharp, 2016)

TABLE 15.1 (Continued)
Summary of the major viral genera/species colonizing the human gut

Viral family	Viral genera/species	Morphology	References
Circoviridae	- Chicken anemia virus	- Viral particle size: 20 nm. - Virion: naked. - Number of capsomers: 12 pentagonal trumpet-shaped pentamer (T = 1). - Capsid symmetry: icosahedral. - Molecular weight of nucleic acid in virion: $1.8–2.1 \times 10^6$	(Breitbart et al., 2017)
Microviridae	- Bdellovibrio phage phiMH2K - Chlamydia phage 1,3,4 - Chlamydia phage CPAR39 - Chlamydia phage CPG1 - Spiroplasma phage 4	- Viral particle size: Isometric (25–27 nm in diameter). - Virion: naked. - Number of capsomers: 12 conspicuous capsomers (T = 1). - Capsid symmetry: icosahedral. - Molecular weight of nucleic acid in virion: 1.7×10^6	(Francki et al., 1991)

dsRNA viral group

Viral family	Viral genera/species	Morphology	References
Picobirnaviridae	- Human picobirnavirus	- Viral particle size: 20–30 nm. - Virion: naked. - Number of capsomers: 32. - Capsid symmetry: icosahedral. - Molecular weight of nucleic acid in virion: $2.3–2.8 \times 10^6$	(Delmas et al., 2019)
Reoviridae	- Human rotavirus	- Viral particle size: 60–80 nm. - Virion: naked. - Capsid symmetry: icosahedral. - Molecular weight of nucleic acid in virion: $12–15 \times 10^6$	(Francki et al., 1991)

(+) ssRNA viral group

Viral family	Viral genera/species	Morphology	References
Astroviridae	- Human astrovirus	- Viral particle size: 28–30 nm. - Virion: naked. - Number of capsomers: 32. - Capsid symmetry: icosahedral. - Molecular weight of nucleic acid in virion: $6.4–7.7 \times 10^6$	(Matsui et al., 2001)
Caliciviridae	- Norwalk virus	- Viral particle size: 35–39 nm. - Virion: naked. - Number of capsomers: 32. - Capsid symmetry: icosahedral. - Molecular weight of nucleic acid in virion: $2.6–2.8 \times 10^6$	(Francki et al., 1991)
Coronaviridae	- Human coronavirus OC43, NL63, HKU1, 229E	- Viral particle size: 80–160 nm. - Virion: enveloped. - Capsid symmetry: unknown or complex. - Molecular weight of nucleic acid in virion: $9–11 \times 10^6$	(Francki et al., 1991)
Picornaviridae	- Aichi virus - Human cosavirus - Human coxsackievirus - Human echovirus - Human enterovirus - Human klassevirus/salivirus - Human parechovirus - Human poliovirus - Saffold cardiovirus	- Viral particle size: 20–30 nm. - Virion: naked. - Number of capsomers: 32. - Capsid symmetry: icosahedral. - Molecular weight of nucleic acid in virion: $2.3–2.8 \times 10^6$	(Francki et al., 1991)
Virgaviridae	- Pepper mild mottle virus - Tobacco mosaic virus	- Viral particle size: helically constructed with a pitch of 2.3–2.5 nm, and an axal canal diameter of 20 nm. - Virion: naked. - Number of capsomers: 2130. - Capsid symmetry: Rod shaped. - Molecular weight of nucleic acid in virion: RNA-1 is 6–7 kb and RNA-2 is 3.5–3.6 kb.	(Adams et al., 2017)

(-) ssRNA viral group
Not documented.

Retroviruses
Not documented.

could potentially help to restore or manipulate the balance of bacteria in the gut. This, in turn, may indirectly affect cancer development or treatment, as the gut microbiota can influence inflammation, immunity, and even response to cancer therapies (Emencheta et al., 2023, Kabwe et al., 2021). (ii) *Modulating immune responses in cancer patients:* Some research suggests that certain phages can influence the host immune response. By manipulating the gut microbiota and consequently the immune system, phage therapy might indirectly affect the body's ability to recognize and respond to cancer cells (Souza et al., 2023, Kabwe et al., 2021). (iii) *Treating bacterial infections in cancer patients:* Cancer patients often have weakened immune systems due to the disease itself or the side effects of cancer treatments. They may be more susceptible to bacterial infections. In such cases, phage therapy could be considered to treat bacterial infections in cancer patients, which can help in managing complications and improving overall health during cancer treatment (Li et al., 2023, Kabwe et al., 2021).

PHAGES USED IN CANCER THERAPY

M13 phage

The M13 phage, one of the Ff phages and a member of the Inoviridae family, is a lysogenic filamentous bacteriophage (temperate phage) composed of circular ssDNA. It has a length of ~880 nm and diameter of ~6 nm and contains five capsid proteins (minor capsid proteins: pIII, pVI, pVII, and pIX and major capsid protein: pVIII). The major capsid protein (pVIII) contains 50 amino acids and constitutes 98% of the total mass of the M13 phage, and is composed of three domains: (i) N-terminal domain (1–20 AA), (ii) intermediate hydrophobic domain (21–39 AA), and (iii) positively charged domain (40–50 AA) that electrostatically interacts with the phage genomic DNA (Wang et al., 2023). M13 phages display high immunogenicity and can precisely target the surface of tumor cells to trigger the penetration of activated innate immune cells and inflammation, resulting in tumor-associated immunosuppression and antitumor immunity promotion (Wang et al., 2023, Murgas et al., 2018).

Several intestinal bacterial species, including *Fusobacterium* spp. (Alon-Maimon et al., 2022), *Streptococcus* spp. (Abdulamir et al., 2011), *Prevotella* spp. (Lo et al., 2022), *Peptostreptococcus* spp. (Gu et al., 2023), *Parvimonas* spp. (Khan et al., 2019), and *Treponema* spp. (Nieminen et al., 2018) play an insidious role in colorectal cancer development. Dong and colleagues (2020) bioengineered the M13 phage to target *Fusobacterium nucleatum*, a bacterium that can selectively increase immunosuppressive myeloid-derived suppressor cells (MDSCs) to hinder the host's anticolorectal cancer immune response.

In this study, silver nanoparticles were electrostatically assembled on the surface of the capsid protein of the *Fusobacterium nucleatum*-binding M13 phage to specifically remove *Fusobacterium nucleatum* and modify the tumor-immune microenvironment. The bioengineered M13 phage was reported to scavenge *Fusobacterium nucleatum* in the gut leading to a significant decrease in MDSC in the tumor site, and activated antigen-presenting cells to promote the activation of the host immune response for colorectal cancer suppression. The investigators concluded that the bioengineered M13 phage in combination with chemotherapeutics (FOLFIRI: folinic acid, fluorouracil, and irinotecan) or checkpoint inhibitors (α-PD1) significantly increased overall survival rate the in orthotopic colorectal cancer mouse model (Dong et al., 2020).

Murgas et al. (2018) targeted the M13 phage to the carcinoembryonic antigen (CEA), a tumor-associated antigen that is highly expressed in individuals with colorectal cancer and reported to promote a broad spectrum of malignant features of colorectal cancer cells. The CEA-specific M13 phages were shown to elicit antitumor T-cell responses through promotion of infiltration of macrophages and neutrophils in tumors as well as dendritic cell maturation in tumor-draining lymph nodes. It was concluded that CEA-specific M13 phages could play a pivotal role in colorectal cancer immunotherapy due to their ability to activate and mediate CD8+ T-cells (Murgas et al., 2018).

The M13 phage also has the potential to identify tumor-targeting agents and can act as carriers of vaccines during breast cancer therapy. A study isolated the F56 anticancer peptide by screening the M13 phage library. The F56 was reported to be antimetastatic and antiangiogenic in mice that were implanted with human BICR-H1 breast cancer cells (An et al., 2004).

T7 phage

The T7 phage, a mature protein-expressing vector belonging to the Podoviridae family, is a virus that infects several strains of *E. coli*. The icosahedral head of the lytic T7 phage, with a diameter of 55 nm, is composed of linear dsDNA and six capsid proteins (gp8, gp10A, gp10B, gp11, gp12 and gp17). The tail length of the T7 phage is 28.5 nm and mostly consists of gp12 and gp11, while the end of the tail consists of gp17 (Yue et al., 2022). The T7 phage can be genetically modified to have targeting motifs that identify cells or tissues with high affinity, allowing it to function as a disease site-homing drug, a vaccine, an antibacterial agent, a gene delivery carrier, and a probe for detecting biomarkers (Yue et al., 2022).

Hwang and Myung (2020) constructed and engineered a potent anticancer T7 phage that displayed a specific peptide that targets murine melanoma cells and harbors cytokine granulocyte macrophage-colony stimulating factor (GM-CSF) in its viral DNA. Thereafter, the engineered phage was transduced to B16F10 melanoma cells *in vitro* and *in vivo* which resulted in GM-CSF being expressed. All mice treated with the engineered T7 phage survived and had significantly increased TNF-α, IL-1α and GM-CSF serum cytokine levels compared to untreated mice which had a 40% survival rate. In addition, the engineered T7 phage inhibited tumor growth by 72% and immunohistochemical analysis revealed infiltration by dendritic cells, macrophages, and CD8+ T-cells in tumor tissue in comparison to untreated mice (Hwang and Myung, 2020).

The V-Ki-ras2 Kirsten rat sarcoma viral oncogene homolog (K-Ras) gene is a prominent growth driver in various types of cancers, and it appears to be one of the most effective anticancer drug targets. Amino-acid mutations of Gly12 (G12C, G12D, G12V) of K-Ras are common in cancer patients, however inhibitors effective against K-Ras mutated individuals with cancer have not been marketed (Sakamoto et al., 2017). A study screened for K-Ras(G12D) inhibitory peptides through biopanning of T7 phage libraries and found KRpep-2 (Ac-RRCPLYISYDPVCRR-NH2) as a consensus sequence, which showed a ten-fold inhibition- and binding-selectivity to K-Ras(G12D). KRpep-2d inhibited the K-Ras(G12D) enzymatic activity, caused ERK-phosphorylation suppression downstream of K-Ras(G12D), and suppressed cancer cell proliferation at 30 μM peptide concentration (Sakamoto et al., 2017).

Roxithromycin is a semisynthetic macrolide antibiotic that displays antiangiogenic activity in solid tumors (Takakusagi et al., 2015). A study aimed to identify the target gene of roxithromycin through biopanning of T7 phage libraries and found the extracellular domain (E458-T596) of angiomotin to be the consensus sequence. It was shown that roxithromycin interacts directly with angiomotin, which also corresponded to the binding site for the endogenous anti-angiogenic inhibitor angiostatin (Takakusagi et al., 2015).

Considering that copper is cytotoxic to cancer cells, a study synthesized nanoparticles using an intact T7 phage as a scaffold to display hexahistidine peptide and cyclic Arginine-Glycine-Aspartic Acid (RGD4C) sequence to capture copper ions and to convert it to copper metal to target integrin and cancer cells. The copper hybridized T7 phage/6His/RGD4C complex was shown to be selectively ingested by MCF-7 cancer cells, with an intake rate of 1000 times higher versus the control group (Dasa et al., 2012). Studies have also shown that T7 phages displaying the RGD motif have a very high degree of affinity to human transferrin (Sakamoto et al., 2006).

T4 phage

The lytic T4 phage, a member of the Myoviridae family of the Caudovirales order, is a virus that infects several strains of *E. coli*. Its elongated icosahedral head contains the 168 kbp dsDNA genome and three capsid proteins (gp23, gp24, and gp20). It also contains two non-essential coat proteins, namely a small outer capsid protein (SOC) and a highly outer capsid protein (HOC). Mature T4 phages have an 850-Å-wide and 1150-Å-long prolate head, and 240-Å-diameter and 925-Å-long contractile tail (Yap and Rossmann, 2014, Ragothaman and Yoo, 2023). One of the most striking feature of T4 phages is their ability to display highly immunogenic foreign antigens on the SOC and HOC proteins, making them highly suitable for drug and vaccine delivery and therapy. The SOC proteins confer stability to the T4 phage capsid; SOC protein play a role in protecting the phage head from enzymes, heat and pH which is beneficial when transporting anticancer drug and vaccines (Ragothaman and Yoo, 2023).

Sanmukh et al. (2017) reported that T4 phage (in addition to the M13 phage mentioned above) play a role in the suppression of HSP90 gene in human prostate cancer cells (PC3); HSP90 play a role in stimulating tumor-promoting signaling pathways, activation of mitosis, DNA repair, and in the inhibition of apoptotic events (Sanmukh et al., 2017). Another study by Sanmukh and colleagues (2021) found both T4 and M13 phages upregulated integrins (*ITGA5*, *ITGB3*, *ITGB5*, and *ITGAV*) gene expression and impaired human PC3 cell migration (Sanmukh et al., 2021). Dysregulated integrin expression plays a therapeutic role in arresting tumor growth, lowering resistance to radiotherapy and chemotherapy, and in the attenuating invasion and metastasis (Bergonzini et al., 2022).

A study constructed the mouse vasculogenic and angiogenic factor and its receptor (VEGFR2) on T4 phage nanometer-particle surface as a recombinant vaccine for lung cancer. Immunotherapy with T4 phage/VEGFR2 recombinant vaccine conferred a protective immunity against lung carcinoma, and it was shown that CD4+ T lymphocytes depletion could neutralize the antitumor activity and autoantibody production of VEGFR2 (Ren et al., 2011).

Hou et al. (2023) developed a T4 phage display technology for improved photodynamic therapy of breast cancer. Hypoxia in tumor tissues can adversely impact the efficacy of photodynamic therapy; to resolve this issue the investigators used the T4 phage as a nanocarrier of the catalase protein to trigger hydrogen peroxide and chemically coupled chlorin e6, a photosensitizer used to generate reactive oxygen species. The bioengineered T4 phage was shown to increase the oxygen concentration and alleviated hypoxia in tumor tissues, resulting in tumor inhibition rate of 86.07% (Hou et al., 2023).

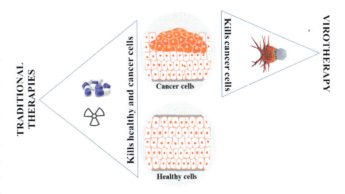

FIGURE 15.2 Traditional cancer therapies are not selective, indiscriminately killing both healthy and cancer cells. Virotherapy uses oncolytic viruses to selectively target cancer cells.

Lambda (λ) phage

The dsDNA lytic/lysogenic λ phage, a member of the Siphoviridae family of the Caudovirales order, is a virus that infects several strains of E. coli. Its icosahedral head, which is 55 nm in diameter and connected to the non-contractile 150-nm-long tail, contains the 48.45 kbp dsDNA genome and consists of 300–600 capsomers arranged in clusters of five and six subunits. The capsid contains two major proteins, namely gpD and gpE (Lander et al., 2008). The λ phages have great potential in acting as gene delivery vehicles due to their physical characteristics, genetic tractability, safety, and low cost (Ghaemi et al., 2010a). Phage-like particles derived from λ phages display physiochemical properties consistent with pharmaceutical standards (Catala et al., 2021).

A study constructed recombinant λ-phage nanobioparticles displaying a mammalian expression cassette encoding the E7 gene of Human Papillomavirus type 16 and enhanced green fluorescent protein (EGFP) gene to evaluate phage-mediated gene transfer and expression in vitro. The nanobioparticles were transduced in fibroblastic (CHO and COS-7) and epithelial (TC-1 and HEK293) cell lines. In addition, the therapeutic antitumor effect of the nanobioparticles was evaluated in a C57BL/6 tumor mouse model. The delivery and expression of the E7 gene and EGFP gene in fibroblastic cells was more efficient than epithelial cells using these nanobioparticles. Mice vaccinated with the nanobioparticles were able to produce potent therapeutic antitumor effects in comparison to the group treated with the wild-type phage. It was concluded that recombinant λ phages have the ability to transduce mammalian cells and could be used in phage-based nanomedicines drug design and discovery (Ghaemi et al., 2010a). Recombinant λ phage constructs displaying Human Papillomavirus type 16 E7 gene were shown to induce E7-specific protective immune responses and were proposed to be a promising therapeutic strategy against Human Papillomavirus-related neoplasia and cervical cancer (Ghaemi et al., 2010b).

Hu et al. (2022) generated spheroids of colorectal carcinoma and fibroblastic cancer cells to model the three-dimensional parenchymal and stromal components of colorectal tumors to investigate the suitable and usefulness of wild-type and epidermal growth factor (EGF)-presenting phage λ in delivering targeted genetic interventions in solid cancers. The EGFR-targeted phage λ was shown to penetrate the model stromal and colorectal carcinoma tissues, was taken up into carcinoma cells, and interfered with the early formation and growth of cancer tissues (Huh et al., 2022). Studies have also shown λ phage-based vaccine constructs against aspartate β-hydroxylase (ASPH) induces antitumor immunity in hepatocellular carcinoma (Iwagami et al., 2017).

Razazan et al. (2019) constructed a λ phage containing a human epidermal growth factor receptor 2 (HER2/neu) (a protooncogene that is overexpressed in human breast cancer)-derived peptide GP2 (a potent immunogenic peptide that acts against HER2/neu overexpressing breast cancers) fused to the gpD capsid protein, and thereafter used this construct as an anticancer vaccine in a BALB/c mouse xenograft tumor model. The λ phage/GP2 vaccine induced a robust cytotoxic T lymphocyte response and displayed prophylactic and therapeutic activities (Razazan et al., 2019). Catala and colleagues (2021) used phage-like particles derived from λ phages for targeted intracellular delivery of trastuzumab (used for the treatment of cancers that overexpress the HER2 protein) to human breast cancer cells. When compared to breast cancer cells treated with trastuzumab, robust internalization of λ phages/trastuzumab nanoparticles resulted in increased intracellular concentrations of trastuzumab, prolonged cell growth inhibition, and controlled regulation of cellular activities associated with HER2 signaling, protein synthesis, metabolism, and proliferation (Catala et al., 2021). λ phage nanobioparticle expressing apoptin (a protein that induces apoptosis in carcinoma cells only) was shown to efficiently aid in the suppression of human breast carcinoma tumor growth (Shoae-Hassani et al., 2013), and the cytotoxic activity of the phage λ-holin protein (holin triggers and regulates the degradation of the host's cell membrane) was shown to reduce tumor growth rates in mammary cancer cell xenograft models (Agu et al., 2006).

MS2 phage

The 3.57-kbp-long ssRNA lytic MS2 phage, a member of the Leviviridae family, is a virus that infects several strains of E. coli. The icosahedral virion is 26 nm in diameter and contains 180 copies of the coat protein, which are organized as 90 dimers, arranged into an icosahedral shell with triangulation number T=3 (Ragothaman and Yoo, 2023).

Sanmukh et al. (2023) found wild-type MS2 phage can interact directly with LNCaP prostate epithelial cells as well as their surface receptors to induce notable changes in gene expression profiles (upregulation of androgen receptor, AKT, integrin α5, integrin β1, MAPK1, MAPK3, PGC1α, and STAT3 genes) which, in turn, severely influenced LNCaP cell viability by reducing androgen signaling and anchorage-dependent survival. It was concluded that MS2 phages utilize caveolin-mediated endocytosis and alter prostate cancer cell signaling pathways (Sanmukh et al., 2023). Kolesanova and colleagues (2019) conjugated the (Gly)3-iRGD peptide, a ligand of integrins found in certain tumor cells and on the endotheliocytes of the tumor tissue neovasculature, to the MS2 phage capsid protein for targeted delivery of thallium (I) ions (Tl+) to breast cancer cells. The modified (Gly)3-iRGD/Tl+ MS2 phage, which exhibited no acute toxicity at a therapeutic dose and showed promise for solid tumor chemotherapy, caused cell death of cultivated human breast cancer cells, and effected necrosis of tumor xenografts in mice (Kolesanova et al., 2019).

TABLE 15.2
Advantages of selected DNA and RNA OVs

	Name of virus	Advantages / Disadvantages
DNA viruses	Adenoviruses Herpes simplex virus (HSV) Parvoviruses Poxviruses	• high genome stability • large transgene insertion capability without compromising viral infection and replication
RNA viruses	Coxsackie virus (CV) Maraba virus Measles virus (MV) Newcastle disease virus (NDV) Poliovirus Reovirus (RV) Retroviruses (RTV) Seneca Valley virus (SVV) Semliki Forest virus (SFV) Vesicular stomatitis virus (VSV) Sindbis virus (SBV)	• limited genome packaging capacity • some can be more immunogenic

Source: Adapted from Rahman and McFadden, 2021, Harrington et al., 2019, Lawler et al., 2017

THERAPEUTIC POTENTIAL OF ONCOLYTIC VIRUSES

What is an Oncolytic Virus?

An oncolytic virus (OV) is a natural/unmodified or genetically modified virus that is recognized for the ability to selectively infect and kill cancer cells without harming normal cells (Rahman and McFadden, 2021, Cao et al., 2020). To qualify as an OV, a virus must be non-pathogenic, able to target and kill cancer cells, and amenable to genetic engineering methods that facilitate the expression of recognizable tumor antigens (Russell et al., 2012, Maroun et al., 2017). Not all viruses are oncolytic, but both DNA and RNA viruses may qualify as an OV (Rahman and McFadden, 2021). Several naturally occurring viruses with the potential to infect cells are being explored for their OV potential (Table 15.2). Moreover, they have different clinical applications in cancer treatment.

The History of OV Use

The observation that some patients go into remission after virus infection prompted researchers to explore the idea of using phages to modulate the composition of the gut microbiome for anticancer purposes. Researchers also started to explore the use of oncolytic viruses to kill cancer cells (Rahman and McFadden, 2021, Bell and McFadden, 2014, Kelly and Russell, 2007). The 1950s–1970s witnessed case reports of various OVs with potential to reduce solid tumors and leukemia. However, the development of technology for genetic modification of viruses has contributed to the explosion of OVs research in the past three decades (Rahman and McFadden, 2021, Macedo et al., 2020). The OV field gained considerable attention after positive results from many clinical trials. Thus far, four OVs have been approved globally.

Mechanism of Anticancer Effect of Oncolytic Virus

Infection of the host cancer cell and subsequent viral replication leads to cell lysis. The accompanying release of tumor antigens after infection may elicit an immune response (Figure 15.3). Selectivity for infection of cancer cells may be conferred by the deletion of disease-causing genes that influence intracellular antiviral responses (Cao et al., 2020, Seymour and Fisher, 2016, Kaufman et al., 2015). Normal cells that are infected will mount an antiviral response to successfully eliminate the infection. However, cancer cells have impaired antiviral mechanisms (Vitiello et al., 2021). They are therefore susceptible to infection and are not able to mount an antiviral response, facilitating undeterred replication of the virus in the cancer cells that will cause cancer cell lysis. The consequent release of cancer antigens will stimulate the immune response (Figure 15.3). In addition, factors that facilitate viral entry or enhance viral gene expression and replication also contribute to increased susceptibility (Cao et al., 2020, Seymour and Fisher, 2016, Kaufman et al., 2015).

Approved OV Therapy

Several oncolytic viruses are in various phases of clinical trials, and four have been approved globally. In 2004, Latvia approved Rigvir (ECHO-7) that used the unmodified Picornavirus derived from the intestine of healthy children to treat melanoma; its registration has since been suspended (Babiker et al., 2017, Rahman and McFadden, 2021, Donina et al., 2015). China followed in 2005 and approved the use

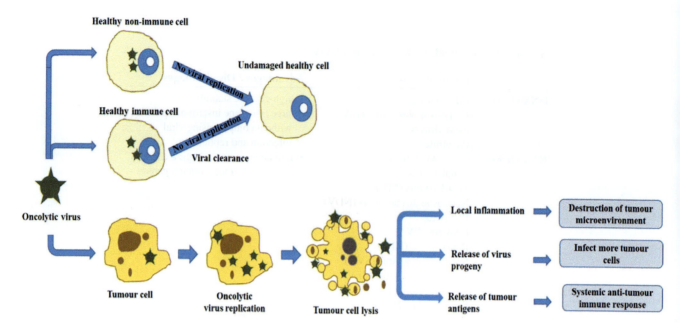

FIGURE 15.3 The role of oncolytic viruses in selectively targeting tumor cells. Oncolytic viruses can infect and replicate in tumor cells, leading to tumor cell lysis and (i) local inflammation which can cause the destruction of the tumor microenvironment, (ii) release of viral progeny to infect more tumor cells, and (iii) release of tumor antigens which can induce antitumor immune response.

of Adenovirus serotype 5 (deleted for viral E1B-55K and with four deletions in viral E3) in Oncorine (H101) to treat head-and-neck cancers; this was the first recombinant drug approved for virotherapy and must be used in combination with chemotherapy (Rahman and McFadden, 2021, Cao et al., 2020, Liang, 2018, Garber, 2006). After a decade-long lag, Talimogene laherparepvec (T-VEC; HSV-1) was approved by the Food and Drug Administration (FDA) in 2015 to treat metastatic melanoma; this genetically modified HSV-1 (deletion of ICP34.5 and ICP47; encoding two copies of human granulocyte-macrophage colony-stimulating factor (GMCSF)) for treating melanoma is the only drug approved by the FDA (Rahman and McFadden, 2021, Cao et al., 2020, Johnson et al., 2015b). Recently, Japan approved the use of DELYTACT serpaturev/G47Δ (HSV-1 with deleted ICP34.5, ICP6 and α47 genes) for malignant glioma or any brain cancer (Rahman and McFadden, 2021). However, there are side effects associated with their use and many present with flu-like symptoms and local reactions at the site of injection (Table 15.3).

ONCOLYTIC VIRUSES IN CLINICAL TRIAL

Genetically modified oncolytic viruses have shown promise for the treatment of multiple tumors (Table 15.3). The DNA OVs in Table 15.3 include Adenovirus, Herpes simplex virus, Vaccinia virus, and Reovirus. Adenovirus is amenable to genetic engineering, commonly at E1, to increase tumor tropism and selectivity, and enhance viral entry and replication. It is therefore frequently employed for its potential for cytolysis and to invoke an immune response (Zhao et al., 2021). The first approved OD in China for the treatment of head-and-neck cancer, adenovirus presents a host of modifications that aid in the treatment of several cancer types including melanoma, lung cancer, colorectal cancer, prostate adenocarcinoma, malignant glioma, ovarian cancer, and solid tumors (Zhu et al., 2023b, Javanbakht et al., 2023, Cejalvo et al., 2022, Zhao et al., 2021, O'Bryan and Mathis, 2018, Lang et al., 2018, Garber, 2006).

Herpes virus is considered a highly efficient virus with capacity to infect and replicate in a range of host cells and tissues. Viral transformation via deletions renders improved efficiency, as demonstrated by its antineoplastic efficacy in melanoma, breast cancer, glioblastoma, colorectal cancer, and other solid tumors (Zhu et al., 2023b, Javanbakht et al., 2023, Cejalvo et al., 2022, Carpenter et al., 2021, Rahman and McFadden, 2021, Cao et al., 2020, O'Bryan and Mathis, 2018, Kooby et al., 1999). The first FDA-approved OV drug, T-VEC, is indicated for the treatment of malignant melanoma (Rahman and McFadden, 2021, Cao et al., 2020, Johnson et al., 2015b). The modified T-VEC virus (ICP34.5 gene deletion) makes it highly selective for tumor cells, but the expression of an immune-activating protein renders the virus more susceptible to immune clearance (Zhu et al., 2023b, Yin et al., 2017, Harrington et al., 2015). Therefore, the additional ICP47 gene deletion was necessary to prevent viral clearance by the immune system (Jin et al., 2021). The Deltyact (testerpaturev/G47 Δ) virus approved by Japan also deleted ICP34.5 and ICP47, but added an ICP6 gene mutation (Zhu et al., 2023b, Frampton, 2022). Insertion of GMCSF was implemented to enhance local immune toxicity (Zhu et al., 2023b).

Vaccinia virus is indicated for smallpox infection, but is advantageous as an OV because it replicates quickly. Gene deletions and insertions have increased selectivity and immunogenicity. Vaccinia virus has demonstrated efficacy as an OV that targets liver cancer, melanoma colorectal cancer,

TABLE 15.3
Natural oncolytic virus infection characteristics and OV therapy indicated for different cancers

Enterovirus type	Group	Features	Characteristics of natural infection / Symptoms	Used for
Adenovirus	I	Double-stranded, linear, DNA (135 kb)	Infection associated with mild, cold-like symptoms including sore throat and fatigue	Breast cancer, liver cancer, malignant glioma, melanoma, lung cancer, colorectal cancer, prostate adenocarcinoma, ovarian cancer, and solid tumors (Zhu et al., 2023b, Javanbakht et al., 2023, Cejalvo et al., 2022, Zhao et al., 2021, O'Bryan and Mathis, 2018, Lang et al., 2018, Garber, 2006)
Herpes simplex virus	I	Double-stranded, linear, DNA (154 kb)	Cold sores / fever sores typically near the mouth	Breast cancer, colorectal cancer, malignant glioma, melanoma (Zhu et al., 2023b, Javanbakht et al., 2023, Cejalvo et al., 2022, Carpenter et al., 2021, Rahman and McFadden, 2021, Cao et al., 2020, O'Bryan and Mathis, 2018, Kooby et al., 1999)
Vaccinia virus	I	Double-stranded, linear, DNA	Vaccinate against and eliminate smallpox	Breast cancer, colorectal cancer, liver cancer, malignant glioma, melanoma (Zhu et al., 2023a, Zhu et al., 2023b, Javanbakht et al., 2023, Crupi et al., 2022, Cejalvo et al., 2022, Carpenter et al., 2021, O'Bryan and Mathis, 2018)
Reovirus	III	Double-stranded, linear, RNA (23 kb)	Affect the gastrointestinal and respiratory tracts in a range of animal species	Breast cancer, colorectal cancer, liver cancer, malignant glioma (Zhu et al., 2023a, Zhu et al., 2023b, Javanbakht et al., 2023, Cejalvo et al., 2022, Carpenter et al., 2021, O'Bryan and Mathis, 2018, Davis, 2015)
Picornavirus virus e.g., Coxsackie virus	IV	Single-stranded RNA (28 kb)	Infects mammals and birds	Advanced melanoma, breast cancer, bladder cancer, myeloma, lung cancer (Zhu et al., 2023b, Javanbakht et al., 2023, Cejalvo et al., 2022, Carpenter et al., 2021, O'Bryan and Mathis, 2018, Davis, 2015)
Poliovirus	IV	Single-stranded, linear, RNA (7.5 kb)		Breast cancer, malignant glioma, melanoma, bladder cancer (Zhu et al., 2023a, Javanbakht et al., 2023, Cejalvo et al., 2022, Carpenter et al., 2021, O'Bryan and Mathis, 2018)
Maraba virus	V	Single-stranded RNA (11 kb)	Infects insects	Breast cancer (Zhu et al., 2023b, Carpenter et al., 2021)
Measles	V	Single-stranded RNA (16 kb)	Infects the respiratory tract, causes measles, very contagious	Breast cancer (Carpenter et al., 2021)
Newcastle Disease Virus	V	Single-stranded, linear, RNA (15 kb)	Mostly infects birds, flu-like symptoms in humans, conjunctivitis	Breast cancer, liver cancer, malignant glioma (Zhu et al., 2023b, Carpenter et al., 2021)
Vesicular stomatitis virus (VSV)	V	Single-stranded RNA (11 kb)	same family as the Maraba virus	Breast cancer, colorectal cancer (Carpenter et al., 2021)
Parvovirus		Single-stranded, linear, DNA (5 kb)	Infects rats, dogs	Malignant glioma (Carpenter et al., 2021)

peritoneal cancer, glioblastoma, and breast cancer, amongst others (Zhu et al., 2023a, Zhu et al., 2023b, Javanbakht et al., 2023, Crupi et al., 2022, Cejalvo et al., 2022, Carpenter et al., 2021, O'Bryan and Mathis, 2018). Reovirus is a RNA virus with oncolytic activity in breast, colorectal, and liver cancer, as well as malignant glioma (Zhu et al., 2023a, Zhu et al., 2023b, Javanbakht et al., 2023, Cejalvo et al., 2022, Carpenter et al., 2021, O'Bryan and Mathis, 2018, Davis, 2015). There is also evidence of antitumor effect in multiple myeloma and lung cancer.

The RNA OVs are also indicated for their oncolytic potential (Table 15.3). Following infection, Coxsackie virus produces symptoms of fever, cough, and cold. British scientists have shown that Coxsackie virus is effective for bladder cancer, melanoma, breast cancer, myeloma, and lung cancer (Zhu et al., 2023b, Javanbakht et al., 2023, Cejalvo et al., 2022, Carpenter et al., 2021, O'Bryan and Mathis, 2018, Davis, 2015), entering cancer cells via intercellular adhesion molecule 1 (CD54), decal accelerating factor (CD55), or connectors that are overexpressed in these cancer cells (Zhu et al., 2023b, Annels et al., 2019). After viral entry and infection, Coxsackie virus will replicate and ultimately destroy cancer cells by cytolysis (Zhu et al., 2023b, Annels et al., 2019). Launched in Latvia in 2004, Rigvir is a naturally occurring OV used to treat melanoma, colorectal cancer, renal carcinoma, lung cancer, uterine cancer, lymphoid sarcoma, gastrointestinal cancer, and other cancers (Zhu et al., 2023b, Javanbakht et al., 2023, Cejalvo et al., 2022, Rahman and McFadden, 2021, O'Bryan and Mathis, 2018, Alberts et al., 2016). It is particularly indicated in advanced melanoma; in this regard, its efficacy has been demonstrated as a therapy in a female patient suffering with a lumbar melanoma who received single treatment with remarkable reduction in tumor size (Zhu et al., 2023a, Alberts et al., 2016).

Other RNA viruses include Poliovirus, Maraba virus, Measles, Newcastle Disease virus, Vesicular stomatitis virus, and Parvovirus (Table 15.3) (Zhu et al., 2023b, Rahman and McFadden, 2021). Researchers have shown that they are able to enter a variety of tumor cell types including malignant glioma, melanoma, bladder cancer, and liver cancer (Zhu et al., 2023a, Zhu et al., 2023b, Javanbakht et al., 2023, Cejalvo et al., 2022, Carpenter et al., 2021, O'Bryan and Mathis, 2018). Although these OVs have demonstrated efficacy, more work is required to reduce potential cytotoxicity.

MANIPULATION OF THE VIROME TO MODULATE ANTITUMOR IMMUNE RESPONSES

The ability of the virome to shape the immune system development and function in health and disease (Cao et al., 2022) provides an entry point for manipulation of the virome for the prevention and reduction of cancer development. This holds potential for cancer immunotherapy and strategies towards personalized cancer therapy (Figure 15.4). Modulation of the immune system for optimal and effective antitumor response provides a much safer and less aggressive alternative to the current cancer treatments like radiation, chemotherapy and surgery which have debilitating side effects.

THERAPEUTIC STRATEGIES TARGETING ANTITUMOR IMMUNITY THROUGH THE GUT VIROME

A variety of cancers have been associated with different viral infections, such as cervical cancer and HPV, Liver cancer and HBV and HCV, Burkitt's lymphoma and nasopharyngeal carcinoma with EBV. Similarly, changes in gut virome have been associated with colorectal cancer (Gao et al., 2021; Nakatsu et al., 2018). The causal relationship occurs through direct virus–host cell/tissue interactions. Other indirect interactions include the virome/phage-bacteria–immune system interactions. The sections below explore possible mechanisms of exploiting the gut virome for enhancing antitumor immunity. However, very limited studies have used gut virome directly in any of the following approaches, therefore, the sections will mostly extrapolate possible adaptations from what has been applied in other viruses or bacterial microbiome.

FECAL VIROME TRANSPLANTATION

Fecal virome transplantation (FVT) can be achieved through a sterile filtrate where bacteria are removed by a series of filters and phages remain (Borin et al., 2023). This strategy can provide feasible clinical practice benefits that are superior to contemporary microbiome therapeutics (including fecal microbiome transplantation (FMT), bacterial probiotics consumption, or antibiotics usage), which may inadvertently introduce opportunistic pathogens and further dysregulate the bacterial microbiome composition that results in an unwanted dysbiosis and health disturbances (Borin et al., 2023). FVT has been successfully done on experimental mice and shown to confer microbiota-associated phenotypes such as obesity, and it is noted that human virome analyses and transplantation studies are limited (Broecker and Moelling, 2021). However, it has been demonstrated that virome transplantation can shape the profile of microbiota phenotypes (Cao et al., 2022). This plus the natural ability of viruses to infect cells, could be adapted to promote the growth of tumoricidal bacteria and enhance an antitumor environment.

Many of the preclinical FMT studies had been done on mice to show differences in gut bacteria from mice that were responding as compared to non-responders to anti-immune checkpoint immunotherapy (programmed cell death-1 (PD-1) treatment) where in the latter therapy responses were restored by transplantation of stool microbiota from the former (Broecker and Moelling, 2021). Similar results have been reported since in human clinical studies, showing differences in composition, diversity, and abundance of different taxa in melanoma patients responsive versus resistant to anti-PD-1 treatment (Gopalakrishnan et al., 2018). Two more clinical studies of patients with metastatic melanoma that was refractory to anti-PD-1 treatment confirmed that FMT from responders can convert-non-responders into responders (Baruch et al., 2021; Davar et al., 2021). The main microbial differences reported were in bacterial populations between responders and non-responders. Increased abundance and diversity of taxa that had been previously shown to be associated with response to anti-PD-1 was noted in non-responders who after FMT showed a response to immunotherapy. A significant immunological shift was an increased CD8$^+$ T cell activation, and decreased frequency of interleukin-8-expressing myeloid cells, which are involved in immunosuppression.

However, the majority of published studies to date have investigated the immunomodulatory effect of FMT, not necessarily the virome specifically. It has been suggested that the phages are transmitted during FMT and in fact stabilize in the donor before the bacterial population establishes itself in a mouse model of fecal virome (Broecker et al., 2017).

An enterococcus phage-specific, MHC-1 restricted T cell epitope enhanced immunotherapy in mice, while its presence in stools of humans with renal and lung cancer, together with cross-reactivity with tumor antigens, correlated with better outcomes of anti-PD-1 therapy. Likewise in melanoma patients, T cell clones recognizing cancer antigens that are cross-reactive with microbial peptides were detected. This T cell epitope has been proposed to induce memory T cells cross-reacting with a tumor antigen. (Fluckiger et al., 2020). This shows promise for development of virome-based tumoricidal immunotherapy enhancement.

ATTENUATING INFLAMMATORY NETWORKS IN CANCER PREVENTION BY INCREASING BUTYRATE-PRODUCING BACTERIA BY USING SPECIFIC PHAGES

Targeting bacteriophages that will enhance specific pathways such as increasing butyrate-producing bacterial populations, as a means to decrease inflammatory networks in the gut, can contribute towards the suppression of oncogenesis. Chronic inflammation increases the rate of destruction of normal healthy cells and increases the risk of cancer development (Multhoff et al., 2012). Butyrate reduces the production of inflammatory cytokines through the modulation of activity of G protein-coupled receptors, NF-κB, JAK/STAT, and other inflammation-related pathways (Segain et al., 2000). Furthermore, butyrate is a potent histone deacetylase inhibitor and promotes the proliferation and activation of regulatory T-cells (Treg cells) (Zhu et al., 2021).

The increase of microbiota-derived butyrate, by transplantation of fecal virome that promotes the growth and multiplication of these bacteria is a feasible clinical strategy for cancer prevention. Borin and colleagues (2023) demonstrated that FVT can shape the bacterial composition and subsequently confer a specific phenotype to recipient mice. In this case the virome transplant determined weight gain or loss in mice. This aptly demonstrates that the virome can be sequenced and used to determine phages that are specific to the target bacteria. Specific viral transplants can be prepared to then adopt this strategy in order to increase the abundance of butyrate- producing phyla and species. Indeed, Gao et al. (2021) showed that colorectal cancer patients had decreased diversity of butyrate-producing and anti-inflammatory bacteria plus Enterobacteria phages compared to healthy controls in a study of the gut virome. This supports the strategy proposed herein for targeting phages that promote the growth of butyrate-producing, anti-inflammatory bacteria for potentiating antitumor immune responses. As indicated, currently no human interventions aimed at manipulating the gut virome to enhance antitumor immunity have been identified.

IMMUNE CHECKPOINT INHIBITION AND ONCOLYTIC VIRUS COMBINATION IMMUNE THERAPY

Immune checkpoint (IC) inhibitors act by blocking the checkpoint proteins such as PD-1 or CTLA-4, from competitively binding to and inhibiting costimulatory molecules such as CD28 (Lao et al., 2022). IC inhibitors can enhance antitumor immune responses through blocking the "off" signal, allowing the T cells to proliferate and kill cancer cells (Lao et al., 2022). This immunotherapy approach has been effective against a variety of tumors. However, as a monotherapy, it is sometimes less effective as some tumor microenvironments inherently evade IC inhibition therapy (Chiu et al., 2020). A classic example is the fact that although ICI was the first class of immunotherapy to be associated with long-term survival of advanced melanoma patients, only a subset of melanoma patients respond to immune checkpoint inhibitors (Rausch and Hastings, 2017). This then highlighted the need to identify biomarkers that are predictive of response and to develop strategies that overcome resistance. Combining IC inhibitors with oncolytic viruses is combination therapy aimed at promoting a robust immune response against cancer cells. Oncolytic viruses lyse tumor cells, releasing tumor antigens to be recognized by the immune system, thus stimulating robust tumor-specific T cell responses, while IC inhibitors attenuate T cell anergy induced by immune checkpoints. This approach promises better outcomes in cancer immunotherapy (Ren et al., 2022).

The phase 3 study combining pembrolizumab (IC inhibitor) with or without Talimogene laherparepvec (T-Vec) (a genetically engineered oncolytic virus) injection showed that there were no new safety concerns with the addition of T-VEC to pembrolizumab, and the safety profile of the combination remained similar to the known safety profile of each drug (Kaufman et al., 2022). Talimogene laherparepvec (T-VEC; IMLYGIC®, Amgen Inc.) is the first oncolytic viral immunotherapy to be approved for the local treatment of inoperable metastatic stage IIIB/C–IVM1a melanoma (Kaufman et al., 2022).

GUT VIROME AS POTENTIAL VIRAL VECTORS FOR CANCER GENE THERAPY

The advances in gene-editing technology have advanced the field for gene therapy and enhanced its safety through reaching base-level editing, using CRISPR/CAS9 (Lu et al., 2020). The natural evolutional capability of viruses to infect cells and insert their genome into the host cells, and tropism of oncolytic viruses, combined with advances in vector manufacture and gene engineering all culminate in the advancement of the field of cancer gene therapy (Bezeljak, 2022). Viral vectors, therefore, offer the advantage of efficient delivery of therapeutic genes to modulate antitumor immune responses. For example, adenoviral vectors can be used to deliver genes that encode cytokines (e.g., interleukin-12) to enhance immune cell activity at the tumor site (Bezeljak, 2022).

Gendicine was the first viral vector approved in 2003 by the China Food and Drug Administration for treatment of head-and-neck cancer (Zhang et al., 2018). The Gendicine immunological mechanism involves transduction of cells to express the wild-type (wt) p53 protein, a tumor suppressor protein that is activated by cellular stress, induces cell cycle arrest, DNA repair or programmed death apoptosis, and/or autophagy, depending upon cellular stress conditions (Zhang et al., 2018). This accomplishment has laid a foundation for more viral vector production and approvals. The extent and clinical application or clinical trials of viral gene therapy against a variety of cancers is reviewed by Bezeljak (2022) and indicates the popularity of the Retrovirus (43.1%), followed by Adenovirus (27.1%), Poxvirus (18.1%), Herpes Simplex Virus (7.4%), and the least used are Adeno-Associated Virus (1.6%) as gene therapy vectors in clinical trials as of October 2021. There are many viral vectors for delivery of target genes for immunomodulation of antitumor responses currently in clinical trial phases (Bezeljak, 2022). Some are monotherapy while others aim at enhancing conventional therapy, such as the combination of surgery and injection of CAR-T antigen into the tumor microenvironment (Vitiello et al., 2021). Other immune enhancement mechanisms use the viral vectors for the targeted delivery of immune checkpoint inhibitors (Reul et al., 2019) and a viral vector (Adenovirus-Associated Virus Type 6) was used to prepare allogenic CAR-T cells and accurately deliver the CRISPR/CAS9 engineered genetic material for allogeneic T cell immune mediation (MacLeod et al., 2017; Eyquem et al., 2017).

In terms of the use of gut virome as vectors for antitumor immune response stimulation, nothing has been published to date. However, the confirmation of the changes in gut virome associated with colorectal cancer and survival (Nakatsu et al., 2018) can be used as a lead for identification of immunogenic viruses, their potential engineering for vector manufacture, and enhancement of antitumor immunity. The three widely tested vector systems, namely adenoviral, lentiviral, or adeno-associated viral vectors can also provide the basis for identifying the gut virome for potential. The CRISPR-based strategies to specifically edit the target genes and also improve the delivery of CRISPR therapeutics directly into the human body using adeno-associated virus vectors (Wang et al., 2020) combined with metagenomic profiling of the gut virome will drive the field of gut virome manipulation for antitumor immune response amplification. Taxonomical identification and standardized protocol development that allows the simultaneous extraction of DNA and RNA in several biological samples (Tamayo-Trujillo et al., 2023) will simplify the characterization of the complex composition of gut virome, possibly down to species level.

PERSONALIZED VIROME IDENTIFICATION FOR PRECISION ONCOLOGY

The composition and diversity of the microbiome is highly variable between individuals and between disease and health in the same individual. In addition, the success of donor microbiome engraftment post transplantation is also highly variable between individuals (Junca et al., 2022). While germ-free or antibiotic-treated mice have been successfully used to demonstrate the feasibility of fecal microbiome transfer between donor and recipients, these experiments cannot be fully inferred and translated to human applicability because of the highly individualized microbiome profiles, in addition to the fact that other factor, such as lifestyle, diet, and geography, determine the profile of the individual microbiome (Junca et al., 2022).

Artificial intelligence (AI) plays a significant role in tailor-making the virome for modulation of immune responses at individual level. The application of AI in virus discovery from viral dark matter, together with metagenomics can be further harnessed for personalized precision oncology purposes (Santiago-Rodriguez and Hollister, 2022). Deep learning, which uses deep artificial neural networks to "learn" features from a given input and predict the output,

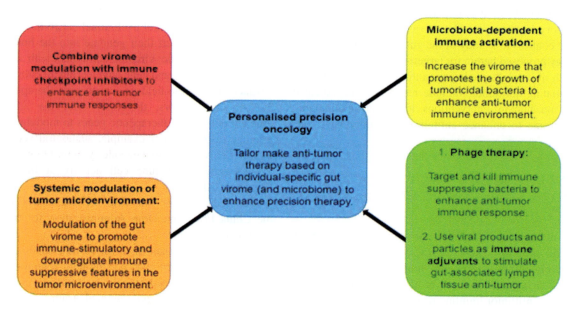

FIGURE 15.4 Approaches to manipulate the virome to modulate antitumor immune responses through combined virome modulation with immune checkpoint inhibitors, systematic modulation of tumor microenvironment, microbiota-dependent immune activation and phage therapy.

has been applied to metagenomic datasets for virus identification and discovery from dark matter (Santiago-Rodriguez and Hollister, 2022).

Deep learning tools such as DeepVirFinder (Ren et al., 2020) and Vibrant (Kieft et al., 2020) have been used successfully and found to be superior compared to other methods to accurately predict viruses. The practical value of these tools will contribute immensely to the still emerging field of virome therapeutics.

THE CHALLENGES ASSOCIATED WITH HARNESSING THE THERAPEUTIC POTENTIAL OF THE GUT VIROME IN PERSONALIZED CANCER THERAPIES

PHAGE THERAPY

Some of the major challenges associated with using phage therapy for cancer treatment include: (i) phages may induce allergic reactions in certain individuals; (ii) some phage particles are unable to display large antigens; (iii) difficulties in precisely displaying a molecule of interest on the phage surface; (iv) endotoxin contamination during phage production; (v) phages require specialized handling and storage; (vi) phages may not be able to reach certain target organs and tumors of interest to offer effective treatment; (vii) phage therapy may not be suitable for immunocompromised patients; (viii) the delivery method used for phage entry in the body influences phage efficacy and treatment outcomes; (ix) phage DNA vaccines must be within the genome length of the virion packing limit; (x) immune rejection and rapid clearance (high phage titers can trigger the release of high amounts of neutralizing antibodies which could hinder the mode of action of phages); (xi) phage treatment needs to undergo more clinical trials to receive regulatory approval; and (xii) lack of awareness of phage therapy due to fear, ignorance, and doubt (Ragothaman and Yoo, 2023, Immadi Siva, 2022).

ONCOLYTIC VIRAL THERAPY

Although OV therapy shows promise as a viable therapeutic option, some factors may contribute to decreased efficacy that requires further investigation. The ideal OV should be susceptible to genetic engineering with minimal cytotoxicity to healthy cells or tissues. To date, several DNA and RNA OV variants have been tested on different cancers. It may be that an ideal OV exists with efficacy for all cancers. Alternatively, there may be organ-specific effects associated with the chosen OV. In addition, individual host factors may limit the therapeutic value of the OV; these may include physical barriers to entry (viral entry should not be dependent of an expressed receptor that is absent on the tumor cell), antiviral signaling pathways activated may restrict viral replication or limit viral spread and adaptive immunity that interfere with viral function directly or indirectly. For clinical roll-out, large-scale production needs to be optimized to maximize the therapeutic potential of the chosen OV. Route of administration may also be a limitation, since tumors may not be accessible for direct injection, and intravenous administration presents further barriers that the OV must overcome.

MANIPULATION OF THE VIROME TO MODULATE ANTITUMOR IMMUNE RESPONSES

(i) *Innate and acquired viral /phage immunity and self-tolerance:* The ubiquity of many viral infections globally confers lifelong immunity. Natural immune responses towards viral vectors therefore hinder progress in large-scale adaptation and use of viral vectors to enhance antitumor immune responses (Bezeljak, 2022). This is compounded by the large number of autoantigens in the tumor microenvironment, and the inherent lifelong self-tolerance, together requiring stringent selection of tumoricidal immune stimulation.

(ii) *Technological limitation in access to sequencing technology:* The gut virome is highly heterogenous between individuals and is also determined by geographic locations, age, diet, and lifestyle. This then warrants highly individualized profiling of virome-based therapy. Screening, for development of highly specific personalized virome-based therapeutics, depends on metagenomic and technology such as AI that uses deep learning technology. On the one hand this will enhance tailor-made personalized and precise therapy, on the other hand, the technology for this is still limited in many areas, particularly in low- and middle-income countries that are in need of all advances in therapy and disease prevention (Cao et al., 2022).

(iii) *Safety, efficacy, and long-term effects of viral based immunotherapy:* The field of virobiome manipulation is still emerging, therefore, many issues regarding safety and long-term effects remain largely unknown risks currently. This therefore requires caution, which may reduce the pace of large-scale implementation of virome- based therapeutics. The efficacy of virome-based therapy across many cancers still needs interrogation. Another issue of concern is the risk of oncogenic potential caused by insertional mutation. However, there are promising improvements to avert this challenge of insertional mutations through use of CRISPR/CAS9 engineering, allogeneic CAR-T generation, and targeted integration of genetic material into a known genomic locus. To further improve the advances in gut virome therapeutics, a collaborative approach between immunologists, virologists, bacteriologists, bioinformatics specialists and microbiome researchers is central for speeding the process to address all the unanswered risk questions.

(iv) *Viral dark matter:* While the viral metagenomic sequence analysis continues to unravel more virome populations, many virus identities and functions still remain unknown—the viral dark matter (Santiago-Rodriguez & Hollister, 2022). With this gap, it is plausible to conclude that the therapeutic capacity of the virome cannot be fully harnessed. The field is therefore still emerging and requires further collaborative research.

CONCLUDING REMARKS

The use of phage therapy in cancer is still in the early stages of research, and its specific applications are not well-established. Most cancer treatments involve surgery, chemotherapy, radiation therapy, immunotherapy, or targeted therapies designed to directly target cancer cells. While phage therapy may have a role in supporting cancer care indirectly through its impact on the microbiota and the immune system, further research is needed to better understand its potential applications in cancer treatment and prevention. Oncolytic virotherapy presents an attractive alternate approach to cancer therapy. Deletion or insertion of genes in OVs harnesses the patients' immune system to enable a simultaneous antiviral and antitumor response. Active research involving optimization and testing of these viruses will contribute to positive antitumor outcomes. While there have been remarkable accomplishments in the various aspects of manipulation of microbiome for cancer immunotherapy, the specific use of gut virome has lagged behind and the field is still emerging. Several techniques such as theshotgun new-generation sequencing for viral metagenomics to identify the millions of taxa at scale, CRISPR/CAS9 gene editing, and AI technologies that have been applied successfully to cancer immunotherapy can be adopted to harness the potential of the gut virome as a potent antitumor immune response enhancer.

REFERENCES

Abdulamir, A. S., Hafidh, R. R. & Abu Bakar, F. 2011. The association of Streptococcus bovis/gallolyticus with colorectal tumors: the nature and the underlying mechanisms of its etiological role. *Journal of Experimental & Clinical Cancer Research*, 30, 11.

Abouelkhair, M. A. & Kennedy, M. 2022. Papillomaviridae and Polyomaviridae. *Veterinary Microbiology*, 4, 484–488.

Adams, M. J., Adkins, S., Bragard, C., Gilmer, D., Li, D., Macfarlane, S. A., Wong, S.-M., Melcher, U., Ratti, C. & Ryu, K. H. 2017. ICTV virus taxonomy profile: Virgaviridae. *Journal of General Virology*, 98, 1999–2000.

Agu, C. A., Klein, R., Schwab, S., König-Schuster, M., Kodajova, P., Ausserlechner, M., Binishofer, B., Bläsi, U., Salmons, B., Günzburg, W. H. & Hohenadl, C. 2006. The cytotoxic activity of the bacteriophage λ-holin protein reduces tumor growth rates in mammary cancer cell xenograft models. *The Journal of Gene Medicine*, 8, 229–241.

Alberts, P., Olmane, E., Brokāne, L., Krastiņa, Z., Romanovska, M., Kupčs, K., Isajevs, S., Proboka, G., Erdmanis, R. & Nazarovs, J. 2016. Long-term treatment with the oncolytic ECHO-7 virus Rigvir of a melanoma stage IV M1c patient, a small cell lung cancer stage IIIA patient, and a histiocytic sarcoma stage IV patient-three case reports. *Journal of Pathology, Microbiology and Immunology - APMIS*, 124, 896–904.

Alon-Maimon, T., Mandelboim, O. & Bachrach, G. 2022. Fusobacterium nucleatum and cancer. *Periodontology 2000*, 89, 166–180.

An, P., Lei, H., Zhang, J., Song, S., He, L., Jin, G., Liu, X., Wu, J., Meng, L., Liu, M. & Shou, C. 2004. Suppression of tumor growth and metastasis by a VEGFR-1 antagonizing peptide identified from a phage display library. *International Journal of Cancer*, 111, 165–73.

Annels, N. E., Mansfield, D., Arif, M., Ballesteros-Merino, C., Simpson, G.R., Denyer, M., Sandhu, S. S., Melcher, A. A., Harrington, K. J. & Davies, B. 2019. Phase I trial of an ICAM-1-targeted immunotherapeutic-coxsackievirus A21 (CVA21) as an oncolytic agent against non muscle-invasive bladder cancer. *Clinical Cancer Research*, 25, 5818–5831.

Babiker, H. M., Riaz, I. B., Husnain, M. & Borad, M. J. 2017. Oncolytic virotherapy including Rigvir and standard therapies in malignant melanoma. *Oncolytic Virotherapy*, 6, 11–18.

Barr, J. J., Youle, M. & Rohwer, F. 2013. Innate and acquired bacteriophage-mediated immunity. *Bacteriophage*, 3, e25857.

Baruch, E.N., Youngster, I., Ben-Betzalel, G., Ortenberg, R., Lahat, A., Katz, L., Adler, K., Dick-Necula, D., Raskin, S., Bloch, N., Rotin, D., Anafi, L., Avivi, C., Melnichenko, J., Steinberg-Silman, Y., Mamtani, R., Harati, H., Asher, N., Shapira-Frommer, R., Brosh-Nissimov, T., Eshet, Y., Ben-Simon, S., Ziv, O., Khan, M. A. W., Amit, M., Ajami, N. J., Barshack, I., Schachter, J., Wargo, J.A., Koren, O., Markel, G. & Boursi, B. 2021 Feb 5. Fecal microbiota transplant promotes response in immunotherapy-refractory melanoma patients. *Science*, 371(6529), 602–609. doi: 10.1126/science.abb5920. Epub 2020 Dec 10. PMID: 33303685.

Bell, J. & McFadden, G. 2014. Viruses for tumor therapy. *Cell host & microbe*, 15, 260–265.

Bergonzini, C., Kroese, K., Zweemer, A. J. M. & Danen, E. H. J. 2022. Targeting Integrins for Cancer Therapy – Disappointments and Opportunities. *Frontiers in Cell and Developmental Biology*, 10, 1–13.

Bezeljak U. 2022 Feb 11. Cancer gene therapy goes viral: Viral vector platforms come of age. *Radiology & Oncology*, 56(1), 1–13. doi: 10.2478/raon-2022-0002. PMID: 35148469; PMCID: PMC8884858.

Borin, J. M., Liu, R., Wang, Y., Wu, T. C., Chopyk, J., Huang, L., et al. 2023. Fecal virome transplantation is sufficient to alter fecal microbiota and drive lean and obese body phenotypes in mice. *Gut Microbes*, 15(1), 1–15. https://doi.org/10.1080/19490976.2023.2236750

Breitbart, M., Hewson, I., Felts, B., Mahaffy, J. M., Nulton, J., Salamon, P. & Rohwer, F. 2003 Oct;18. Metagenomic analyses of an uncultured viral community from human feces. *Journal of Bacteriology* 5(20), 6220–3. doi: 10.1128/JB.185.20.6220-6223.2003. PMID: 14526037; PMCID: PMC225035.

Breitbart, M., Delwart, E., Rosario, K., Segalés, J., Varsani, A. & Consortium, I. R. 2017. ICTV virus taxonomy profile: Circoviridae. *Journal of General Virology*, 98, 1997–1998.

Broecker F. & Moelling K. 2021 Dec 8. The roles of the virome in cancer. *Microorganisms*, 9(12), 2538. doi: 10.3390/microorganisms9122538. PMID: 34946139; PMCID: PMC8706120.

Broecker F., Russo G., Klumpp J. & Moelling K. Stable core virome despite variable microbiome after fecal transfer. *Gut Microbes*, 8(3), 214–220. doi: 10.1080/19490976.2016.1265196. Epub 2016 Dec 9. PMID: 27935413; PMCID: PMC5479397.

Cao Z., Sugimura N., Burgermeister E, Ebert M. P., Zuo T. & Lan P. 2022 Jul, The gut virome: A new microbiome component in health and disease. *EBioMedicine*, 81,104113. doi: 10.1016/j.ebiom.2022.104113. Epub 2022 Jun 23. PMID: 35753153; PMCID: PMC9240800.

Cao, G. D., He, X. B., Sun, Q., Chen, S., Wan, K., Xu, X., Feng, X., Li, P. P., Chen, B. & Xiong, M. M. 2020. The oncolytic virus in cancer diagnosis and treatment. *Frontiers in Oncology*, 10, 1786.

Carpenter, A. B., Carpenter, A. M., Aiken, R. & Hanft, S. 2021. Oncolytic virus in gliomas: a review of human clinical investigations. *Annals of Oncology*, 32, 968–982.

Catala, A., Dzieciatkowska, M., Wang, G., Gutierrez-Hartmann, A., Simberg, D., Hansen, K. C., D'alessandro, A. & Catalano, C. E. 2021. Targeted intracellular delivery of trastuzumab using designer phage lambda nanoparticles alters cellular programs in human breast cancer cells. *ACS Nano*, 15, 11789–11805.

Cejalvo, J. M., Falato, C., Villanueva, L., Tolosa, P., Gonzalez, X., Pascal, M., Canes, J., Gavila, J., Manso, L., Pascual, T., Prat, A. & Salvador, F. 2022. Oncolytic viruses: A new immunotherapeutic approach for breast cancer treatment? *Cancer Treatment Reviews*, 106, 102392.

Chiu, M., Armstrong, E., Jennings, V., Foo, S., CrespoRodriguez, E., Bozhanova, G., Patin, E., McLaughli, M., Mansfield, D., Baker, G., Grove, L., Pedersen, M., Kyula, J., Roulstone, V.,Wilkins, A., McDonald, F., Harrington, K. & Melcher, A. 2020. Combination therapy with oncolytic viruses and immune checkpoint inhibitors. *Expert Opinion on Biological Therapy*, DOI: 10.1080/14712598.2020.1729351.

Crupi, M. J. F., Taha, Z., Janssen, T. J. A., Petryk, J., Boulton, S., Alluqmani, N., Jirovec, A., Kassas, O., Khan, S. T., Vallati, S., Lee, E., Huang, B. Z., Huh, M., Pikor, L., He, X., Marius, R., Austin, B., Duong, J., Pelin, A., Neault, S., Azad, T., Breitbach, C. J., Stojdl, D. F., Burgess, M. F., Mccomb, S., Auer, R., Diallo, J. S., Ilkow, C. S. & Bell, J. C. 2022. Oncolytic virus driven T-cell-based combination immunotherapy platform for colorectal cancer. *Frontiers in Immunology*, 13, 1029269.

Dasa, S. S., Jin, Q., Chen, C. T. & Chen, L. 2012. Target-specific copper hybrid T7 phage particles. *Langmuir*, 28, 17372–17380.

Davar, D., Dzutsev, A. K., McCulloch, J. A., Rodrigues, R. R., Chauvin, J. M., Morrison, R. M., Deblasio, R. N., Menna, C., Ding, Q., Pagliano, O., Zidi, B., Zhang, S., Badger, J.H., Vetizou, M., Cole, A.M., Fernandes, M.R., Prescott, S., Costa, R. G. F., Balaji, A. K., Morgun, A., Vujkovic-Cvijin, I., Wang, H., Borhani, A. A., Schwartz, M. B., Dubner, H. M., Ernst, S.J., Rose, A., Najjar, Y. G., Belkaid, Y., Kirkwood, J.M., Trinchieri, G. & Zarour, H. M. Fecal microbiota transplant overcomes resistance to anti-PD-1 therapy in melanoma patients. *Science*, 371(6529), 595–602. doi: 10.1126/science.abf3363. PMID: 33542131; PMCID: PMC8097968.

Davis, D. 2015. Application of Oncolytic Viruses for Cure of Colorectal Cancer. Cancer Research Journal, 3, 76.

Delmas, B., Attoui, H., Ghosh, S., Malik, Y. S., Mundt, E., Vakharia, V. N. & Consortium, I. R. 2019. ICTV virus taxonomy profile: Picobirnaviridae. *Journal of General Virology*, 100, 133–134.

Dion, M. B., Oechslin, F. & Moineau, S. 2020. Phage diversity, genomics and phylogeny. *Nature Reviews Microbiology*, 18, 125–138.

Dong, X., Pan, P., Zheng, D. W., Bao, P., Zeng, X. & Zhang, X. Z. 2020. Bioinorganic hybrid bacteriophage for modulation of intestinal microbiota to remodel tumor-immune microenvironment against colorectal cancer. *Science Advances*, 6, eaba1590.

Donina, S., Strele, I., Proboka, G., Auziņš, J., Alberts, P., Jonsson, B., Venskus, D. & Muceniece, A. 2015. Adapted ECHO-7 virus Rigvir immunotherapy (oncolytic virotherapy) prolongs survival in melanoma patients after surgical excision of the tumour in a retrospective study. *Melanoma research*, 25, 421–426.

Emencheta, S. C., Olovo, C. V., Eze, O. C., Kalu, C. F., Berebon, D. P., Onuigbo, E. B., Vila, M. M. D. C., Balcão, V. M. & Attama, A. A. 2023. The Role of Bacteriophages in the Gut Microbiota: Implications for Human Health. *Pharmaceutics*, 15, 2416.

Eyquem, J., Mansilla-Soto, J., Giavridis, T., van der Stegen, S.J.C., Hamieh, M., Cunanan, K.M., et al. 2017. Targeting a CAR to the TRAC locus with CRISPR/Cas9 enhances tumour rejection. *Nature*, 543, 113–117. doi: 10.1038/nature21405.

Fluckiger, A., Daillère, R., Sassi, M., Sixt, B.S., Liu, P., Loos, F., Richard, C., Rabu, C., Alou, M. T., Goubet, A.G., Lemaitre, F., Ferrere, G., Derosa, L., Duong, C. P. M., Messaoudene, M., Gagné, A., Joubert, P., De, Sordi L., Debarbieux, L., Simon, S., Scarlata, C. M., Ayyoub, M., Palermo, B., Facciolo, F., Boidot, R., Wheeler, R., Boneca, I. G., Sztupinszki, Z., Papp, K., Csabai, I., Pasolli, E., Segata, N., Lopez-Otin, C., Szallasi, Z., Andre, F., Iebba, V., Quiniou, V., Klatzmann, D., Boukhalil, J., Khelaifia, S., Raoult, D., Albiges, L., Escudier, B., Eggermont, A., Mami-Chouaib, F., Nistico, P., Ghiringhelli, F., Routy, B., Labarrière, N., Cattoir, V., Kroemer, G. & Zitvogel, L. . 2020 Aug 21. Cross-reactivity between tumor MHC class I-restricted antigens and an enterococcal bacteriophage. *Science*; 369(6506), 936–942. doi: 10.1126/science.aax0701. PMID: 32820119.

Frampton, J. E. 2022. Teserpaturev/G47Δ: first approval. *BioDrugs*, 36, 667–672.

Francki, R. I. B., Fauquet, C. M., Knudson, D. L. & Brown, F. 1991. Descriptions of virus families sad groups. *In*: Francki, R. I. B., Fauquet, C. M., Knudson, D. L. & Brown, F. (eds.) *Classification and Nomenclature of Viruses: Fifth Report of the International Committee on Taxonomy of Viruses. Virology Division of the International Union of Microbiological Societies.* Vienna: Springer Vienna.

Gao, R., Zhu, Y., Kong, C., Xia, K., Li, H., Zhu, Y., Zhang X, Liu Y, Zhong H, Yang R, Chen C, Qin N, Qin H. 2021. Alterations, Interactions, and Diagnostic Potential of Gut Bacteria and Viruses in Colorectal Cancer. *Frontiers in Cellular and Infection Microbiology*, 06 July 2021 Sec. *Microbiome in Health and Disease,* 11, 2021. https://doi.org/10.3389/fcimb.2021.657867

Garber, K. 2006. China approves world's first oncolytic virus therapy for cancer treatment. *Journal of the National Cancer Institute*, 98, 298–300.

Ghaemi, A., Soleimanjahi, H., Gill, P., Hassan, Z. M., Razeghi, S., Fazeli, M. & Razavinikoo, S. M. H. 2010b. Protection of Mice by a λ-Based Therapeutic Vaccine against Cancer Associated with Human Papillomavirus Type 16. *Intervirology*, 54, 105–112.

Ghaemi, A., Soleimanjahi, H., Gill, P., Hassan, Z., Jahromi, S. R. & Roohvand, F. 2010a. Recombinant lambda-phage nanobioparticles for tumor therapy in mice models. *Genetic Vaccines and Therapy*, 8, 3.

Gogokhia, L., Buhrke, K., Bell, R., Hoffman, B., Brown, D. G., Hanke-Gogokhia, C., Ajami, N. J., Wong, M. C., Ghazaryan, A., Valentine, J. F., Porter, N., Martens, E., O'Connell, R., Jacob, V., Scherl, E., Crawford, C., Stephens, W. Z., Casjens, S. R., Longman, R. S. & Round, J. L. 2019. Expansion of Bacteriophages Is Linked to Aggravated Intestinal Inflammation and Colitis. *Cell Host & Microbe*, 25, 285–299. e8.

Gopalakrishnan, V., Spencer, C.N., Nezi, L., Reuben, A., Andrews, M. C., Karpinets, T. V., Prieto, P. A., Vicente, D., Hoffman, K., Wei, S. C., Cogdill, A. P., Zhao, L., Hudgens, C. W., Hutchinson, D., Manzo, T., Petaccia, de Macedo M., Cotechini, T., Kumar, T., Chen, W. S., Reddy, S. M., Szczepaniak, Sloane R., Galloway-Pena, J., Jiang, H., Chen, P. L., Shpall, E. J., Rezvani, K., Alousi, A. M., Chemaly, R. F., Shelburne, S., Vence, L. M., Okhuysen, P. C., Jensen, V. B., Swennes, A. G., McAllister, F., Marcelo, Riquelme Sanchez E., Zhang, Y., Le, Chatelier E., Zitvogel, L., Pons, N., Austin-Breneman, J. L., Haydu, L. E., Burton, E. M., Gardner, J. M., Sirmans, E., Hu, J., Lazar, A.J., Tsujikawa, T., Diab, A., Tawbi, H., Glitza, I. C., Hwu, W. J., Patel, S. P., Woodman, S. E., Amaria, R. N., Davies, M. A., Gershenwald, J. E., Hwu, P., Lee, J. E., Zhang, J., Coussens, L. M., Cooper, Z. A., Futreal, P.A., Daniel, C. R., Ajami, N. J., Petrosino, J. F., Tetzlaff, M. T., Sharma, P., Allison, J.P., Jenq, R. R. & Wargo J. A. 2018 Jan 5. Gut microbiome modulates response to anti-PD-1 immunotherapy in melanoma patients. *Science*, 359(6371), 97–103. doi: 10.1126/science.aan4236. Epub 2017 Nov 2. PMID: 29097493; PMCID: PMC5827966.

Górski, A., Międzybrodzki, R., Borysowski, J., Dąbrowska, K., Wierzbicki, P., Ohams, M., Korczak-Kowalska, G., Olszowska-Zaremba, N., Łusiak-Szelachowska, M., Kłak, M., Jończyk, E., Kaniuga, E., Gołaś, A., Purchla, S., Weber-Dąbrowska, B., Letkiewicz, S., Fortuna, W., Szufnarowski, K., Pawełczyk, Z., Rogóż, P. & Kłosowska, D. 2012. Phage as a modulator of immune responses: Practical implications for phage therapy. *Advances in Virus Research*, 83, 41–71.

Gu, J., Lv, X., Li, W., Li, G., He, X., Zhang, Y., Shi, L. & Zhang, X. 2023. Deciphering the mechanism of Peptostreptococcus anaerobius-induced chemoresistance in colorectal cancer: The important roles of MDSC recruitment and EMT activation. *Frontiers in Immunology*, 14, 1230681.

Harrington, K., Freeman, D. J., Kelly, B., Harper, J. & Soria, J. -C. 2019. Optimizing oncolytic virotherapy in cancer treatment. Nature Reviews Drug discovery, 18, 689–706.

Harrington, K. J., Puzanov, I., Hecht, J. R., Hodi, F. S., Szabo, Z., Murugappan, S. & Kaufman, H. L. 2015. Clinical development of talimogene laherparepvec (T-VEC): A modified herpes simplex virus type-1–derived oncolytic immunotherapy. Expert Review of Anticancer Therapy, 15, 1389–1403.

Hou, X. -L., Xie, X. -T., Tan, L. -F., Zhang, F., Fan, J. -X., Chen, W., Hu, Y. -G., Zhao, Y. -D., Liu, B. & Xu, Q. -R. 2023. T4 phage display technology for enhanced photodynamic therapy of breast cancer. *ACS Materials Letters*, 5, 2270–2281.

Huh, H., Chen, D. W., Foldvari, M., Slavcev, R. & Blay, J. 2022. EGFR-targeted bacteriophage lambda penetrates model stromal and colorectal carcinoma tissues, is taken up into carcinoma cells, and interferes with 3-dimensional tumor formation. *Frontiers in Immunology*, 13, 957233.

Hwang, Y. J. & Myung, H. 2020. Engineered bacteriophage T7 as a potent anticancer agent in vivo. *Frontiers in Microbiology*, 11, 1–11.

Immadi Siva, R. 2022. Phage therapy: Challenges and opportunities. *Fine Focus*, 8, 12–35.

Iwagami, Y., Casulli, S., Nagaoka, K., Kim, M., Carlson, R. I., Ogawa, K., Lebowitz, M. S., Fuller, S., Biswas, B., Stewart, S., Dong, X., Ghanbari, H. & Wands, J. R. 2017. Lambda phage-based vaccine induces antitumor immunity in hepatocellular carcinoma. *Heliyon*, 3, e00407.

Javanbakht, M., Tahmasebzadeh, S., Cegolon, L., Gholami, N., Kashaki, M., Nikoueinejad, H., Mozafari, M., Mozaffari, M., Zhao, S., Khafaei, M., Izadi, M., Fathi, S. & Akhavan-Sigari, R. 2023. Oncolytic viruses: A novel treatment strategy for breast cancer. *Genes & Diseases*, 10, 430–446.

Jin, K. -T., Tao, X. -H., Fan, Y. -B. & Wang, S. -B. 2021. Crosstalk between oncolytic viruses and autophagy in cancer therapy. *Biomedicine & Pharmacotherapy*, 134, 110932.

Johnson, C. H., Dejea, C. M., Edler, D., Hoang, L. T., Santidrian, A. F., Felding, B. H., Ivanisevic, J., Cho, K., Wick, E. C., Hechenbleikner, E. M., Uritboonthai, W., Goetz, L., Casero, R. A. Jr, Pardoll, D. M., White, J. R., Patti, G. J., Sears, C. L., Siuzdak, G. 2015a. Metabolism links bacterial biofilms and colon carcinogenesis. Cell Metabolism., 21(6), 891–897. doi: 10.1016/j.cmet.2015.04.011. Epub 2015 May 7. PMID: 25959674; PMCID: PMC4456201.

Johnson, D. B., Puzanov, I. & Kelley, M. C. 2015b. Talimogene laherparepvec (T-VEC) for the treatment of advanced melanoma. Immunotherapy, 7, 611–619.

Junca, H., Pieper, D. H. & Medina, E. 2022 Jan 19. The emerging potential of microbiome transplantation on human health interventions. *Computational and Structural Biotechnology Journal*. 20, 615–627. doi: 10.1016/j.csbj.2022.01.009. PMID: 35140882; PMCID: PMC8801967.

Kabwe, M., Dashper, S., Bachrach, G. & Tucci, J. 2021. Bacteriophage manipulation of the microbiome associated with tumour microenvironments-can this improve cancer therapeutic response? *FEMS Microbiology Reviews*, 45, 1–19.

Kaufman, H. L., Kohlhapp, F. J. & Zloza, A. 2015. Oncolytic viruses: A new class of immunotherapy drugs. *Nature Reviews Drug Discovery*, 14, 642–662.

Kaufman, H.L., Shalhout, S.Z. and Iodice, G., 2022. Talimogene laherparepvec: Moving from first-in-class to best-in-class. *Frontiers in Molecular Biosciences*, 9, p.834841.

Kelly, E. & Russell, S.J. 2007. History of oncolytic viruses: Genesis to genetic engineering. *Molecular Therapy*, 15, 651–659.

Khan, M. S., Ishaq, M., Hinson, M., Potugari, B. & Rehman, A. U. 2019. Parvimonas micra bacteremia in a patient with colonic carcinoma. *Caspian Journal of Internal Medicine*, 10, 472.

Kieft, K., Zhou, Z. & Anantharaman, K. VIBRANT: Automated recovery, annotation and curation of microbial viruses, and evaluation of viral community function from genomic sequences. *Microbiome* 8, 90 (2020). https://doi.org/10.1186/s40168-020-00867-0

Kolesanova, E. F., Melnikova, M. V., Bolshakova, T. N., Rybalkina, E. Y. & Sivov, I. G. 2019. Bacteriophage MS2 as a tool for targeted delivery in solid tumor chemotherapy. *Acta Naturae*, 11, 98–101.

Kooby, D. A., Carew, J. F., Halterman, M. W., Mack, J. E., Bertino, J. R., Blumgart, L. H., Federoff, H. J. & Fong, Y. 1999. Oncolytic viral therapy for human colorectal cancer and liver metastases using a multi-mutated herpes simplex virus type-1 (G207). *FASEB Journal*, 13, 1325–1334.

Lander, G. C., Evilevitch, A., Jeembaeva, M., Potter, C. S., Carragher, B. & Johnson, J. E. 2008. Bacteriophage lambda stabilization by auxiliary protein gpD: timing, location, and mechanism of attachment determined by cryo-EM. *Structure*, 16, 1399–1406.

Lang, F. F., Conrad, C., Gomez-Manzano, C., Yung, W. K. A., Sawaya, R., Weinberg, J. S., Prabhu, S. S., Rao, G., Fuller, G. N., Aldape, K. D., Gumin, J., Vence, L.M., Wistuba, I., Rodriguez-Canales, J., Villalobos, P. A., Dirven, C. M. F., Tejada, S., Valle, R. D., Alonso, M. M., Ewald, B., Peterkin, J. J., Tufaro, F. & Fueyo, J. 2018. Phase I study of DNX-2401 (Delta-24-RGD) oncolytic adenovirus: Replication and immunotherapeutic effects in recurrent malignant glioma. *Journal of Clinical Oncology*, 36, 1419–1427.

Lao, Y., Shen, D., Zhang, W., He, R., Jiang, M. 2022. Immune checkpoint inhibitors in cancer therapy-how to overcome drug resistance? Cancers (Basel), 4(15), 3575. doi: 10.3390/cancers14153575.

Lawler, S.E., Speranza, M.-C., Cho, C.-F. & Chiocca, E.A. 2017. Oncolytic viruses in cancer treatment: A review. *JAMA Oncology*, 3, 841–849.

Li, J., Zheng, H. & Leung, S. S. Y. 2023. Potential of bacteriophage therapy in managing Staphylococcus aureus infections during chemotherapy for lung cancer patients. *Scientific Reports*, 13, 9534.

Liang, G. & Bushman, F. D. The human virome: Assembly, composition and host interactions. *Nature Reviews Microbiology*., 19(8),514–527. doi: 10.1038/s41579-021-00536-5. Epub 2021 Mar 30. PMID: 33785903; PMCID: PMC8008777.

Liang, M. 2018. Oncorine, the world first oncolytic virus medicine and its update in China. *Current Cancer Drug Targets*, 18, 171–176.

Lo, C. -H., Wu, D. -C., Jao, S. -W., Wu, C. -C., Lin, C.- Y., Chuang, C. -H., Lin, Y. -B., Chen, C. -H., Chen, Y. -T., Chen, J. -H., Hsiao, K. -H., Chen, Y. -J., Chen, Y .-T., Wang, J. -Y. & Li, L. -H. 2022. Enrichment of prevotella intermedia in human colorectal cancer and its additive effects with Fusobacterium nucleatum on the malignant transformation of colorectal adenomas. *Journal of Biomedical Science*, 29, 88.

Lu, Y., Xue, J., Deng, T., Zhou, X., Yu, K., Deng, L., Huang, M., Yi, X., Liang, M., Wang, Y., Shen, H., Tong, R., Wang, W., Li, L., Song, J., Li, J., Su, X., Ding, Z., Gong, Y., Zhu, J., Wang, Y., Zou, B., Zhang, Y., Li, Y., Zhou, L., Liu, Y., Yu, M., Wang, Y., Zhang, X., Yin, L., Xia, X., Zeng, Y., Zhou, Q., Ying, B., Chen, C., Wei, Y., Li, W., Mok, T. 2020 May. Safety and feasibility of CRISPR-edited T cells in patients with refractory non-small-cell lung cancer. *Nature Medicine.*, 26(5), 732–740. doi: 10.1038/s41591-020-0840-5. Epub 2020 Apr 27. Erratum in: Nat Med. 2020 Jul;26(7), 1149. PMID: 32341578.

Macedo, N., Miller, D.M., Haq, R. & Kaufman, H.L. 2020. Clinical landscape of oncolytic virus research in 2020. *Journal for Immunotherapy of Cancer*, 8, 1–14.

MacLeod, D.T., Antony, J., Martin, A.J., Moser, R.J., Hekele, A., Wetzel, K.J., et al. 2017. Integration of a CD19 CAR into the TCR alpha chain locus streamlines production of allogeneic gene-edited CAR T cells. *Molecular Therapy*, 25, 949–961. doi: 10.1016/j.ymthe.2017.02.005.

Maroun, J., Muñoz-Alía, M., Ammayappan, A., Schulze, A., Peng, K. -W. & Russell, S. 2017. Designing and building oncolytic viruses. *Future Virology*, 12, 193–213.

Matsui, S. M., Kiang, D., Ginzton, N., Chew, T. & Geigenmüller-Gnirke, U. Molecular biology of astroviruses: Selected highlights. *Gastroenteritis Viruses: Novartis Foundation Symposium*, 238, 2001. Wiley Online Library, 219–236.

Multhoff, G., Molls, M. & Radons, J. 2012 Jan 12. Chronic inflammation in cancer development. *Frontiers in Immunology*, 2, 98. doi: 10.3389/fimmu.2011.00098. PMID: 22566887; PMCID: PMC3342348.

Murgas, P., Bustamante, N., Araya, N., Cruz-Gómez, S., Durán, E., Gaete, D., Oyarce, C., López, E., Herrada, A. A., Ferreira, N., Pieringer, H. & Lladser, A. 2018. A filamentous bacteriophage targeted to carcinoembryonic antigen induces tumor regression in mouse models of colorectal cancer. *Cancer Immunology & Immunotherapy*, 67, 183–193.

Nakatsu, G., Zhou, H., Wu, WKK., Wong, SH., Coker, OO., Dai, Z., Li, X., Szeto, CH., Sugimura, N., Lam, TY., Yu, AC., Wang, X., Chen, Z., Wong, MC., Ng, SC., Chan, MTV., Chan, PKS., Chan, FKL., Sung, JJ., Yu, J. Alterations in enteric virome are associated with colorectal cancer and survival outcomes. *Gastroenterology*. 2018 Aug;155(2), 529–541. e5. doi: 10.1053/j.gastro.2018.04.018. Epub 2018 Apr 22. PMID: 29689266.

Nayfach, S., Páez-Espino, D., Call, L., Low, S. J., Sberro, H., Ivanova, N. N, Proal AD, Fischbach MA, Bhatt AS, Hugenholtz P., Kyrpides N. C. Metagenomic compendium of 189,680 DNA viruses from the human gut microbiome. *Nature Microbiology*, 6(7), 960–970. doi: 10.1038/s41564-021-00928-6. Epub 2021 Jun 24. PMID: 34168315; PMCID: PMC8241571.

Nicklin, S. A., Wu, E., Nemerow, G. R. & Baker, A. H. 2005. The influence of adenovirus fiber structure and function on vector development for gene therapy. *Molecular Therapy*, 12, 384–393.

Nieminen, M. T., Listyarifah, D., Hagström, J., Haglund, C., Grenier, D., Nordström, D., Uitto, V. J., Hernandez, M., Yucel-Lindberg, T., Tervahartiala, T., Ainola, M. & Sorsa, T. 2018. Treponema denticola chymotrypsin-like proteinase may contribute to orodigestive carcinogenesis through immunomodulation. *British Journal of Cancer*, 118, 428–434.

O'Bryan, S. & Mathis, J. 2018. Oncolytic virotherapy for breast cancer treatment. *Current Gene Therapy*, 18, 192–205.

Popgeorgiev, N., Temmam, S., Raoult, D. & Desnues, C. 2013. Describing the silent human virome with an emphasis on giant viruses. *Intervirology*, 56, 395–412.

Ragothaman, M. & Yoo, S. Y. 2023. Engineered phage-based cancer vaccines: Current advances and future directions. *Vaccines (Basel)*, 11, 1–18.

Rahman, M. M. & McFadden, G. 2021. Oncolytic viruses: Newest frontier for cancer immunotherapy. *Cancers (Basel)*, 13.

Rausch, M. P. and Hastings, K. T., 2017. Immune checkpoint inhibitors in the treatment of melanoma: From basic science to clinical application. *Exon Publications*, 121–142.

Razazan, A., Nicastro, J., Slavcev, R., Barati, N., Arab, A., Mosaffa, F., Jaafari, M. R. & Behravan, J. 2019. Lambda bacteriophage nanoparticles displaying GP2, a HER2/neu derived peptide, induce prophylactic and therapeutic activities against TUBO tumor model in mice. *Scientific Reports*, 9, 2221.

Ren, J., Song, K., Deng, C., Ahlgren, N. A., Fuhrman J. A., Li, Y, Xie X, Poplin R, Sun F. Identifying viruses from metagenomic data using deep learning. *Quantitative Biology*, 8(1), 64–77. doi: 10.1007/s40484-019-0187-4. PMID: 34084561; PMCID: PMC8172088.

Ren, S., Zuo, S., Zhao, M., Wang, X., Wang, X., Chen, Y., Wu, Z. & Ren, Z. 2011. Inhibition of tumor angiogenesis in lung cancer by T4 phage surface displaying mVEGFR2 vaccine. *Vaccine*, 29, 5802–5811.

Ren, Y., Miao, J. M., Wang, Y. Y., Fan, Z., Kong, X. B., Yang, L. & Cheng, G., 2022. Oncolytic viruses combined with immune checkpoint therapy for colorectal cancer is a promising treatment option. *Frontiers in Immunology*, 13, p.961796.

Reul, J., Frisch, J., Engeland, C. E., Thalheimer, F. B., Hartmann, J., Ungerechts, G., Buchholz, C. J. 2019 Feb 14. Tumor-specific delivery of immune checkpoint inhibitors by engineered AAV vectors. *Frontiers in Oncology*, 9, 52. doi: 10.3389/fonc.2019.00052. PMID: 30838171; PMCID: PMC6382738.

Russell, S. J., Peng, K. -W. & Bell, J. C. 2012. Oncolytic virotherapy. *Nature Biotechnology*, 30, 658–670.

Sakamoto, K., Ito, Y., Mori, T. & Sugimura, K. 2006. Interaction of human lactoferrin with cell adhesion molecules through RGD motif elucidated by lactoferrin-binding epitopes. *Journal of Biological Chemistry*, 281, 24472–8.

Sakamoto, K., Kamada, Y., Sameshima, T., Yaguchi, M., Niida, A., Sasaki, S., Miwa, M., Ohkubo, S., Sakamoto, J. I., Kamaura, M., Cho, N. & Tani, A. 2017. K-Ras(G12D)-selective inhibitory peptides generated by random peptide T7 phage display technology. *Biochemical & Biophysical Research Communications*, 484, 605–611.

Sanmukh, S. G., Dos Santos, N. J., Barquilha, C. N., De Carvalho, M., Dos Reis, P. P., Delella, F. K., Carvalho, H. F., Latek, D., Fehér, T. & Felisbino, S. L. 2023. Bacterial RNA virus MS2 exposure increases the expression of cancer progression genes in the LNCaP prostate cancer cell line. *Oncology Letters*, 25, 86.

Sanmukh, S. G., Santos, N. J., Barquilha, C. N., Dos Santos, S. A. A., Duran, B. O. S., Delella, F. K., Moroz, A., Justulin, L. A., Carvalho, H. F. & Felisbino, S. L. 2021. Exposure to bacteriophages T4 and M13 increases integrin gene expression and impairs migration of human PC-3 prostate cancer cells. *Antibiotics (Basel)*, 10.

Sanmukh, S., Dos Santos, S. & Felisbino, S. 2017. Natural bacteriophages T4 and M13 down-regulates Hsp90 gene expression in human prostate cancer cells (PC-3) representing a potential nanoparticle against cancer. *Virology Research Joutnal* 2017; 1 (1), 21–23.

Santiago-Rodriguez, T. M., Hollister, E. B. Unraveling the viral dark matter through viral metagenomics. *Frontiers in Immunology*. 2022 Sep 16;13, 1005107. doi: 10.3389/fimmu.2022.1005107. PMID: 36189246; PMCID: PMC9523745.

Segain, J. P., Raingeard de la Blétière, D., Bourreille, A., Leray, V., Gervois, N., Rosales, C., Ferrier, L., Bonnet, C., Blottière, H. M. & Galmiche, J. P. Butyrate inhibits inflammatory responses through NF kappaB inhibition: implications for Crohn's disease. *Gut*. 2000 Sep;47(3), 397–403. doi: 10.1136/gut.47.3.397. PMID: 10940278; PMCID: PMC1728045.

Seymour, L. W. & Fisher, K. D. 2016. Oncolytic viruses: Finally delivering. *British Journal of Cancer*, 114, 357–361.

Sharma, S., Chatterjee, S., Datta, S., Prasad, R., Dubey, D., Prasad, R. K. & Vairale, M. G. 2017. Bacteriophages and its applications: an overview. *Folia Microbiologica*, 62, 17–55.

Shkoporov, A. N., Clooney, A. G., Sutton, T. D., Ryan, F. J., Daly, K. M., Nolan, J. A., Mcdonnell, S. A., Khokhlova, E. V., Draper, L. A. & Forde, A. 2019. The human gut virome is highly diverse, stable, and individual specific. *Cell Host & Microbe*, 26, 527–541. e5.

Shoae-Hassani, A., Keyhanvar, P., Seifalian, A. M., Mortazavi-Tabatabaei, S. A., Ghaderi, N., Issazadeh, K., Amirmozafari, N. & Verdi, J. 2013. λ Phage nanobioparticle expressing apoptin efficiently suppress human breast carcinoma tumor growth in vivo. *PLoS One*, 8, e79907.

Simmonds, P. & Sharp, C. P. 2016. Anelloviridae. In: Richman D. D., Whitley R. J., Hayden F. J. (eds.) *Clinical Virology*,. Chapter 31, pp. 701–711. 10.1128/9781555819439.ch31.

Sinha, A. & Maurice, C. F. 2019. Bacteriophages: Uncharacterized and dynamic regulators of the immune system. *Mediators of Inflammation*, 2019, 3730519.

Souza, E. B. D., Pinto, A. R. & Fongaro, G. 2023. Bacteriophages as potential clinical immune modulators. *Microorganisms*, 11, 2222.

Takakusagi, K., Takakusagi, Y., Suzuki, T., Toizaki, A., Suzuki, A., Kawakatsu, Y., Watanabe, M., Saito, Y., Fukuda, R., Nakazaki, A., Kobayashi, S., Sakaguchi, K. & Sugawara, F. 2015. Multimodal biopanning of T7 phage-displayed peptides reveals angiomotin as a potential receptor of the anti-angiogenic macrolide roxithromycin. *European Journal of Medicinal Chemistry*, 90, 809–21.

Tamayo-Trujillo, R., Guevara-Ramírez, P., Cadena-Ullauri, S, Paz-Cruz, E., Ruiz-Pozo, V. A., Zambrano, A.K. 2023 Mar. Human virome: Implications in cancer. *Heliyon*. ;9(3), e14086. doi: 10.1016/j.heliyon.2023.e14086. Epub 2023 Feb 25. PMID: 36873548; PMCID: PMC9957661.

Umakanthan, S., Bukelo, M. M. 2021 Jun 22. Molecular genetics in Epstein-Barr virus-associated malignancies. *Life (Basel)*. 11(7), 593. doi: 10.3390/life11070593. PMID: 34206255; PMCID: PMC8306230.

Van Belleghem, J. D., Dąbrowska, K., Vaneechoutte, M., Barr, J. J. & Bollyky, P. L. 2019. Interactions between bacteriophage, bacteria, and the mammalian immune system. *Viruses*, 11, 10.

Vitiello, G. A. F., Ferreira, W. A. S., Cordeiro, de Lima V. C., Medina, T. D. S. 2021 Dec 2. Antiviral responses in cancer: Boosting antitumor immunity through activation of interferon pathway in the tumor microenvironment. *Frontiers in Immunology* 12, 782852. doi: 10.3389/fimmu.2021.782852. PMID: 34925363; PMCID: PMC8674309.

Wang D, Zhang F, Gao G. CRISPR-based therapeutic genome editing: Strategies and in vivo delivery by AAV vectors. *Cell*, 181(1), 136–150. doi: 10.1016/j.cell.2020.03.023. PMID: 32243786; PMCID: PMC7236621.

Wang, R., Li, H. D., Cao, Y., Wang, Z. Y., Yang, T. & Wang, J. H. 2023. M13 phage: a versatile building block for a highly specific analysis platform. *Analytical & Bioanalytical Chemistry*, 415, 3927–3944.

Xu, H. M., Xu, W. M. & Zhang, L. 2022. Current status of phage therapy against infectious diseases and potential application beyond infectious diseases. *International Journal of Clinical Practice*, 2022, 4913146.

Yap, M. L. & Rossmann, M. G. 2014. Structure and function of bacteriophage T4. *Future Microbiology*, 9, 1319–1327.

Yin, J., Markert, J. M. & Leavenworth, J. W. 2017. Modulation of the intratumoral immune landscape by oncolytic herpes simplex virus virotherapy. *Frontiers in Oncology*, 7, 136.

Yue, H., Li, Y., Yang, M. & Mao, C. 2022. T7 Phage as an Emerging Nanobiomaterial with Genetically Tunable Target Specificity. *Advanced Science (Weinh)*, 9, e2103645.

Zhang, W. W., Li, L., Li, D., Liu, J., Li, X., Li W, Xu, X., Zhang, M. J., Chandler, L. A., Lin, H., Hu, A., Xu, W., Lam, D. M.. 2018 Feb. The first approved gene therapy product for cancer Ad-p53 (Gendicine): 12 Years in the clinic. *Human*

Gene Therapy 29(2),160–179. doi: 10.1089/hum.2017.218. PMID: 29338444.

Zhang, Y. & Wang, R. 2023. The human gut phageome: Composition, development, and alterations in disease. *Frontiers in Microbiology*, 14, 1–9.

Zhao, G., Droit, L., Gilbert, M. H., Schiro, F. R., Didier, P. J., Si, X., Paredes, A., Handley, S. A., Virgin, H. W. & Bohm, R. P. 2019. Virome biogeography in the lower gastrointestinal tract of rhesus macaques with chronic diarrhea. *Virology*, 527, 77–88.

Zhao, Y., Liu, Z., Li, L., Wu, J., Zhang, H., Zhang, H., Lei, T. & Xu, B. 2021. Oncolytic adenovirus: Prospects for cancer immunotherapy. *Frontiers in Microbiology*, 12, 707290.

Zhu LB, Zhang YC, Huang HH, Lin J. 2021 Sep 9. Prospects for clinical applications of butyrate-producing bacteria. *World Journal of Clinical Pediatrics*, 10(5), 84–92. doi: 10.5409/wjcp.v10.i5.84. PMID: 34616650; PMCID: PMC8465514.

Zhu, L., Lei, Y., Huang, J., An, Y., Ren, Y., Chen, L., Zhao, H. & Zheng, C. 2023a. Recent advances in oncolytic virus therapy for hepatocellular carcinoma. Frontiers in Oncology, 13, 1172292.

Zhu, X., Fan, C., Xiong, Z., Chen, M., Li, Z., Tao, T. & Liu, X. 2023b. Development and application of oncolytic viruses as the nemesis of tumor cells. *Frontiers in Microbiology*, 14, 1–19.

16 Microbiome-Based Cancer Therapeutics

Thifhelimbilu Luvhengo, Thabiso Victor Miya, Demetra Demetriou, Kim R.M Blenman, and Zodwa Dlamini

INTRODUCTION

Measures to increase life expectancy among adults should include prevention and early treatment of non-communicable diseases as they have replaced bacterial and viral infections as the leading cause of fatalities, globally. Non-communicable diseases that have become increasingly more predominant in the world include solid and hematological malignancies (Xia et al., 2022). Commonly occurring malignancies include breast, colon, cervix, gastric, hematological, liver, lung, prostate, skin, soft tissue tumor, and thyroid cancer (Jaye et al., 2021; Ugare et al., 2022; Xia et al., 2022). Prevalent malignancies particularly in Africa are as follows: In Northern Africa, bladder, liver, and breast cancers are the most prevalent types of cancer. In Southern Africa, lung, colorectal, and prostate cancers are common. On the other hand, cervical and esophageal cancers are prevalent in East Africa (Hamdi et al., 2021). The rate of occurrence of most of the malignancies mentioned above is increasing, especially among young adults and adolescents (Ugare et al., 2022). Some of the factors implicated in the rise in the rate of occurrence of cancers are exposure to environmental carcinogens and cancer-predisposing lifestyles such as tobacco use, chronic inflammation, alcohol consumption, etc. (Georgiou et al., 2021).

Surgical excision, chemotherapy, and/or radiotherapy are key strategies for the curative management of the majority of cancers. However, despite the advances some of the cancers such as anaplastic carcinoma of the thyroid, glioblastoma, pancreatic adenocarcinoma, and triple-negative breast cancer remain difficult to treat (Cullin et al., 2021; Dono et al., 2022; Puig-Saenz et al., 2023). Furthermore, some cancers that usually have a favorable prognosis may behave aggressively and be resistant to standard treatment or develop resistance during follow-up (Wang et al., 2019a). The heterogeneity of cancers and the tumor microenvironment (TME) necessitate the delivery of individualized management strategies (Stefańska et al., 2023).

INFLUENCE OF TUMOR MICROENVIRONMENT ON CLINICAL BEHAVIOR AND PROGNOSIS OF CANCERS

The poor outcomes associated with the management of some of the cancers persist despite an improvement in comprehension of cancer initiation and progression (Rahman et al., 2022). Until recently, malignant cells were the only target during cancer treatment with radiotherapy, chemotherapy, targeted therapy, or surgery (Liu et al., 2021). Recent studies have demonstrated that the main determinant of outcomes in cancer patients is not the malignant cells themselves but the nature of the TME (Pickup et al., 2014; Wang et al., 2018a; Laplane et al., 2019; Sepich-Poore et al., 2021; Reinfeld et al., 2022; Zhang et al., 2022; Stefańska et al., 2023). Treatment strategies targeting components of the TME have led to an improvement in cancer response to therapy, reversal of resistance, or reduction of recurrence (Mohan et al., 2020). The TME cellular and non-cellular components comprise tumor-associated macrophages, lymphocytes, dendritic cells, natural killer cells, fibroblast, endothelial cells, and the extracellular matrix, just to name a few (Wang et al., 2018b; Faubert et al., 2020; D'Angelo et al., 2021; Zhang et al., 2022) (Figure 16.1).

The majority of cancers in adults are linked with a state of low-grade chronic systemic inflammation, deranged immunity, altered hormonal milieu, and a change in the level of metabolites (Zhang et al., 2022). The hormonal milieu in and around the tumor also includes intra-tumoral bacteria (Dono et al., 2022; Huang et al., 2022; Kabwe et al., 2022). The tumor-associated bacteria are usually derived from the gut and are often found inside some of the cancer cells (Zhang et al., 2022; Oliva et al., 2021). The tumor-associated bacteria and the gut microbiome (GM) can have an effect on the status of the TME, tumor organismal environment (TOE), and immunity on the progression including metastasis and response of cancer to treatment (Laplane et al., 2019). The TOE can be described as all the parts of the organism that are not inside the tumor or near it but have an impact on the development of cancer. Tumor-induced systemic environment, tumor metabolic environment, tumor immune microenvironment, and tumor-dependent endocrine environment are examples of the elements that make up the TOE, which stands for the participation of the body as a whole in carcinogenesis (Dieterich and Bikfalvi, 2020). Among the changes that tumor-associated bacteria can induce is down- or upregulation of immunity against the cancer cells.

The discovery of the significant influence of the gut and tumor-based microbiome in carcinogenesis, progression, and response to treatment, has generated interest in the possibility of incorporating measures to manipulate microbiota composition during the management of cancer (Zhao et al., 2023). Among the commonly used strategies to reverse dysbiosis is treatment with antibiotics, prebiotics, probiotics,

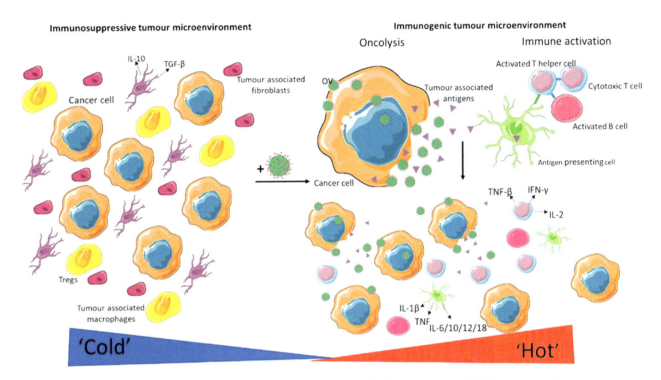

FIGURE 16.1 **The cellular composition of a tumor microenvironment (TME).** Two types of TMEs exist, namely, immunosuppressive TME and immunogenic TME.

synbiotics, postbiotics, and fecal microbial transplant (FMT) (Fong et al., 2020). Newer to reverse dysbiosis is the use of synthetic antimicrobial peptides, genetic engineering, and oncolytic virotherapy (Kuroda and Caputo, 2013; Gan et al., 2021; Kwan et al., 2021; Sugimura et al., 2019).

THE ROLE OF THE GM IN CARCINOGENESIS, PROGRESSION, AND TREATMENT OF CANCER

All the body sites that interact with the external environment are inhabited by symbiotic, commensal, and pathogenic organisms, and the majority of organisms in the microbiota in the body are found in the gastrointestinal (GI) tract (Garrett, 2015; Gilbert et al., 2018). The microbiota of the gut includes bacteria, fungi, viruses, and parasites (Garrett, 2015). Various microbes together with their products and their genes make up the GM (Mendes and Vale, 2023). The GM composition is impacted by the availability of nutrients and antimicrobial activities of peptides synthesized by either the intestinal epithelial cells or commensal bacteria (Riquelme et al., 2019; Mohan et al., 2020; Rulten et al., 2023). Certain resident viruses and fungi also participate in the regulation of the GM composition (Sugimura et al., 2022). Failure to regulate the microbiota may result in dysbiosis (Wu et al., 2019; Georgiou et al., 2021; Dono et al., 2022).

Dysbiosis of the GM is pivotal in the pathogenesis of most of the commonly occurring malignancies such as lung, colon, breast, liver, pancreas, prostate, skin, and prostate cancer (Saus Martínez et al., 2019; Wu et al., 2019; Cullin et al., 2021; Georgiou et al., 2021;Matson et al., 2021; Cai et al., 2022; Makaranka et al., 2022; Mekadim et al., 2022). The influence of gut microbiota dysbiosis is more significant in inherently aggressive cancers or aggressive subtypes of common malignancies (Mekadim et al., 2022; Geller et al., 2017). Dysbiosis may lead to the dominance of bacterial phyla or the production of metabolites that either make the tumor aggressive or responsive to the treatment (Makaranka et al., 2022). The influence of dysbiosis on cancer is not limited to tumorigenesis as it can also modify the TME, immune response to the tumor, and the effectiveness of treatment (Georgiou et al., 2021; Bultman and Jobin, 2014; Park et al., 2022; Chrysostomou et al., 2023; Tripodi et al., 2023; Zhao et al., 2023) (Figure 16.2).

Among the pathological basis of increased cancer in individuals with dysbiosis of gut microbiota are induction of DNA damage, immunosuppression, chronic inflammation, and production of oncogenic metabolites (Li et al., 2022; Li et al., 2023).

OPTIONS FOR MANIPULATION OF THE GUT MICROBIOME TO PREVENT OR REVERSE DYSBIOSIS

Strategies for manipulation of the GM may be selective or non-selective (Fong et al., 2020). Ideally, selective strategies should be used to reduce the risk of overgrowth of other pathogenic species or the development of resistance to antimicrobials. Antibiotics may be used intentionally to alter GM but are non-selective which is likely to encourage the development of resistance (Furfaro et al., 2018). Other options commonly

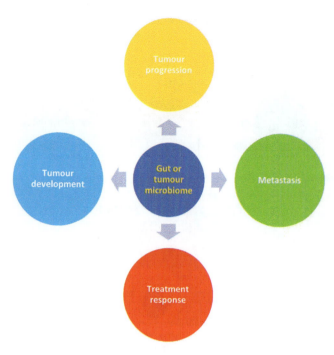

FIGURE 16.2 A schematic diagram showing various influences the gut or tumor microbiome has on cancers. These are tumor progression, metastasis, treatment response, and tumor development.

used for manipulation of the gut microbiota are alteration of diet, intake of probiotics, prebiotics, synbiotics, postbiotics, change of lifestyle, and FMT (Saus Martínez et al., 2019; D'Angelo et al., 2021; Brevi et al., 2022; Kumar et al., 2022; Matsushita et al., 2023).

MICROBIOME-BASED CANCER THERAPEUTICS AND MICROBIOME MANIPULATION STRATEGIES

ANTIBIOTHERAPY

The prevention of MALT lymphoma and gastric carcinoma by eradicating *Helicobacter pylori* is the only indication for antibiotics-induced microbial elimination of cancer (Cheung and Leung, 2018; Kamboj et al., 2017; Selgrad and Malfertheiner, 2008). Universal eradication is still disputed even in this situation considering that *H. pylori* is a commensal that is typically not linked to the development of cancer (Kakiuchi et al., 2021; Watanabe et al., 2021). Recently, experimental antibiotics against intratumoral bacteria capable of metabolizing gemcitabine have been developed to restore the effectiveness of gemcitabine in model mice that were injected with MC-26 carcinoma cells, subcutaneously (Geller et al., 2017). This application is being evaluated as a pancreatic ductal adenocarcinoma (PDAC) therapy in a recent phase III research (Guenther et al., 2020). Nevertheless, the use of broad-spectrum antibiotics can also have detrimental consequences on the development of tumors. Antibiotics induced the loss of *Akkermansia* spp. or *Bifidobacterium* spp. and were linked to the depletion of microbial metabolites like short-chain fatty acids (SCFA). These factors collectively attenuated treatment efficacy in patients exposed to allogeneic hematopoietic cell transfer therapy for immune checkpoint inhibitors (ICIs) in advanced melanomas (Elkrief et al., 2019) and hematologic malignancies (Shono et al., 2016). Similar to non-treated patients or patients exposed to antibiotics at a later period, cancer patients who received broad-spectrum antibiotics up to 30 days prior to the start of ICI had a significantly lower overall survival (Pinato et al., 2019). Strategies are being developed to reduce the impact of antibiotics on the local microbiome because they are frequently prescribed to cancer patients as a life-saving therapy for battling an infection. Colon-targeted antibiotic adsorbents are one such experimental method that is currently being evaluated in a phase III trial in patients with myelodysplastic syndrome or acute myeloid leukemia (De Gunzburg et al., 2018). Given their indiscriminate effects on the local microbiome, which could result in negative effects, the occurrence of resistant strains, and unpredictable effects on disease prognosis and efficacy of the therapy, antibiotics will only be used in limited circumstances to eradicate cancer-promoting pathobionts. An area of active study involves developing new techniques that allow for the targeted eradication of commensals that promote cancer while having no negative effects on the microbiome (Cullin et al., 2021).

DIET

New objectives for nutrition research in cancer patients are being shaped by the GM's expanding significance in tailored cancer therapy. There are no specific or scientifically supported dietary recommendations to offer patients after their diagnosis. This is despite frequent requests and the widespread perception that diet plays a crucial role in health (McQuade et al., 2019). A lack of prospective innovative dietary research demonstrating changes in cancer response and survival outcomes, as well as poor dietary data collecting in clinical trials and cohorts, are some of the contributing factors to this gap (World Cancer Research Fund International, 2018). Although varying bacterial taxa shared certain similarities in their associations to upstream dietary components and downstream pathways, certain bacterial taxa vary in responders to immune checkpoint blockade in numerous studies (with *Akkermansia muciniphila*, *Bifidobacterium longum*, *Faecalibacterium prausnitzii*, and *Clostridium* genera members identified across the cohorts) (Valdes et al., 2018).

Numerous foods (like processed meats) and food ingredients (like dietary fiber) have been found to either raise or lessen the risk of getting cancer (World Cancer Research Fund International, 2018). However, it seems to be less and less probable that nutrients, foods, or other bioactive compounds derived from food are significant independent factors in mediating or inhibiting cancer. Instead, various dietary patterns work together to produce an inflammatory and metabolic state that is more or less favorable to tumor progression. Healthy eating index scores and the Mediterranean diet score, for example, are linked with a significantly reduced risk of carcinogenesis and dying from cancer (World Cancer

Research Fund International, 2018). They were also associated with decreased inflammation and improved immune function through T-helper and cytotoxic cells (Oude Griep et al., 2013). Nevertheless, there is still a lot of curiosity about whether certain food elements might improve the microbiome. Randomized controlled trials examining the addition of certain foods or nutrients—for instance, switching from refined to whole grains—have revealed only minor alterations in the microbiota and immune system (Vanegas et al., 2017; Roager et al., 2019). Nevertheless, multiple short-term dietary research studies using endpoints for the GM have demonstrated that drastic dietary changes, such as switching from a vegetarian to a meat-based dietary intake or imposing an energy restriction of more than 30%, can have an equally drastic impact on the microbiome and cancer biomarkers like cell proliferation (Ou et al., 2013; David et al., 2014; O'Keefe et al., 2015; Zhao et al., 2018). However, if dietary modifications are not sustained, these microbiome changes are just as quickly reversible. Therefore, regular dietary adjustment is required to increase beneficial bacteria in the gut and alter its microbial composition; yet, altering deeply ingrained dietary habits is notoriously challenging. Understanding of the significance of diet-induced modifications on the makeup and function of the GM and the impact of these alterations on response to cancer therapy will be improved by well-designed and controlled studies (McQuade et al., 2019).

PREBIOTICS

Prebiotics, which are described as fermentable, non-digestible substrates or substances that encourage the growth of a particular type of bacteria and, as a result, a diversified and "healthy" microbiota, are another method for specifically modifying the microbiome (Raman et al., 2013). When compared to using microbiotics directly, the administration of prebiotics is intended to provide beneficial microbes a selection advantage. These prebiotics mostly consist of carbohydrates that enter the large intestine undigested and are processed there by commensal bacteria. SCFA is synthesized during this fermentation, resulting in reduced pH levels in the intestine. In return, this prolongs the proliferation of beneficial microorganisms like *Lactobacillus* and *Bifidobacterium* (McLoughlin et al., 2017). Resistant starch, which is one of the most researched prebiotics, can mediate the development of bacteria that participate in the generation of butyrate. According to preclinical investigations, prebiotics may support therapeutic efficacy. Taper and colleagues found that adding oligofructose or inulin to liver cancer mouse models' basal diets significantly increased the therapeutic efficacy of six cytotoxic drugs, including 5-FU, doxorubicin, cyclophosphamide, methotrexate, cytarabine, and vincristine which are all commonly used chemotherapeutic agents (Taper and Roberfroid, 2005).

Patients with gynecological cancer receiving radiation therapy participated in a randomized, placebo-controlled, double-blind experiment to examine the impact of a blend of fiber (50% fructo-oligosaccharide and 50% percent inulin) on microbiota (Guarner et al., 2012). Two weeks after completing radiation therapy, the group taking the prebiotic mixture recovered more quickly than the placebo group in terms of *Bifidobacterium* spp. and *Lactobacillus* spp. counts (Guarner et al., 2012), which improved the consistency of their stools (Garcia-Peris et al., 2016). In 140 perioperative patients with colorectal cancer, a double-blind, randomized clinical trial examined the impact of prebiotics (resistant dextrin, fructooligosaccharides, polydextrose, xylooligosaccharides) on GM and immune function (Xie et al., 2019). When compared to placebo, prebiotic ingestion increased the abundance of *Enterococcus* and *Bifidobacterium* and decreased the abundance of *Bacteroides* counts in the preoperative time. Compared to the prebiotic group, the control group had higher levels of *Bacillus, Enterococcus, Streptococcus,* and *Lactococcus* during the postoperative period. Furthermore, after consuming prebiotics during the recovery phase, the quantity of innocuous *Escherichia-Shigella* bacteria rose. Particularly, the non-prebiotic group's intestinal microbiota's richness declined from preoperative to postoperative periods. Prebiotic consumption had a major effect on immunologic indices throughout both the preoperative and postoperative phases in terms of immunological markers. When compared to controls, prebiotics significantly raised serum levels of immunoglobulin (Ig)M, IgG, and transferrin in the preoperative period, and IgA, IgG, suppressor/cytotoxic T cells (CD3+, CD8+), and total B lymphocytes in the postoperative time (Xie et al., 2019).

Notably, most of the research found that prebiotics had positive impacts on immune system enhancement through regulating the expression of pro- or anti-inflammatory cytokines. As evidenced by a reduced ratio of IFN-γ to IL-10 in mesenteric lymph nodes (mLNs), butyrate synthesis, which is accelerated by RS, dramatically suppresses the synthesis of proinflammatory cytokines interleukin (IL)-2 and interferon (IFN)-γ in rats (Looijer–Van Langen and Dieleman, 2009). Other researchers have also backed the prebiotic combination of the aforementioned and oligofructose and inulin, which can considerably reduce cecal proinflammatory IL-1β expression after being added to rats' drinking water (Herfel et al., 2011; Cani et al., 2009). Prebiotics' ability to regulate the host immune system suggests a possible therapeutic role in cancer immunotherapy, and this topic is currently being explored in clinical investigations. For instance, pilot research is being conducted to evaluate the impact of giving resistant starch to patients receiving dual ICI therapy for solid tumors on their gut flora. The rate of known adverse events associated with ICI treatment will be contrasted to the previous incidence (NCT04552418). Additionally, it has been discovered that the gut microbiota's purine nucleoside inosine contributes to the control of immunotherapy responses. Mager and colleagues have discovered inosine to be a metabolite made by *Bifidobacterium pseudolongum* that enhances the effectiveness of ICI-induced antitumor responses in germ-free animals with a variety of tumor forms, including melanoma, bladder cancer, and colorectal cancer. Further research demonstrated that the action of inosine depends on the adenosine A_2A

receptor expression and it specifically needs co-stimulation in T lymphocytes (Mager et al., 2020).

Recently, the analysis of lipids was undertaken to find out how probiotics affected the physiology of the host. A study was undertaken to determine changes in the composition of the lipids in the hosts and bacteria. It was discovered that variations in phosphatidylcholine and phosphatidylglycerol levels could affect nematode host physiology (Schifano et al., 2020). Furthermore, when cultivating *Enterococcus durans* (probiotic strain) with prebiotic fructooligosaccharides, a quantitative proteomics approach was utilized. The findings showed that *E. durans* was stimulated to synthesize clinically significant cancer therapeutics, namely, arginine deiminase and L-asparaginase (Comerlato et al., 2020).

PROBIOTICS

Probiotics can be described as live bacteria which provide health benefits to the host to whom they are delivered. Probiotics are present in supplements or fermented foods (like miso, kefir, yogurt, sauerkraut, kombucha, or kimchi). Probiotic supplements have the advantages of being simple to use and widely available, but there are significant problems and variations with standardization, quality control, bioavailability, and target modification (Kristensen et al., 2016). Single strains of easy-to-grow bacteria from food sources, like the lactic acid bacilli *Lactobacillus* and *Bifidobacterium*, were the first commercially available probiotic supplements. With varied degrees of clinical efficacy data in terms of certain disorders, these probiotics have been thoroughly investigated in terms of several gastrointestinal ailments (Hempel et al., 2012; Goldenberg et al., 2017). Probiotics vary in their capacity to withstand stomach acids and colonize the intestines, depending on the species, dosage, and preparation used as well as the host's microbiome (Sanders, 2011; Kristensen et al., 2016; Maldonado-Gómez et al., 2016; Sheflin et al., 2017).

The remarkable effectiveness of single-strain probiotics in model mice for ameliorating the antitumor immune response bolsters the case for clinical trials in cancer cohorts (Sivan et al., 2015; Routy et al., 2018). Probiotic colonization in a human with a rich natural gut environment, however, is far more difficult (Zmora et al., 2018). According to a study, probiotics may lessen the reconstruction of a varied microbial ecosystem following antibiotics (Suez et al., 2018). Therefore, these strategies must be carefully evaluated in clinical trials even though antibiotic ablation may be utilized as a gut conditioning mechanism to elevate colonization. Considering the gaps in terms of the comprehension of how these microbes may alter the immune system and therapeutic outcomes, off-trial usage of probiotics in terms of immunotherapy must be discouraged. Furthermore, investigations have demonstrated that quality might differ significantly because these supplements are mostly unregulated in the United States and EU. This variability is particularly concerning in a vulnerable patient cohort, like those with cancer, as it can impair the efficacy and safety of these medications (De Simone, 2019).

Synthetic stools or designer probiotics have aimed to combine the advantages of FMT in giving a diversified environment with the ability to create such a product at scale with little lot-to-lot variation (i.e., consistent composition). Early results show that engrafting a diverse microbial population steadily is encouraged when employing these products to treat recurrent *C. difficile* infections (Khanna et al., 2016). The continued development of commensal bacteria that are typically uncultivable into probiotics has also been made possible by technological advancements. One example is an obligate anaerobe bacteria called *F. prausnitzii*. This bacteria ferments fiber and was linked to a positive response to immunotherapy (Khan et al., 2014; Chaput et al., 2017; Gopalakrishnan et al., 2018). Testing of postbiotics, which are described as metabolic byproducts from microorganisms with advantageous biological activities, like butyrate, was also suggested, as discussed below. However, there is a dearth of reliable data to support this strategy (McQuade et al., 2019).

POSTBIOTICS

Postbiotics can be described as metabolic products released by probiotics, which are living bacteria like *Bifidobacterium* (*B.*) and *Lactobacillus* (*L.*). These bacteria use prebiotics as nutritional sources, e.g., oligosaccharides and dietary fiber (Nataraj et al., 2020). As previously mentioned, probiotics metabolize in the gut and offer health benefits (Batista et al., 2020). Postbiotics research has recently been extensively pursued using these benefits. According to reports, postbiotics have health-promoting properties like immunomodulation, hypolipidemic, anticancer, and antihypertensive attributes (Fang et al., 2014; Aguilar-Toalá et al., 2020; Engevik et al., 2021). For high-risk individuals or patients with underlying disorders who find it difficult to use live probiotic strains, postbiotics have lately become a viable alternative to probiotics. Compared to probiotics, postbiotics have qualities including a safe profile, nontoxicity, known chemical structure, a longer shelf life, resistance to hydrolysis, and resilience to conditions in the digestive system, making them potential anticancer treatments (Nataraj et al., 2020).

SYNBIOTICS

Synbiotics are a mixture of prebiotics and probiotics (Sędzikowska and Szablewski, 2021). There have been few investigations into the role of synbiotics in cancer therapeutics. In a prospective, double-blind trial, the use of synbiotics in patients having surgery for periampullary neoplasms (PNs) was investigated. Furthermore, the impact of these agents on survival, length of hospital stay, antibiotic use, nutritional condition, and postoperative complications was assessed. For a total of 14 days, patients were randomized to receive prebiotics and probiotics—synbiotics—group S (fructooligosaccharides (FOS) 100 mg, *Lactobacillus acidophilus* HS 111, 1×10^9

CFU, *Bifidobacterium bifidum*, 1 × 10⁹ CFU, *Lactobacillus rhamnosus* HS 111, 1 × 10⁹ CFU, and *Lactobacillus casei* 10, 1 × 10⁹ CFU) or placebo-controls, group C. These treatments were administered twice daily. For each group, 23 patients were assigned. Compared to group C (16 of 23 patients, 69.6%), group S (6 of 23 patients, 26.1%) had a considerably decreased incidence of postoperative infection (P= 0.00) (Sommacal et al., 2015). Nevertheless, additional research is warranted to ascertain the effectiveness of pre- and synbiotics in cancer treatment (Villéger et al., 2019).

Fecal Microbial Transplant (FMT)

FMT is one method for changing the makeup of the GM. FMT involves transfer of the fecal material from a donor to a recipient through a nasogastric tube, enema, nasojejunal tube, colonoscopy, upper tract endoscopy, or as a prepared capsule (Chervin and Gajewski, 2020). The Infectious Diseases Society of America and the Society for Healthcare Epidemiology of America have included the transfer of fecal material from healthy donors in their *Clostridium difficile* infection management guidelines because it was demonstrated to be efficacious in treating recurrent infections with *C. difficile* (Merchante Gutiérrez et al., 2022; Van Nood et al., 2013; Cohen et al., 2010). Additionally, FMT was researched in clinical studies for treating irritable bowel syndrome, ulcerative colitis, and other gastrointestinal diseases (Tian et al., 2019; Costello et al., 2019; Cammarota and Ianiro, 2019; Xu et al., 2019; Aroniadis et al., 2019; Wang et al., 2018b; Rohlke and Stollman, 2012). In preclinical studies, microbiota from a patient was gavage-transferred into germ-free mice (GFM), demonstrating the therapeutic ability of FMT in cancer immunotherapy. When compared to GFM colonized with FMT from non-responder patients, those colonized with FMT from responder patients showed slower tumorigenesis (Matson et al., 2018). Additionally, anti-PD-L1 therapy was more successful when GFM was reconstituted with responder-derived FMT compared to mice with FMT derived from non-responders. In a different group of epithelial tumor patients, mice treated with broad-spectrum antibiotics or given FMT from non-responders had their therapeutic response to anti-PD-1 therapy eliminated (Routy et al., 2018). FMT transfer from either non-responder-derived FMT or responder-derived FMT enriched with *A. muciniphila* might then be used to restore response to anti-PD-1 therapy. Mice exposed to FMT combined with *Faecalibacterium* spp. also showed better antitumor responses (Gopalakrishnan et al., 2018). These findings point to a potential functional relationship between the GM and the effectiveness of anti-PD-1 immunotherapy as well as the possibility of a therapeutic manipulation capsule (Chervin and Gajewski, 2020).

Currently, several independent research teams are examining how well FMT can improve the clinical response to anti-PD-1 therapy. A clinical trial at the University of Pittsburgh Hillman Cancer Center is investigating the administration of FMT in conjunction with pembrolizumab in melanoma patients who have not responded to anti-PD1 therapy (NCT03341143). The ability of FMT from donor patients who responded to PD-1 blockade to ameliorate therapeutic results in anti-PD-1-resistant melanoma patients is being investigated in phase II feasibility research. The adaptive and innate immune systems' functional and phenotypic alterations will be investigated concurrently. In 2019, Giorgio Trinchieri reported that two of three melanoma patients who had FMT and immune checkpoint therapy saw stable disease or tumor regression (G, 2019). A phase I clinical trial is being carried out at the Sheba Medical Center in Israel to assess FMT from responder patients being transferred through colonoscopy, followed by anti-PD-1 retreatment and administration of stool-microbiota capsules in patients suffering from metastatic melanoma resistant to PD-1 therapy (NCT03353402) (Baruch et al., 2019). The preliminary findings for the first three patients were reported. One patient had remission of the disease at the time of the initial imaging but progressed on later scans. Another patient had a 45% reduction in disease load and was still alive after eight months. Following treatment, intratumoral CD8⁺ and CD68⁺ cells increased in the tumor biopsies taken from these patients, pointing to a change in the tumor microenvironment. Given the exceedingly small sample sizes and the heterogeneity of the patients under investigation (for example, refractory to ICI therapy vs. relapse post-initial response), these data should be interpreted cautiously. Clinical trial designs will need to consider these variations in patient characteristics because some patients with recurrent anti-PD-1-resistant cancers may respond to follow-up anti-PD-1 therapy even without a microbiome-based intervention. However, these preliminary findings so far indicate the viability and safety of FMT combined with anti-PD-1 therapy (Chervin and Gajewski, 2020).

Although FMT is one method for altering the GM to improve clinical responses to immunotherapy, certain dangers and unknowns that are associated with its application exist. Safety is the first primary concern since asymptomatic donors may contain parasites and bacteria that are harmful to humans. Furthermore, multi-drug resistant organisms (multi-drug resistant microorganisms) may be colonizing them. In June 2019, the US Food and Drug Administration (FDA) released a safety letter alerting medical practitioners to the possibility of infections that could be fatal after exploratory FMT (Hourigan et al., 2021). This safety warning was issued due to two patients who acquired significant bacterial infections after exposure to FMT, one of whom died. One of the participants was taking part in an FMT clinical study for hepatic encephalopathy treatment. The other participant was getting an allogeneic stem cell transplant for treating myelodysplastic syndrome (DeFilipp et al., 2019). These were undoubtedly complicated instances with other coexisting medical issues, but despite that, these occurrences raise concerns about FMT in patients bearing advanced cancer. Due to a lack of methods to adequately describe these species, FMT entails the transfer of not only commensal bacteria but also fungus, protozoa, viruses, and archaea (Cho and Blaser, 2012; Peterson et al., 2009). There is mounting evidence that these microbial populations as a whole have an impact on the emergence of lung diseases (Arrieta et al., 2015), neurological disorders (Vendrik et al., 2020), metabolic disorders (Yu et al., 2020; Qin et al., 2012; Le Chatelier et al., 2013;;Ridaura et al., 2013), cardiovascular diseases (Kazemian et al., 2020, Sanchez-Rodriguez et al., 2020), and psychiatric conditions (Hsiao et al., 2013). Theoretically, fecal microbiota transfer could result in undetected transmission and propensity to certain chronic health diseases, necessitating more careful donor selection and additional research to better understand the long-term health effects of FMT (Alang and Kelly, 2015; de Clercq et al., 2019). Only 3% of stool donors would meet strict criteria, according to a recent comprehensive analysis of stool donors as candidates for FMT protocols, who had undergone extensive screening for the presence of infectious pathogens subclinically in the specimen, medical conditions, or the detection of antibiotic-resistant bacteria (Kassam et al., 2019). Therefore, FMT is still under investigation, and it is predicted that future studies will require thorough donor screening (Chervin and Gajewski, 2020).

ANTIMICROBIAL PEPTIDES

The lack of new antibacterial medications and the resistance to antibiotics increased the risk of serious infections in patients receiving medical care. Antibacterial peptides (AMPs) have demonstrated considerable promise in the search for novel antibacterial approaches (Luong et al., 2020). AMPs have been extensively investigated for potential medicinal uses as well as their methods of action (Mookherjee et al., 2020; Magana et al., 2020). Until recently, most clinical studies have concentrated on its antibacterial characteristics and the possibility of topical administration. Nevertheless, numerous recent investigations suggested that AMPs have promising properties for wound healing, novel cosmetic components, and anticancer (Pfalzgraff et al., 2018; Alencar-Silva et al., 2018; da Silva et al., 2018).

Cancer cells differ structurally from healthy cells in several ways, including having a membrane with a larger negative charge because they include anionic substances including the phospholipid phosphatidylserine (PS), sialylated gangliosides, heparin sulfate, and O-glycosylated mucins. Additionally, cancer cells have fluid membranes compared to normal mammalian cells. These characteristics create a large window for anticancer peptides to act on tumor cell membranes selectively and effectively, leading to fast rupture, pore creation, ion channel alteration, and penetration (Baxter et al., 2017). Although there are many different tertiary structures, including α-helical, β-sheet, and combinations, most anticancer peptides share a few common characteristics, such as a positively charged, amphipathic structure (Ciumac et al., 2019). The mechanism underlying the selective anticancer therapy of Na-D1, derived from *Nicotiana alata*, is reported to be explained by the interaction of cationic anticancer peptides with specific lipids such as a plasma membrane phospholipid called phosphatidylinositol 4,5-bisphosphate. This binding rapidly leads the tumor cells to bleb, which results in their death (Poon et al., 2014). Additionally, Polybia-MP1 was thoroughly examined for its interactions with PS on the membrane, and it was discovered that PS affected MP1's lytic characteristics (Alvares et al., 2017a). According to a different study, MP1 might create a pore on a cell's membrane with the help of a mixture of phosphatidylethanolamine (PE) and PS lipids (Leite et al., 2015), which have a mutually beneficial interaction and together can change cancer cells' membrane (Ishii et al., 2005). The analysis of AMP and the cell membrane is efficiently aided by analyzing the interaction of AMP and artificial lipid bilayer vesicles with various lipid compositions. These investigations provided numerous insights into the real-world circumstances for developing AMPs as anticancer medications (dos Santos Cabrera et al., 2011; Alvares et al., 2017b; dos Santos Cabrera et al., 2012).

On the other hand, AMPs can internalize cells, interact with intracellular structures like mitochondria, and trigger cell apoptosis (Deslouches and Di, 2017). In addition to killing cancer cells through programmed cell death, the peptide m2386 from the lactic acid bacterium *L. casei* ATCC334 increased the expression of TRAILR1 and Fas death receptors on the cell surface of treated SW480 cells (Tsai et al., 2015). In addition, exposure to Parasporin, a non-insecticidal crystalline protein of *Bacillus thuringiensis* (Chubicka et al., 2018), Hexokinase II-derived cell-penetrating peptide (Woldetsadik et al., 2017), and other substances increased the apoptosis in cancer cells. In addition to killing cancer cells, LTX-315, a cationic antimicrobial peptide with oncolytic attributes, has been shown to alter the TME by reducing the frequency of myeloid-derived suppressor cells and immunosuppressive Tregs and elevating the frequency of polyfunctional T helper type 1/type 1 cytotoxic T cells. This finding is very encouraging for the development of anticancer immunotherapy (Yamazaki et al., 2016). Immunotherapy for cancer treatment is nearing clinical application, and AMPs are emerging as a significant part of evolutionary biology (Roudi et al., 2017; Liu et al., 2018).

VIROTHERAPY

Bacteriophage technology

Bacteriophages can be described as *Duplodnaviria* viruses that attack, infect, and reproduce inside bacteria (Rogovski et al., 2021). The therapeutic use of bacteriophages and viruses to improve ICI efficacy or reduce immune-related adverse effects (irAEs) has already been advocated, but primarily from a theoretical standpoint (Veeranarayanan et al., 2021; Foglizzo and Marchiò, 2021; Petrov et al., 2022). The production of human phage-derived anti-PD1 antibodies (Ghaderi et al., 2022) or the delivery of specific tumor antigens by manufactured phage systems (Dong et al., 2022) are two recent examples of novel efforts to build an effective adjuvant treatment platform for ICI. The growth of the MCA205 cell-line sarcoma was reported to be suppressed by the tail length tape measure protein (TMP1) in a recent study. However, this was only when *E. hirae* 13144 was treated in conjunction with cyclophosphamide or PD1 inhibitors in mice models

(Fluckiger et al., 2020; Wong et al., 2021). A current clinical trial (NCT04495153) hypothesizes that CAN-2409 viral immunotherapy may encourage T cells to enter tumor cells more deeply and subsequently increase PD-L1, improving ICI therapy.

Phage therapy has gained popularity in recent years, primarily for the treatment of serious or recurrent GI infections and the elimination of antibiotic-resistant strains of bacteria (Araya et al., 2010; Chen et al., 2017; Federici et al., 2021; Mu et al., 2021). As additional potential immunomodulatory agents, bacteriophages have been developed to increase cellular immunity and antigen recognition to provide adjuvanticity (Sartorius et al., 2015; Won et al., 2018). Despite the increasing number of initiatives in the area, there has not been any direct research on gut microbiota alteration about ICI-related irAEs and efficacy undertaken yet. Phage-mediated microbiome engineering (Paule et al., 2018; Barr, 2019; Baaziz et al., 2022) is a promising therapeutic strategy that should be prioritized in the future due to the existence of a technical platform. Hematological and metastatic cancers, as well as other forms of cancer, have all benefited from ICI treatment. A better comprehension of the function of individual bacteria will give crucial insight into GM's ever-expanding role. The control of the gut microbiota has the prospect of optimizing anticancer medicines and improving patient care as its developing impacts on immunotherapy become more apparent (Dora et al., 2023).

Oncolytic virotherapy

Oncolytic virotherapy has gained recognition as a novel potential cancer treatment in recent years. Oncolytic viruses occur naturally or they can be genetically modified to proliferate only in cancer cells and kill them without harming the healthy cells (Fukuhara et al., 2016). The notion of utilizing viruses to treat patients suffering from cancer first emerged in the 1950s (Kelly and Russell, 2007). Oncolytic viral formulations were utilized to treat a large number of cancer patients. Some of these patients had tumor shrinkage over a variety of time scales (Southam, 1960). In a study from Osaka University, treatment with non-attenuated mumps virus resulted in tumor regressions in 37 of 90 patients with terminal cancer (Asada, 1974). Researchers have since been increasingly interested in oncolytic viruses for cancer therapy. Oncolytic virotherapy encompasses two major components: (1) post infection, oncolytic viruses inhibit cancer cell protein synthesis and destroy infected cancer cells through virus self-replication; and (2) by encouraging the release of a significant amount of tumor cytokines and antigens, oncolytic viruses attract and activate immune cells that have infiltrated tumors, triggering potent anticancer immune responses (Figure 16.3) (Kaufman et al., 2015; Bai et al., 2019; Gujar et al., 2019).

Oncolytic virotherapy is a novel strategy for treating cancer and has enormous potential and offers cancer sufferers new hope (Li et al., 2020). Newcastle disease virus, herpes simplex virus type 1 (HSV-1), oncolytic pox virus, oncolytic adenovirus, and reovirus are currently the most frequently used oncolytic viruses. Numerous naturally occurring and genetically altered oncolytic viruses have been created and are currently in the clinical research stages (Russell et al., 2012). However, biosafety concerns continue to be significant. The main issue with oncolytic virotherapy is the possibility of unchecked reproduction *in vivo* and transmission to patients' contacts, including medical professionals, and other patients (Robilotti et al., 2019). The following three factors could be considered to increase the biosafety of oncolytic virotherapy:

1) The first strategy entails choosing viruses that do not infect healthy tissues. Since rats are the parvovirus's natural host, its anticellulosic selectivity renders it non-pathogenic to humans, with minimal selectivity for benign human tumor cells. The overexpression of transcription factors and cytokines in tumor cells can activate a metabolic pathway that controls the function of Non-structural protein 1 (NS1), a necessary protein for viral gene expression, DNA replication, and cytotoxic effects. In return, these factors can make parvoviruses more tumor-selective (Geletneky et al., 2012; Angelova et al., 2015). Furthermore, reovirus has little to no pathogenicity in people, and continuous subculturing can lessen its toxicity in normal cells (Comins et al., 2010; Yamaguchi and Uchida, 2018). According to Kaid and colleagues, ZIKVBR has the potential to treat CNS embryonal tumors because it can specifically and efficiently kill CNS tumor cells without harming healthy cells or other types of tumor cells. In clinical trials, ZIKVBR also produced moderate infectious cases involving adults and infants (Kaid et al., 2018).

2) The second strategy, which has been employed in numerous research, entails genetically modifying oncolytic viruses to lessen their pathogenicity to normal cells. The ICP-34.5 gene in HSV1716, which is a neurovirulence factor of HSV, was removed to develop oncolytic HSV-1 medicines, such as T-VEC and G207, which reduce HSV's infectivity in normal neurons (Varghese et al., 2001; Maroun et al., 2017; Lundstrom, 2018; Wang et al., 2019b; Kelly et al., 2008). The H10 and Onyx-015 viruses were genetically modified to include a mutation or deletion of the E1 gene, which can decrease the selectivity of healthy cells against adenoviruses (Kimball et al., 2010; Wei et al., 2009). Furthermore, to increase the oncolytic adenovirus's infectivity in tumor cells, the arg-gly-asp (RGD) sequence was inserted into the HI loop of the adenovirus capsid protein through genetic modification (Kimball et al., 2010; Jung et al., 2015). It was reported that the binding of coagulation factor (F) × to hypervariable regions (HVR) may be the source of the amplified liver infection caused by adenovirus. Therefore, oncolytic adenovirus liver tropism can be greatly decreased by introducing mutations into the FX-binding domain of the HVR and swapping them out with HVRs from different serotypes of the original adenovirus (Yamamoto et al., 2017). It is possible to

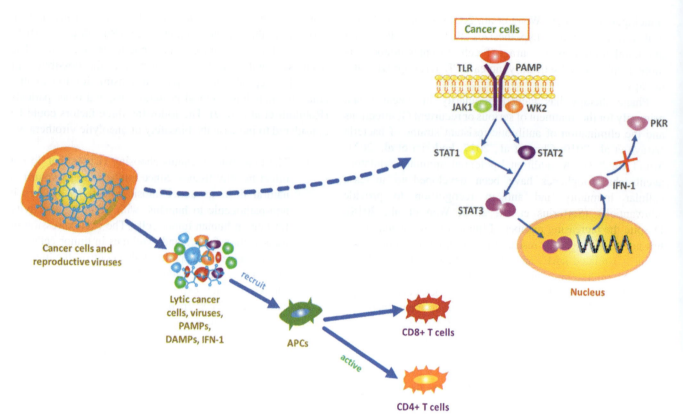

FIGURE 16.3 **The oncolytic virotherapy mechanism.** When oncolytic viruses infect a healthy cell, they engage with TLRs and PAMPs to activate the NF-kB or JAK-STAT pathways, which results in the production and release of IFN-1. Subsequently, PKR is triggered by IFN-1 and plays an important role in controlling aberrant cell division and natural defense mechanisms against viruses. On the other hand, interferon signaling, and PKR activity are suppressed when oncolytic viruses target cancer cells; as a result, virus clearance is impeded, permitting virus reproduction. Majority of oncolytic viruses can trigger cell death after virus replication, thereby producing viral PAMPs, extracellular DAMPs, and cytokines in addition to tumor-linked antigens that can stimulate an adaptive immune response. These secreted chemicals attract and facilitate the maturation of APCs, which in turn triggers antigen-specific CD8+ and CD4+ T cell responses. This allows CD8+ T cells to proliferate into cytotoxic effector cells, subsequently inducing antitumor immunity. APCs, Antigen-presenting cells; TLRs, Toll-like receptors; PAMPs, pathogen-associated molecular patterns; IFN-1, Type 1 interferon; PKR, interferon-induced double-stranded RNA-dependent protein kinase; DAMPs, danger-associated molecular pattern signals; JAK1, Janus kinase 1; STAT, signal transducer and activator of transcription.

significantly lessen the virulence of the oncolytic pox virus in normal cells by deleting genes including TK, VGF, hemagglutinin, and B18R (Waters et al., 2016; Zeh et al., 2015; Futami et al., 2017).

3) The third strategy entails the therapeutic recombination of various oncolytic virus types. Newcastle disease virus (NDV) and vesicular stomatitis virus (VSV) were combined to create recombinant VSV-NDV (rVSV-NDV), which was not harmful to developing eggs and significantly decreased cytotoxicity in healthy hepatocytes and neurons. The VSV's structure is preserved in the rVSV-NDV. However, hemagglutinin-neuraminidase (HN) and the NVD envelope proteins take the place of its glycoprotein. The substitution of the glycoprotein considerably reduced the unfavorable events brought on by the off-target effects in the brain and liver that were noted during the trials of wild-type VSV (Abdullahi et al., 2018). Recombinant oncolytic viral therapies, like those based on adenovirus-coxsackie virus and adenovirus parvovirus, frequently involve adenoviruses (Coughlan et al., 2012). Recombinant parvoviruses and adenoviruses attack tumor cells while sparing healthy cells by maintaining the parvovirus' harmlessness and the adenovirus' infectivity in healthy cells (Marchini et al., 2015).

Three oncolytic virus therapeutics have so far been authorized for use in cancer treatment. In 2004, the unmodified Echo virus called Rigvir (also known as the Rigvir virus) was given the green light for treating melanoma (Alberts et al., 2018). In China and the rest of the world, Oncorine, an attenuated adenovirus, was the first oncolytic virus to receive clinical approval in 2005. This was for the treatment of head and neck malignancies in conjunction with chemotherapy (Russell and Peng, 2018). The European Union later approved T-VEC which is a recombinant human HSV-1 that is used to treat locally advanced or metastatic cutaneous melanoma.

T-VEC was initially licensed by the US FDA in 2015 for treating unresectable metastatic melanoma (Bommareddy et al., 2017). Clinical research is actively addressing the efficacy of oncolytic viruses on different types of cancers, including lung, pancreatic, liver, breast, ovarian, prostate, and bladder cancer, although nothing is known about it (Russell et al., 2012). Oncolytic virotherapy is effective against several refractory malignant tumors, including triple-negative breast cancer and glioblastoma, according to recent clinical research (Delwar et al., 2018; Bourgeois-Daigneault et al., 2018; Martikainen and Essand, 2019).

Recent advances in genetic engineering and synthetic biology have resulted in the introduction of newer and more selective strategies for use to modify gut microbiota (Sugimura et al., 2022). Among the newer strategies are gene editing (Cullin et al., 2021), DNA conjugation technology (Dorado-Morales et al., 2023), synthetic polymers (Kuroda and Caputo, 2013), nanomedicines (Lee et al., 2021), bacterial vaccine (Anderson et al., 2019), phage therapy (Soendergaard et al., 2014), and virotherapy (Kwan et al., 2021). Conjugation-based manipulation of gut microbiota involves mixing the DNA of bacteria by transferring it from one bacterium to another (Dorado-Morales et al., 2023). Manipulation of dysbiosis of the local or GM is especially useful during the management of cancers that were historically not treatable or have acquired resistance to standard treatment. Figure 16.4 below summarizes strategies that are available for use to manipulate the microbiome.

Overall, microbiomes may play a critical role in the development, progression, and response to treatment of some cancers. Manipulation of the microbiota of the gut and the local tumor environment may be helpful during management of the commonly occurring cancers, especially their aggressive variants, which are resistant to surgery, immunotherapy, chemotherapy, and targeted therapy. Manipulation of the microbiome and/or oncolytic virotherapy is also useful as an adjuvant to standard cancer therapy.

PROSPECTS AND CHALLENGES FOR THE STUDY OF MICROBIOMES IN CANCER

Opportunities to enhance patient care at distinct phases of the cancer journey, such as diagnosis, screening, and risk assessment before and during treatment, may be provided by the GM. A crucial need for more thorough and standardized multi-omics studies is highlighted by the inconsistent beneficial microbiome signatures across studies and the growing understanding of the processes underlying the interactions between the metabolome, microbiome, and host immune system. Interventional trials to control the GM and enhance responses in ICI patient groups have been prompted by several ICI studies. However, additional research is needed

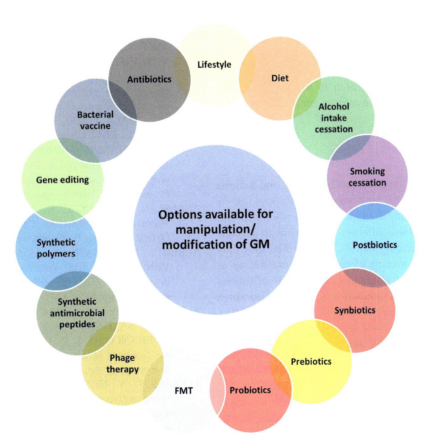

FIGURE 16.4 A schematic diagram showing various strategies that can be utilized to manipulate or modify the GM. These include diet, prebiotics, probiotics, synbiotics, postbiotics, fecal microbial transplant (FMT), etc.

to address other tumor subtypes, including those with fewer established connections to the GM. Large-scale prospective clinical trials with nutritional evaluations are certainly required (Lee et al., 2021).

Considering the extremely individualized reactions to diet that are observed across individuals (Berry et al., 2020), as well as the strong correlation between diet and GM, a tailored approach based on the GM composition of individual patients would be necessary. Finding very accurate prediction microbial biosignatures for different disease states has been the holy grail of onco-microbial research. The individual microbial composition has received more attention in the investigation of GM in relation to human disease than the functional output, especially when it comes to cancer. Metabolomics is expected to become more important in microbiome science in the upcoming years, since the identification of important metabolic markers and pathways may indicate the functional output of the GM (Lee et al., 2021).

Modifications to the gut microbiota's composition may make individuals more vulnerable to certain health issues. There is growing evidence of a connection between the gut, the intestinal microbiota, and the central nervous system. FMT from a healthy person to a person with a mental illness can be therapeutically beneficial. Nevertheless, the opposite may also be true, carrying a danger of unintentionally increasing the likelihood that an FMT recipient will experience a mental consequence or, in the worst-case scenario, cause one. Furthermore, the gastrointestinal system is the site of origin for numerous infections in immunocompromised and neutropenic patients. The pathogenesis of these diseases is frequently unknown, but it begins with their modification or disruption due to antibiotic use and host immune impairment. It is still clear that additional clinical research is warranted to fully understand how GM modulation affects immunosuppression (Lee et al., 2021).

CONCLUSION

Microorganisms such as fungi, viruses, protozoa, and bacteria reside on every surface of the body and impact multiple facets of host physiology, including immune system development and metabolism. They might use different mechanisms to advance or play a dual role in treating tumors. Specifically, they may facilitate or hinder the growth of tumors by preventing or encouraging pro-tumor inflammation, in turn. Modifications in the environment or the host can result in dysbiosis, which affects the occurrence and course of diseases like cancer. The utilization of antibiotics without discrimination exacerbates the risk of cancer development and progression by lowering microbial diversity, encouraging pathogen colonization, and eradicating beneficial bacteria. Therefore, it is advantageous to maintain the ideal microbiota composition by restoring normal flora through the utilization of probiotic supplements or other dietary strategies. Additionally, the development of novel anti-bacterial techniques (e.g. nanomedicine) and more pathogen-specific antibiotics with restricted spectrums contribute to the preservation of eubiosis (Bhatt et al., 2017; Chaurasia et al., 2016).

There is a bidirectional link between the gastrointestinal microbiota and the development of some cancers. This means that the microbiota of the tumor influences the growth of the tumor and vice versa. Therefore, it would be beneficial to look into the microbial community as a predictor of carcinogenesis and response to therapy, regardless of whether the dysbiosis in the gut is the result of cancer or its cause. Furthermore, any modifications to the diversity or population of microflora may have an impact on the clinical results of anticancer therapies since they may be involved in influencing the curative efficacy of these treatments and mitigating their side effects. Despite extensive study in this area, only a limited number of prospective research studies have demonstrated the causal role of microbiota in tumorigenesis. Therefore, further research is warranted to ascertain the mechanisms by which bacteria contribute to carcinogenesis and subsequently inhibit it. Despite tremendous progress in the area, not all patients react to cancer treatment in the same way. These differences may, at least in part, be explained by the variety of the microbial community. Therefore, improving the therapeutic response can involve identifying the bacterial species implicated and modifying the microbiome by dietary changes, FMT, and antibiotic administration.

REFERENCES

ABDULLAHI, S., JÄKEL, M., BEHREND, S. J., STEIGER, K., TOPPING, G., KRABBE, T., COLOMBO, A., SANDIG, V., SCHIERGENS, T. S. & THASLER, W. E. 2018. A novel chimeric oncolytic virus vector for improved safety and efficacy as a platform for the treatment of hepatocellular carcinoma. *Journal of Virology,* 92, 10.1128/jvi. 01386–18.

AGUILAR-TOALÁ, J., HALL, F., URBIZO-REYES, U., GARCIA, H., VALLEJO-CORDOBA, B., GONZÁLEZ-CÓRDOVA, A., HERNÁNDEZ-MENDOZA, A. & LICEAGA, A. 2020. In silico prediction and in vitro assessment of multifunctional properties of postbiotics obtained from two probiotic bacteria. *Probiotics and Antimicrobial Proteins,* 12, 608–622.

ALANG, N. & KELLY, C. R. 2015. *Weight Gain after Fecal Microbiota Transplantation. Open Forum Infectious Diseases,* Oxford University Press, ofv004.

ALBERTS, P., TILGASE, A., RASA, A., BANDERE, K. & VENSKUS, D. 2018. The advent of oncolytic virotherapy in oncology: The Rigvir® story. *European Journal of Pharmacology,* 837, 117–126.

ALENCAR-SILVA, T., BRAGA, M. C., SANTANA, G. O. S., SALDANHA-ARAUJO, F., POGUE, R., DIAS, S. C., FRANCO, O. L. & CARVALHO, J. L. 2018. Breaking the frontiers of cosmetology with antimicrobial peptides. *Biotechnology Advances,* 36, 2019–2031.

ALVARES, D. S., NETO, J. R. & AMBROGGIO, E. E. 2017a. Phosphatidylserine lipids and membrane order precisely regulate the activity of Polybia-MP1 peptide. *Biochimica et Biophysica Acta (BBA)-Biomembranes,* 1859, 1067–1074.

ALVARES, D. S., WILKE, N., NETO, J. R. & FANANI, M. L. 2017b. The insertion of Polybia-MP1 peptide into phospholipid monolayers is regulated by its anionic nature and phase state. *Chemistry and Physics of Lipids,* 207, 38–48.

ANDERSON, K. J., CORMIER, R. T. & SCOTT, P. M. 2019. Role of ion channels in gastrointestinal cancer. *World Journal of Gastroenterology,* 25, 5732.

ANGELOVA, A. L., GELETNEKY, K., NÜESCH, J. P. & ROMMELAERE, J. 2015. Tumor selectivity of oncolytic parvoviruses: from in vitro and animal models to cancer patients. *Frontiers in Bioengineering and Biotechnology,* 3, 55.

ARAYA, D. V., QUIROZ, T. S., TOBAR, H. E., LIZANA, R. J., QUEZADA, C. P., SANTIVIAGO, C. A., RIEDEL, C. A., KALERGIS, A. M. & BUENO, S. M. 2010. Deletion of a prophage-like element causes attenuation of Salmonella enterica serovar Enteritidis and promotes protective immunity. *Vaccine,* 28, 5458–5466.

ARONIADIS, O. C., BRANDT, L. J., ONETO, C., FEUERSTADT, P., SHERMAN, A., WOLKOFF, A. W., KASSAM, Z., SADOVSKY, R. G., ELLIOTT, R. J. & BUDREE, S. 2019. Faecal microbiota transplantation for diarrhoea-predominant irritable bowel syndrome: a double-blind, randomised, placebo-controlled trial. *The Lancet Gastroenterology & Hepatology,* 4, 675–685.

ARRIETA, M.-C., STIEMSMA, L. T., DIMITRIU, P. A., THORSON, L., RUSSELL, S., YURIST-DOUTSCH, S., KUZELJEVIC, B., GOLD, M. J., BRITTON, H. M. & LEFEBVRE, D. L. 2015. Early infancy microbial and metabolic alterations affect risk of childhood asthma. *Science Translational Medicine,* 7, 307ra152–307ra152.

ASADA, T. 1974. Treatment of human cancer with mumps virus. *Cancer,* 34, 1907–1928.

BAAZIZ, H., BAKER, Z. R., FRANKLIN, H. C. & HSU, B. B. 2022. Rehabilitation of a misbehaving microbiome: Phages for the remodeling of bacterial composition and function. *Iscience.*

BAI, Y., HUI, P., DU, X. & SU, X. 2019. Updates to the antitumor mechanism of oncolytic virus. *Thoracic Cancer,* 10, 1031–1035.

BARR, J. J. 2019. Precision engineers: bacteriophages modulate the gut microbiome and metabolome. *Cell Host & Microbe,* 25, 771–773.

BARUCH, E. N., YOUNGSTER, I., ORTENBERG, R., BEN-BETZALEL, G., KATZ, L. H., LAHAT, A., BARSHACK, I., DICK-NECULA, D., MAMTANI, R. & BLOCH, N. 2019. Abstract CT042: fecal microbiota transplantation (FMT) and re-induction of anti-PD-1 therapy in refractory metastatic melanoma patients-preliminary results from a phase I clinical trial (NCT03353402). *Cancer Research,* 79, CT042-CT042.

BATISTA, V. L., DA SILVA, T. F., DE JESUS, L. C. L., COELHO-ROCHA, N. D., BARROSO, F. A. L., TAVARES, L. M., AZEVEDO, V., MANCHA-AGRESTI, P. & DRUMOND, M. M. 2020. Probiotics, prebiotics, synbiotics, and paraprobiotics as a therapeutic alternative for intestinal mucositis. *Frontiers in Microbiology,* 11, 544490.

BAXTER, A. A., LAY, F. T., POON, I. K., KVANSAKUL, M. & HULETT, M. D. 2017. Tumor cell membrane-targeting cationic antimicrobial peptides: novel insights into mechanisms of action and therapeutic prospects. *Cellular and Molecular Life Sciences,* 74, 3809–3825.

BERRY, S. E., VALDES, A. M., DREW, D. A., ASNICAR, F., MAZIDI, M., WOLF, J., CAPDEVILA, J., HADJIGEORGIOU, G., DAVIES, R. & AL KHATIB, H. 2020. Human postprandial responses to food and potential for precision nutrition. *Nature medicine,* 26, 964–973.

BHATT, A. P., REDINBO, M. R. & BULTMAN, S. J. 2017. The role of the microbiome in cancer development and therapy. *CA: A Cancer Journal for Clinicians,* 67, 326–344.

BOMMAREDDY, P. K., PATEL, A., HOSSAIN, S. & KAUFMAN, H. L. 2017. Talimogene laherparepvec (T-VEC) and other oncolytic viruses for the treatment of melanoma. *American Journal of Clinical Dermatology,* 18, 1–15.

BOURGEOIS-DAIGNEAULT, M.-C., ROY, D. G., AITKEN, A. S., EL SAYES, N., MARTIN, N. T., VARETTE, O., FALLS, T., ST-GERMAIN, L. E., PELIN, A. & LICHTY, B. D. 2018. Neoadjuvant oncolytic virotherapy before surgery sensitizes triple-negative breast cancer to immune checkpoint therapy. *Science Translational Medicine,* 10, eaao1641.

BREVI, A., COGROSSI, L. L., LORENZONI, M., MATTORRE, B. & BELLONE, M. 2022. The insider: Impact of the gut microbiota on cancer immunity and response to therapies in multiple myeloma. *Frontiers in Immunology,* 13, 845422.

BULTMAN, S. J. & JOBIN, C. 2014. Microbial-derived butyrate: an oncometabolite or tumor-suppressive metabolite? *Cell Host & Microbe,* 16, 143–145.

CAI, J., SUN, L. & GONZALEZ, F. J. 2022. Gut microbiota-derived bile acids in intestinal immunity, inflammation, and tumorigenesis. *Cell Host & Microbe,* 30, 289–300.

CAMMAROTA, G. & IANIRO, G. 2019. FMT for ulcerative colitis: closer to the turning point. *Nature Reviews Gastroenterology & Hepatology,* 16, 266–268.

CANI, P. D., POSSEMIERS, S., VAN DE WIELE, T., GUIOT, Y., EVERARD, A., ROTTIER, O., GEURTS, L., NASLAIN, D., NEYRINCK, A. & LAMBERT, D. M. 2009. Changes in gut microbiota control inflammation in obese mice through a mechanism involving GLP-2-driven improvement of gut permeability. *Gut,* 58, 1091–1103.

CHAPUT, N., LEPAGE, P., COUTZAC, C., SOULARUE, E., LE ROUX, K., MONOT, C., BOSELLI, L., ROUTIER, E., CASSARD, L. & COLLINS, M. 2017. Baseline gut microbiota predicts clinical response and colitis in metastatic melanoma patients treated with ipilimumab. *Annals of Oncology,* 28, 1368–1379.

CHAURASIA, A. K., THORAT, N. D., TANDON, A., KIM, J.-H., PARK, S. H. & KIM, K. K. 2016. Coupling of radiofrequency with magnetic nanoparticles treatment as an alternative physical antibacterial strategy against multiple drug resistant bacteria. *Scientific Reports,* 6, 33662.

CHEN, F., JIANG, R., WANG, Y., ZHU, M., ZHANG, X., DONG, S., SHI, H. & WANG, L. 2017. Recombinant phage elicits protective immune response against systemic S. globosa infection in mouse model. *Scientific Reports,* 7, 42024.

CHERVIN, C. S. & GAJEWSKI, T. 2020. Microbiome-based interventions: therapeutic strategies in cancer immunotherapy. *Immuno-Oncology Technology,* 8, 12–20.

CHEUNG, K.-S. & LEUNG, W. K. 2018. Risk of gastric cancer development after eradication of Helicobacter pylori. *World Journal of Gastrointestinal Oncology,* 10, 115.

CHO, I. & BLASER, M. J. 2012. The human microbiome: at the interface of health and disease. *Nature Reviews Genetics,* 13, 260–270.

CHRYSOSTOMOU, D., ROBERTS, L. A., MARCHESI, J. R. & KINROSS, J. M. 2023. Gut microbiota modulation of efficacy and toxicity of cancer chemotherapy and immunotherapy. *Gastroenterology*, 164, 198–213.

CHUBICKA, T., GIRIJA, D., DEEPA, K., SALINI, S., MEERA, N., RAGHAVAMENON, A. C., DIVYA, M. K. & BABU, T. D. 2018. A parasporin from Bacillus thuringiensis native to Peninsular India induces apoptosis in cancer cells through intrinsic pathway. *Journal of Biosciences*, 43, 407–416.

CIUMAC, D., GONG, H., HU, X. & LU, J. R. 2019. Membrane targeting cationic antimicrobial peptides. *Journal of Colloid and Interface Science*, 537, 163–185.

COHEN, S. H., GERDING, D. N., JOHNSON, S., KELLY, C. P., LOO, V. G., MCDONALD, L. C., PEPIN, J. & WILCOX, M. H. 2010. Clinical practice guidelines for Clostridium difficile infection in adults: 2010 update by the society for healthcare epidemiology of America (SHEA) and the infectious diseases society of America (IDSA). *Infection Control & Hospital Epidemiology*, 31, 431–455.

COMERLATO, C. B., ZHANG, X., WALKER, K., BRANDELLI, A. & FIGEYS, D. 2020. Comparative proteomic analysis reveals metabolic variability of probiotic Enterococcus durans during aerobic and anaerobic cultivation. *Journal of Proteomics*, 220, 103764.

COMINS, C., SPICER, J., PROTHEROE, A., ROULSTONE, V., TWIGGER, K., WHITE, C. M., VILE, R., MELCHER, A., COFFEY, M. C. & METTINGER, K. L. 2010. REO-10: A phase I study of intravenous reovirus and docetaxel in patients with advanced cancer. *Clinical Cancer Research*, 16, 5564–5572.

COSTELLO, S. P., HUGHES, P. A., WATERS, O., BRYANT, R. V., VINCENT, A. D., BLATCHFORD, P., KATSIKEROS, R., MAKANYANGA, J., CAMPANIELLO, M. A. & MAVRANGELOS, C. 2019. Effect of fecal microbiota transplantation on 8-week remission in patients with ulcerative colitis: a randomized clinical trial. *Jama*, 321, 156–164.

COUGHLAN, L., VALLATH, S., GROS, A., GIMÉNEZ-ALEJANDRE, M., VAN ROOIJEN, N., THOMAS, G. J., BAKER, A. H., CASCALLÓ, M., ALEMANY, R. & HART, I. R. 2012. Combined fiber modifications both to target αvβ6 and detarget the coxsackievirus–adenovirus receptor improve virus toxicity profiles in vivo but fail to improve antitumoral efficacy relative to adenovirus serotype 5. *Human Gene Therapy*, 23, 960–979.

CULLIN, N., ANTUNES, C. A., STRAUSSMAN, R., STEIN-THOERINGER, C. K. & ELINAV, E. 2021. Microbiome and cancer. *Cancer Cell*, 39, 1317–1341.

D'ANGELO, C. R., SUDAKARAN, S. & CALLANDER, N. S. 2021. Clinical effects and applications of the gut microbiome in hematologic malignancies. *Cancer*, 127, 679–687.

DA SILVA, A. M. B., SILVA-GONÇALVES, L. C., OLIVEIRA, F. A. & ARCISIO-MIRANDA, M. 2018. Pro-necrotic activity of cationic mastoparan peptides in human glioblastoma multiforme cells via membranolytic action. *Molecular Neurobiology*, 55, 5490–5504.

DAVID, L. A., MAURICE, C. F., CARMODY, R. N., GOOTENBERG, D. B., BUTTON, J. E., WOLFE, B. E., LING, A. V., DEVLIN, A. S., VARMA, Y. & FISCHBACH, M. A. 2014. Diet rapidly and reproducibly alters the human gut microbiome. *Nature*, 505, 559–563.

DE CLERCQ, N. C., FRISSEN, M. N., DAVIDS, M., GROEN, A. K. & NIEUWDORP, M. 2019. Weight gain after fecal microbiota transplantation in a patient with recurrent underweight following clinical recovery from anorexia nervosa. *Psychotherapy and Psychosomatics*, 88, 58–60.

DE GUNZBURG, J., GHOZLANE, A., DUCHER, A., LE CHATELIER, E., DUVAL, X., RUPPÉ, E., ARMAND-LEFEVRE, L., SABLIER-GALLIS, F., BURDET, C. & ALAVOINE, L. 2018. Protection of the human gut microbiome from antibiotics. *The Journal of Infectious Diseases*, 217, 628–636.

DE SIMONE, C. 2019. The unregulated probiotic market. *Clinical Gastroenterology and Hepatology*, 17, 809–817.

DEFILIPP, Z., BLOOM, P. P., TORRES SOTO, M., MANSOUR, M. K., SATER, M. R., HUNTLEY, M. H., TURBETT, S., CHUNG, R. T., CHEN, Y.-B. & HOHMANN, E. L. 2019. Drug-resistant E. coli bacteremia transmitted by fecal microbiota transplant. *New England Journal of Medicine*, 381, 2043–2050.

DELWAR, Z. M., KUO, Y., WEN, Y. H., RENNIE, P. S. & JIA, W. 2018. Oncolytic virotherapy blockade by microglia and macrophages requires STAT1/3. *Cancer research*, 78, 718–730.

DESLOUCHES, B. & DI, Y. P. 2017. Antimicrobial peptides with selective antitumor mechanisms: prospect for anticancer applications. *Oncotarget*, 8, 46635.

DIETERICH, L. C. & BIKFALVI, A. The tumor organismal environment: Role in tumor development and cancer immunotherapy. *Seminars in cancer biology*, 2020. Elsevier, 197–206.

DONG, H., QI, Y., KONG, X., WANG, Z., FANG, Y. & WANG, J. 2022. PD-1/PD-L1 inhibitor-associated myocarditis: epidemiology, characteristics, diagnosis, treatment, and potential mechanism. *Frontiers in Pharmacology*, 13, 835510.

DONO, A., NICKLES, J., RODRIGUEZ-ARMENDARIZ, A. G., MCFARLAND, B. C., AJAMI, N. J., BALLESTER, L. Y., WARGO, J. A. & ESQUENAZI, Y. 2022. Glioma and the gut–brain axis: opportunities and future perspectives. *Neuro-Oncology Advances*, 4, vdac054.

DORA, D., BOKHARI, S. M. Z., ALOSS, K., TAKACS, P., DESNOIX, J. Z., SZKLENÁRIK, G., HURLEY, P. D. & LOHINAI, Z. 2023. Implication of the Gut Microbiome and Microbial-Derived Metabolites in Immune-Related Adverse Events: Emergence of Novel Biomarkers for Cancer Immunotherapy. *International Journal of Molecular Sciences*, 24, 2769.

DORADO-MORALES, P., LAMBÉRIOUX, M. & MAZEL, D. 2023. Unlocking the potential of microbiome editing: A review of conjugation-based delivery. *Molecular Microbiology* 00, 1–11.

DOS SANTOS CABRERA, M. P., ALVARES, D. S., LEITE, N. B., MONSON DE SOUZA, B., PALMA, M. S., RISKE, K. A. & RUGGIERO NETO, J. O. 2011. New insight into the mechanism of action of wasp mastoparan peptides: lytic activity and clustering observed with giant vesicles. *Langmuir*, 27, 10805–10813.

DOS SANTOS CABRERA, M. P., ARCISIO-MIRANDA, M., GORJAO, R., LEITE, N. B., DE SOUZA, B. M., CURI, R., PROCOPIO, J., RUGGIERO NETO, J. & PALMA, M. S. 2012. Influence of the bilayer composition on the binding and membrane disrupting effect of Polybia-MP1, an antimicrobial mastoparan peptide with leukemic T-lymphocyte cell selectivity. *Biochemistry*, 51, 4898–4908.

ELKRIEF, A., DEROSA, L., KROEMER, G., ZITVOGEL, L. & ROUTY, B. 2019. The negative impact of antibiotics on outcomes in cancer patients treated with immunotherapy: a new independent prognostic factor? *Annals of Oncology,* 30, 1572–1579.

ENGEVIK, M. A., RUAN, W., ESPARZA, M., FULTZ, R., SHI, Z., ENGEVIK, K. A., ENGEVIK, A. C., IHEKWEAZU, F. D., VISUTHRANUKUL, C. & VENABLE, S. 2021. Immunomodulation of dendritic cells by Lactobacillus reuteri surface components and metabolites. *Physiological Reports,* 9, e14719.

FANG, S.-B., SHIH, H.-Y., HUANG, C.-H., LI, L.-T., CHEN, C.-C. & FANG, H.-W. 2014. Live and heat-killed Lactobacillus rhamnosus GG upregulate gene expression of pro-inflammatory cytokines in 5-fluorouracil-pretreated Caco-2 cells. *Supportive Care in Cancer,* 22, 1647–1654.

FAUBERT, B., SOLMONSON, A. & DEBERARDINIS, R. J. 2020. Metabolic reprogramming and cancer progression. *Science,* 368, eaaw5473.

FEDERICI, S., NOBS, S. P. & ELINAV, E. 2021. Phages and their potential to modulate the microbiome and immunity. *Cellular & Molecular Immunology,* 18, 889–904.

FLUCKIGER, A., DAILLERE, R., SASSI, M., SIXT, B. S., LIU, P., LOOS, F., RICHARD, C., RABU, C., ALOU, M. T. & GOUBET, A.-G. 2020. Cross-reactivity between tumor MHC class I–restricted antigens and an enterococcal bacteriophage. *Science,* 369, 936–942.

FOGLIZZO, V. & MARCHIÒ, S. 2021. Bacteriophages as therapeutic and diagnostic vehicles in cancer. *Pharmaceuticals,* 14, 161.

FONG, W., LI, Q. & YU, J. 2020. Gut microbiota modulation: A novel strategy for prevention and treatment of colorectal cancer. *Oncogene,* 39, 4925–4943.

FUKUHARA, H., INO, Y. & TODO, T. 2016. Oncolytic virus therapy: A new era of cancer treatment at dawn. *Cancer science,* 107, 1373–1379.

FURFARO, L.L., PAYNE, M.S., CHANG, B.J. Bacteriophage Therapy: Clinical Trials and Regulatory Hurdles. Frontiers in Cellular and Infection Microbiology 2018, 8, 376.

FUTAMI, M., SATO, K., MIYAZAKI, K., SUZUKI, K., NAKAMURA, T. & TOJO, A. 2017. Efficacy and safety of doubly-regulated vaccinia virus in a mouse xenograft model of multiple myeloma. *Molecular Therapy-Oncolytics,* 6, 57–68.

G, T. 2019. *The microbiome in cancer therapy.* AACR Annual Meeting 2019, 01 April 2019 2019 Atlanta, Georgia. AACR.

GAN, B. H., GAYNORD, J., ROWE, S. M., DEINGRUBER, T. & SPRING, D. R. 2021. The multifaceted nature of antimicrobial peptides: Current synthetic chemistry approaches and future directions. *Chemical Society Reviews,* 50, 7820–7880.

GARCIA-PERIS, P., VELASCO, C., HERNANDEZ, M., LOZANO, M., PARON, L., DE LA CUERDA, C., BRETON, I., CAMBLOR, M. & GUARNER, F. 2016. Effect of inulin and fructo-oligosaccharide on the prevention of acute radiation enteritis in patients with gynecological cancer and impact on quality-of-life: a randomized, double-blind, placebo-controlled trial. *European Journal of Clinical Nutrition,* 70, 170–174.

GARRETT, W. S. 2015. Cancer and the microbiota. *Science,* 348, 80–86.

GELETNEKY, K., HUESING, J., ROMMELAERE, J., SCHLEHOFER, J. R., LEUCHS, B., DAHM, M., KREBS, O., VON KNEBEL DOEBERITZ, M., HUBER, B. & HAJDA, J. 2012. Phase I/IIa study of intratumoral/intracerebral or intravenous/intracerebral administration of Parvovirus H-1 (ParvOryx) in patients with progressive primary or recurrent glioblastoma multiforme: ParvOryx01 protocol. *BMC Cancer,* 12, 1–9.

GELLER, L. T., BARZILY-ROKNI, M., DANINO, T., JONAS, O. H., SHENTAL, N., NEJMAN, D., GAVERT, N., ZWANG, Y., COOPER, Z. A. & SHEE, K. 2017. Potential role of intratumor bacteria in mediating tumor resistance to the chemotherapeutic drug gemcitabine. *Science,* 357, 1156–1160.

GEORGIOU, K., MARINOV, B., FAROOQI, A. A. & GAZOULI, M. 2021. Gut microbiota in lung cancer: where do we stand? *International Journal of Molecular Sciences,* 22, 10429.

GHADERI, S. S., RIAZI-RAD, F., QAMSARI, E. S., BAGHERI, S., RAHIMI-JAMNANI, F. & SHARIFZADEH, Z. 2022. Development of a human phage display-derived anti-PD-1 scFv antibody: An attractive tool for immune checkpoint therapy. *BMC Biotechnology,* 22, 1–12.

GILBERT, J. A., BLASER, M. J., CAPORASO, J. G., JANSSON, J. K., LYNCH, S. V. & KNIGHT, R. 2018. Current understanding of the human microbiome. *Nature Medicine,* 24, 392–400.

GOLDENBERG, J. Z., YAP, C., LYTVYN, L., LO, C. K. F., BEARDSLEY, J., MERTZ, D. & JOHNSTON, B. C. 2017. Probiotics for the prevention of Clostridium difficile-associated diarrhea in adults and children. *Cochrane Database of Systematic Reviews,* 12(12), 1–156.

GOPALAKRISHNAN, V., SPENCER, C. N., NEZI, L., REUBEN, A., ANDREWS, M., KARPINETS, T., PRIETO, P., VICENTE, D., HOFFMAN, K. & WEI, S. C. 2018. Gut microbiome modulates response to anti–PD-1 immunotherapy in melanoma patients. *Science,* 359, 97–103.

GUARNER, F., HERNÁNDEZ, M., GARCÍA-PERIS, P., VELASCO, C., LOZANO, M., MORENO, Y., PARON, L., DE LA CUERDA, C., BRETÓN, I. & CAMBLOR, M. 2012. Effect of a mixture of inulin and fructo-oligosaccharide on lactobacillus and bifidobacterium intestinal microbiota of patients receiving radiotherapy; a randomised, double-blind, placebo-controlled trial. *Nutricion Hospitalaria,* 27, 1908–1915.

GUENTHER, M., HAAS, M., HEINEMANN, V., KRUGER, S., WESTPHALEN, C. B., VON BERGWELT-BAILDON, M., MAYERLE, J., WERNER, J., KIRCHNER, T. & BOECK, S. 2020. Bacterial lipopolysaccharide as negative predictor of gemcitabine efficacy in advanced pancreatic cancer–translational results from the AIO-PK0104 Phase 3 study. *British Journal of Cancer,* 123, 1370–1376.

GUJAR, S., BELL, J. & DIALLO, J.-S. 2019. SnapShot: cancer immunotherapy with oncolytic viruses. *Cell,* 176, 1240–1240. e1.

HAMDI, Y., ABDELJAOUED-TEJ, I., ZATCHI, A. A., ABDELHAK, S., BOUBAKER, S., BROWN, J. S. & BENKAHLA, A. 2021. Cancer in Africa: the untold story. *Frontiers in Oncology,* 11, 650117.

HEMPEL, S., NEWBERRY, S. J., MAHER, A. R., WANG, Z., MILES, J. N., SHANMAN, R., JOHNSEN, B. & SHEKELLE, P. G. 2012. Probiotics for the prevention and treatment of antibiotic-associated diarrhea: a systematic review and meta-analysis. *Jama,* 307, 1959–1969.

HERFEL, T. M., JACOBI, S. K., LIN, X., FELLNER, V., WALKER, D. C., JOUNI, Z. E. & ODLE, J. 2011. Polydextrose enrichment of infant formula demonstrates prebiotic characteristics by altering intestinal microbiota, organic acid concentrations, and cytokine expression in suckling piglets. *The Journal of Nutrition,* 141, 2139–2145.

HOURIGAN, S.K., NICHOLSON, M.R., KAHN, S.A., KELLERMAYER, R. 2021. Updates and Challenges in Fecal Microbiota Transplantation for Clostridioides difficile Infection in Children. *Journal of Pediatric Gastroenterology and Nutrition* 73(4), 430–432.

HSIAO, E. Y., MCBRIDE, S. W., HSIEN, S., SHARON, G., HYDE, E. R., MCCUE, T., CODELLI, J. A., CHOW, J., REISMAN, S. E. & PETROSINO, J. F. 2013. Microbiota modulate behavioral and physiological abnormalities associated with neurodevelopmental disorders. *Cell*, 155, 1451–1463.

HUANG, J., LIU, D., WANG, Y., LIU, L., LI, J., YUAN, J., JIANG, Z., JIANG, Z., HSIAO, W. W. & LIU, H. 2022. Ginseng polysaccharides alter the gut microbiota and kynurenine/tryptophan ratio, potentiating the antitumour effect of antiprogrammed cell death 1/programmed cell death ligand 1 (anti-PD-1/PD-L1) immunotherapy. *Gut*, 71, 734–745.

WORLD CANCER RESEARCH FUND INTERNATIONAL. 2018. *Diet, nutrition, physical activity and cancer: A global perspective. Third annual report.*

ISHII, H., MORI, T., SHIRATSUCHI, A., NAKAI, Y., SHIMADA, Y., OHNO-IWASHITA, Y. & NAKANISHI, Y. 2005. Distinct localization of lipid rafts and externalized phosphatidylserine at the surface of apoptotic cells. *Biochemical and Biophysical Research Communications*, 327, 94–99.

JAYE, K., LI, C. G. & BHUYAN, D. J. 2021. The complex interplay of gut microbiota with the five most common cancer types: From carcinogenesis to therapeutics to prognoses. *Critical Reviews in Oncology/Hematology*, 165, 103429.

JUNG, S.-J., KASALA, D., CHOI, J.-W., LEE, S.-H., HWANG, J. K., KIM, S. W. & YUN, C.-O. 2015. Safety profiles and antitumor efficacy of oncolytic adenovirus coated with bioreducible polymer in the treatment of a CAR negative tumor model. *Biomacromolecules*, 16, 87–96.

KABWE, M., DASHPER, S. & TUCCI, J. 2022. The Microbiome in Pancreatic Cancer-Implications for Diagnosis and Precision Bacteriophage Therapy for This Low Survival Disease. *Frontiers in Cellular and Infection Microbiology*, 12, 871293.

KAID, C., GOULART, E., CAIRES-JÚNIOR, L. C., ARAUJO, B. H., SOARES-SCHANOSKI, A., BUENO, H. M., TELLES-SILVA, K. A., ASTRAY, R. M., ASSONI, A. F. & JÚNIOR, A. F. 2018. Zika virus selectively kills aggressive human embryonal CNS tumor cells in vitro and in vivo. *Cancer Research*, 78, 3363–3374.

KAKIUCHI, T., YAMAMOTO, K., IMAMURA, I., HASHIGUCHI, K., KAWAKUBO, H., YAMAGUCHI, D., FUJIOKA, Y. & OKUDA, M. 2021. Gut microbiota changes related to Helicobacter pylori eradication with vonoprazan containing triple therapy among adolescents: a prospective multicenter study. *Scientific Reports*, 11, 755.

KAMBOJ, A. K., COTTER, T. G. & OXENTENKO, A. S. 2017. Helicobacter pylori: the past, present, and future in management. *Mayo Clinic Proceedings*, Elsevier, 599–604.

KASSAM, Z., DUBOIS, N., RAMAKRISHNA, B., LING, K., QAZI, T., SMITH, M., KELLY, C. R., FISCHER, M., ALLEGRETTI, J. R. & BUDREE, S. 2019. Donor screening for fecal microbiota transplantation. *The New England Journal of Medicine*, 381, 2070–2072.

KAUFMAN, H. L., KOHLHAPP, F. J. & ZLOZA, A. 2015. Oncolytic viruses: a new class of immunotherapy drugs. *Nature Reviews Drug Discovery*, 14, 642–662.

KAZEMIAN, N., MAHMOUDI, M., HALPERIN, F., WU, J. C. & PAKPOUR, S. 2020. Gut microbiota and cardiovascular disease: opportunities and challenges. *Microbiome*, 8, 1–17.

KELLY, E. & RUSSELL, S. J. 2007. History of oncolytic viruses: genesis to genetic engineering. *Molecular Therapy*, 15, 651–659.

KELLY, K. J., WONG, J. & FONG, Y. 2008. Herpes simplex virus NV1020 as a novel and promising therapy for hepatic malignancy. *Expert Opinion on Investigational Drugs*, 17, 1105–1113.

KHAN, M. T., VAN DIJL, J. M. & HARMSEN, H. J. 2014. Antioxidants keep the potentially probiotic but highly oxygen-sensitive human gut bacterium Faecalibacterium prausnitzii alive at ambient air. *PLoS One*, 9, e96097.

KHANNA, S., PARDI, D. S., KELLY, C. R., KRAFT, C. S., DHERE, T., HENN, M. R., LOMBARDO, M. -J., VULIC, M., OHSUMI, T. & WINKLER, J. 2016. A novel microbiome therapeutic increases gut microbial diversity and prevents recurrent Clostridium difficile infection. *The Journal of Infectious Diseases*, 214, 173–181.

KIMBALL, K. J., PREUSS, M. A., BARNES, M. N., WANG, M., SIEGAL, G. P., WAN, W., KUO, H., SADDEKNI, S., STOCKARD, C. R. & GRIZZLE, W. E. 2010. A phase I study of a tropism-modified conditionally replicative adenovirus for recurrent malignant gynecologic diseases. *Clinical Cancer Research*, 16, 5277–5287.

KRISTENSEN, N. B., BRYRUP, T., ALLIN, K. H., NIELSEN, T., HANSEN, T. H. & PEDERSEN, O. 2016. Alterations in fecal microbiota composition by probiotic supplementation in healthy adults: a systematic review of randomized controlled trials. *Genome Medicine*, 8, 1–11.

KUMAR, P., BRAZEL, D., DEROGATIS, J., VALERIN, J. B. G., WHITESON, K., CHOW, W. A., TINOCO, R. & MOYERS, J. T. 2022. The cure from within? a review of the microbiome and diet in melanoma. *Cancer and Metastasis Reviews*, 41, 261–280.

KURODA, K. & CAPUTO, G. A. 2013. Antimicrobial polymers as synthetic mimics of host-defense peptides. *Wiley Interdisciplinary Reviews: Nanomedicine and Nanobiotechnology*, 5, 49–66.

KWAN, A., WINDER, N. & MUTHANA, M. 2021. Oncolytic virotherapy treatment of breast cancer: barriers and recent advances. *Viruses*, 13, 1128.

LAPLANE, L., DULUC, D., BIKFALVI, A., LARMONIER, N. & PRADEU, T. 2019. Beyond the tumour microenvironment. *International Journal of Cancer*, 145, 2611–2618.

LE CHATELIER, E., NIELSEN, T., QIN, J., PRIFTI, E., HILDEBRAND, F., FALONY, G., ALMEIDA, M., ARUMUGAM, M., BATTO, J.-M. & KENNEDY, S. 2013. Richness of human gut microbiome correlates with metabolic markers. *Nature*, 500, 541–546.

LEE, K., LUONG, M., SHAW, H., NATHAN, P., BATAILLE, V. & SPECTOR, T. 2021. The gut microbiome: What the oncologist ought to know. *British journal of cancer*, 125, 1197–1209.

LEITE, N. B., AUFDERHORST-ROBERTS, A., PALMA, M. S., CONNELL, S. D., NETO, J. R. & BEALES, P. A. 2015. PE and PS lipids synergistically enhance membrane poration by a peptide with anticancer properties. *Biophysical Journal*, 109, 936–947.

LI, L., LIU, S., HAN, D., TANG, B. & MA, J. 2020. Delivery and biosafety of oncolytic virotherapy. *Frontiers in oncology*, 10, 475.

LI, S., LIU, J., ZHENG, X., REN, L., YANG, Y., LI, W., FU, W., WANG, J. & DU, G. 2022. Tumorigenic bacteria in colorectal cancer: mechanisms and treatments. *Cancer Biology & Medicine,* 19, 147.

LI, Z., FEIYUE, Z., GAOFENG, L. & HAIFENG, L. 2023. Lung cancer and oncolytic virotherapy——enemy's enemy. *Translational Oncology,* 27, 101563.

LIU, J., LIU, C. & YUE, J. 2021. Radiotherapy and the gut microbiome: facts and fiction. *Radiation Oncology,* 16, 1–15.

LIU, X., WU, F., JI, Y. & YIN, L. 2018. Recent advances in anticancer protein/peptide delivery. *Bioconjugate chemistry,* 30, 305–324.

LOOIJER–VAN LANGEN, M. A. & DIELEMAN, L. A. 2009. Prebiotics in chronic intestinal inflammation. *Inflammatory bowel diseases,* 15, 454–462.

LUNDSTROM, K. 2018. New frontiers in oncolytic viruses: optimizing and selecting for virus strains with improved efficacy. *Biologics: Targets and Therapy,* 43–60.

LUONG, H. X., THANH, T. T. & TRAN, T. H. 2020. Antimicrobial peptides–Advances in development of therapeutic applications. *Life Sciences,* 260, 118407.

MAGANA, M., PUSHPANATHAN, M., SANTOS, A. L., LEANSE, L., FERNANDEZ, M., IOANNIDIS, A., GIULIANOTTI, M. A., APIDIANAKIS, Y., BRADFUTE, S. & FERGUSON, A. L. 2020. The value of antimicrobial peptides in the age of resistance. *The lancet infectious diseases,* 20, e216-e230.

MAGER, L. F., BURKHARD, R., PETT, N., COOKE, N. C., BROWN, K., RAMAY, H., PAIK, S., STAGG, J., GROVES, R. A. & GALLO, M. 2020. Microbiome-derived inosine modulates response to checkpoint inhibitor immunotherapy. *Science,* 369, 1481–1489.

MAKARANKA, S., SCUTT, F., FRIXOU, M., WENSLEY, K. E., SHARMA, R. & GREENHOWE, J. 2022. The gut microbiome and melanoma: A review. *Experimental Dermatology,* 31, 1292–1301.

MALDONADO-GÓMEZ, M. X., MARTÍNEZ, I., BOTTACINI, F., O'CALLAGHAN, A., VENTURA, M., VAN SINDEREN, D., HILLMANN, B., VANGAY, P., KNIGHTS, D. & HUTKINS, R. W. 2016. Stable engraftment of Bifidobacterium longum AH1206 in the human gut depends on individualized features of the resident microbiome. *Cell host & microbe,* 20, 515–526.

MARCHINI, A., BONIFATI, S., SCOTT, E. M., ANGELOVA, A. L. & ROMMELAERE, J. 2015. Oncolytic parvoviruses: from basic virology to clinical applications. *Virology journal,* 12, 1–16.

MAROUN, J., MUÑOZ-ALÍA, M., AMMAYAPPAN, A., SCHULZE, A., PENG, K.-W. & RUSSELL, S. 2017. Designing and building oncolytic viruses. *Future virology,* 12, 193–213.

MARTIKAINEN, M. & ESSAND, M. 2019. Virus-based immunotherapy of glioblastoma. *Cancers,* 11, 186.

MATSON, V., CHERVIN, C. S. & GAJEWSKI, T. F. 2021. Cancer and the microbiome—influence of the commensal microbiota on cancer, immune responses, and immunotherapy. *Gastroenterology,* 160, 600–613.

MATSON, V., FESSLER, J., BAO, R., CHONGSUWAT, T., ZHA, Y., ALEGRE, M.-L., LUKE, J. J. & GAJEWSKI, T. F. 2018. The commensal microbiome is associated with anti–PD-1 efficacy in metastatic melanoma patients. *Science,* 359, 104–108.

MATSUSHITA, M., FUJITA, K., HATANO, K., DE VELASCO, M. A., TSUJIMURA, A., UEMURA, H. & NONOMURA, N. 2023. Emerging relationship between the gut microbiome and prostate cancer. *The World Journal of Men's Health,* 41.

MCLOUGHLIN, R. F., BERTHON, B. S., JENSEN, M. E., BAINES, K. J. & WOOD, L. G. 2017. Short-chain fatty acids, prebiotics, synbiotics, and systemic inflammation: a systematic review and meta-analysis. *The American Journal of Clinical Nutrition,* 106, 930–945.

MCQUADE, J. L., DANIEL, C. R., HELMINK, B. A. & WARGO, J. A. 2019. Modulating the microbiome to improve therapeutic response in cancer. *The Lancet Oncology,* 20, e77-e91.

MEKADIM, C., SKALNIKOVA, H. K., CIZKOVA, J., CIZKOVA, V., PALANOVA, A., HORAK, V. & MRAZEK, J. 2022. Dysbiosis of skin microbiome and gut microbiome in melanoma progression. *BMC microbiology,* 22, 1–19.

MENDES, I. & VALE, N. 2023. How can the microbiome induce carcinogenesis and modulate drug resistance in cancer therapy? *International Journal of Molecular Sciences,* 24, 11855.

MERCHANTE GUTIÉRREZ, N., CHICO, P., MÁRQUEZ-SAAVEDRA, E., RIERA, G., HERRERO, R., GONZÁLEZ DE LA ALEJA, P. & MERINO, E. 2022. Impact of COVID19 pandemic on the incidence of health-care associated Clostridioides difficile infection. *Anaerobe,* 75, 102579.

MOHAN, V., DAS, A. & SAGI, I. 2020. *Emerging roles of ECM remodeling processes in cancer. Seminars in cancer biology.* Elsevier, 192–200.

MOOKHERJEE, N., ANDERSON, M. A., HAAGSMAN, H. P. & DAVIDSON, D. J. 2020. Antimicrobial host defence peptides: functions and clinical potential. *Nature Reviews Drug discovery,* 19, 311–332.

MU, A., MCDONALD, D., JARMUSCH, A. K., MARTINO, C., BRENNAN, C., BRYANT, M., HUMPHREY, G. C., TORONCZAK, J., SCHWARTZ, T. & NGUYEN, D. 2021. Assessment of the microbiome during bacteriophage therapy in combination with systemic antibiotics to treat a case of staphylococcal device infection. *Microbiome,* 9, 1–8.

NATARAJ, B. H., ALI, S. A., BEHARE, P. V. & YADAV, H. 2020. Postbiotics-parabiotics: The new horizons in microbial biotherapy and functional foods. *Microbial Cell Factories,* 19, 1–22.

O'KEEFE, S. J., LI, J. V., LAHTI, L., OU, J., CARBONERO, F., MOHAMMED, K., POSMA, J. M., KINROSS, J., WAHL, E. & RUDER, E. 2015. Fat, fibre and cancer risk in African Americans and rural Africans. *Nature Communications,* 6, 1–14.

OLIVA, M., MULET-MARGALEF, N., OCHOA-DE-OLZA, M., NAPOLI, S., MAS, J., LAQUENTE, B., ALEMANY, L., DUELL, E. J., NUCIFORO, P. & MORENO, V. 2021. Tumor-associated microbiome: where do we stand? *International Journal of Molecular Sciences,* 22, 1446.

OU, J., CARBONERO, F., ZOETENDAL, E. G., DELANY, J. P., WANG, M., NEWTON, K., GASKINS, H. R. & O'KEEFE, S. J. 2013. Diet, microbiota, and microbial metabolites in colon cancer risk in rural Africans and African Americans. *The American Journal of Clinical Nutrition,* 98, 111–120.

OUDE GRIEP, L. M., WANG, H. & CHAN, Q. 2013. Empirically derived dietary patterns, diet quality scores, and markers of inflammation and endothelial dysfunction. *Current Nutrition Reports,* 2, 97–104.

PARK, E. M., CHELVANAMBI, M., BHUTIANI, N., KROEMER, G., ZITVOGEL, L. & WARGO, J. A. 2022. Targeting the gut and tumor microbiota in cancer. *Nature Medicine,* 28, 690–703.

PAULE, A., FREZZA, D. & EDEAS, M. 2018. Microbiota and phage therapy: future challenges in medicine. *Medical Sciences*, 6, 86.

PETERSON, J., GARGES, S., GIOVANNI, M., MCINNES, P., WANG, L., SCHLOSS, J. A., BONAZZI, V., MCEWEN, J. E., WETTERSTRAND, K. A. & DEAL, C. 2009. The NIH human microbiome project. *Genome Research*, 19, 2317–2323.

PETROV, G., DYMOVA, M. & RICHTER, V. 2022. Bacteriophage-Mediated Cancer Gene Therapy. *International Journal of Molecular Sciences*, 23, 14245.

PFALZGRAFF, A., BRANDENBURG, K. & WEINDL, G. 2018. Antimicrobial peptides and their therapeutic potential for bacterial skin infections and wounds. *Frontiers in Pharmacology*, 9, 281.

PICKUP, M. W., MOUW, J. K. & WEAVER, V. M. 2014. The extracellular matrix modulates the hallmarks of cancer. *EMBO reports*, 15, 1243–1253.

PINATO, D. J., HOWLETT, S., OTTAVIANI, D., URUS, H., PATEL, A., MINEO, T., BROCK, C., POWER, D., HATCHER, O. & FALCONER, A. 2019. Association of prior antibiotic treatment with survival and response to immune checkpoint inhibitor therapy in patients with cancer. *JAMA oncology*, 5, 1774–1778.

POON, I. K., BAXTER, A. A., LAY, F. T., MILLS, G. D., ADDA, C. G., PAYNE, J. A., PHAN, T. K., RYAN, G. F., WHITE, J. A. & VENEER, P. K. 2014. Phosphoinositide-mediated oligomerization of a defensin induces cell lysis. *Elife*, 3, e01808.

PUIG-SAENZ, C., PEARSON, J. R., THOMAS, J. E. & MCARDLE, S. E. 2023. A holistic approach to hard-to-treat cancers: The future of immunotherapy for glioblastoma, triple negative breast cancer, and advanced prostate cancer. *Biomedicines*, 11, 2100.

QIN, J., LI, Y., CAI, Z., LI, S., ZHU, J., ZHANG, F., LIANG, S., ZHANG, W., GUAN, Y. & SHEN, D. 2012. A metagenome-wide association study of gut microbiota in type 2 diabetes. *Nature*, 490, 55–60.

RAHMAN, M. M., ISLAM, M. R., SHOHAG, S., AHASAN, M. T., SARKAR, N., KHAN, H., HASAN, A. M., CAVALU, S. & RAUF, A. 2022. Microbiome in cancer: Role in carcinogenesis and impact in therapeutic strategies. *Biomedicine & Pharmacotherapy*, 149, 112898.

RAMAN, M., AMBALAM, P., KONDEPUDI, K. K., PITHVA, S., KOTHARI, C., PATEL, A. T., PURAMA, R. K., DAVE, J. & VYAS, B. 2013. Potential of probiotics, prebiotics and synbiotics for management of colorectal cancer. *Gut Microbes*, 4, 181–192.

REINFELD, B. I., RATHMELL, W. K., KIM, T. K. & RATHMELL, J. C. 2022. The therapeutic implications of immunosuppressive tumor aerobic glycolysis. *Cellular & Molecular Immunology*, 19, 46–58.

RIDAURA, V. K., FAITH, J. J., REY, F. E., CHENG, J., DUNCAN, A. E., KAU, A. L., GRIFFIN, N. W., LOMBARD, V., HENRISSAT, B. & BAIN, J. R. 2013. Gut microbiota from twins discordant for obesity modulate metabolism in mice. *Science*, 341, 1241214.

RIQUELME, E., ZHANG, Y., ZHANG, L., MONTIEL, M., ZOLTAN, M., DONG, W., QUESADA, P., SAHIN, I., CHANDRA, V. & SAN LUCAS, A. 2019. Tumor microbiome diversity and composition influence pancreatic cancer outcomes. *Cell*, 178, 795–806. e12.

ROAGER, H. M., VOGT, J. K., KRISTENSEN, M., HANSEN, L. B. S., IBRÜGGER, S., MÆRKEDAHL, R. B., BAHL, M. I., LIND, M. V., NIELSEN, R. L. & FRØKIÆR, H. 2019. Whole grain-rich diet reduces body weight and systemic low-grade inflammation without inducing major changes of the gut microbiome: a randomised cross-over trial. *Gut*, 68, 83–93.

ROBILOTTI, E. V., KUMAR, A., GLICKMAN, M. S. & KAMBOJ, M. 2019. Viral oncolytic immunotherapy in the war on cancer: Infection control considerations. *Infection Control & Hospital Epidemiology*, 40, 350–354.

ROGOVSKI, P., CADAMURO, R. D., DA SILVA, R., DE SOUZA, E. B., BONATTO, C., VIANCELLI, A., MICHELON, W., ELMAHDY, E. M., TREICHEL, H. & RODRÍGUEZ-LÁZARO, D. 2021. Uses of Bacteriophages as Bacterial Control Tools and Environmental Safety Indicators. *Frontiers in Microbiology*, 12, 3756.

ROHLKE, F. & STOLLMAN, N. 2012. Fecal microbiota transplantation in relapsing Clostridium difficile infection. *Therapeutic Advances in Gastroenterology*, 5, 403–420.

ROUDI, R., SYN, N. L. & ROUDBARY, M. 2017. Antimicrobial peptides as biologic and immunotherapeutic agents against cancer: a comprehensive overview. *Frontiers in Immunology*, 8, 1320.

ROUTY, B., LE CHATELIER, E., DEROSA, L., DUONG, C. P., ALOU, M. T., DAILLÈRE, R., FLUCKIGER, A., MESSAOUDENE, M., RAUBER, C. & ROBERTI, M. P. 2018. Gut microbiome influences efficacy of PD-1–based immunotherapy against epithelial tumors. *Science*, 359, 91–97.

RULTEN, S. L., GROSE, R. P., GATZ, S. A., JONES, J. L. & CAMERON, A. J. 2023. The Future of Precision Oncology. *International Journal of Molecular Sciences*, 24, 12613.

RUSSELL, L. & PENG, K.-W. 2018. The emerging role of oncolytic virus therapy against cancer. *Chinese Clinical Oncology*, 7, 16.

RUSSELL, S. J., PENG, K.-W. & BELL, J. C. 2012. Oncolytic virotherapy. *Nature Biotechnology*, 30, 658–670.

SANCHEZ-RODRIGUEZ, E., EGEA-ZORRILLA, A., PLAZA-DÍAZ, J., ARAGÓN-VELA, J., MUÑOZ-QUEZADA, S., TERCEDOR-SÁNCHEZ, L. & ABADIA-MOLINA, F. 2020. The gut microbiota and its implication in the development of atherosclerosis and related cardiovascular diseases. *Nutrients*, 12, 605.

SANDERS, M. E. 2011. Impact of probiotics on colonizing microbiota of the gut. *Journal of Clinical Gastroenterology*, 45, S115-S119.

SARTORIUS, R., D'APICE, L., TROVATO, M., CUCCARO, F., COSTA, V., DE LEO, M. G., MARZULLO, V. M., BIONDO, C., D'AURIA, S. & DE MATTEIS, M. A. 2015. Antigen delivery by filamentous bacteriophage fd displaying an anti-DEC-205 single-chain variable fragment confers adjuvanticity by triggering a TLR 9-mediated immune response. *EMBO Molecular Medicine*, 7, 973–988.

SAUS MARTÍNEZ, E., IRAOLA GUZMAN, S., WILLIS, J. R., BRUNET-VEGA, A. & GABALDÓN ESTEVAN, J. A. 2019. Microbiome and colorectal cancer: Roles in carcinogenesis and clinical potential. *Mol Aspects Med.* 2019; 69: 93–106.

SCHIFANO, E., CICALINI, I., PIERAGOSTINO, D., HEIPIEPER, H. J., DEL BOCCIO, P. & UCCELLETTI, D. 2020. In vitro and in vivo lipidomics as a tool for probiotics evaluation. *Applied Microbiology and Biotechnology*, 104, 8937–8948.

SĘDZIKOWSKA, A. & SZABLEWSKI, L. 2021. Human gut microbiota in health and selected cancers. *International Journal of Molecular Sciences*, 22, 13440.

SELGRAD, M. & MALFERTHEINER, P. 2008. New strategies for Helicobacter pylori eradication. *Current Opinion in Pharmacology*, 8, 593–597.

SEPICH-POORE, G. D., ZITVOGEL, L., STRAUSSMAN, R., HASTY, J., WARGO, J. A. & KNIGHT, R. 2021. The microbiome and human cancer. *Science,* 371, eabc4552.

SHEFLIN, A. M., BORRESEN, E. C., KIRKWOOD, J. S., BOOT, C. M., WHITNEY, A. K., LU, S., BROWN, R. J., BROECKLING, C. D., RYAN, E. P. & WEIR, T. L. 2017. Dietary supplementation with rice bran or navy bean alters gut bacterial metabolism in colorectal cancer survivors. *Molecular Nutrition & Food Research,* 61, 1500905.

SHONO, Y., DOCAMPO, M. D., PELED, J. U., PEROBELLI, S. M., VELARDI, E., TSAI, J. J., SLINGERLAND, A. E., SMITH, O. M., YOUNG, L. F. & GUPTA, J. 2016. Increased GVHD-related mortality with broad-spectrum antibiotic use after allogeneic hematopoietic stem cell transplantation in human patients and mice. *Science Translational Medicine,* 8, 339ra71-339ra71.

SIVAN, A., CORRALES, L., HUBERT, N., WILLIAMS, J. B., AQUINO-MICHAELS, K., EARLEY, Z. M., BENYAMIN, F. W., MAN LEI, Y., JABRI, B. & ALEGRE, M.-L. 2015. Commensal Bifidobacterium promotes antitumor immunity and facilitates anti–PD-L1 efficacy. *Science,* 350, 1084–1089.

SOENDERGAARD, M., NEWTON-NORTHUP, J. R. & DEUTSCHER, S. L. 2014. In vivo phage display selection of an ovarian cancer targeting peptide for SPECT/CT imaging. *American Journal of Nuclear Medicine and Molecular Imaging,* 4, 561.

SOMMACAL, H. M., BERSCH, V. P., VITOLA, S. P. & OSVALDT, A. B. 2015. Perioperative synbiotics decrease postoperative complications in periampullary neoplasms: a randomized, double-blind clinical trial. *Nutrition and Cancer,* 67, 457–462.

SOUTHAM, C. M. 1960. Division of microbiology: present status of oncolytic virus studies. *Transactions of the New York Academy of Sciences,* 22, 657–673.

STEFAŃSKA, K., JÓZKOWIAK, M., ANGELOVA VOLPONI, A., SHIBLI, J. A., GOLKAR-NARENJI, A., ANTOSIK, P., BUKOWSKA, D., PIOTROWSKA-KEMPISTY, H., MOZDZIAK, P. & DZIĘGIEL, P. 2023. The Role of Exosomes in Human Carcinogenesis and Cancer Therapy—Recent Findings from Molecular and Clinical Research. *Cells,* 12, 356.

SUEZ, J., ZMORA, N., ZILBERMAN-SCHAPIRA, G., MOR, U., DORI-BACHASH, M., BASHIARDES, S., ZUR, M., REGEV-LEHAVI, D., BRIK, R. B.-Z. & FEDERICI, S. 2018. Post-antibiotic gut mucosal microbiome reconstitution is impaired by probiotics and improved by autologous FMT. *Cell,* 174, 1406–1423. e16.

SUGIMURA, N., LI, Q., CHU, E. S. H., LAU, H. C. H., FONG, W., LIU, W., LIANG, C., NAKATSU, G., SU, A. C. Y. & COKER, O. O. 2022. Lactobacillus gallinarum modulates the gut microbiota and produces anti-cancer metabolites to protect against colorectal tumourigenesis. *Gut,* 71, 2011–2021.

SUGIMURA, N., OTANI, K., WATANABE, T., NAKATSU, G., SHIMADA, S., FUJIMOTO, K., NADATANI, Y., HOSOMI, S., TANAKA, F. & KAMATA, N. 2019. High-fat diet-mediated dysbiosis exacerbates NSAID-induced small intestinal damage through the induction of interleukin-17A. *Scientific Reports,* 9, 16796.

TAPER, H. S. & ROBERFROID, M. B. 2005. Possible adjuvant cancer therapy by two prebiotics-inulin or oligofructose. *In Vivo,* 19, 201–204.

TIAN, Y., ZHOU, Y., HUANG, S., LI, J., ZHAO, K., LI, X., WEN, X. & LI, X.-A. 2019. Fecal microbiota transplantation for ulcerative colitis: a prospective clinical study. *BMC Gastroenterology,* 19, 1–12.

TRIPODI, L., FEOLA, S., GRANATA, I., WHALLEY, T., PASSARIELLO, M., CAPASSO, C., COLUCCINO, L., VITALE, M., SCALIA, G. & GENTILE, L. 2023. Bifidobacterium affects antitumor efficacy of oncolytic adenovirus in a mouse model of melanoma. *Iscience,* 26, 107668.

TSAI, T.-L., LI, A.-C., CHEN, Y.-C., LIAO, Y.-S. & LIN, T.-H. 2015. Antimicrobial peptide m2163 or m2386 identified from Lactobacillus casei ATCC 334 can trigger apoptosis in the human colorectal cancer cell line SW480. *Tumor Biology,* 36, 3775–3789.

UGARE, U., BOMBIL, I. & LUVHENGO, T. 2022. Early-onset malignant solid tumours in young adult South Africans–an audit based on histopathological records of patients seen at the three academic hospitals in Johannesburg. *South African Journal of Surgery,* 60, 134–140.

VALDES, A. M., WALTER, J., SEGAL, E. & SPECTOR, T. D. 2018. Role of the gut microbiota in nutrition and health. *Bmj,* 361.

VAN NOOD, E., VRIEZE, A., NIEUWDORP, M., FUENTES, S., ZOETENDAL, E. G., DE VOS, W. M., VISSER, C. E., KUIJPER, E. J., BARTELSMAN, J. F. & TIJSSEN, J. G. 2013. Duodenal infusion of donor feces for recurrent Clostridium difficile. *New England Journal of Medicine,* 368, 407–415.

VANEGAS, S. M., MEYDANI, M., BARNETT, J. B., GOLDIN, B., KANE, A., RASMUSSEN, H., BROWN, C., VANGAY, P., KNIGHTS, D. & JONNALAGADDA, S. 2017. Substituting whole grains for refined grains in a 6-wk randomized trial has a modest effect on gut microbiota and immune and inflammatory markers of healthy adults. *The American Journal of Clinical Nutrition,* 105, 635–650.

VARGHESE, S., NEWSOME, J. T., RABKIN, S. D., MCGEAGH, K., MAHONEY, D., NIELSEN, P., TODO, T. & MARTUZA, R. L. 2001. Preclinical safety evaluation of G207, a replication-competent herpes simplex virus type 1, inoculated intraprostatically in mice and nonhuman primates. *Human Gene Therapy,* 12, 999–1010.

VEERANARAYANAN, S., AZAM, A. H., KIGA, K., WATANABE, S. & CUI, L. 2021. Bacteriophages as solid tumor theragnostic agents. *International Journal of Molecular Sciences,* 23, 402.

VENDRIK, K. E., OOIJEVAAR, R. E., DE JONG, P. R., LAMAN, J. D., VAN OOSTEN, B. W., VAN HILTEN, J. J., DUCARMON, Q. R., KELLER, J. J., KUIJPER, E. J. & CONTARINO, M. F. 2020. Fecal microbiota transplantation in neurological disorders. *Frontiers in Cellular and Infection Microbiology,* 10, 98.

VILLÉGER, R., LOPÈS, A., CARRIER, G., VEZIANT, J., BILLARD, E., BARNICH, N., GAGNIÈRE, J., VAZEILLE, E. & BONNET, M. 2019. Intestinal microbiota: a novel target to improve anti-tumor treatment? *International Journal of Molecular Sciences,* 20, 4584.

WANG, J.-J., LEI, K.-F. & HAN, F. 2018a. Tumor microenvironment: recent advances in various cancer treatments. *European Review for Medical & Pharmacological Sciences,* 22.

WANG, X., ZHANG, H. & CHEN, X. 2019a. Drug resistance and combating drug resistance in cancer. *Cancer Drug Resistance,* 2, 141.

WANG, Y., WIESNOSKI, D. H., HELMINK, B. A., GOPALAKRISHNAN, V., CHOI, K., DUPONT, H. L., JIANG, Z. -D., ABU-SBEIH, H., SANCHEZ, C. A. & CHANG, C.-C. 2018b. Fecal microbiota transplantation for refractory immune checkpoint inhibitor-associated colitis. *Nature Medicine*, 24, 1804–1808.

WANG, Y., ZHOU, X., WU, Z., HU, H., JIN, J., HU, Y., DONG, Y., ZOU, J., MAO, Z. & SHI, X. 2019b. Preclinical safety evaluation of oncolytic herpes simplex virus type 2. *Human Gene Therapy*, 30, 651–660.

WATANABE, T., NADATANI, Y., SUDA, W., HIGASHIMORI, A., OTANI, K., FUKUNAGA, S., HOSOMI, S., TANAKA, F., NAGAMI, Y. & TAIRA, K. 2021. Long-term persistence of gastric dysbiosis after eradication of Helicobacter pylori in patients who underwent endoscopic submucosal dissection for early gastric cancer. *Gastric Cancer*, 24, 710–720.

WATERS, A. M., FRIEDMAN, G. K., RING, E. K. & BEIERLE, E. A. 2016. Oncolytic virotherapy for pediatric malignancies: future prospects. *Oncolytic Virotherapy*, 73–80.

WEI, N., FAN, J. K., GU, J. F., HE, L. F., TANG, W. H., CAO, X. & LIU, X. Y. 2009. A double-regulated oncolytic adenovirus with improved safety for adenocarcinoma therapy. *Biochemical and Biophysical Research Communications*, 388, 234–239.

WOLDETSADIK, A. D., VOGEL, M. C., RABEH, W. M. & MAGZOUB, M. 2017. Hexokinase II–derived cell-penetrating peptide targets mitochondria and triggers apoptosis in cancer cells. *The FASEB Journal*, 31, 2168.

WON, G., EO, S. K., PARK, S.-Y., HUR, J. & LEE, J. H. 2018. A Salmonella Typhi ghost induced by the E gene of phage φX174 stimulates dendritic cells and efficiently activates the adaptive immune response. *Journal of Veterinary Science*, 19, 536–542.

WONG, M. K., BARBULESCU, P., COBURN, B. & REGUERA-NUÑEZ, E. 2021. Therapeutic interventions and mechanisms associated with gut microbiota-mediated modulation of immune checkpoint inhibitor responses. *Microbes and Infection*, 23, 104804.

WU, Y., LI, R. W., HUANG, H., FLETCHER, A., YU, L., PHAM, Q., YU, L., HE, Q. & WANG, T. T. 2019. Inhibition of tumor growth by dietary indole-3-carbinol in a prostate cancer xenograft model may be associated with disrupted gut microbial interactions. *Nutrients*, 11, 467.

XIA, C., DONG, X., LI, H., CAO, M., SUN, D., HE, S., YANG, F., YAN, X., ZHANG, S. & LI, N. 2022. Cancer statistics in China and United States, 2022: profiles, trends, and determinants. *Chinese Medical Journal*, 135, 584–590.

XIE, X., HE, Y., LI, H., YU, D., NA, L., SUN, T., ZHANG, D., SHI, X., XIA, Y. & JIANG, T. 2019. Effects of prebiotics on immunologic indicators and intestinal microbiota structure in perioperative colorectal cancer patients. *Nutrition*, 61, 132–142.

XU, D., CHEN, V. L., STEINER, C. A., BERINSTEIN, J. A., ESWARAN, S., WALJEE, A. K., HIGGINS, P. D. & OWYANG, C. 2019. Efficacy of fecal microbiota transplantation in irritable bowel syndrome: A systematic review and meta-analysis. *The American Journal of Gastroenterology*, 114, 1043.

YAMAGUCHI, T. & UCHIDA, E. 2018. Oncolytic virus: Regulatory aspects from quality control to clinical studies. *Current Cancer Drug Targets*, 18, 202–208.

YAMAMOTO, Y., NAGASATO, M., YOSHIDA, T. & AOKI, K. 2017. Recent advances in genetic modification of adenovirus vectors for cancer treatment. *Cancer science*, 108, 831–837.

YAMAZAKI, T., PITT, J., VÉTIZOU, M., MARABELLE, A., FLORES, C., REKDAL, Ø., KROEMER, G. & ZITVOGEL, L. 2016. The oncolytic peptide LTX-315 overcomes resistance of cancers to immunotherapy with CTLA4 checkpoint blockade. *Cell Death & Differentiation*, 23, 1004–1015.

YU, E. W., GAO, L., STASTKA, P., CHENEY, M. C., MAHABAMUNUGE, J., TORRES SOTO, M., FORD, C. B., BRYANT, J. A., HENN, M. R. & HOHMANN, E. L. 2020. Fecal microbiota transplantation for the improvement of metabolism in obesity: The FMT-TRIM double-blind placebo-controlled pilot trial. *PLoS medicine*, 17, e1003051.

ZEH, H. J., DOWNS-CANNER, S., MCCART, J. A., GUO, Z. S., RAO, U. N., RAMALINGAM, L., THORNE, S. H., JONES, H. L., KALINSKI, P. & WIECKOWSKI, E. 2015. First-in-man study of western reserve strain oncolytic vaccinia virus: safety, systemic spread, and antitumor activity. *Molecular Therapy*, 23, 202–214.

ZHANG, C.-Y., LIU, S. & YANG, M. 2022. Clinical diagnosis and management of pancreatic cancer: Markers, molecular mechanisms, and treatment options. *World Journal of Gastroenterology*, 28, 6827–6845.

ZHAO, L.-Y., MEI, J.-X., YU, G., LEI, L., ZHANG, W.-H., LIU, K., CHEN, X.-L., KOŁAT, D., YANG, K. & HU, J.-K. 2023. Role of the gut microbiota in anticancer therapy: from molecular mechanisms to clinical applications. *Signal Transduction and Targeted Therapy*, 8, 201.

ZHAO, L., ZHANG, F., DING, X., WU, G., LAM, Y. Y., WANG, X., FU, H., XUE, X., LU, C. & MA, J. 2018. Gut bacteria selectively promoted by dietary fibers alleviate type 2 diabetes. *Science*, 359, 1151–1156.

ZMORA, N., ZILBERMAN-SCHAPIRA, G., SUEZ, J., MOR, U., DORI-BACHASH, M., BASHIARDES, S., KOTLER, E., ZUR, M., REGEV-LEHAVI, D. & BRIK, R. B.-Z. 2018. Personalized gut mucosal colonization resistance to empiric probiotics is associated with unique host and microbiome features. *Cell*, 174, 1388–1405. e21.

17 Gut Microbiome Engineering for Cancer Therapies

Talent Chipiti, Elisa Marie Ledet, Amanda Skepu, and Zodwa Dlamini

INTRODUCTION

Cancer is one of the most common causes of death globally. Research has indicated that microorganisms could potentially contribute to approximately 15–20% of cancer cases. The correlation between gut microbiota and overall health has been linked to the constituents of the microbiota and the microbes that may be implicated in the increase of cancer. Despite this, the exact nature of the correlation between gut microbiota and cancer remains incompletely understood (Viswanathan et al., 2023). The composition and particular bacteria implicated in disease development are frequently connected to associations between gut microbiota and illness. The link between gut microbiota and cancer is yet unknown (Gurbatri et al., 2022).

The human body is a complicated network composed of both human and microbial cells that collaborate for mutual benefit. There are around 100 trillion bacteria in the body, including the gastrointestinal system, which is considered the body's second genome. These microorganisms have genomes 150 times bigger than the host cell and play an important role in health maintenance, but they can also contribute to illness. Thanks to advancements in sequencing techniques, researchers have been able to identify dysbiotic microbial signatures that can affect the progression of various diseases, including cancer. Extensive research shows that the composition and regulation of the microbiome and the specific microbes present can trigger tumor formation and promote tumor growth in the body (Fernandes et al., 2022; Gurbatri et al., 2022).

The microbiota can affect cancer development in three ways. For instance, it can upset the equilibrium of cell proliferation and death by stimulating cell growth. This is accomplished by influencing the host's *Wnt/-catenin* pathway, which is crucial for maintaining cell polarity and proliferation and has been associated with cancer progression. FadA (*Fusobacterium nucleatum*), Avra (*Salmonella typhi*), and CagA (*Helicobacter pylori*) are proteins that activate *Wnt-catenin* and are linked to the development of colorectal, hepatobiliary, and stomach cancer, respectively (Gurbatri et al., 2022) Additionally, bacterial toxins can cause double-stranded DNA breaks, leading to cellular DNA damage and carcinogenesis. Colibactin from *Enterococaceae*, *Bacteroides fragilis* toxin (BFT) from *B. fragilis*, and cytolethal expansive toxin (CDT) from various proteobacteria are examples of such toxins (Viswanathan et al., 2023).

This chapter explores the gut microbiome's role in cancer development and immunotherapy. It highlights how the microbiome regulates the immune system, promotes inflammation, and influences the host's metabolism, all contributing to cancer development.

Gut microbiota plays a crucial role in cancer treatment effectiveness and side effects, but can also promote inflammation and contribute to tumor progression. Some gut microbes can protect the tumor microenvironment and regulate the immune response. Recent studies suggest using bacteria as a synthetic biology tool for tumor-specific delivery systems, with modified immunogenicity and local payload generation. This chapter explores the engineering of relationships among bacteria, cancer cells, and immune cells, and how bacteria can be combined with other cancer treatments for more effective therapy. This advances the idea of using synthetic biology to design interactions among programmable medications.

Scientists have recognized bacteria's potential for treating cancer since the 19th century. Early experiments showed tumor regression in patients with *Streptococcus pyogenes* and *Serratia marcescens* (MacCarthy, 2006). However, it wasn't until the 20th century that bacteria possess immunostimulatory properties and can thrive in hypoxic and immunosuppressive tumor microenvironments. Various genera, including *Salmonella*, *Escherichia*, *Clostridium*, *Bifidobacterium*, *Proteus*, and *Lactobacillus*, have demonstrated these properties (Duong et al., 2019). Bacteria can target various cell types in the tumor microenvironment, and their agents can interact with imaging methods like MRI and focused ultrasound (FUS) for bacterial identification and activation (Fernandes et al., 2022; Gurbatri et al., 2022). Synthetic biology can now be used to fine-tune bacterial interactions and manage their growth and release of payloads (Gurbatri et al., 2022).

APPLICATION OF VARIOUS ENGINEERING TOOLS IN GUT MICROBES TOWARDS EFFICIENT CANCER TREATMENT

Engineering technologies, such as gene modification (GM) techniques, allow us to conduct studies that help us understand the interactions between gut microorganisms, nutrition, the host, and other members of the community. They also allow us to develop transgenic strains for illness diagnosis and treatment. Genetically modified bacteria provide various benefits for in vivo use over conventional approaches such as FMT, synthetic microbial consortia, and species-targeted antibiotics (Zhou et al., 2018). The use of genetic modification tools enables the engineering of bacterial cells capable of creating intricate and intelligent circuits that can promptly detect and respond to changes within the gut microenvironment. Such advancements have numerous benefits, including enhanced clinical safety as it minimizes disturbance to the host gut microenvironment, increased accessibility for producing desired prebiotic, metabolite, or drug quantities in situ, and broader availability of advanced synthetic biology tools. In the following section, we will delve into how these tools can be utilized to engineer bacteria as biosensors, metabolic regulators, or drug delivery agents (Chen et al., 2023). Figure 17.1 below summarizes various approaches to microbiota engineering, which can be achieved through the use of live therapeutic bacteria.

ENGINEERING THE BACTERIA-TUMOR INTERFACE

USE OF BACTERIA IN TUMOR LOCALIZATION

Tumoral environments are hypoxic and favorable for bacterial growth. Studies have shown bacterial growth up to 10,000-fold in tumors compared to other tissue (Forbes, 2010; Kasinskas and Forbes, 2007). Some of these bacterial strains can be engineered to make them less virulent and less endotoxic and make them inhabit healthy cells and organs. A good example is the *S. typhimurium* VNP20009 strain, which was engineered to produce an attenuated version with this reduced systemic inflammation (Low et al., 1999). One way to enhance cancer treatment is to modify bacteria so that

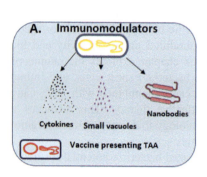
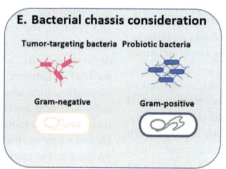
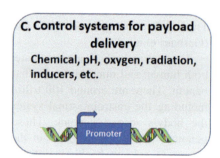
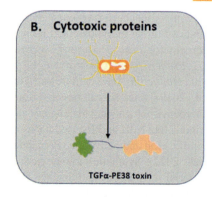
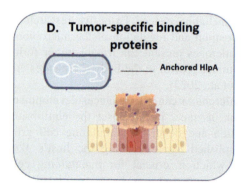

FIGURE 17.1 Components of engineered live therapeutic bacteria. The human gut microbiota is made up of trillions of microorganisms that reside in our gastrointestinal tract. This microbiota can be modified or engineered to develop innovative approaches for fighting various types and stages of cancer. This field of research holds the promise of creating new and effective treatments for cancer, which could significantly improve patient outcomes and survival rates. The approaches, as illustrated above include: (A) bacteria deliver immunomodulators like cytokines, small molecules, and immune checkpoint nanobodies, stimulating antitumor responses and leukocyte migration. Live cancer vaccines also present tumor-associated antigens on bacterial surface for adaptive immune response; (B) toxin delivery by bacteria, such as fusion transforming growth factor (TGF)-PE38; (C) inducible systems that are activated by chemicals, pH, radiation exposure, and oxygen levels can regulate the expression and delivery of therapeutic payloads; (D) therapeutic bacteria can have binding proteins like HlpA anchored on their surface to improve their binding to malignancies; (E) different categories of bacteria, including tumor-targeting, probiotic, and Gram-positive and Gram-negative bacteria, are suitable for delivering cancer therapeutics due to their unique qualities that make them suitable for this purpose (Chen et al., 2023).

they display tumor-targeting antigens and adhesion peptides on their surface membranes (Sieow et al., 2021). Scientists have modified *Salmonella* bacteria to improve their ability to target tumor cells. This was accomplished by combining the bacterial outer membrane protein A with a tumor-homing arginine-glycine-aspartate (RGD) peptide (OmpA). As a result, adhesion peptides can connect to integrins such as v3, which are overexpressed by tumor cells. This permits the bacteria to bind to tumor cells more efficiently than healthy cells (Duong et al., 2019).

It is possible to modify bacteria so that they can regulate genetic circuits that connect bacterial growth with tumor markers such as high levels of lactate, low oxygen levels, and low pH. These sensing circuits work by controlling the expression of important genes for bacterial growth through bacterial promoters that respond to environmental signals. This limits bacterial growth to tumors and provides a potential method of treatment (Chien et al., 2022). To enhance the effectiveness of bacterial therapies for cancer treatment, the sensing circuits can be combined using AND logic gates. This is because some signals may also be present in other tissues, reducing the specificity of the therapy and increasing the likelihood of bacterial mutational escape. By using AND gates, the bacteria can deliver therapeutic payloads to specific locations within the tumor, resulting in longer-term biocontainment (Chien et al., 2022). This approach, which is promising, has resulted in the emergence of the field of Theranostics.

Theranostics is a way of creating individualized remedies for various ailments by combining medicine and diagnostics. It examines patients for possible medication reactions and tailors therapy depending on test results (Pene et al., 2009). This strategy is critical for economics since it results in more cost-effective therapy, and more efficient medical processes, and aids in preclinical drug development or clinical trial eligibility (Idée et al., 2013). Theranostics are diagnostic biomarkers used in cancer treatment to identify and eliminate cancer cells. They use molecular imaging, analogous to positron emission tomography (PET), to follow radioactive drugs through the body in order to target specific cancer cells (Pruis et al., 2020). This kind of highly concentrated radiation is less harmful to neighboring healthy tissues.

When the bacteria infiltrate the tumor, they have the ability to transport different types of payloads to specific areas with concentrated effectiveness. These payloads, which comprise various therapeutic targets and molecule types, are designed to be optimally suited for these locations. Small molecules can reach their destinations by passive diffusion or membrane transport, but bigger payloads such as nucleic acids need intracellular delivery into the cytoplasm or nucleus, and some proteins require extracellular localization to act on receptors (Gurbatri et al., 2022).

TARGETING THE INTRACELLULAR SPACE

For a long time, getting chemicals into cells has been difficult. To access intracellular targets, many approaches such as viral and nanoparticle delivery platforms have been developed.

Bacteria can manage themselves, feel and respond to the internalization process, and then release the cargo since they are living medicines. This makes intracellular delivery useful since it may target proteins and processes that have historically been difficult to investigate (Stewart et al., 2016).

Gram-negative bacteria such as *S. typhimurium* use a specific secretion system called type 3 secretion system (T3SS) for direct injection of effector proteins into the host cell cytoplasm. This system has been engineered to optimize the delivery of various cargo into tumor cells such as human cervix adenocarcinoma, and human colorectal carcinoma cells. The T3SS delivery system has been improved to efficiently deliver macromolecules, including monobodies and synthetic proteins such as Designed Ankyrin Repeat Proteins (DARPins). Several studies have focused on enhancing the T3SS delivery system for targeted and precise delivery of therapeutic molecules into the cells (Chabloz et al., 2020). A good example is the pCASP-hyperinvasive locus A (HilA) vector which is a generalized secretion system. The effectiveness of this delivery system was verified through an in vitro study. The study involved using a bacterial system to deliver various DARPins and monobodies that inhibit the RAS signaling pathway, which is typically difficult to treat. The delivery successfully transported these inhibitors to the cytosol of human colon cancer cells. The study confirmed that this system functionally inhibits RAS signaling (Chabloz et al., 2020; Widmaier et al., 2009).

When *Salmonella typhimurium* enters a host cell, it has the ability to reproduce within a *Salmonella*-containing vacuole (SCV) once it has been engulfed. However, *Salmonella* T3SS needle complexes can puncture the SCV membrane and release proteins into the host cytosol, which can impede the transportation of additional bacterial content through the SCV. To overcome this challenge, scientists have explored methods to actively break down the SCV. They have taken cues from escape strategies used by other intracellular species like *Listeria monocytogenes* and *Shigella flexneri* to enhance *S. typhimurium* efficiency in escaping the vacuole (Gurbatri et al., 2022; Weiss and Krusch, 2001). The invasin protein, a molecule produced by the inv gene in *Yersinia pseudotuberculosis*, possesses a unique ability to interact with 1-integrins found in a variety of cell lines. As a result of this interaction, extracellular bacteria such as *E. coli* can be engulfed by phagosomes. This process plays a crucial role in the pathogenesis of *Y. pseudotuberculosis* infections and sheds light on the fascinating mechanisms by which bacteria can invade host cells (Anderson et al., 2006). Diaminopimelate auxotrophic *E. coli* strains, which are unable to make a cell wall, can be engineered to increase bacterial cell lysis upon entering mammalian cells (Gurbatri et al., 2022; Widmaier et al., 2009).

TARGETING THE EXTRACELLULAR SPACE

In order to target therapeutic areas like tumor cell receptors, extracellular delivery methods are often necessary. An extracellular delivery method is a simpler approach to delivering medication as it is not dependent on physical proximity to the tumor cells. Bacteria can grow in high densities in the extracellular spaces, allowing for more of their payload to be produced and diffuse throughout the tumor space. The probiotic strain *E. coli* Nissle 1917 (EcN) is a non-invasive bacterium that can be employed for extracellular delivery strategies. These bacteria can be modified to encode a *Shigella*-derived type 3 secretion apparatus, which generates a modified version of the system called PROT3EcT. This system secretes anti-TNF-α nanobodies that are equally effective as antibodies delivered systemically in reducing inflammation in a preclinical mouse model of colitis (Lynch et al., 2022). Quorum sensing (QS)-dependent genetic circuits have the potential to effectively synchronize bacterial behaviors in the extracellular environment of tumors, resulting in a consistent and prolonged administration of curative agents. Nevertheless, utilizing QS-based techniques may present certain challenges. For instance, obtaining the necessary bacterial concentration may not be feasible for all tumor sizes, and the application of lysis genes derived from bacteriophages may exert significant evolutionary pressure for mutations (Gurbatri et al., 2022; Kim et al., 2021).

REWIRING OF THE IMMUNE SYSTEM

When bacteria invade a host body, they typically trigger a response from the immune system. This results in a connection being established between the bacteria and the immune cells, which is summarized in Figure 17.2. Bacteria, which are not native to the human body, naturally activate the immune system by activating innate immune receptors, secreting immunostimulatory metabolites, and injecting effector proteins. When immune components destroy and phagocytize bacteria and bacterial lysis products are generated within the tumor core, the immune system is activated (Harimoto et al., 2022). This stimulation leads to an increase in the immune response against the bacteria, as illustrated in Figure 17.2.

Apart from their inherent immunostimulatory features, synthetic biology techniques can be utilized to engineer bacteria for targeted delivery of cargo that can act at different stages of the antitumor immune response. This approach has the potential to boost the therapeutic efficacy of bacterial cancer treatments against a variety of tumor types such as syngeneic CT26 colorectal cancer model, genetically engineered spontaneous breast cancer model (MMTV-PyMT), and orthotopic breast cancer (mammary fat pad 4T1) in conjunction with the bacteria innate immune activation properties (Gurbatri et al., 2022; Harimoto et al., 2022). In the early stages of tumor growth, bacterial ligands can stimulate the immune system to recruit and activate immune cells like monocytes, macrophages, and neutrophils. These cells contribute to the destruction of tumor-colonizing microorganisms and the production of inflammatory cytokines. To further enhance this response, scientists have engineered a strain of *S. typhimurium* to produce a more potent type of flagellin called FlaB, which stimulates the immune system through the activation of Toll-like receptors TLR4 and TLR5 (Zheng et al., 2017). This leads to the infiltration of immune cells into the tumor microenvironment and a shift in macrophages from a protumor to an antitumor state, resulting in delayed tumor growth and inhibition of metastases in animal models (Gurbatri et al., 2022).

Antigen-presenting cells (APCs) can activate an adaptive immune response by presenting new antigens after engulfing cells. In the case of melanoma tumors derived from patients, melanoma cells and infiltrating APCs can present antigens from intracellular bacteria in the tumor microbiome, leading to adaptive immunity (Kalaora et al., 2021). The utilization of attenuated *S. typhimurium* is an established alternative to *Listeria*-based strategies for delivering neoantigen peptides into tumorous tissues. A matrix metalloproteinase (MMP) target sequence is employed to anchor multiple neoantigen peptides to the outer membrane of *S. typhimurium*. This approach is known to be effective and efficient in delivering neoantigen peptides to tumor sites (Shahabi et al., 2008). Once engineered bacteria are home to tumors, proteases present in the tumor cleave neoantigens from bacteria and release them into the tumor microenvironment, where they can recruit and activate lymphocytes. This treatment increased the levels of proinflammatory cytokines and tumor-infiltrating lymphocytes in murine colorectal tumors (Hyun et al., 2021; Selvanesan et al., 2023). The presence of microorganisms within a tumor has been shown to exert a profound influence on the tumor microenvironment (TME), thereby enhancing the adaptive immune response through metabolic regulation. Among these microorganisms, *Escherichia coli* Nissle (EcN) has been found to be particularly noteworthy, owing to its ability to convert ammonia, a metabolic waste product commonly found within tumors, into l-arginine as depicted in Figure 17.2. This metabolic conversion has the potential to significantly alter the tumor microenvironment, thereby impacting the immune response in profound ways. Injecting this L-arginine-producing strain directly into the tumor can result in better formation of tumor-infiltrating lymphocytes (TILs) and an overall improvement in therapeutic effectiveness when combined with checkpoint blocking (Canale et al., 2021).

ENGINEERING MICROBIAL INTERFACES

Bacteria can interact with external materials and technologies such as ultrasound and magnetic-based methods to influence their behavior outside the tumor and engage with immune cells in the tumor microenvironment (TME). These technologies also help in visualizing the tumor and controlling the release of therapeutics at specific times and locations. Nanoparticles, radiation therapy, and their cargo can alter the TME and affect how bacteria interact with the immune system. An interrelated

Gut Microbiome Engineering for Cancer Therapies

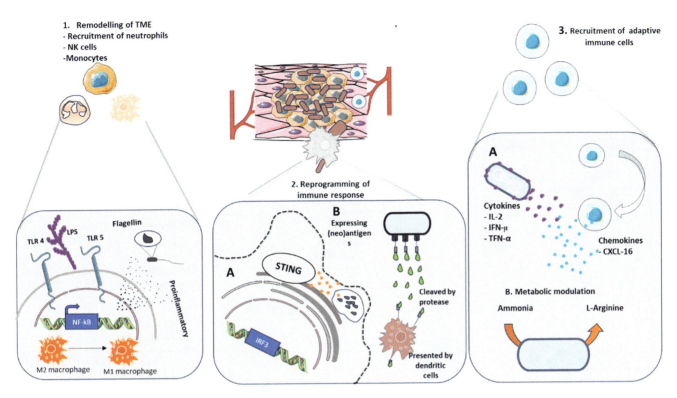

FIGURE 17.2 Reprogrammed bacteria-immune interface. As the immune response advances, Antigen-Presenting Cells (APCs) infiltrate the tumor and consume deceased tumor cells and intertumoral bacteria, which can enhance the immune response. One promising method involves utilizing a bacterial strain known as *EcN* that has been modified to provide STING agonists directly to APCs as highlighted in (A and B). This approach has been effective in producing long-lasting antitumor immunity and tumor regression in animal models, as reported by Kalaora et al. in 2021. Currently, a particular strain is undergoing phase 1 clinical trials to determine its effectiveness in treating patients with advanced solid tumors and lymphomas. Another bacterial strain known as STACT is also in clinical development. It has been engineered to activate the STING pathway upon uptake by tumor-resident APCs, which could ultimately lead to tumor regression (Gurbatri et al., 2022; Zheng et al., 2017). Recent research has revealed that bacteria can be altered to carry a variety of substances, which activate and recruit immune cells. This process enhances the antitumor immune response. Cytokines such as IL-2, IL-18, and CCL-21 work in conjunction to stimulate immune functions against cancer cells (Duong et al., 2019). When EcN is modified to produce C-X-C chemokine ligand 16 (CXCL16) as shown in (**3A**), it promotes the chemotaxis of cytotoxic T cells to tumors, which results in tumor regression. These findings suggest that by utilizing the natural structure of the immune response, we can modify the interactions between bacteria and immune cells. By producing different substances at different stages of the immune response, bacteria can communicate with specific immune cells and reprogram the antitumor response to be more effective (Duong et al., 2019; Gurbatri et al., 2022).

illustration of these combinations is illustrated in Figure 17.3. When combined, these approaches create a system of living and non-living therapies that work together to improve overall outcomes by overcoming each other limitations (Duong et al., 2019; Gurbatri et al., 2022).

Medical imaging methods like PET and MRI have been utilized for cancer detection and visualization for a long time. They may additionally work with naturally occurring or genetically created bacteria to improve tumor detection and bacterial localization in situ (Kang and Min, 2021). Certain types of cancer, such as prostate cancer, adult pheochromocytoma, paraganglioma, and neuroendocrine cancer, are treated using theranostic drugs (Sheikhbahaei et al., 2021). FDA-approved medicines include PLUVICTOTM (Lu-PSMA-617) for advanced prostate-specific membrane antigen-positive metastatic castration-resistant prostate cancer, AzedraR for those 12 and older with local, advanced, or metastatic pheochromocytomas and paragangliomas, and LutatheraR for neuroendocrine cancer (Hennrich and Eder, 2022). These drugs work by sticking to cancer cells and causing radiation damage.

Furthermore, bacteria can create molecules that are detectable through urine, blood, and stool, leading to non-invasive diagnoses. When equipped with bacterium-based sensors and circuits, engineered bacteria can also offer information on tumor existence, burden, and microenvironmental conditions (Danino et al., 2015). *In vivo*, external manipulation can interact with bacteria. FUS technique penetrates tissues precisely, allowing for specific visualization and manipulation of bacteria (Abedi et al., 2022). The use of acoustic reporter genes enables the visualization of *E. coli* and *S. typhimurium* in the gastrointestinal tract

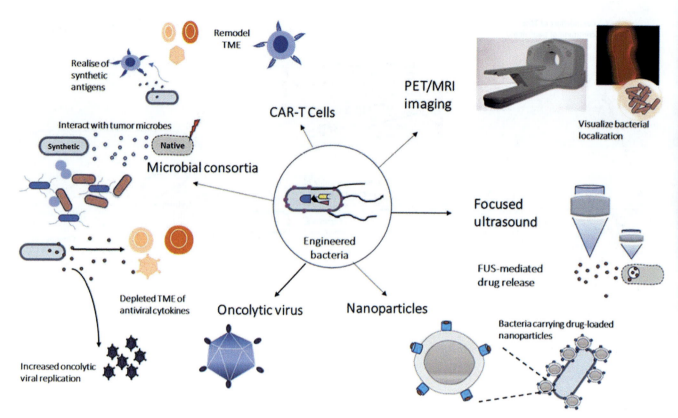

FIGURE 17.3 Interaction of engineered bacteria with other cancer treatment modalities. Combining bacteria with living and non-living technologies can enhance diagnostic and therapeutic outcomes. Advanced imaging techniques like MRI, PET, and FUS can monitor and visualize bacteria delivered systemically. By encoding bacteria with acoustic reporter genes or thermal switches, FUS can activate therapeutic release (Kang and Min, 2021; Gurbatri et al., 2022). Drug-loaded nanoparticles that are coupled to microorganisms can penetrate tumor depths. Researchers are looking into ways to engineer interactions between replicating or living modalities, such as modifying tumor microenvironments for oncolytic virus therapy, collaborating with synthetic consortia for predictable immune responses, and activating CAR-T cells to respond to synthetic antigens released by bacteria (Gurbatri et al., 2022).

and TME. By manipulating these genes, FUS can accurately detect the presence of bacteria and create a map of their location, providing valuable insights into their behavior and potential impact on human health. This innovative approach to bacterial detection and mapping holds great promise for advancing the field of microbiology and improving our understanding of the complex microbial communities that inhabit our bodies (Bourdeau et al., 2018).

Since the turn of the century, ultrasound technology (US) has been utilized in medicine to diagnose malignancies in brain tissue based on tissue density. Its uses have since grown to include cancer detection. The power of diagnostic ultrasound is in using high-intensity focused ultrasound (HIFU) which was first proposed in 1942. FUS is often used to treat various ailments by causing tissue damage, increasing membrane permeability, and boosting medicine absorption and cytotoxicity. It has been shown to trigger tumor cell death in malignant tissues (Chen et al., 2022). In 2022, Chen et al. detailed a fascinating discovery: bacteria can be genetically modified to produce immune checkpoint inhibitors, cytotoxic agents, or cytokines in response to FUS heat. As highlighted in Table 17.1, which shows various molecules that can be produced from engineering bacteria in cancer therapy.

Moreover, FUS can be employed for bacterium-encoded mechanotherapy, wherein bacteria are engineered to transport micrometer-scale cavitating bubbles that generate potent local mechanical impacts. These impacts can aid in destroying tissue and cells, lysing bacteria, and administering therapeutic agents (Bar-Zion et al., 2021). Several studies have attempted to enhance the penetration of customized strains of bacteria into the hypoxic cores of tumors by combining them with magnetic guidance. Many of these studies have utilized the magneto-aerotactic property of *Magnetococcus marinus*, which suggests that wireless control of bacteria carrying liposomal cargo can be achieved using external magnetic torque-driven actuation, thereby improving bacterial concentration deep within the tumor microenvironment (Felfoul et al., 2016).

In addition, the use of magnetic nanoparticles and chemotherapeutic-encapsulating nanoliposomes coated on the surface of *E. coli* has allowed bacteria to be steered magnetically through three-dimensional materials. The bacteria can be directed to an externally supplied magnetic field and to release their cargo in vitro (Akolpoglu et al., 2023).

Utilizing therapeutic techniques like radiation can heighten the efficacy of nanoparticle and bacteria therapies by promoting interactions between bacteria and immune cells.

TABLE 17.1
Engineered bacteria and the antitumor agent produced

Genus of engineered bacteria	Antitumor agents produced	References
	Cytokines	
Clostridium, Salmonella	IL-2 (A signaling molecule that modulates lymphocyte activity)	(Al-Ramadi et al., 2009; Chen et al., 2022)
Salmonella	CCL21 (A chemokine that modulates T, DC, and NK cell migration)	(Loeffler et al., 2009)
Salmonella	IL-18 (An IFNγ inducer factor that boosts cytokine production in both T and NK cells)	(Loeffler et al., 2008, Chen et al., 2022)
Clostridium	IL-12 (An anticancer cytokine that stimulates IFN-c production)	(Zhang et al., 2014)
	Cytotoxic agents and regulator	
Salmonella	TRAIL (Induces apoptosis in cancer cells)	(Zhang et al., 2014)
Salmonella	Endostatin (Inhibits angiogenesis)	(Liang et al., 2018)
Salmonella, Escherichia	Cytolysin A (Pro-apoptotic molecule)	(Nguyen et al., 2010)
Salmonella	FasL (Tumor necrosis factor-α(TNF-α))	(Loeffler et al., 2008, Chen et al., 2022)

The process involves coating weakened *S. typhimurium* with positively charged polyamidoamine dendrimer nanoparticles, which facilitate the attraction of negatively charged antigens through electrostatic interactions. When tumors that hinder the immune system are subjected to radiation therapy, they release tumor antigens that the modified bacteria can transport to functional dendritic cells situated at the tumor perimeter. This leads to a robust systemic immune response against the tumor (Wang et al., 2022).

ENGINEERING COMMUNITIES OF PROGRAMMABLE MEDICINES

The scientific community is recognizing the collaborative potential of bacteria in enhancing therapeutic outcomes. This is achieved through the modification of the tumor microenvironment to create a more hospitable setting for other microbial and cellular therapies. A prime example is the use of non-pathogenic *E. coli* carrying an IFN-I antagonist, B18R, to aid vesicular stomatitis virus (VSV) replication within the tumor by preventing immune system clearance (Cronin et al., 2014). Two types of microbes, when used alone, do not exhibit significant antitumor efficacy. However, when used together, they provide an improved antitumor response and increased survival outcomes in murine cancer models (Guo et al., 2022). Similarly, combining attenuated bacterial strains like *Brucella melitenis* with chimeric antigen receptor (CAR)-T cell therapies can promote proinflammatory M1 polarization of tumor macrophages and increase the frequency of CD8+ T cells within tumors (Gurbatri et al., 2022). Direct connection between modified bacteria and cellular treatments has the potential to improve therapeutic outcomes. Probiotic-guided CAR-T cells (ProCARs) carry a synthetic antigen that CAR-T cells recognize, enabling more precise regulation of CAR activation within tumor areas. ProCARs, which are released by tumor-colonizing bacteria, dramatically delay tumor development in mice with human tumor xenografts, outperforming a combination of bacteria vehicle and CAR-T cell therapy (Vincent et al., 2021).

Bacteria can be genetically modified to identify and destroy microbes that promote the growth of tumors by producing antimicrobial substances. Another strategy is to utilize small groups of microbes as medical treatments (Sepich-Poore et al., 2021). For example, researchers have discovered an 11-strain commensal consortium of bacteria within the gut microbiome that can boost the immune response by triggering the production of IFNγ+ CD8+ T cells and cytotoxic T cell immunity. This can help improve the effectiveness of an immune checkpoint blockade in preventing tumor growth. Synthetic biology can be used to create synthetic communities of bacteria that work together or against each other to enhance the therapeutic efficacy of cancer treatments (Tanoue et al., 2019).

EFFICIENT DRUG DELIVERY IN CANCER THERAPY THROUGH ENGINEERING OF THE GUT MICROBIAL CHASSIS

With the use of technology tools like engineering, microbes have provided a potent method that enables the large-scale manufacturing of biological compounds and medications. Through genetic modification, microbes can be fine-tuned to create enhanced chassis by either removing or enhancing their natural features. This results in improved safety, targetability, and colonization, which has paved the way for remarkable progress. One such breakthrough is the use of virulence-deficient GM strains of pathogens such as *Salmonella typhi*, *Clostridium novyi*, and *Listeria monocytogenes*. These strains have been instrumental in cancer treatment and the precise delivery of therapeutic payloads (Chen et al., 2023). Antitumor therapeutic compounds, including cytotoxic drugs, prodrug-converting enzymes, and immunomodulators, such as cytokines and tumor antigens, can be delivered by gut commensals (Chen et al., 2023; Zhou et al., 2018).

One impressive instance is the way EcN has been engineered to create nanobodies that target PD-L1 and CTLA-4. This method works by blocking crucial immune checkpoints during cancer treatment. By utilizing the QS-controlled autolysis circuit, the engineered EcN can deliver a payload of antibodies directly to tumors, resulting in an effective treatment option for immunotherapy against CRC. The approach of combining these techniques leads to synergistic effects (Gurbatri et al., 2020). Recent studies have shown that the gut commensal *Bifidobacterium longum* can be transformed with a plasmid that expresses the WT1 protein, making it a potential vaccination against castration-resistant prostate cancer (CRPC). This makes it one of the most promising tumor-associated antigens. Furthermore, combining GM gut bacteria with nanomedicine and cellular immunotherapy has shown promising potential in tumor therapy (Holay et al., 2021).

Studies have ascertained that specific gut commensals, like *Akkermansia muciniphila* (Cani et al., 2022) and *Faecalibacterium* spp. (Lopez-Siles et al., 2017), possess the ability to impede tumor growth and boost the immune response to therapy. Nevertheless, the lack of genetic modification methods for these bacteria has impeded the required strides towards creating secure and efficient live bacterial therapeutics (LBTs). The field of biotechnology is poised for rapid acceleration thanks to cutting-edge engineering tools like the CRISPR-Cas toolkit. By harnessing the power of probiotic strains, we may soon see the emergence of dependable, precisely defined, and reproducible therapeutics that could overcome the limitations of current treatments such as FMT. At present, FMT is limited to treating a select few types of cancer, including melanoma, and requires extensive donor screening to prevent the transmission of harmful microorganisms (Chen et al., 2023).

CHALLENGES AND LIMITATIONS TO THE ENGINEERING OF GUT MICROBIOTA IN CANCER THERAPY

Much progress has been achieved in the field of gut microbiota engineering and genetic manipulation, yet substantial gaps and hurdles have also been recognized. One example is the precise targeting of transgenic microbes to diverse local microenvironments in vivo. The progress of gut microbiota engineering is impeded due to the absence of an accurate delivery method for foreign DNA. In addition, the host cells plasmid replication and the integration of supplied genetic material into the genome also pose significant challenges. Engineering gut microbiota for cancer therapy is a complex task with several challenges. The lack of a standardized technique for detecting microbial signatures in gut microbiota-based therapeutics is a major impediment, resulting in inconsistencies in sample selection, collection, technology, data quality, and resource analysis. Sample management, DNA extraction, bioinformatics, and data gathering are all critical technical variables. NGS or third-generation sequencing may yield high-throughput data, however interpretation might be difficult owing to resource variety.

While there is a growing body of evidence supporting the potential of microbial targets for cancer therapy, their full application remains underdeveloped. The intricate nature of the disease, coupled with variations in individual susceptibility to microbial pathogens, presents a challenge in determining the optimal treatment course. It is unclear whether incorporating such therapies into current cancer management practices would yield significant antitumor benefits. Additional preclinical research and clinical trials are necessary to identify potential roadblocks and explore possible solutions. There are various factors that could hinder the widespread use of microbial methods, aside from technical difficulties. Individual differences in biology, such as genetics, dietary habits, age, gender, existing medical conditions, and geographical location, can all affect the makeup of a person microbiota. One of the main challenges in applying discoveries related to microbiota to other regions is the geographic diversity of human microbiota. For instance, while certain bacteria may serve as useful non-invasive diagnostic markers for colorectal cancer (CRC), it may not be applicable to other diseases.

CONCLUSION

The gut microbiota has enormous promise for generating tailored anticancer therapies. However, numerous issues have to be solved, including effective biocontainment and precision targeting. Despite this, there is an increasing interest in researching the makeup and function of gut bacteria. According to research, depending on the kind of cancer and experimental participants, the gut microbiota can play a dual function in cancer development. The efficiency of anticancer treatment can be increased while lowering side effects and increasing prognosis by integrating gut microbiota with established antitumor treatment regimens and including probiotics, FMT, and dietary management. Furthermore, the importance of the gut microbiota in cancer diagnosis and prediction is becoming clear. Eventually, by providing a scientific foundation for building more effective anticancer therapy regimens, regulating gut microbiota can progress cancer treatment and promote precision medicine. The use of the gut microbiota to build tailored anticancer therapy has considerable promise. However, other issues remain to be solved, such as effective biocontainment and precision targeting.

Nonetheless, there is growing interest in understanding the makeup and function of the gut microbiota. Recent study has shown that the gut microbiota can play a dual role in cancer development, depending on the disease type and experimental participants. By integrating gut microbiota with established antitumor therapy regimens and including probiotics, FMT, and dietary management, anticancer treatment efficacy can be increased while minimizing adverse effects and increasing prognosis. Furthermore, the importance of the gut microbiota in cancer diagnosis and prediction is becoming increasingly apparent. Finally, managing the gut microbiota can progress cancer treatment and promote precision medicine by providing a scientific foundation for building more effective anticancer treatment strategies.

Although there are still obstacles to overcome, it is crucial to recognize the significance and untapped potential of gut microbiota when it comes to creating innovative anticancer methods. Thus investigating a holistic strategy that incorporates microbial modulation treatment into the present cancer care system is essential.

REFERENCES

Abedi, M.H., Yao, M.S., Mittelstein, D.R., Bar-Zion, A., Swift, M.B., Lee-Gosselin, A., Barturen-Larrea, P., Buss, M.T., Shapiro, M.G., 2022. Ultrasound-controllable engineered bacteria for cancer immunotherapy. Nature Communications 13, 1585.

Akolpoglu, M.B., Alapan, Y., Dogan, N.O., Baltaci, S.F., Yasa, O., Aybar Tural, G., Sitti, M., 2023. Magnetically steerable bacterial microrobots moving in 3D biological matrices for stimuli-responsive cargo delivery Science Advances 8, eabo6163.

Al-Ramadi,B.K., Fernandez-Cabezudo,M.J.,El-Hasasna,H., AlSalam,S., Bashir, G., Chouaib, S. (2009). Potent anti-tumor activity of systemically-administered IL-2-expressing salmonella correlates with decreased angiogenesis and enhanced tumor apoptosis. Clinical Immunology 130 (1)89–97.

Anderson, J.C., Clarke, E.J., Arkin, A.P., Voigt, C.A., 2006. Environmentally Controlled Invasion of Cancer Cells by Engineered Bacteria. Journal of Molecular Biology 355, 619–627.

Bar-Zion, A., Nourmahnad, A., Mittelstein, D.R., Shivaei, S., Yoo, S., Buss, M.T., Hurt, R.C., Malounda, D., Abedi, M.H., Lee-Gosselin, A., Swift, M.B., Maresca, D., Shapiro, M.G., 2021. Acoustically triggered mechanotherapy using genetically encoded gas vesicles. Nature Nanotechnology 16, 1403–1412.

Bourdeau, R.W., Lee-Gosselin, A., Lakshmanan, A., Farhadi, A., Kumar, S.R., Nety, S.P., Shapiro, M.G., 2018. Acoustic reporter genes for noninvasive imaging of microorganisms in mammalian hosts. Nature 553, 86–90.

Canale, F.P., Basso, C., Antonini, G., Perotti, M., Li, N., Sokolovska, A., Neumann, J., James, M.J., Geiger, S., Jin, W., Theurillat, J.-P., West, K.A., Leventhal, D.S., Lora, J.M., Sallusto, F., Geiger, R., 2021. Metabolic modulation of tumours with engineered bacteria for immunotherapy. Nature 598, 662–666.

Cani, P.D., Depommier, C., Derrien, M., Everard, A., de Vos, W.M., 2022. Akkermansia muciniphila: paradigm for next-generation beneficial microorganisms. Nature Reviews Gastroenterology & 19, 625–637.

Chabloz, A., Schaefer, J. V, Kozieradzki, I., Cronin, S.J.F., Strebinger, D., Macaluso, F., Wald, J., Rabbitts, T.H., Plückthun, A., Marlovits, T.C., Penninger, J.M., 2020. Salmonella-based platform for efficient delivery of functional binding proteins to the cytosol. Communications Biology 3, 342.

Chen J, Li T, Liang J, Huang Q, Huang JD, Ke Y. 2022. Current status of intratumor microbiome in cancer and engineered exogenous microbiota as a promising therapeutic strategy. *Biomedicine & Pharmacotherapy* 145:112443.

Chen, Z., Jin, W., Hoover, A., Chao, Y., Ma, Y., 2023. Decoding the microbiome: advances in genetic manipulation for gut bacteria. Trends Microbiology. 31(11):1143–1161.

Chien, T., Harimoto, T., Kepecs, B., Gray, K., Coker, C., Hou, N., Pu, K., Azad, T., Nolasco, A., Pavlicova, M., Danino, T., 2022. Enhancing the tropism of bacteria via genetically programmed biosensors. Nature Biomedical Engineering 6, 94–104.

Cronin, M., Le Boeuf, F., Murphy, C., Roy, D.G., Falls, T., Bell, J.C., Tangney, M., 2014. Bacterial-Mediated Knockdown of Tumor Resistance to an Oncolytic Virus Enhances Therapy. Molecular Therapy. 22, 1188–1197.

Danino, T., Prindle, A., Kwong, G.A., Skalak, M., Li, H., Allen, K., Hasty, J., Bhatia, S.N., 2015. Programmable probiotics for detection of cancer in urine. Science Translational Medicine 7, 289ra84–289ra84.

Duong, M.T.-Q., Qin, Y., You, S.-H., Min, J.-J., 2019. Bacteria-cancer interactions: bacteria-based cancer therapy. Experimental & Molecular Medicine 51, 1–15.

Felfoul, K. O., Mohammadi, M., Taherkhani, S., de Lanauze, D., Zhong Xu, Y., Loghin, D., Essa, S., Jancik, S., Houle, D., Lafleur, M., Gaboury, L., Tabrizian, M., Kaou, N., Atkin, M., Vuong, T., Batist, G., Beauchemin, N., Radzioch, D., Martel, S., 2016. Magneto-aerotactic bacteria deliver drug-containing nanoliposomes to tumour hypoxic regions. Nature Nanotechnology 11, 941–947.

Fernandes, M.R., Aggarwal, P., Costa, R.G.F., Cole, A.M., Trinchieri, G., 2022. Targeting the gut microbiota for cancer therapy. Nature Reviews Cancer 22, 703–722.

Forbes, N.S., 2010. Engineering the perfect (bacterial) cancer therapy. Nature Reviews 10, 785-794.

Guo, F., Das, J.K., Kobayashi, K.S., Qin, Q.M., A Ficht, T., Alaniz, R.C., Song, J., Figueiredo, P. De, 2022. Live attenuated bacterium limits cancer resistance to CAR-T therapy by remodeling the tumor microenvironment. The Journal for ImmunoTherapy of Cancer.10(1):e003760

Gurbatri, C.R., Arpaia, N., Danino, T., 2022. Engineering bacteria as interactive cancer therapies. Science 378, 858-864.

Gurbatri, C.R., Lia, I., Vincent, R., Coker, C., Castro, S., Treuting, P.M., Hinchliffe, T.E., Arpaia, N., Danino, T., 2020. Engineered probiotics for local tumor delivery of checkpoint blockade nanobodies. Science Translational Medicine 12, eaax0876.

Harimoto, T., Hahn, J., Chen, Y.-Y., Im, J., Zhang, J., Hou, N., Li, F., Coker, C., Gray, K., Harr, N., Chowdhury, S., Pu, K., Nimura, C., Arpaia, N., Leong, K.W., Danino, T., 2022. A programmable encapsulation system improves delivery of therapeutic bacteria in mice. Nature Biotechnology 40, 1259-1269.

Hennrich, U., Eder, M., 2022. [177Lu]Lu-PSMA-617 (PluvictoTM): The First FDA-Approved Radiotherapeutical for Treatment of Prostate Cancer. Pharmaceuticals (Basel). 15(10): 1292.

Holay, M., Guo, Z., Pihl, J., Heo, J., Park, J.H., Fang, R.H., Zhang, L., 2021. Bacteria-inspired nanomedicine. ACS Applied Bio Materials 4, 3830-3848.

Hyun, J., Jun, S., Lim, H., Cho, H., You, S.-H., Ha, S.-J., Min, J.-J., Bang, D., 2021. Engineered attenuated salmonella typhimurium expressing neoantigen has anticancer effects. ACS Synthetic Biology 10, 2478-2487.

Idée, J.-M., Louguet, S., Ballet, S., Corot, C., 2013. Theranostics and contrast-agents for medical imaging: a pharmaceutical company viewpoint. Quantitative Imaging in Medicine and Surgery 3, 292.

Kalaora, S., Nagler, A., Nejman, D., Alon, M., Barbolin, C., Barnea, E., Ketelaars, S.L.C., Cheng, K., Vervier, K., Shental, N., Bussi, Y., Rotkopf, R., Levy, R., Benedek, G., Trabish, S., Dadosh, T., Levin-Zaidman, S., Geller, L.T., Wang, K., Greenberg, P., Yagel, G., Peri, A., Fuks, G., Bhardwaj, N., Reuben, A., Hermida, L., Johnson, S.B., Galloway-Peña, J.R., Shropshire, W.C., Bernatchez, C., Haymaker, C., Arora, R., Roitman, L., Eilam, R., Weinberger, A., Lotan-Pompan, M., Lotem, M., Admon, A., Levin, Y., Lawley, T.D., Adams, D.J., Levesque, M.P., Besser, M.J., Schachter, J., Golani, O., Segal, E., Geva-Zatorsky, N., Ruppin, E., Kvistborg, P., Peterson, S.N., Wargo, J.A., Straussman, R., Samuels, Y., 2021. Identification of bacteria-derived HLA-bound peptides in melanoma. *Nature* 592, 138-143.

Kang, S.-R., Min, J.-J., 2021. Recent progress in the molecular imaging of tumor-treating bacteria. Nuclear Medicine and Molecular Imaging 55, 7-14.

Kasinskas, R.W., Forbes, N.S., 2007. Salmonella typhimurium lacking ribose chemoreceptors localize in tumor quiescence and induce apoptosis. Cancer Research 67, 3201-3209.

Kim, T., Weinberg, B., Wong, W., Lu, T.K., 2021. Scalable recombinase-based gene expression cascades. Nature Communications 12, 2711.

Liang, K., Liu, Q., Li, P., Han, Y., Bian, X., Tang, Y.,Kong, Q. ((2018). Endostatin gene therapy delivered by attenuated Salmonella typhimurium in murine tumor models. Cancer Gene Therapy.167-183

Loeffler, M., Le Negrate,G., Krajewska,M., Reed, J.C. (2008). IL-18-producing salmonella inhibit tumor growth Cancer Gene Therapy., 15 (12)787-794.

Loeffler, M., Le Negrate,G., Krajewska,M., Reed, J.C. (2009). Salmonella typhimurium engineered to produce CCL21 inhibit tumor growth Cancer Immunol. Journal of Immunotherapy., 58 (5)769-775.

Lopez-Siles, M., Duncan, S.H., Garcia-Gil, L.J., Martinez-Medina, M., 2017. Faecalibacterium prausnitzii: from microbiology to diagnostics and prognostics. ISME Journal: Multidisciplinary Journal of Microbial 11, 841-852.

Low, K.B., Ittensohn, M., Le, T., Platt, J., Sodi, S., Amoss, M., Ash, O., Carmichael, E., Chakraborty, A., Fischer, J., Lin, S.L., Luo, X., Miller, S.I., Zheng, L., King, I., Pawelek, J.M., Bermudes*, D., 1999. Lipid A mutant Salmonella with suppressed virulence and TNFα induction retain tumor-targeting in vivo. Nature Biotechnology Nat Biotechnol 17, 37-41.

Lynch, J.P., Goers, L., Lesser, C.F., 2022. Emerging strategies for engineering—Escherichia coli—Nissle 1917-based therapeutics. Trends Journal of Pharmacological Sciences Pharmacol Sci 43, 772-786.

MacCarthy, E.F., 2006. The Toxins of William B. Coley and the Treatment of Bone and Soft-Tissue Sarcomas. Iowa Orthopedic Journal 26, 154-158.

Nguyen, V.H., Kim, H., Ha, J., Hong, Y., Choy, H.E., Min, J. (2010). Genetically engineered salmonella typhimurium as an imageable therapeutic probe for cancer. Cancer Research., 70 (1)18-23.

Pene, F., Courtine, E., Cariou, A., Mira, J.-P., 2009. Toward theragnostics. Critical Care Medicine 37, S50-S58.

Pruis, I.J., van Dongen, G.A.M.S., Veldhuijzen van Zanten, S.E.M., 2020. The added value of diagnostic and theranostic PET imaging for the treatment of CNS tumors. International Journal of Molecular Sciences 21(3):1029

Selvanesan, B.C., Chandra, D., Quispe-Tintaya, W., Jahangir, A., Patel, A., Meena, K., Alves Da Silva, R.A., Friedman, M., Gabor, L., Khouri, O., Libutti, S.K., Yuan, Z., Li, J., Siddiqui, S., Beck, A., Tesfa, L., Koba, W., Chuy, J., McAuliffe, J.C., Jafari, R., Entenberg, D., Wang, Y., Condeelis, J., DesMarais, V., Balachandran, V., Zhang, X., Lin, K., Gravekamp, C., 2023. Listeria delivers tetanus toxoid protein to pancreatic tumors and induces cancer cell death in mice. Science Translational Medicine 14, eabc1600.

Sepich-Poore, G.D., Zitvogel, L., Straussman, R., Hasty, J., Wargo, J.A., Knight, R., 2021. The microbiome and human cancer. Science. 371(6536):eabc4552

Shahabi Kang, S.-R., Min, J.-J., 2021. Recent Progress in the Molecular Imaging of Tumor-Treating Bacteria. Nuclear Medicine and Molecular Imaging. 55, 7-14.

Sheikhbahaei, S., Sadaghiani, M.S., Rowe, S.P., Solnes, L.B., 2021. Neuroendocrine Tumor Theranostics: An Update and Emerging Applications in Clinical Practice. American Journal of Roentgenology 217, 495-506.

Sieow, B.F.L., Wun, K.S., Yong, W.P., Hwang, I.Y., Chang, M.W., 2021. Tweak to Treat: Reprograming Bacteria for Cancer Treatment. Trends Cancer. 7(5):447-464

Stewart, M.P., Sharei, A., Ding, X., Sahay, G., Langer, R., Jensen, K.F., 2016. In vitro and ex vivo strategies for intracellular delivery. Nature 538, 183-192.

Tanoue, T., Morita, S., Plichta, D.R., Skelly, A.N., Suda, W., Sugiura, Y., Narushima, S., Vlamakis, H., Motoo, I., Sugita, K., Shiota, A., Takeshita, K., Yasuma-Mitobe, K., Riethmacher, D., Kaisho, T., Norman, J.M., Mucida, D., Suematsu, M., Yaguchi, T., Bucci, V., Inoue, T., Kawakami, Y., Olle, B., Roberts, B., Hattori, M., Xavier, R.J., Atarashi, K., Honda, K., 2019. A defined commensal consortium elicits CD8 T cells and anti-cancer immunity. Nature 565, 600-605.

Vincent, R.L., Gurbatri, C.R., Redenti, A., Coker, C., Arpaia, N., Danino, T., 2021. Probiotic-guided CAR-T cells for universal solid tumor targeting. bioRxiv 2021.10.10.463366.

Viswanathan, S., Parida, S., Lingipilli, B.T., Krishnan, R., Podipireddy, D.R., Muniraj, N., 2023. Role of Gut Microbiota in Breast Cancer and Drug Resistance. Pathogens. 12(3):468

Wang, W., Xu, H., Ye, Q., Tao, F., Wheeldon, I., Yuan, A., Hu, Y., Wu, J., 2022. Systemic immune responses to irradiated tumours via the transport of antigens to the tumour periphery by injected flagellate bacteria. Nature Biomedical Engineering Nat Biomed Eng 6, 44-53.

Weiss, S., Krusch, S., 2001. Bacteria-Mediated Transfer of Eukaryotic Expression Plasmids into Mammalian Host Cells. Journal of Biological Chemistry 382(4):533-41

Widmaier, D.M., Tullman-Ercek, D., Mirsky, E.A., Hill, R., Govindarajan, S., Minshull, J., Voigt, C.A., 2009. Engineering the Salmonella type III secretion system to export spider silk monomers. Molecular Systems Biology 5, 309.

Zhang, Y.L., Lu, R., Chang, Z.S., Zhang, W.Q., Wang, Q.B., Ding, S.Y., Zhao, W. (2014). Clostridium sporogenes delivers interleukin-12 to hypoxic tumours, producing antitumour activity without significant toxicity. Letters in Applied Microbiology. 59(6):580-6.

Zheng, J.H., Nguyen, V.H., Jiang, S.-N., Park, S.-H., Tan, W., Hong, S.H., Shin, M.G., Chung, I.-J., Hong, Y., Bom, H.-S., Choy, H.E., Lee, S.E., Rhee, J.H., Min, J.-J., 2017. Two-step enhanced cancer immunotherapy with engineered Salmonella typhimurium secreting heterologous flagellin. Science Translational Medicine. 9(376):eaak9537.

Zhou, S., Gravekamp, C., Bermudes, D., Liu, K., 2018. Tumour-targeting bacteria engineered to fight cancer. Nature Reviews Cancer 18, 727-743.

18 Conclusion, Future Perspectives, and Challenges in Gut Microbiome Cancer Research

Zodwa Dlamini, Rodney Hull, Serwalo Ramagaga, and Alexandre Kokoua

GUT MICROBIOME DYSBIOSIS AND CANCER

The revelations regarding gut microbiome dysbiosis and its pivotal role in cancer development underscore the profound impact of microbial ecology on human physiology. The recognition of specific bacterial species as influencers in cancer risk and progression marks a paradigm shift, emphasizing the importance of understanding the molecular underpinnings of host-microbiome interactions. The revolution in characterizing gut microbial communities, facilitated by "next-generation" sequencing, has propelled the field forward, revealing the intricate relationship between the microbiota and the human immune system. Dysbiosis, influenced by environmental and genetic factors, emerges as a critical player in the emergence and dissemination of cancer (Figure 18.1).

GUT MICROBIOME AND CANCER TREATMENT RESPONSE

The chapter on the gut microbiome and cancer treatment response brings forth a paradigmatic shift—from a mere association to a discernible cause and effect relationship. The manipulative potential demonstrated in animal model studies suggests a transformative avenue for positively altering cancer outcomes. However, the transition from preclinical insights to clinical application demands meticulous exploration of critical pathways in the gut-tumor microbial axis (Figure 18.1). The imperative for standardized microbial analysis becomes evident, particularly considering the geographical and regional variations in the human gut microbiome.

GUT MICROBIOME MODULATION FOR PERSONALIZED CANCER THERAPIES

Recognition of disturbances in commensal microbiota as contributors to various diseases, including cancer, sets the stage for personalized precision antimicrobial cancer therapy. The chapter delves into strategies to modulate the gut microbiome, emphasizing the need for personalized precision antimicrobial cancer therapy, an approach tailored to individual microbial variations. A call for collaborative research at every stage, from basic to translational and clinical investigations, resonates through the narrative, highlighting the intricate balance between promoting a healthy gut microbial composition and the challenges posed by individual variability.

GUT MICROBIOME AND IMMUNOTHERAPY RESISTANCE

Immunotherapy, a beacon of hope in medical oncology, encounters a bottleneck in resistance, intricately linked to the composition and diversity of the gut microbiome. The potential role of Fecal Microbiota Transplantation (FMT) in overcoming immunotherapy resistance is explored, acknowledging safety concerns and cancer-specific variations in microbiota composition. The prospect of incorporating diet and lifestyle to support desired microbiota growth adds a layer of complexity and opportunity to enhance immunotherapeutic effects (Figure 18.1).

GUT MICROBIOME AND CHEMOTHERAPY RESISTANCE

The interplay between chemotherapeutic agents and the gut microbiota unfolds a narrative of chemotherapy-induced dysbiosis, influencing chemoresistance or sensitivity (Figure 18.1). The impact of antibiotics on microbial modulation in promoting or inhibiting chemosensitivity adds a layer of complexity to the delicate balance between protective and harmful microbes.

GUT MICROBIOME BIOMARKERS FOR CANCER DIAGNOSIS AND PROGNOSIS

The emergence of the gut microbiome as a fundamental colorectal cancer (CRC) risk factor introduces the concept of microbial signatures as diagnostic and prognostic markers. While strides in next-generation sequencing (NGS) techniques have been made (Figure 18.1), challenges such as data inconsistency and microbial variations across cancer types necessitate a shift toward long-read sequencers for improved accuracy. Identifying key variables is deemed essential to bridge the translational gap in CRC diagnostic and prognostic utility.

Conclusion, Future Perspectives, and Challenges

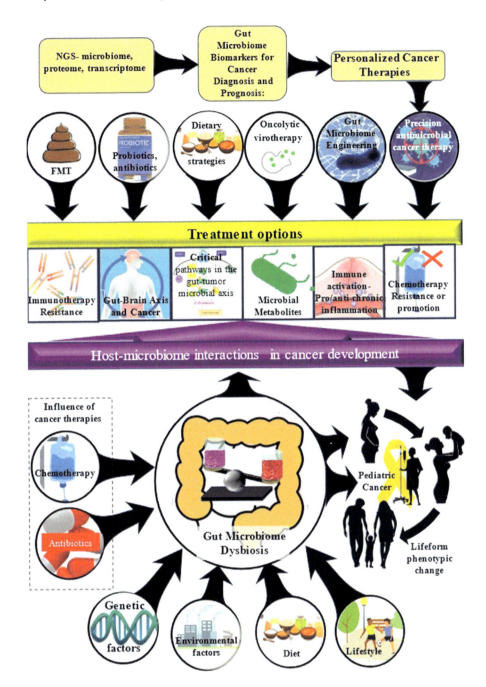

FIGURE 18.1 **A summary of the roles the gut microbiome plays in cancer and cancer therapy.** Dysbiosis is central to the role that the gut microbiome can play in cancer. This can be caused by a myriad of environmental and lifestyle factors as well as genetic factors. Certain cancer therapies such as chemotherapy or the use of antibiotics to prevent secondary infections can also lead to dysbiosis. Dysbiosis can lead to changes in the interactions between the host and their microbiome that can lead to the promotion of carcinogenesis. In infants this can result from dysbiosis within the mother or at later stages due to environmental factors. This can result in the development of pediatric cancers or lifetime phenotypic changes due to the importance of the microbiome in the development of the child. Changes in the interaction between the gut microbiome and the host can also lead to changes in the response to cancer therapy. This can result in increased resistance or sensitivity to chemotherapy and immunotherapy resistance. They can also promote cancer development through promoting changes in neurogenesis and immune signaling in the central nervous system through the gut brain axis, changes in immune induced inflammation, changes in cancer signaling pathways, and alter the secretion of bacterial metabolites, which can have a pro- or anticarcinogenic activity. Restoring the balance of the gut microbiome can be used as a therapeutic approach to treat or prevent cancer. Alternately specific microbes can be used to target cancer cells (oncolytic viruses and engineered microbes). Finally, analysis of the transcriptome, proteome, and microbiome as well as the metabolome can be used to identify microbial biomarkers for prognostic and diagnostic applications. This will help promote the development of personalized medicine and allow for the development of targeted antimicrobial cancer therapy.

MICROBIAL METABOLITES AND CANCER

The intricate association between microbial metabolites and cancer progression unfolds a narrative of regulatory mechanisms influencing the tumor microenvironment, immune function, and signaling pathways. The paradoxical functions of certain microbial metabolites and the context-dependent nature of their roles underscore the complexity of this nascent field. Therapeutic approaches exploring microbial metabolites for cancer treatment offer a promising frontier but necessitate a deeper insight into specific bacterial species and their function.

GUT–BRAIN AXIS AND CANCER

The profound influence of the gut microbiome on the nervous system, immune responses, and cancer development underscores the therapeutic potential of altering the gut–brain axis. Strategies involving probiotics, fecal transplants, and antibiotics aim to restore a diverse microbial population (Figure 18.1) but are faced with challenges in the variability of individual microbiomes. The intricate balance between environmental factors, socioeconomic factors, especially diet, immune status, and the need for personalized therapeutic solutions, emerges as a focal point for future research.

GUT MICROBIOME AND CANCER-RELATED INFLAMMATION

The chapter on gut microbiome and cancer-related inflammation elucidates the dual role of microbiota in promoting local chronic inflammation and inhibiting tumor growth through immune activation (Figure 18.1). The realization of the NF-kβ signaling pathway's exaggerated role in various cancers underscores the potential therapeutic application of gut microbiota in correcting dysbiosis and enhancing cancer treatment outcomes.

DIET, LIFESTYLE, AND THE GUT MICROBIOME

A detailed overview of how dietary patterns and lifestyle profoundly affect human health via modulation of the gut microbiota sets the stage for preventive measures against cancer. Despite considerable advances, the challenge lies in determining the precise roles of microorganisms in maintaining tissue integrity and understanding the factors influencing microbial populations. The shift toward a new food culture, centered on restricting dietary excess and favoring locally grown, fresh, and natural foods, holds promise for microbiota-associated health improvements.

GUT MICROBIOME AND PEDIATRIC CANCER

The challenges in understanding the relationship between the gut microbiome and pediatric tumors, exacerbated by small patient cohorts and intensive anticancer therapies, underscore the need for prospective research involving larger cohorts. The potential of microbiomes as biomarkers in pediatric cancer treatment is a tantalizing prospect, but the unresolved question of whether dysbiosis promotes or results from neoplasms, remains a critical area for investigation.

GUT MICROBIOME AND SYSTEMIC SIDE EFFECTS OF CANCER THERAPIES

Knowledge concerning the gut microbiome's role in mediating systemic side effects of cancer therapies, emphasizes its significance in cancer survivorship. The imperative for clinical trials involving a substantial number of cancer survivors becomes evident, pointing toward microbiota-mediated therapeutics to mitigate long-term negative effects. The need for personalized biomarkers to detect dysbiotic situations associated with poor cancer therapy outcomes adds another layer of complexity to the landscape.

GUT MICROBIOME AND PRECISION MEDICINE IN CANCER

Exploration of the gut microbiome as a cornerstone in precision medicine for cancer, showcases its potential in designing specific treatment modalities. The integration of proteomics, microbiomics, and precision medicine promises a personalized approach to colorectal cancer and beyond (Figure 18.1). The utilization of machine learning-based genetic engineering and rational donor selection in fecal microbiome transplant, represents the forefront of innovation in enhancing treatment efficacy.

THERAPEUTIC POTENTIAL OF THE GUT VIROME IN CANCER

The exploration of the therapeutic potential of the gut virome in cancer introduces the nascent field of phage therapy. While oncolytic virotherapy demonstrates promise, further research is essential to understand its applications and harness the immune potential of the gut virome for potent antitumor responses. Cutting-edge technologies like shotgun new generation sequencing and CRISPR/CAS gene editing hold the key to unlocking the therapeutic potential of the gut virome.

MICROBIOME-BASED CANCER THERAPEUTICS

Microbial communities, spanning fungi, viruses, protozoa, and bacteria, showcase the bidirectional link between the gastrointestinal microbiota and carcinogenesis. The emphasis on maintaining the ideal microbiota composition through antibiotic use, dietary strategies, and probiotic supplements introduces novel avenues for cancer prevention and treatment (Figure 18.1). The nuanced understanding of microbial roles in various cancers serves as a foundation for targeted therapeutic approaches.

GUT MICROBIOME ENGINEERING FOR CANCER THERAPIES

Gut microbiome engineering emerges as a ground-breaking strategy for enhancing cancer therapies (Figure 18.1). The amalgamation of traditional antitumor treatments with gut microbiota interventions promises to improve treatment efficacy and prognosis. Challenges in biocontainment and precision targeting necessitate innovative solutions, pushing the boundaries of biotechnological applications for personalized anticancer strategies.

FUTURE PERSPECTIVES AND CHALLENGES

The synthesis of knowledge in this extensive exploration paves the way for future research endeavors. The imperative for standardization and collaboration echoes through every facet of microbiome research. Mechanistic studies at the molecular level are essential to identify precise bacterial species and unravel their functions in mediating the effects of anticancer treatment. The recognition of microbial variability across diverse populations urges the exploration of ways to account for inter-individual microbial variations per population and area. Bridging the translational gap from preclinical insights to clinical applications, demands large-scale clinical trials for validating findings from animal model studies. Longitudinal studies tracking changes in the gut microbiome over time promise insights into the dynamic nature of the microbiome following cancer treatment.

The identification of microbial biomarkers for cancer diagnosis and prognosis necessitates addressing challenges such as data inconsistency, microbial variations across cancer types, and limitations of current sequencing techniques. Personalized precision antimicrobial cancer therapy stands at the forefront of future research, demanding a deeper understanding of individual microbial profiles for tailoring interventions. The safety concerns associated with interventions like FMT, and phage therapy necessitate rigorous screening of donor microbiota, improved processing methods, and ethical considerations regarding personalized cancer therapies.

The integration of disciplines, ranging from genetics and microbiology to artificial intelligence, emerges as a necessity for unraveling the complexity of the gut microbiome and its interactions with cancer. Machine learning-based approaches hold the potential to enhance donor selection in fecal microbiome transplants, contributing to the precision of microbiome-based therapies. Overcoming challenges related to biocontainment and precision targeting in gut microbiome engineering requires advancements in technology. Innovations in delivery methods and targeting specific bacterial strains will be crucial for the success of engineered therapies.

The response to cancer treatment is variable. Many factors have been repeatedly investigated in the literature, from genetic variability, metabolic status, generalized immune status, and functional status, affecting treatment response to cancer. However, there is paucity in the literature regarding the impact of the gut microbiome in tumorigenesis, prevention, and treatment. The judicious use of antibiotics has changed many facets of medicine, including the fast-emerging crisis of antibiotic resistance to an increasing number of cancer patients. It is, indeed, a subject worth paying attention to.

In conclusion, while "Exploring the Gut Microbiome in Cancer: From Biomarkers to Personalized Therapies" provides a comprehensive overview of the current state of research, the outlined future perspectives and challenges underscore the need for continued interdisciplinary collaboration and technological advancements. The intricacies of the gut microbiome's involvement in cancer beckon researchers to venture into uncharted territories, with the promise of unraveling new dimensions in personalized cancer therapeutics.

Index

16S rDNA 182
16S rRNA sequencing 76.128
5-Fluorouracil (5-FU) 5, 41, 45, 170
5-hydroxy tryptamine (5-HT), 109
53 BP1 29
ß-Glucuronidase 75
β-catenin pathway 98, 126
β-hydroxybutyrate 142
β-glucan 138
β-glucuronidase 33, 170
B-lapachone 5
B-linear fructans 135
γ-Aminobutyric acid (GABA) 95

A

ABC transporter proteins 72
ABCG2 71
Aberrant signaling pathways 29
Acetate 20
Acetitomaculum 134
Acetylcholine 113
Acetylcholine receptor 3 (M3R3) 113
Acetylcholine receptor M 113
Acinetobacter baylyi 87
Actinomyces ondontolyticus 182
Acoustic reporter genes 232
Actinobacteria 70, 122, 129, 140, 142, 153
Actinomyces 128
Activated antigen-presenting cells 192
Active immune cells 107
Acute gastrointestinal toxicity 169
Acute lymphoblastic leukemia (ALL) 155, 160, 161
Adaptive immune function compounds 155
Adeno-associated virus 200
Adenoma-carcinoma sequence 84
Adenomatous polyposis coli (APC) 85, 98
Adenoviral 200
Adenoviridae 188
Adenovirus 196
Adenovirus-Associated Virus Type 6 200
Adenovirus serotype 5 196
Adenylate cyclase toxin 59
Adhesion protein α2β1 integrin 99
Adipocyte 136
Adjunct to cancer treatment (microbiome) 6
Adoptive T-cell therapy 19
Advanced glycation end-products 42
Adverse effects of using the microbiome to reduce cancer incidence 33
Africa (Paleolithic era) 142
AGT16L 96
Akkermansia muciniphila 4, 127, 144, 184, 234
Akkermansia spp. 210
Akkermansia muciniphila 60, 140, 142, 213
Akt/ mTOR signaling 62
AKY pathway 2
Alcohol consumption 140
Alistipes spp. 75
Alkylating agents 153, 170
Allergic reactions 154, 201
Alloprevotella spp. 75
Alpha-diversity 140, 158, 171
Alzheimer's disease 100

American Cancer Society 14
Amgen Inc 199
Amniotic fluid microbiota 159
AMP characteristics 214
Anaerobic colon-dwelling bacteria 19
Anaerophaga spp. 134
Anaerosporobacter spp. 76
Anaerostipes caccae 136
Anchorage-dependent survival 195
AND logic gates 229
Anelloviridae 188
Angiogenesis 15, 100, 107
Angiogenic substances 27
Angiopoietin-like 4 (ANGPTL4) 172
Anthracyclines, 5
Anti-inflammatory cytokines 57, 142, 211
Anti-oxidative 142
Anti-PD-1 refractory melanoma 62
Antibiotherapy 210
Antibiotic bacterial ablation 46, 47
Antibiotic treatment of infants 154
Antibiotics 137
Anticancer drugs Effect of microbes on) 162
Anticancer therapy toxicity 169
Antigen-presenting cells (APCs) 230
Antimetabolite agents 170
Antimicrobial protein 140, 214
Antimicrotubule agents 171
Anti-PD-1/PD-L1 monoclonal antibodies 19
Antitumor immune function 110
Antitumor immunity through the gut virome 198
Anxiety 136
Anxiolytic, antidepressant, and nociceptive action 43
Apcmin/ + mice 85
APCMin/ + MSH2-/ -mice colonocytes 94
Apoptin 194
Application of microbial maximal extractable values (MEVs) 182
Approved oncolytic viral therapies 196
Arbotoxicity 143
Arginine-Glycine-Aspartic Acid (RGD4C) 193
ArgR 100
Artificial intelligence (AI) 179, 201
Aspartate β-hydroxylase (ASPH) 194
Asthma, 154
Astroviridae 188
ATM 29
Atopobium parvulum 182
ATP-binding cassette (ABC) 71
ATP-dependent group of proteins 70
Attenuating inflammatory networks 199
Autism 142
Autoimmunity. 17
Autonomic nervous system (ANS) 107
Autophagy 73
Autophagy-related genes (ATGs) 73
Avra 227
AzedraR 231

B

B-lactam antibiotics, m 47
B16-OVA melanoma 172

B16F10 melanoma cells 193
B18R 216, 233
Bacillus spp. 211
Bacillus clausii 171
Bacillus-derived QSPs 181
Bacillus polyfermenticus 42
Bacillus thuringiensis 214
Bacteria quorum-sensing peptides (QSPs) 181
Bacteria that induce cancer in humans 125
Bacteria tumor interface 229
Bacterial consortium transplantation 21
Bacterial engineering 6
Bacterial outer membrane protein A (OmpA) 229
Bacterial ß-glucuronidases 5
Bacterial translocation 140, 184
Bacterial vaccine 217
Bacteriophage 48, 188, 189, 214
Bacteroidaceae 142, 171
Bacteroidales 6
Bacteroides 5, 14, 20, 75, 76, 159, 171, 211
Bacteroides fragilis 2, 4, 15, 27, 58, 59, 76, 108, 110, 126, 129, 142, 153, 161, 181–183 227
Bacteroides fragilis toxin (BFT) 227
Bacteroides ovatus 32
Bacteroides thetaiotaomicron 4, 76, 172
Bacteroides xylanisolvens 32
Bacteroides intestinalis 33
Bacteroidetes 70, 129, 140, 142, 153, 155, 160
Baculoviral IAP Repeat Containing 3 (BIRC3) 5
BAK 99
BALB/ c mice 75, 194
Barcoded spots 18
Barnesiella intestini hominis 74
Bartonella spp. 32, 74, 126
BCL2-associated agonist of cell death (Bad) to 98
Beta-diversity 158
BICR-H1 breast cancer cells 192
Bifidobacterium spp. 3, 4, 20, 34, 45, 100, 110, 114, 127, 135, 140, 155, 163, 171, 183, 184, 210, 211, 212
Bifidobacterium animalis 179, 184
Bifidobacterium animalis subsp. *lactis* 143
Bifidobacterium bifidum G9-1 44
Bifidobacterium infantum 42
Bifidobacterium lactis Bb12 45
Bifidobacterium longum 113, 143, 211, 234
Bifidobacterium longum (BB536) 129
Bifidobacterium pseudolongum 183, 212
Bifidobacterium thetaiotaomicron 143
Bile acid binding 138
Bile acid composition 20
Bile acid metabolism 20
Bioactive microbial metabolites 94
Biocontainment 229
Biofilms 189
Biogeographical maternal microbiota 158
Biomarkers 57, 82, 83, 85, 114, 128
Bio panning 193
Biosafety concerns of viral therapy 215
Biosynthesis of genotoxic and toxic metabolites 15
BIRC3 75
Birth 154

243

Bladder cancer 19
Blauti spp. 75
Blood Brain Barrier (BBB) 4, 107, 110
Blood samples 6, 58
Bordetella pertussis 59
Brain-derived neurotrophic factor (BDNF) 111, 113
Branched chain hydroxy acids (BCHA) 143
Breast cancer (BC) 27, 93
Breast cancer resistance protein (BCRP) 71
Breast feeding 3, 114, 154, 155
Breast milk 155
Brucella melitenis 233
BTBRT+ tf/j mouse model 142
Bunge extract 41
Burkholderia cepacia 183
Burkholderiales 4
Burkina Faso 134
Butyrate 20, 96, 109, 142, 199
Butyrate effect on oxaliplatin 32
Butyrate-producing bacterial populations 199

C

C-reactive protein (CRP) 141
C57BL/ 6 tumor mouse model 74, 76, 194
Cachexia 3
Caesarean section 3, 154
CagA 2, 27, 29, 227
CagA-MET pathway 126
Caliciviridae 188
Caloric consumption 41
Campylobacter 159
Campylobacter jejuni 111
CAN-2409 viral immunotherapy 215
Cancer-associated fibroblasts 172
Cancer cell membrane structure 214
Cancer gene therapy 199
Cancer gene therapy using viral vectors 199
Cancer signaling pathways 84
Cancer stem cells (CSC) 69
Candida albicans 137
Candida spp. 27
Capnocytophaga gingivalis 128
Capsid proteins 192, 193
CAR-T antigen 200
Carcinoembryonic antigen (CEA) 192
Carcinogenesis 181
Carcinogenesis relayed to the gut microbiome 31
Carcinogenic classification of microbes 2
Cardiovascular (influenced by dysbiosis) 14
CART 201
castration-resistant prostate cancer (CRPC) 234
Catecholamine 113
Caudovirales 193, 194
Caveolin-mediated endocytosis 195
Chemotherapy related cognitive impairment (CRCI) 52
CD3+ T-cell infiltration 27
CD31 111
CD83 129
CEA-specific M13 phages 192
Cell cycle arrest 2, 41
Cell death 15
Cell surface receptors 98, 111
Cellular processes prompting CRC 84
Central nervous system 16, 107, 108
Cervical cancer 29

Cervical squamous epithelial cells (GPR81) receptor 93
Check-point inhibitors 127, 169
Chemically coupled chlorin e6 193
Chemotherapeutic-encapsulating nanoliposomes 233
Chemotherapy 74, 170
Chemotherapy (Effects on the gut microbiome) 70, 71, 161
Chemotherapy induced cognitive impairment (CICI) 114
Chemotherapy resistance 5, 70, 77, 240
Chemotherapy side effects 51
Childhood development 154
Childhood microbiome 3
Childhood versus adult microbiome 156
Children targeted treatments 160
Chimeric antigen receptor (CAR)-T cell therapies 233
Chlamydia pneumonia 126
Chlamydia trachomatis 29
CHO cells 194
Cholecystokinin (CCK) 109
Choline 95
Christensenella minuta 44
(Chrm1) muscarinic receptors 113
Chromatin remodeling 28, 72
Chromosomal instability 2
Chronic and acute stress 139
Chronic gastritis 125
Chronic inflammation 17, 125
Chronic infections 122
Chronic superficial gastric inflammation 125
CIN3+ 62
Ciprofloxacin 5
Circoviridae 188
Circulating tumor DNA (ctDNA) 83
Circulatory system 17, 107
Cisplatin 6, 74, 171
Cladribine 5
Claudins 29, 93
Clonorchis sinensis 1
Clostridia spp. 184
Clostridiacea 129, 161
Clostridiales Cluster XIVa 160
Clostridioides 128, 155, 158
Clostridium 5, 75, 170, 171
Clostridium butyricum 6
Clostridium butyricum (LCs) 171
Clostridium cluster XIVa 171
Clostridium decile 29, 47, 76, 143
Clostridium dificile with reduced microbial diversity 180
Clostridium novyi 234
Clostridium perfringens 143, 172
Clostridium perfringens enterotoxin (CPE) 29
Clostridium spp. 45, 127, 211
Clostridium tyrobutyricum 110
CNS native immune cells 111
Coagulation factor (F) × to hypervariable regions (HVR) 216
Codex Alimentarius Commission 138
Cognitive function 108, 171
Colibactin 2, 28, 153, 182, 227
Colitis 169
Colitis-associated colorectal cancer (CAC) 17, 60
Collinsella spp. 140

Collinsella aerofaciens 143
Colonization of the mucosa 127
Colony stimulating factor-1 (CSF-1) 124
Colony stimulating factor 1 receptor (CSF1R) 111
Colorectal cancer 2. 14
Co-metabolism of pharmacologicals 40
Commensal microbiota 18
Complete response 171
Components of engineered live therapeutic bacteria 228
Composition of gut phages by family 189
Conjugation based manipulation 217
Conserved intracellular bacterial profile 27
Contact-independent effects 27
Contamination if microbial samples 114
Continuous replication 15
Coprococcus spp. 74
Coriobacteriaceae 139
Coronaviridae, 188
COS-7 cells 194
Coxsackie virus 198
CpG oligodeoxynucleotides 5
CRC and IBD 123
CRISPR/ CAS9 199, 200, 201, 234
Crohn's disease 140
Cronobacter spp. 142
CT26 colorectal cancer model 230
CTLA-4 inhibitor 43
C-X-C motif ligand 9 (CXCL9) 32
Cyclooxygenase-2 (COX-2) 17, 59
Cyclophosphamide (CTX) 5, 74, 170
Cytidine deaminase (CDD) 5, 75
Cyto-lethal distending toxin 2
Cyto-lethal expansive toxin (CDT) 227
Cytotoxic drugs 211
Cytotoxic T lymphocyte-associated protein 4 (CTLA-4) 4, 19, 30, 32, 33, 43, 47, 59, 53, 199, 234
Cytotoxic T lymphocyte-associated protein 4 (CTLA4) inhibitors 110

D

DARPins 229
Daunorubicin 5
Deep learning, 201
DeepVirFinde 201
Deltyact (testerpaturev/G47 %) 197
DELYTACT serpaturev/ G47 196
Deoxycholic acid (DCA) 27, 93, 95, 100, 137
Designed Ankyrin Repeat Proteins (DARPins) 229
Designer probiotics 212
Desulfovibrio genera 128
Desulfovibrio, 58
Detoxification (role of the microbiota in) 17
Development of malignancies (effect of dysbiosis) 16
Diagnostic biomarker 6, 19, 59, 229
Dialister pneumosintes 1
Diet 3, 134, 210, 211, 240
Diet (salt) 138
Diet African rural children 134
Diet and Prebiotics 184
Diet developed nations 134
Diet Western children 134
Dietary components 135

Index

Dietary fat 137
Dietary fiber 135, 138
Dietary interventions 41, 134, 141, 144, 211
Digestion (role of the microbiota in) 17
Dihydrotanshinone I 41
Disease site-homing drug 193
Displaying large antigens 201
Distal mucosal site 17
Distribution of microbiota in the body 123
DNA alkylation 2
DNA conjugation technology 217
DNA damage 2, 15, 28. 29, 74, 82, 83, 96, 100, 109, 123, 126, 164, 210, 227
DNA damage in colonic epithelial cell 28
DNA damage response pathway 2, 15, 28
DNA double strand breaks 2, 72, 70, 75
DNA methylation 28, 72, 125
DNA repair 41, 72
DNA replication and integrity 2
DNA topoisomerase I (Top1) inhibitor 75
DNA topology 170
Docetaxel 171
Dopamine 113
Dopaminergic neurons 113
Doxorubicin 5
Drug delivery 233
Drug metabolism 100, 162
Drug resistance 93
Drug transportation 70
Drugbug database 183
dsRNA viral families 188
Duodenibacillus massiliensis 171
Duplodnaviria viruses 214
Dysbiosis 1, 3, 14, 16, 26, 169, 209, 238

E

E1 gene 215
E6 61
E7 61
E7 194
E7-specic protective immune responses 194
Early-onset colorectal cancer (EOCRC) 41
Ebb and flow effect 189
E-cadherin pathway 2, 83, 126
EGFR 86
Electron microscopy (TEM) 76
Elimination phase (Action of immune system against tumors) 17
Eluding immune surveillance 30
Emotional state (effect on digestion) 16
Endocrine systems (influenced by dysbiosis) 14
Endotoxin 128
Endotoxin contamination 201
Engineered bacteria 184, 228, 232, 233
Engineering microbial interfaces 231
Engineering the gut microbiome 234
Enhanced green fluorescent protein (EGFP) 194
Enteric nervous system 16, 108
Enterobacter 75, 170
Enterobacteria phages 199
Enterobacteriaceae 15, 143, 171, 227
Enterococcus durans 212
Enterococcus faecalis 27, 58, 83, 100, 172
Enterococcus hirae 4, 74
Enterococcus hirae 13144 215
Enterococcus spp. 27, 32, 128, 87, 211
Enterorhabdus spp. 140

Enterotoxigenic 15
Enterotoxigenic Bacteroides fragilis (ETBF), 85
Environmental factors 20, 127
Enzymatic degradation 70, 171
EOC cell line 74
EPIC research study 141
Epidermal growth factor (EGF) 194
Epigenetic alteration 28
Epigenetics 28, 41, 72, 153
Epithelial mesenchymal-like 181
Epithelial-mesenchymal transition (EMT) 27, 72
Epstein-Barr virus 1
Equilibrium phase 17
ErbB2 86
ErbB3 86
Erysipelotrichaceae 139
Escherichia coli 2, 58, 75, 100, 153, 171, 172, 179
Escherichia coli phage fusion proteins 192
Escherichia spp. 75, 76, 134, 155, 211
Escherichia. coli Nissle 1917 (EcN) 230
Esophageal SCC 126
Esophagogastroduodenoscopy (EGD) 64
Ethics of child dietary studies 154
Etoposide 5
Eubacterium eligens 143
Eubacterium rectale 136
Eukaryotic viruses 188
Evolutionary medicine 142
Exercise effect on gut microbiome 139
Extracellular matrix (ECM) 72
Extracellular polysaccharides 45
Extracellular space 230

F

F56 anticancer peptide 192
FadA 227
FadA adhesin 180
FadA 2
Faecalibacterium 6, 127, 134, 161
Faecalibacterium prausnitzi 135, 140, 171, 184, 211
Faecalibacterium spp. 58, 87, 98, 142, 213, 234
Fap2 cell adhesion story 110
Farnesoid X receptor 99
Fasting 144
Fasting-induced adipose factor (FIAF) 172
Fat-to-carbohydrate ratio 137
Fecal and blood microbiomes 84
Fecal donor selection 47
Fecal microbiota transplant (FMT) 6, 46, 100, 129, 163. 171, 184, 213
Fecal microbiota transplant effect on diseases 214
Fecal microbiota transplant effect on immunotherapy 213
Fecal microbiota transplant quality control 214
Fecal samples 6
Fecal virome transplantation (FVT) 198
Feeding tube 64
Fermented foods 143
Ff phages 192
FIAF 171
Fiber fermentability 138
Fiber solubility 138
Fiber viscosity 138
Finegoldia spp. 158

Firmicutes 70, 122, 140, 144, 153, 155
Firmicutes/ Bacteroidetes ratio 142
Fluoropyrimidine analogs 74
Focused ultrasound (FUS) 227
Food additives 14
Forkhead box P3 17
Formula-feeding 154
Free fatty acid receptor 3 (FFAR3) 97
Free radicals and DNA damage 126
Fructo-oligosaccharides (FOS) 19, 45, 135, 212
Functional plasticity 40
Fungal-derived metabolites 100
FUS technique 232
Fusobacteria species 70, 76, 82, 122, 192
Fusobacterium nucleatum 2, 15, 27, 47, 58, 69, 76, 100, 110, 126, 127, 128, 129, 159, 172, 181, 182, 192, 227
Fusobacterium nucleatum (Bacteriophage against) 48
Fusobacterium nucleatum as a diagnostic marker 180
Fusobacterium nucleatum, FadA 181

G

G protein coupled receptors (GPCRs) 111
Galactooligosaccharides (GOS) 19, 135
Gallbladder carcinoma 126
Gamma-aminobutyric acid (GABA) 113
Gamma proteobacteria 32, 75
Gastric cancer 125
Gastric mucosa 126
Gastric mucosa-associated lymphoid tissue (MALT) 123
Gastric surgery 34
Gastro-intestinal tract GIT 69
Gemcitabine 75, 210
Gendicin 200
Gene amplification 72
Gene editing 217
Gene modification (GM) 228
Genetic engineering 6, 49, 87
Genetic makeup 6
Genome instability 2, 15, 41
Genomic DNA mutations 124
Genotoxic compounds from bacteria like 28
Genotoxic *Escherichia coli* 15
Genotoxic stress 19
Genotoxin 153
Germ-free (GF) animal models 108
Gestational periods 154
GLOBOCAN 2020 69
GLP-1 136
Gly3-iRGD peptide 195
Glycolysis (reduction of) 142
Glycosylated MUC2 mucin expression 192
GM-CSF 193, 196
Gordonibacter spp. 140
Gp capsid proteins 193, 194
GPR109a/ HCAR2 109
GPR41/ FFAR3 109
GPR43/ FFAR2 109
G-protein coupled receptors 99
Gram-negative bacteria 134
Granulocyte macrophage-colony stimulating factor (GMCSF) 193
GRB2 29
Group 1 carcinogens 1

Group 2A carcinogens 1
Growth inhibitory mechanisms 15
Grp109a 96
Gut Brain axis 4, 16, 108, 240
Gut-derived microbial metabolites 95
Gut fatty acid receptors 20
Gut functionality 16
Gut hormones regulation 20
Gut microbial enzymes 20
Gut microbiome 14, 180, 182, 210
Gut microbiome and chemotherapy 170
Gut microbiome and immunotherapy 62, 169, 183
Gut microbiome and radiotherapy 171
Gut microbiome and systemic side effects of cancer therapies 170
Gut microbiome modulation 30, 49, 51, 77, 159, 162, 238
Gut microbiome of children who are breastfed 160
Gut microbiota produces metabolites 170
Gut-associated lymphoid tissue (GALT) 30
Gut-tumor microbiome axis 30
Gynecological cancer receiving radiation therapy 211

H

H10 virus 215
Hadza hunter-gatherer population 134, 142
Hallmarks of cancer 1, 15, 16
HCT116 human colon carcinoma cell line 75, 96
HDACi ketone body 142
Head and neck cancer 18, 50, 60, 196, 199
HEK293 cells 194
Helicobacter hepaticus 111
Helicobacter pylori 29, 69, 86, 122, 123, 125, 126, 210, 227
Helicobacter pylori-induced gastritis 123
Helicobacter pylori-induced HCC 123
Helicobacter pylori-induced hepatitis, 123
Hemagglutinin-neuraminidase (HN) 216
Hemagglutinin, 216
Hepatitis and cancer risk 124
Hepatitis B virus 1
Hepatitis C virus 1
Hepatitis D virus 1
Hepatocellular carcinoma 41, 72
Herpes simplex virus type 1 (HSV-1) 215
Herpesviridae 188
Hexahistidine peptide 193
Hexokinase II-derived cell-penetrating peptide 214
HI loop of the adenovirus capsid protein 216
High cholesterol diet 138
High fat diet (HFD) 137
High intake of processed meat 19
High-intensity focused ultrasound (HIFU) 232
High protein diet bacterial composition 135
High-salt diet (HSD 41
High sugar diet 14
Highly fermentable fibers 138
Highly outer capsid protein (HOC) 193
Hippo/ yes-associated protein (YAP) signaling 98
Histone deacetylases (HDACs) 93, 100, 109
Histone modification 72
Histone posttranslational modification 28
History of oncolytic viruses 195

HLA class I genes 99
Holin protein 194
Homeostasis in gut microbiome 128
Homologous recombination (HR) 29
Horizontal translocation of gut microbiome. 6
Hormonal and immunological signaling 16
Hospitalization at birth 3
Host lifestyle 127
HPV high-risk types 61
HPV-Related immunotherapeutic resistance 61
HSP90 193
HSV1716 215
Human cytomegalovirus 1
Human epidermal growth factor receptor 2 (HER2/ neu) 194
human granulocyte-macrophage colony- stimulating factor 196
Human gut virome 188
human immunodeficiency virus-1 1
HUMAN PAPILLOMAVIRUS (HPV) 1, 61
Human Papillomavirus type 16 61, 194
Human phage-derived anti-PD1 antibodies 215
Human T-cell lymphotropic virus 1
Hungatella hathewayi 28
Hydrogen peroxide 193
Hygiene 14
Hyperglycemia 143
Hyperinsulinemia 143
Hypermethylation 28
Hypothalamic-pituitary-adrenal axis (HPA 107
Hypothalamic-pituitary-adrenocortical (HPA) axis 139
Hypoxia 20, 193

I

Icosahedral head of the lytic T7 phage 193
ICP-34.5 gene 215
ICP47 gene deletion 197
Idarubicin 5
IGF1 99
IIIB/ C– IVM1a melanoma 199
IKKß kinase 98
IL-12 110
Immune agonist antibodies (IAAs) 33
Immune checkpoint blockade 15
immune checkpoint inhibitors 4, 7, 11, 18, 19, 30, 199, 200, 210, 232
Immune modulationt 57, 58
Immune regulation (role of the microbiota in) 17
Immune rejection 201
Immune-related side effects 169
Immune response 15, 169
Immune response (effect of dysbiosis) 16
Immune system development 26
Immune system in children 155
Immune system rewiring 230
Immune tolerance 17
Immunocompromised patients 201
Immunological escape phase (Action of immune system against tumors) 17
Immunological molecules and compounds 158
Immunological shift 198
Immunomodulation of antitumor responses 70, 200
Immunomodulators 18, 171
Immunosuppression 6, 27, 29, 127
immunotherapeutic responses (role of microbiota) 58

Immunotherapy 4, 18, 169, 189, 198, 212
Immunotherapy resistance 238
Impact of bioactive metabolites 96
Indole compounds 29, 93, 140
induction of apoptosis 93
Infant gut microbiome 137, 154
Infantile refractory epilepsy 142
Infections (role of the microbiota in) 17
Inflammation 16, 123, 124, 140, 240
inflammation anergy 17
Inflammations induced by grains and legumes 142
inflammatory bowel disease 17, 124
Inflammatory cytokines 76, 140, 170
Inflammatory mediators 125, 128
Inhibitors of apoptosis 5
Inhibitory effects of gut microbial metabolites 94
Inosine 95
Inoviridae family 188, 192
Insertional mutation 201
insulin 19, 141
Integrin response to phages 193
Interferon I 111
Interferon regulatory factors (IRF), 17
Interleukin signaling 17, 88, 99
International Agency for Research on Cancer (IARC) 1
Intestinal antigen-presenting cells 17
Intestinal barrier disruption 142
Intestinal barrier l 14
intestinal gluconeogenesis 20
Intestinal mucositis 161, 171
Intestinal permeability (IP) 140
Intestinal phages 189
Intracellular space 229
Intraepithelial neoplasia 111
Intratumoral bacteria 27
Inulin 45, 135
inv gene 229
Invasion and metastasis 15
Ipilimumab 4
Iridoviridae 188
irinotecan 5, 41, 75
Irinotecan gastrointestinal toxicity 33
Irritable bowel syndrome 139, 213
Italian diet 134, 135

J

JAK2-STAT3 98, 111

K

K-Ras amino-acid mutations 193
K-Ras(G12D) inhibitory peptides 193
Kaposi sarcoma virus 1
Ketogenetic diet 134, 141
kidney cancer 19
KRAS 99
KRpep-2d 193
Kynurenic acid (KYNA) 93, 95

L

L-carnitine 95
Lachnospiraceae spp. 74–76, 86, 129, 140, 142, 183
Lactic acid bacteria (LAB) 143, 217
Lactobacillus acidophilus 42
Lactobacillus casei 42

Index

Lactobacillus casei ATCC334 214
Lactobacillus fermentum BR11 44
Lactobacillus gallinarum 69
Lactobacillus johnsonii 74
Lactobacillus johnsonii (La1) 129
Lactobacillus lactis 42
Lactobacillus murinus 74
Lactobacillus plantarum 42
Lactobacillus reuteri 6, 93, 95. 144, 171
Lactobacillus rhamnaosus 42, 161
Lactobacillus rhamnosus GG strain (LG 45, 129
Lactobacillus salivarius 42
Lactobacillus spp. 3, 5, 34, 45, 46, 75, 113, 127, 140, 141, 163, 184, 211, 212, 227
Lactococcus 76, 211
Lambda phage 194
Lambda phage/ GP2 vaccine 194
L-arginine levels 44
Laser scanning confocal microscopy (LSCM) 76
Later stage milk production 155
LBPs 44
LEfSe algorithm 76
Lentisphaerae phyla 139
Lentiviral, 200
Leukemia 153
Leviviridae family 194
Lifestyle effects on the gut microbiome 6, 14, 139, 240
Ligand-gated ion channels (LGICs) 111
Lipopolysaccharide 86
Liquid biopsy 182
Liquid phase biopsy 182
Listeria monocytogenes 86, 229, 234
Lithocholic acid (LCA) 93
Living biosensor 88
Lactic acid bacteria 136
Lipoteichoic acid (LTA) 27
LNCaP cell viability 195
LNCaP prostate epithelial cells 194
lncRNA urothelial cancer associated 1 (UCA1) 72
Low carbohydrate diet 143
Low fat diet (LFD) 137
LTX-315 214
Lung cancer 6
Lung Resistance-Related Protein 72
LutatheraR 231
Lymphatic system 107
Lymphocyte cell activity 160
Lymphoid cells 111
Lymphoid enhancer binding factor 1 (LEF-1) 98
Lymphoid nodules 17
Lymphoid organs 29
Lymphoma 19
Lymphomagenesis 126
Lynch Syndrome 153
Lysogenic conversion 189
Lytic phages 189

M

M1 macrophages differentiation 127
M1 phenotype 60
M13 phage 48, 192
M2-macrophage 4
M2 phenotype 58–60
m2386 214
Machine learning (ML) 179. 183

Macrophage activation by phages 192
Magnetic guidance 232
Magnetic nanoparticles 233
Magneto aerotactic 232
Magnetococcus marinus 232
Major vault protein (MVP) 71
Malassezia species 27
Manipulation of the gut microbiome 210
Manipulation of the gut virome 198, 201
Manumycin A 95, 97
MAPK pathway 86, 97
Marseilleviridae 188
Mass spectroscopy 6, 180
Maternal microbiota during pregnancy 158
Maternal-milk microbiome 155
Matrix metalloproteinase (MMP-9) activation 87
Matrix metalloproteinase (MMP) target sequence 230
MC-26 mice 75
MCA205 cell line sarcoma 74, 215
MCF-7 98, 193
MCT1/ SLC16A1; SMCT1/ SLC5A8 109
Mechanical stress 27
Mechanism of autophagy in response to cellular stress I 73
Mechanism of chemoresistance 70
Medical imaging 231
Mediterranean diet 134, 141
Mediterranean diet bacterial composition 135
Megasphaera 128
MEK-ERK1/ 2 111
Melanoma 19
MELRESIST 64
Mesenchymal stem cells (MSCs) 69
Metabolic biomarkers 180
Metabolic byproduct) 26, 41
Metabolic flexibility 144
Metabolism (effect of dysbiosis) 14, 16
Metabolism 171
Metabolites and cancer treatment 100
Metabolomic research 181
Metabolomics 179, 183
Metastasis, and therapeutic resistance 40
MHC-1 restricted T cell epitope enhanced immunotherapy 199
MHC class I– restricted antigens 59
Microbe-enteric nervous system 108
Microbe in tumor suppression 28, 29
Microbe produced lactate 93
Microbial and immune cells in cancer 127
Microbial colonization 27
Microbial composition (Adults) 109, 155
Microbial composition (first years of life) 155
Microbial Ecosystem Therapeutic 4 (MET4) 62
Microbial Ecosystem Therapeutics 62
Microbial effect on immunotherapy 30, 124, 126
Microbial extracellular vesicles (MEVs) 182
Microbial-host-irinotecan axis imbalance 170
Microbial invasion 27
Microbial metabolite 4-ethylphenyl sulfate 100
Microbial Metabolites 2, 93, 97–100, 169, 241
Microbial proliferation 27
Microbial toxicity 114
Microbial transplantation (safety and efficacy) 63
Microbial tumorigenesis 28
Microbial-inspired drug delivery systems 30
Microbiome based biomarkers 84, 88, 240

Microbiome based interventions for pediatric patients 162
Microbiome diversity 33
Microbiome effects on chemotherapy 30, 32
Microbiome effects on radiation therapy 30, 32
Microbiome effects on surgery 30
Microbiome engineering 241
Microbiome features 181
Microbiome in cancer therapy 35, 210, 241
Microbiome in tumor onset 180
Microbiome induced chemoresistance 74
Microbiome modulation 218
microbiome modulation effect on immunotherapy 65
Microbiota-accessible carbohydrates 142
microbiota-associated phenotypes 198
microbiota-depleting antibiotics 123
Microbiota-derived molecules 17
Microbiota factors influencing cancer therapy effectiveness 32
Microbiota taxonomy in healthy children 154
Microbiota variations within individuals 156
Microbiotic ecosystem 20
Microinvasive adenocarcinoma 111
Micrometer-scale cavitating bubbles 232
Microorganism-associated molecular patterns (MAMP) 82
Microsatellite instability (MSI) 27, 59
Microviridae 188, 189
Microbiome neural interactions 113
Milk oligosaccharides 155
Minimal residual disease (MRD) 83
Minor capsid proteins 192
miR-134 72
miR-206-3p 113
miR-487b 72
miR-655 72
miRNA 125
miRNA expression changes 18
Mismatch repair-proficient 59
Mitochondrial uncoupling in colon cancer 141, 144
Mitogen-activated protein kinases (MAPK) 17, 29
Mitoxantrone resistance protein (MXR1) MCF-7/ MX cell line 71
MKN45 cell lines 95
Mitoxantrone 5
Modification of the central nervous system 42
Modulation of gut microbiome as a potential tool to circumvent anti-ICI resistance 64
MOLI-SANI trial 141
Monobodies 229
Monocytes differentiate into macrophages 127
Morganella morganii 28
Mothers' dietary intake 114
Mouse model 122
MP 2
MRE11 29
MRI 228
MRN complex 29
mRNAs 113
MS2 phage 194
*MSH*2 gene 153
Mucin 2 95
Mucin-degrading 34
Mucispirillum schaedleri 86
Mucispirillum 75
Mucosal dysfunction 182

Mucosal immunity 4, 140
Mucosal thickness 140
Mucositis 161
Mucositis diarrhea 70
Multimodal therapeutic concept microbiome in oncologics 40
Multiparametric functions of the gut 40
Multiple sclerosis 142
Murine melanoma cells 193
Mutagens (bacterial) 83
Mutation-prone DNA repair 126
Mycobacterium avium subspecies *paratuberculosis* 143
Mycoplasma 75
Mycoplasma hyorhinis 75
MyD88 adaptor proteins pathway 15, 17, 192
Myelodysplastic syndrome or acute myeloid leukemia 210
Myeloid leukemia cell differentiation protein 1 (MCL1) 29
Myeloid-derived suppressor cells (MDSCs) 29, 127
Myoviridae family 188, 193
Myxcoccus fulvus 98

N

n-3 PUFAs 142
N-nitroso compounds 41
Nanocarrier of the catalase protein 193
Nanomedicines 217
Nanotechnology 47
Natural oncolytic virus 197
NC101 *Escherichia* 123
NCT02858310 62
NCT0334114 213
NCT03341143 62
NCT03353402 213
NCT04116775 52
NCT04495153 215
NCT04552418 212
NCT05032014 52
NCT05032027 52
Nephrotoxicity 6
Nervous-immune system 110
Neurogenesis 4, 113
Neuroinflammation 114
Neuromusculoskeletal (influenced by dysbiosis) 14
Neurotransmitters 111, 112
Neurotransmitters (linked to sleep) 139
Newcastle disease virus (NDV) 216
Next generation sequencing 6, 179, 234
Niacin 95, 96
Nicotiana alata 214
Nitrates ad nitrites 41
Nitric oxide (NO) 125
NK cell cytotoxicity 160
NK4 A136 75
NLRP3 inflammasome 96
Nod1 KO mice 123
NOD-like 58
non-coding RNA 28, 72
Non-small cell lung carcinoma (NSCLC) 19, 60, 72
Non-structural protein 1 (NS1) 215
Non-viscous, soluble fibers 138
Nonhomologous end-joining (NHEJ) 29

Nonsolid biological tissue 182
Norepinephrine signaling 113
Nuclear factor erythroid 2-related factor 2 (Nrf2) 98
Nuclear factor kappa B signaling (NFκB) 98, 126
Nucleotide-binding oligomerization (NOD)-like receptor (NLR) 17, 127
Nutrition (effect on gut microbiome) 19, 26, 158
Nutrition in shaping the gut microbiome in pre- and postnatal stages 160
Nutrition research in cancer patients 210
Nutrition synthesis (role of the microbiota) 17
Nutritional glucosinolate 44

O

Obesity 41
Odoribacter spp. 129
Oligofructose 45
Omics in the gut microbiome 180
Oncogenic potential 201
Oncolytic adenovirus 216
Oncolytic phages 2
oncolytic pox virus 216
Oncolytic viral formulations 215
Oncolytic viral therapy 197, 201, 215–217
Oncolytic virus 195, 196
Oncolytic viruses and immune checkpoint inhibitors 199
Oncolytic viruses in clinical trials 196
Oncomicrobiome 40, 45
Oncorine 217
Oncorine (H101) 196
Onyx-015 virus 215
Opisthorchis felineus 1
Opisthorchis viverrini 1
Optimal ancestral microbiome 142
Oral bacteria and cancer 128
oral squamous cell carcinoma (SC) 126, 128
Organogenesis 18
Orthotopic breast cancer (mammary fat pad 4T1) 230
Oscillospira 58
Outer membrane vesicles 27
Overcoming immunotherapy resistance 62
Oxaliplatin 74, 171

P

P-glycoprotein (P-gp) 71
p53 protein 28, 199
p70 ribosomal S6 protein kinase (p70A6K) 98
Paclitaxel 171
Pediatric cancers 150, 240
Paleolithic diets 134, 142
Pancreatic ductal adenocarcinoma (PDAC) 32, 61, 210
Parasporin 214
Parasutteralla spp. 76
Parasympathetic nervous system (PNS) 113
Parvimonas micra 1
Parvimonas spp. 76, 192
Parvovirus 216
Pasteurella stomatis 1
Pathobiont microbial networks 35
Pathogen-associated molecular patterns (PAMPs) 110, 189
Pattern recognition receptors (PRRs) 17
PAX5 gene 153

pCASP-hyperinvasive locus A (HilA) vector 229
PD-L1 blockade 114
PDAC chemotherapy 48
Pectin 138
Pediatric treatments 160
Pediatric oncology patient outcomes 161
Pembrolizumab 62, 199
Peptostreptoccaceae and neuroticism 139
Peptostreptococcus anaerobius 85, 182
Peptostreptococcus spp. 76, 128, 192
Periampullary neoplasms (PNs) 213
Perineural invasion (PNI) 113
Periodontal disease 128
Peroxisome proliferator 172
Personalized medicine 6, 7, 40, 49, 179, 183, 184, 238
Personalized virome 200
Pervotella spp. 142
Peyer's patch 192
PGE2 59
Phage DNA vaccines 201
Phage entry 201
Phage reversal of drug resistance 189
Phage therapy 21, 189, 192, 217
Phage-mediated immune responses 189, 192
Phages as an epithelial defense 189
Pharmacodynamics 160
Pharmacomicrobiomics 34, 40
Phosphatase D 2
Phosphate 5
Photodynamic therapy 193
Physicochemical features of fibers 138
PI3K-Akt-mTOR signaling 98
PI3K/ AKT PATHWAY 85, 98
PI3K/ protein kinase 62
Picobirnaviridae 188
Picornavirus 196
Placenta microbiota 159
Plasma endotoxin 140
Platinum-based agents 74, 171
PLUVICTOTM (Lu-PSMA-617) 231
Podoviridae family 188, 193
Polyamidoamine dendrimer nanoparticles 233
Polybia-MP1 214
Polyketide synthase (pks) 153, 182
Polyomaviridae 188
Polysaccharide A (PSA) 110
Porphyromonas gingivalis 86, 128
Positron emission tomography (PET) 229
Post infection oncolytic viruses 215
Postbiotic composition 212
Postbiotics 5, 44, 45, 184, 212
Postoperative anastomotic leaks 34
Postoperative ileus (POI) 87
Postpartum colostrum 155
Poxviridae 188
Prebiotics 5, 19, 21, 44, 45, 123, 135, 163, 184, 211
Prebiotics in beverages 136
precisely displaying a molecule of interest 201
Precision medicine 184, 240
Precision oncology 179, 200
Prevalent malignancies in Africa 208
Prevotella spp. 14, 76, 108, 128, 142, 155, 192
Prevotella/ Bacteroides ratio of 129
Prevotellaceae 142
Principal component analysis or hierarchical clustering 180

Index

Probiotic guided CAR-T cells (ProCARs) 233
Probiotics 5, 21, 41, 42, 43, 52, 113, 129, 134, 136, 163, 184, 212
Probiotics' potential risks 43
Prognostic biomarkers (microbiome) In CRC 86
Programmed cell death 1 (PD-1) 19
Programmed cell death ligand 1 (PD-L1) 19
Progression and treatment of cancer 209
Proinflammatory cytokines 17, 44, 59, 83, 99, 110, 124, 140
Proinflammatory microorganisms 143
Proliferative and survival pathways 2
Proliferative signaling 15
Prominent phyla 14
Propionate 20, 93
Propionibacterium 20, 158
Prospects for microbiomes in cancer 217
Prostaglandin E2 4
prostate cancer 19
PROT3EcT 230
Protein-expressing vector 193
Protein rich diet 140
Proteobacteria 70, 140, 142, 155
Proteolytic enzymes to ensure EC invasion 100
Proteomic signatures 114
Proteomics 183
Proteus 227
Pseudomonas aeruginosa 29, 87
Pseudoxanthomonas 171
PSMA castration-resistant prostate cancer 231
Psychobiotic bacterial species 139
Psychosocial stress 127
Psyllium 138

Q

Quorum sensing (QS)-dependent genetic circuits 230

R

(Rac1)/p21 protein-activated kinase 1 (PAK1 signaling system 98
Radiation enteropathy 33
Radiotherapy 171
Radiotherapy and the gut microbiome bidirectional link 33
Raoultella planticola 5
Ras-related C3 botulinum toxin substrate 1 (Rac1)/p21 98
RAS signaling pathway 229
Reactive oxygen species (ROS) 5, 17, 28, 33, 58, 74, 83, 96, 101, 124, 141, 171, 194
Recombinant oncolytic viral therapies 216
Rectal enema 64
Red sage 41
Reduced diversity 171
Reduced diversity resulting from chemotherapy 70
Regulatory T (Treg) cells 17
Reinforcement learning 179
Reoviridae 188
Reovirus 196
Reprogrammed bacteria-immune interface 231
Respiratory tract infections 128
Response to cancer treatment 238
RIG-IFN-1 signaling 30
Rigvir (ECHO-7) 196, 198, 217
Rikenella spp. 75
Rikenellaceae spp. 171
RKO human colon carcinoma cell line 75
RNA sequencing (RNA-seq) 18
RNA viruses (oncolytic) 198
Role of the gut microbiome in cancer 209, 239
Role of the gut microbiome in cancer therapy 239
Roseburia spp. 74
Roseburia hominis 140
Roseburia intestinalis 136
Route of administration 201
Roxithromycin 193
Ruminobacter 134
Ruminococcaceae 61, 129, 140, 142
Ruminococcus 14, 108

S

s-equol 95, 98
Saccharomyces spp. 184
Saccharopolyspora 171
sagA 100
Saliva 58
Salmonella 127, 229
Salmonella enterica str 44
Salmonella oncolytic strain VNP20009 49
Salmonella typhi 1, 29, 126, 227, 234
Salmonella typhimurium 29, 229, 230, 232
Salmonella typhimurium VNP20009 strain 229
Salmonella-containing vacuole (SCV) 229
Salvia miltiorrhiza 41
Satiety signals 20
Saturated fat 137
Schistosoma haematobium 1
Schistosoma mansonii 1
Scientific Association for Probiotics and Prebiotics (ISAPP) 143
Secretory vesicles 26
Seesaw effect 189
Selectivity of cancer therapy 194
Senescent associated secretory phenotype (SASP) 100
Sensation and emotion 136
Sentinel cells 17
Serotonin (5-hydroxy tryptamine) 111
Serratia marcescens 227
Serratia species 107
Serum glucose levels 136
Serum LDL-cholesterol and 136
Sheba Medical Centre 213
Shigella flexneri 2, 229
Shigella spp. 75, 76, 134, 211
Shigella-derived type 3 secretion apparatus 230
Short chain fatty acids (SCFAs) 3, 20, 45, 93, 95, 109, 111, 135, 141, 182, 210
Side effects of chemotherapy 144
Signal transducer and activator of transcription 3 (STAT3) 97
Signature gut microbiota 129
Silver nanoparticles (AgNPs) 48, 192
Single-strand breaks (SSBs) 72
Siphoviridae family 188, 189, 194
Sleep effect on the gut microbiome 139
SMAD 86
Small groups of microbes as medical treatments 233
Small outer capsid protein (SOC) 193
SN38 5
SN38G 75
SNU-484 cells 96
SNU-216 cell lines 95
Society for Healthcare Epidemiology of America 213
Soybean oligosaccharides (SBOSs) 135
Spatial transcriptomics 18
Splenic DC 17
Spodoptera exigua 1
Spontaneous breast cancer model (MMTV-PyMT) 230
ssDNA viral families 188
ssRNA viral families 188
standard operating procedure (SOP) 34
Staphylococcus 5, 75, 76, 87
STAT3 59, 111
Stool 58
Stool bank 47
Streptococcaceae spp. 161
Streptococcus anginosus 1
Streptococcus bovis 83, 182
Streptococcus faecalis 46
Streptococcus gallolyticus 58, 182
Streptococcus pyogenes 227
Streptococcus spp. 27, 34, 76, 107, 128, 142, 158, 192, 211
Streptococcus thermophilus 69, 183
Streptomyces 5, 171
Stress and anxiety tests 114
Stress-and mood-related conditions 114
Stress effect on the gut microbiome 139
Supervised learning 179
Supplements 113
Surface modification 49
Surgical site infections (SSI) 87
SW480 cells 214
symbiotic microbial communities 35
Symbiotics 5, 21, 44, 184, 213
Sympathetic nervous system (SNS) 113
synchronized lysis circuit 44
Synthetic antimicrobial peptides 209
Synthetic biology 227, 233
Synthetic polymers 217
Synthetic stools 212
Systemic metabolic pathways 17

T

T cell factor (TCF) 29
T cell factor 4 (TCF-4) 98
T cell homeostasis 86
T cell immunoglobulin mucin-3 61
T-cell immunoreceptor tyrosine-based inhibitory motif domains (TIGIT) 110
T cell receptor (TCR) 62
T4 phage 193
T4 phage/ VEGFR2 recombinant vaccine 193
T7 phage 193
Tail length tape measure protein (TMP1) 59, 215
Talimogene laherparepvec (T-VEC) 196, 199, 215, 217
Targeting microbial metabolites 100
Taurine 95
Tauro deoxycholic acid (TDCA) 137
Taxanes 171
Taxonomic variation 26, 135
Taxonomical identification and standardized protocol development 200
TC-1 cells 194

TC-1 lung/ cervical cancer 172
Temperate phages 189
TGF-β Signaling pathway 86
Thallium (I) ions 195
The Infectious Diseases Society of America 213
Theodor Escherich 179
Theragnostic 229
Third-generation sequencing 234
Thymosin ß4 72
TIGIT (limiter of innate and adaptive immunity) 29, 127, 181
TIMER 70, 86, 171
TIR-domain-containing adapter-inducing interferon β 17
Tissue samples 6
TK 216
TME cellular and non-cellular components 208
Tobacco 140
TOE components 209
Toll like receptors 17, 18, 110, 127
Toll oligomerization (NOD)-like receptor (NLR) 17
Topoisomerase I inhibitor 170
TP53, cancer cell-autonomous effects, 123
Trans fats 137
Transcriptomics 18, 114, 183
Transforming growth factor receptor 2 (TGFR2 86
Transforming growth factor-β (TGF-β) type II receptor 86
Translocation of bacteria from bowel to systemic circulation 70
Translocation 171
Trastuzumab 194
Traumatic brain injuries 113
Treatment of infants with antibiotics 4
Treatment plans 18
Tregs 111
Treponema spp. 134, 192
Trimethylamine (TMA) 20
Trimethylamine N-oxide 95
Tryptophan-derived metabolite, KYNA 97
Tryptophan metabolite 3-IAA (indole-3-acetic acid (3-IAA) 76
Tumor antigens 199
Tumor associated macrophages 59
Tumor cytokines release by oncolytic viruses 215

Tumor-elicited inflammation 123
Tumor heterogeneity 18
Tumor-infiltrating lymphocytes (TILs) 59, 61
Tumor microenvironment (TME) 26, 72, 78, 208, 231
Tumor microenvironment cellular composition 209
Tumor mutational burden 58
Tumor organismal environment (TOE) 208
Tumor resistance to chemotherapy 181
Tumor-specific T cell responses 199
Tumor-homing arginine-glycine-aspartate (RGD) peptide 229
Tumor-specific delivery systems 227
Tumor immune evasion 57
Tumor localization using bacteria 229
Tumorigenesis 28
Type 3 secretion system (T3SS) 229
Tyrosine kinase inhibitors 30

U

ULK1-FIP200-ATG13 complex 73
Umbilical cord microbiota 159
Unsaturated fat 137
Unsupervised learning 179
Urban diets 134
Urine 58
urolithin A 41, 95
Urolithin B 95, 98
Ursodeoxycholic acid (UDCA) 95

V

V-Ki-ras2 Kirsten rat sarcoma viral oncogene homolog (K-Ras) 193
Vaccines 19
Vaccinia virus 196, 197
Vaginal birth 154
Vaginal microbiota 3, 155
Vagus nerve 4, 109
Varied microbial ecosystem 212
Varying gut microbiota composition in children and adults 158
Vascular endothelial growth factor (VEGF) 72
Vascular endothelial growth factor receptor 2 27, 193

Vascular endothelial growth factor receptor A (VEGA) 96
Vascular tumor formation 126
Veillonella spp. 128, 155
Veillonellaceae spp. 129, 134
Verrucomicrobia 70, 139
Vertical translocation of gut microbiome. 6
Vesicular stomatitis virus (VSV) 216, 233
VGF 216
Vidarabine 5, 201
Viral dark matter 202
Viral effects om chemotherapy 215
Viral gene therapy 200
Viral genera in the human gut 190
Viral immunotherapy 189
Viral vectors 199
Virgaviridae 188
Virion packing limit 201
Virome 2, 188, 241
Virome diversity 188
Virome manipulation 200
Virotherapy 214
Virulence gene A 2
virulent strains and inflammation 122
VSL#3 probiotic 44

W

Warburg effect 144
Washed microbiota transplantation (WMT) 184
Western diet 134, 137, 138, 141, 142, 144, 145, 159
Whole grain 138, 211, 141
Wild-type (wt) p53 protein 28, 199
William Coley 107
Wnt pathway 29, 85, 93
Wnt/-catenin pathway 125, 227

X

Xenografts 15

Y

Yacon syrup 136
Yersinia pseudotuberculosis 229

Z

ZIKVBR 215

9781032706429